The Guide to
Community Preventive Services

D0331648

The Guide to
Community

Preventive Services

What Works to Promote Health?

Task Force on Community Preventive Services

Stephanie Zaza, Project Co-Director
Peter A. Briss, Project Co-Director
Kate W. Harris, Managing Editor

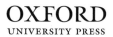
UNIVERSITY PRESS

2005

OXFORD
UNIVERSITY PRESS

Oxford   New York
Auckland   Bangkok   Buenos Aires   Cape Town   Chennai
Dar es Salaam   Delhi   Hong Kong   Istanbul   Karachi   Kolkata
Kuala Lumpur   Madrid   Melbourne   Mexico City   Mumbai   Nairobi
São Paolo   Shanghai   Taipei   Tokyo   Toronto

Copyright © 2005 by Oxford University Press

Published by Oxford University Press, Inc.
198 Madison Avenue, New York, New York 10016

http://www.oup.com

Oxford is a registered trademark of Oxford University Press

Library of Congress Cataloging-in-Publication Data
The guide to community preventive services : what works to promote health? / Task Force
on Community Preventive Services ; edited by Stephanie Zaza, Peter A. Briss, Kate W. Harris.
p.   cm.
Includes bibliographical references and index.
ISBN-13 978-0-19-515108-4; 978-0-19-515109-1 (pbk.)
ISBN 0-19-515108-9; 0-19-515109-7 (pbk.)
1. Community health services—United States.   2. Preventive health services—United States.
3. Health promotion—United States.   I. Zaza, Stephanie.   II. Briss, Peter A.
III. Harris, Kate W.   IV. Task Force on Community Preventive Services (U.S.)
RA445.G785 2005
362.1′0425′0973—dc22   2004050129

9   8   7   6   5   4   3   2   1

Printed in the United States of America
on acid-free paper

Task Force on Community Preventive Services

CHAIR

Jonathan E. Fielding, MD, MPH, MBA (Member since 1996;
  Chair since 2001)
Los Angeles Department of Health Services
Los Angeles, California

MEMBERS

Ross Brownson, PhD (1996–2003)
St. Louis University School of Public Health
St. Louis, Missouri

Patricia A. Buffler, PhD, MPH (1996–2001)
School of Public Health
University of California, Berkeley

Noreen Morrison Clark, PhD (2003–present)
University of Michigan School of Public Health
Ann Arbor, Michigan

John Clymer (2002–present)
Partnership for Prevention
Washington, D.C.

Mary Jane England, MD (1996–2001)
Regis College
Weston, Massachusetts

Caswell A. Evans, Jr., DDS, MPH (Chair of the Task Force, 1996–2001)
National Oral Health Initiative, Office of the U.S. Surgeon General
Rockville, Maryland

David W. Fleming, MD (1996–2000)
The Gates Foundation
Seattle, Washington

Mindy Thompson Fullilove, MD (1996–2004)
New York State Psychiatric Institute and Columbia University
New York, New York

Fernando A. Guerra, MD, MPH (1996–2002)
San Antonio Metropolitan Health District
San Antonio, Texas

Alan R. Hinman, MD, MPH (1996–present)
Task Force for Child Survival and Development
Atlanta, Georgia

George J. Isham, MD (1996–2004)
HealthPartners
Minneapolis, Minnesota

Robert L. Johnson, MD (2003–present)
New Jersey Medical School, Department of Pediatrics
Newark, New Jersey

Garland H. Land, MPH (1997–present)
Missouri Department of Health
Jefferson City, Missouri

Charles S. Mahan, MD (1996–2002)
University of South Florida College of Public Health
Tampa, Florida

Patricia Dolan Mullen, DrPH (1996–2004)
University of Texas–Houston School of Public Health
Houston, Texas

Patricia A. Nolan, MD, MPH (2001–present)
Rhode Island Department of Health
Providence, Rhode Island

Dennis E. Richling, MD (2002–present)
Union Pacific Railroad
Omaha, Nebraska

Barbara K. Rimer, DrPH (2003–present)
School of Public Health, University of North Carolina
Chapel Hill, North Carolina

Susan C. Scrimshaw, PhD (1996–2003)
University of Illinois School of Public Health
Chicago, Illinois

Steven M. Teutsch, MD, MPH (2001–present)
Merck & Company, Inc.
West Point, Pennsylvania

Robert S. Thompson, MD (1996–2003)
Group Health Cooperative of Puget Sound
Seattle, Washington

CONSULTANTS

Robert S. Lawrence, MD (1996–present)
Bloomberg School of Public Health
Johns Hopkins University
Baltimore, Maryland

J. Michael McGinnis, MD (1996–present)
Robert Wood Johnson Foundation
Princeton, New Jersey

Lloyd F. Novick, MD, MPH (1996–present)
Onondaga County Department of Health
Syracuse, New York

Sylvie Stachenko, MD, Msc (1996–1999)
Health Canada
Ottawa, Ontario

Steven M. Teutsch, MD, MPH (1998–2001)
Merck & Company, Inc.
West Point, Pennsylvania

Foreword

It is a great pleasure to present this landmark first edition of *The Guide to Community Preventive Services (Community Guide)*. This *Community Guide* is the product of eight years of work by the Task Force on Community Preventive Services. At its inception in 1996, the Task Force was charged with developing recommendations for interventions that promote health and prevent diseases in our nation's communities and healthcare systems. These recommendations were to be based on systematically derived scientific evidence of their effectiveness. At that time, some deemed the task impossible and maintained that complex community-based interventions could not be evaluated systematically, would not stand up to scientific scrutiny, and could not benefit from focusing on what works. In contrast to those reservations, the *Community Guide's* research into scientific studies has illuminated and helped clarify what we know about what works to promote health and prevent disease, and what we still need to learn. The *Community Guide* is a credible, practical, and essential reference. It is important for helping public health, healthcare provider, academic, business, community planning and advocacy, and research audiences select effective interventions for their communities and for expanding the science base underlying public health practice.

The work of this Task Force follows in the footsteps of the U.S. Preventive Services Task Force, which developed and continues to update the *Guide to Clinical Preventive Services*. The *Clinical Guide* is an important reference providing recommendations for clinical (i.e., individual) prevention interventions. The *Community Guide* complements this work and recommends interventions to improve the performance of healthcare systems; interventions implemented in community settings such as schools, worksites, and community organizations; and interventions applied to entire communities (e.g., laws, regulations, enforcement, mass media, and environmental changes). Together, these two guides provide recommendations that address the needs of both our health and public health systems.

The Task Force on Community Preventive Services is ably supported by staff at the Department of Health and Human Services (led by HHS's Centers for Disease Control and Prevention), other federal agencies, major health organizations, state and local health departments, managed care and other healthcare delivery organizations, academic centers, and voluntary organizations. These broad collaborations are essential to ensure that the approach taken in each chapter—the interventions selected for review, the reviews of evidence, and the recommendations—are accurate, meaningful, and useful. I congratulate the Task Force for this productive collaboration and the example it sets for all of us as we work to improve our nation's health and well-being.

As a nation, we have set challenging goals for improving the health of all Americans. Only by working together—as clinicians, healthcare executives, employers, public health professionals, researchers, policymakers, and community health workers—will we meet those sweeping goals. *The Guide to Community Preventive Services* will surely help us move toward a healthier nation and world, and I recommend this report to all of you.

Julie Louise Gerberding, MD, MPH
Director, Centers for Disease Control and Prevention

Preface

What do we know, how do we know it, and how can we use what we know to improve the public's health? These questions sparked the creation of the Task Force on Community Preventive Services.

Anybody who makes or influences decisions that can affect the health of populations deserves ready access to the best evidence on what works, for what purpose, and at what cost, in order to make good choices among policies and to consider alternative uses of resources. This perceived need in personal healthcare led to the establishment of the U.S. Preventive Services Task Force and similar efforts to make available the best scientific evidence to support decisions in various fields of medicine. Fundamental to all of these efforts was the development of standard approaches to search the literature for evidence; to identify and synthesize the subset of best evidence; and to translate it into specific recommendations for practitioners.

Despite the success of this approach in improving medical care, some doubted whether a complementary effort to assess interventions aimed at populations could succeed. Did high quality evidence exist in the broad domain that constitutes public health? If so, could that evidence be harnessed to support decision making?

In 1996, the Department of Health and Human Services (HHS) acknowledged these concerns and committed to assessing and improving the quality of knowledge about what works to improve population health by establishing the Task Force on Community Preventive Services. This action placed a solemn responsibility in the hands of a 15-member panel of experts and established a special relationship between the Task Force and the Centers for Disease Control and Prevention (CDC), an agency of HHS. CDC provides the research teams that gather and evaluate evidence on the effectiveness of a wide array of public health interventions; the Task Force reviews this evidence and uses it to makes decisions and recommendations. Other federal agencies, voluntary organizations, and many national experts also make important contributions to fulfilling the charge of the Task Force. CDC and other partners also are working to ensure the wide dissemination and use of the results.

This book, a milestone reflecting important new work, is but one aspect of the combined work of the Task Force, CDC, and our many partners. Over the past eight years, we have learned much about which public health interventions are effective, but to do this we had to develop credible, reproducible methods to amass and weigh evidence. First, we developed, tested, and refined a standard methodology to search for and sift through evidence from a wide range of studies reflecting many disciplinary perspectives. Second, the Task Force determined which topics and interventions to address initially, according to the perceived value to practitioners and decision makers. Third, we applied the methods to topics as diverse as immunization, physical activity, diabetes, motor vehicle occupant safety, and housing. Fourth, we developed an approach to translating the evidence into recommendations. Not only were we interested in reaching conclusions, we also wanted to help provide methods that others could use in similar pursuits.

The material found in this guide, in related publications, and on our website, provides a transparent record that allows users to evaluate, from their own perspectives, the credibility and prudency of the recommendations.

The Task Force makes recommendations when enough good quality evidence is available. Unfortunately, in many areas the available evidence is sparse. A major benefit of our efforts in developing the guide has been our ability to identify the gaps in our knowledge. Expanding public health research is critical to improving health and reducing health disparities in the future. The research needs reflected by this process assist CDC and others in deciding what kinds of research to support. Over time, use of this research agenda can lead to better evidence and can provide answers that support sound public health policy.

This first edition of the guide summarizes an enormous body of work, yet it is just the beginning of a longer journey. Continued investment will be needed, as we move ahead in our exploration of the topics already chosen, addressing new interventions and, as evidence becomes available, updating our findings.

The authors wish to acknowledge the enormous contributions of all who have participated in this collective effort. We thank you, and hope that you will continue to work with us as we pursue our goals of contributing to improving the health of all Americans and reducing the persistent health disparities that affect our communities.

Jonathan E. Fielding, MD, MPH, MBA
Chair, Task Force on Community Preventive Services

Acknowledgments

This book is the result of years of research, conducted by many people. From those who first proposed the idea of a Guide to Community Preventive Services in the early 1990s to those who continue to work every day to expand the science base of the *Community Guide,* we express our thanks. If we left anyone off this list, our sincere apologies.

EARLY CONTRIBUTORS TO THE FORMATION OF THE COMMUNITY GUIDE

Claude Earl Fox, MD, MPH—Johns Hopkins Urban Health Institute, Baltimore, MD

Kristine M. Gebbie, DrPH, RN—Columbia University, New York, NY

Catherine Gordon, MD—Centers for Disease Control and Prevention, Washington, DC

William Harlan—National Institute of Mental Health, Bethesda, MD

Alan R. Hinman, MD, MPH—Task Force for Child Survival and Development, Atlanta, GA

Douglas B. Kamerow, MD, MPH—Editor, *BMJ USA*

Douglas S. Lloyd, MD, MPH—Health Resources and Services Administration, Bureau of Health Professions, Rockville, MD

J. Michael McGinnis, MD—Robert Wood Johnson Foundation, Princeton, NJ

David Satcher, MD, PhD—National Center for Primary Care, Morehouse School of Medicine, Atlanta, GA

Steven M. Teutsch, MD, MPH—Merck & Co. Inc., West Point, PA

Randy Wykoff, MD, MPH, TM—Project HOPE, Millwood, Virginia (formerly Deputy Assistant Secretary for Health—Disease Prevention and Health Promotion)

INTERNAL CDC EXECUTIVE ADVISORY COMMITTEE

Edward L. Baker, MD, MPH—Current affiliation, Public Health Leadership Institute, University of North Carolina

Claire V. Broome, MD

Jeffrey R. Harris, MD, MPH—Current affiliation, University of Washington

Dixie E. Snider, Jr., MD, MPH

Stephen B. Thacker, MD, MSc

CDC WORKGROUP ON THE *COMMUNITY GUIDE*

Lynda A. Anderson, PhD
Sevgi O. Aral, PhD
Peter A. Briss, MD, MPH
Blake Caldwell, MD, MPH
Nancy E. Cheal, PhD
José F. Cordero, MD, MPH
Scott D. Deitchman, MD, MPH
Alan R. Hinman, MD, MPH
Deane A. Johnson
Wilma Johnson, MS
Alison Kelly, MPIA
Richard Keenlyside, MD
Kenneth G. Keppel, PhD
Raymond M. (Bud) Nicola, MD, MHSA
Phil Nieburg, MD, MPH
Marguerite Pappaioanou, DVM, PhD
Joseph A. Reid, PhD
John S. Santelli, MD, MPH
Steven L. Solomon, MD
Daniel M. Sosin, MD, MPH
Janet Stansell
Terrie Stirling, PhD

SENIOR ADVISORS

Michael H. Hennessey, PhD, MPH
David V. McQueen, ScD—National Center for Chronic Disease Prevention and Health Promotion, CDC
Lance E. Rodewald, MD—National Immunization Program, CDC
David A. Sleet, PhD, MA—National Center for Injury Prevention and Control, CDC
Michael A. Stoto, PhD—RAND, Arlington, VA
Steven M. Teutsch, MD, MPH—Merck & Co., Inc., West Point, PA

TASK FORCE LIAISONS CURRENT AND PAST

Jacqelyn Admire-Borgelt, MSPH—American Academy of Family Physicians, Leawood, KS
J. Frederick Agel—National Association of Local Boards of Health, Atlanta, GA

David Atkins, MD, MPH—Agency for Healthcare Research and Quality, Rockville, MD

Ronald Bialek, MPP—Public Health Foundation, Washington, DC

Hudson H. Birden, Jr., MPH—Northern Rivers University Department of Rural Health, University of Sydney, Australia

Daniel S. Blumenthal, MD, MPH—Association of Teachers of Preventive Medicine

Mary B. Burdick, PhD, RN—Department of Veterans Affairs, Durham, NC

Bill Calvert, MS, MPH, MBA—U.S. Navy Environmental Health Center, Portsmouth, VA

Joseph Chin, MD, MS—Centers for Medicare and Medicaid Services, Baltimore, MD

Nathaniel Cobb, MD—Indian Health Service, Albuquerque, NM

Arthur B. Elster, MD—American Medical Association

Jessie Gruman, PhD—Center for the Advancement of Health, Washington, DC

Tom Houston, MD—American Medical Association

James D. Leeper, PhD—American Public Health Association

Rose Martinez, ScD—Institute of Medicine, Washington, DC

Robert J. McNellis, MPH, PA-C—American Academy of Physician Assistants, Alexandria, VA

Emmeline Ochiai, MPH—Office of Disease Prevention and Health Promotion, Washington, DC

Bob Rehm, MBA—American Association of Health Plans, Washington, DC

Jordan H. Richland, MPH—American College of Preventive Medicine, Washington, DC

Elizabeth S. Safran, MD, MPH—American Association of Public Health Physicians

Ruth Sanchez-Way, PhD—Substance Abuse and Mental Health Services Administration, Rockville, MD

James H. Scully, Jr., MD—National Association of State Mental Health Program Directors

Harrison Spencer, MD—Association of Schools of Public Health, Washington, DC

Col. Linda Spencer, PhD, RN—U.S. Army

Kristy Straits-Troster, PhD—V.A. National Center for Health Promotion and Disease Prevention, Durham, NC

Jonathan B. VanGeest, PhD—American Medical Association

Martina Vogel-Taylor, MT(ASCP)—National Institutes of Health, Bethesda, MD

Deborah Willis-Fillinger, MD, MPH—Health Resources and Services Administration, Rockville, MD

Steven H. Woolf, MD, MPH—American College of Preventive Medicine, Fairfax, VA

OTHER COMMUNITY GUIDE PARTNERS

Scott Grosse, PhD—Centers for Disease Control and Prevention
Kenji Hayashi, MD—Institute of Public Health, Japan
Hazel K. Keimowitz, MA—retired from Agency for Healthcare Research and Quality
Sally Herndon Malek, MPH—North Carolina Department of Health and Human Services, Raleigh
James L. Nichols, PhD—retired from National Highway Transportation Safety Administration, Washington, DC
C. Tracy Orleans, PhD—Robert Wood Johnson Foundation
Deborah S. Porterfield, MD, MPH—Department of Social Medicine, University of North Carolina at Chapel Hill

CONSULTANTS FOR THE SYSTEMATIC REVIEWS

Each team of consultants is listed at the end of the chapter to which they lent their expertise.

COMMUNITY GUIDE STAFF—CURRENT

Peter A. Briss, MD, MPH (Branch Chief—*Community Guide*)
Sajal K. Chattopadhyay, PhD (Branch Chief—Prevention Effectiveness)
Brad Myers, MPH

Laurie M. Anderson, PhD, MPH
Roy C. Baron, MD, MPH
Carolyn Beeker, PhD
Dawna S. Fuqua-Whitley, MA
Robert A. Hahn, PhD, MPH
Kate W. Harris, BA
David P. Hopkins, MD, MPH
Gail R. Janes, PhD, MS
Stella Kozlova, MPH
Amy Lovvorn, MPH
Angela K. McGowan, JD, MPH
Tarra K. McNally, MA, MPH
Tony Pearson-Clarke, MS
Cornelia K. White, PhD
Gail A. Wilson

OTHER AUTHORS, RESEARCHERS, AND STAFF WHO HAVE BEEN
PART OF THE COMMUNITY GUIDE INITIATIVE

Georgina Agyekum, MPH
Femi Alao, PhD
Tara J. Balsley, MPH
Oleg Bilukha, MD, PhD
Rosalind Breslow, PhD, MPH
S. Scott Brown, MPH
William Callaghan, MD
Vilma G. Carande-Kulis, PhD, MS (Branch Chief—Prevention Effectiveness:
    2001–2004)
Linda Carnes, DrPA
Juanita Chukwara
Joan Cioffi, PhD
Phaedra Corso, PhD
Debjani Das, MPH
Tanisha Denny, MPH
Tho Bella Dinh-Zarr, PhD, MPH
April Dixon
Erica Dunbar, MPH
Randy W. Elder, PhD
Erin Finley, BA
Adele Franks, MD
Nisha Gandhi, MPH
Prethibha George, MPH
Lynn Gibbs, MPH
Kathleen Green-Raleigh, PhD
Kathy W. Grooms, BS
Prakash L. Grover, PhD, MPH
Donna Higgins, PhD
Krista Hopkins, MPH
Angela B. Hutchinson, PhD
Kimberly Jackson-Smith, PhD
Lisa Jeannotte, MA
Evelyn Johnson, PhD
Ping Johnson, MD, PhD, CHES
Emily B. Kahn, PhD, MPH
Karol Kumpfer, PhD
Amy Levinson
Jessica Lowy, MPH, CHES

Cynthia C. Lyons
Mike V. Maciosek, PhD
Rika Maeshiro, MD, MPH
Julie M. Magri, MD, MPH
Melissa McPheeters, PhD, MPH
Wasseem Mina, MA
Gerald A. Mumma, PhD
Serigne Ndiaye, PhD
Phyllis J. Nichols, MPH
Enrique Nieves, MS (Deputy Branch Chief—*Community Guide:* 2001–2003)
Susan L. Norris, MD, MPH
Marguerite Pappaioanou, DVM, PhD (Branch Chief, *Community Guide:* 1996–
   1999)
Jeri D. Pickett, MS
Mummy Warda Rajab, MS
Leigh T. Ramsey, PhD
Vicki Rathel
David Rebanal, MPH, CHES
Connie Ricard, MPH, CHES
Kristi Riccio, CHES
Idania Rodriguez
J. Niels Rosenquist, BS
Joseph (Jay) Roth, MPH
Joseph St. Charles, MPA
Elena Saldanha, BS
Mona Saraiya, MD, MPH
Amanda Schofield, MPH
Julie Schuitema, MPH, MSW
Cheryl L. Scott, MD, MPH
Detrice Sherman, MPH
Carolynne Shinn, MS
Ruth A. Shults, PhD, MPH
Pomeroy Sinnock, PhD
Lynne T. Smith, PhD, MPH, RD
Nancy Smith, MHPA
S. Jay Smith, MIS, MS
Susan R. Snyder, PhD
Jonathan Stevens
Glenda A. Stone, PhD
Iddrisu Sulemana, MPH
Bernice Tannor, MPH
Craig Thomas, PhD

Benedict I. Truman, MD, MPH
Karen Taylor Valverde, MA
Julie A. Wasil
Carla D. Waye
Lori L. Westphal, MA, MPH
Linda Wright-De Agüero, PhD, MPH
Linda C. Yarbrough, BS
Patrice Young-Curtis, MSHCA
Stephanie Zaza, MD, MPH (Branch Chief—*Community Guide:* 1999–2003)

Contents

Part III: Methodological Background

Conventions Used in This Book

What do you want to find in this book? Here's where to look.

FIND RECOMMENDED INTERVENTIONS IN A TOPIC AREA

Chapters 1–9 each cover a specific topic area. Each chapter follows this pattern:

- *Title page,* listing all interventions and findings included in the chapter, when the research was conducted, and where this information has been published.
- *Introduction* to the topic area, including the public health burden it poses.
- *Recommendations from other advisory groups,* including *Healthy People 2010* goals and objectives in this topic area, as well as information from other groups and agencies.
- *Methods:* a brief summary of methods used in this topic area to evaluate the effectiveness of interventions.
- *Economic efficiency:* a brief summary of methods used to determine the economic efficiency of all recommended interventions.
- *Recommendations and findings:* the bulk of the chapter is in this section.
- Interventions are grouped under strategies (e.g., in Tobacco, the three strategies reviewed are Reducing Tobacco Use Initiation, Increasing Tobacco Use Cessation, and Reducing Exposure to Environmental Tobacco Smoke).
- One or two paragraphs give a general introduction to the strategy.
- A summary of the published findings is provided for each intervention (see Table C–1).
- *Using these recommendations:* additional considerations for deciding if use of a particular intervention is appropriate to your situation.
- *Conclusion:* summary of the interventions reviewed in this area and the recommendations or findings.

SEE ALL RECOMMENDATIONS AND FINDINGS
OF THE TASK FORCE LISTED ALPHABETICALLY BY TOPIC

The Appendix provides this list.

GET A BETTER UNDERSTANDING OF *COMMUNITY GUIDE* METHODS AND PROCESSES

The Introduction, "How to Use *The Guide to Community Preventive Services,*" serves as an orientation to the *Community Guide,* discussing various aspects of this book, as well as related publications and our website, www.thecommunityguide.org.

Table C–1. How Reviews of Interventions Are Presented in This Book

Intervention Name, Recommendation or Finding,
and Strength of Evidence for Recommended Interventions

One or two short paragraphs describing this type of intervention

• Bulleted list of key findings on effectiveness and, as appropriate, applicability, other effects, economic efficiency, and/or barriers to implementation

One or two paragraphs describing specific characteristics of the interventions studied for this review

Findings of the systematic review in the following order:

Effectiveness

Applicability to other populations and situations[a]

Other (positive or negative) effects of the intervention[b]

Economic findings[a]

Potential barriers to implementation[a]

Conclusion—summary of key findings

[a]Information on applicability, economic efficiency, and potential barriers to implementation is included only for recommended interventions.

[b]If no other effects have been found, this section is not included.

Chapter 10, "Methods Used for Reviewing Evidence and Linking Evidence to Recommendations in the *Community Guide*," explains the basics of the methodology used to select topic areas for review, as well as the systematic review methods used to evaluate interventions and the ways in which evidence is linked to Task Force recommendations.

Chapter 11, "Understanding and Using the Economic Evidence Provided in the *Community Guide*," provides an orientation to the kinds of economic analyses used in the *Community Guide* to evaluate public health interventions, as well as general information about how the economic reviews for the *Community Guide* are conducted.

Chapter 12, "Continuing Research Needs: Scientific Challenges and Opportunities," discusses the implications of the finding that available evidence is insufficient to determine the effectiveness of an intervention and that additional research is needed.

UNDERSTAND OUR TERMINOLOGY

In the Glossary, we define terms as they are used in the *Community Guide*.

Introduction: How to Use
The Guide to Community Preventive Services

WHAT IS THE *COMMUNITY GUIDE?*

The *Community Guide* (our shorthand for *The Guide to Community Preventive Services*) is a resource to help you select interventions to improve health and prevent disease in your state, community, community organization, business, healthcare organization, or school. It is designed to answer three questions:

1. What has worked for others and how well?
2. How can I select among interventions with proven effectiveness?
3. What might this intervention cost, and what am I likely to achieve through my investment?

The *Community Guide* is also a resource for researchers and research funders to identify important gaps in what we know and to determine how to allocate scarce research funds.

The *Community Guide* reviews evidence about interventions designed to improve health across a wide range of topics. Interventions that combat such risky behaviors as tobacco use, physical inactivity, and violence are included. Other reviewed interventions address specific health conditions such as cancer, diabetes, vaccine-preventable diseases, and motor vehicle injuries. Interventions that address the broad social determinants of health such as education, housing, and access to care are also reviewed in the *Community Guide.* Even with this broad scope, the *Community Guide* is not comprehensive. These initial topics were chosen because together they address the health behaviors, diseases, injuries, and social factors that impose the greatest burden of suffering and that offer the broadest range of intervention opportunities.[1] Intervention reviews are underway for a number of additional topics including nutrition, improving pregnancy outcomes, and reducing depression. In addition, we are updating and expanding most of the chapters in this book.

For each of these broad topics, interventions that promise to improve important health outcomes are reviewed. (For criteria used to select interventions for review, see Chapter 10, Methods Used for Reviewing Evidence and Linking Evidence to Recommendations in the *Community Guide.*) The interventions are applicable to groups, communities, or other populations and include strategies such as healthcare system changes, public laws, workplace and school programs and policies, and community-based programs. All of the

interventions are intended to improve health directly; prevent or reduce risky behaviors, disease, injuries, complications, or detrimental environmental or social factors; or promote healthy behaviors and environments. Diagnostic and treatment interventions are not covered in the *Community Guide,* nor are the clinical preventive services provided by a healthcare professional to an individual patient. Clinical preventive services are reviewed in the *Guide to Clinical Preventive Services.*[2] Together, the *Clinical Guide* and the *Community Guide* provide information on a broad range of preventive services applicable to individuals and populations.

WHO DEVELOPS THE *COMMUNITY GUIDE?*

The *Community Guide* is part of the Department of Health and Human Services' committed effort to strengthen the scientific basis for public health practice. The *Community Guide* is led by the independent Task Force on Community Preventive Services (the Task Force), composed of nonfederal experts from diverse backgrounds. The work of the Task Force is supported by staff at the Centers for Disease Control and Prevention and by numerous other federal and nonfederal experts.

NOT JUST ANY SET OF GUIDELINES

The *Community Guide* uses a technique known as a *systematic review* to provide scientific evidence of the effectiveness of interventions. Recommendations are explicitly linked to this evidence and are therefore evidence-based. Systematic reviews are conducted according to methods and processes intended to be comprehensive and to minimize bias in the review process. The methods, processes, and rationale for *Community Guide* systematic reviews are provided in Chapter 10. Systematic reviews have undergone considerable development in the social sciences, statistics, epidemiology, medicine, and other disciplines since the 1960s as tools to improve the quality of scientific literature synthesis.[3] They are increasingly popular for summarizing information on the efficacy of medical treatments[4] and clinical preventive services,[2,4] and are sometimes used as the foundation for developing clinical practice guidelines. The systematic review is also a useful methodology for summarizing the effectiveness of public health and population-based interventions. The *Community Guide* initiative is a large, high-profile, well-regarded example of the application of systematic review methods to population-oriented health interventions in the United States. The use of systematic reviews to support decision making for population health is an important step in bringing "public health to the same level of scientific scrutiny" as clinical care.[5]

A FAMILY OF PRODUCTS

The *Community Guide* is a family of products that provides systematic review findings, recommendations, and other types of information in different formats.

The Guide to Community Preventive Services: What Works to Promote Health?

This book provides a snapshot of the information available through late 2003. Following this chapter, the intervention reviews are organized into two parts: (*1*) Changing Risk Behaviors and Addressing Environmental Challenges and (*2*) Reducing Disease, Injury, and Impairment. Each part contains chapters about specific topics, and each chapter covers about 5–20 different interventions.

As mentioned, all topics of importance in public health are not yet addressed directly (e.g., cardiovascular disease or HIV/AIDS). However, many chapters contain information directly relevant to these two and other critical health issues (e.g., the chapters on tobacco and physical activity are relevant for reducing cardiovascular disease). As you consult this book, keep in mind that interventions in one or more chapters might be useful to achieve related objectives (e.g., the chapters on tobacco, cancer, and physical activity might be used together to achieve a cancer reduction goal).

Journal Articles

Because book publications can provide information available at only one point in time, *Community Guide* reviews are published in journals as they are completed. In addition, journal publication has allowed for rapid dissemination of the Task Force's findings in advance of publication in book format. Summaries of *Community Guide* reviews and recommendations are published in the *Morbidity and Mortality Weekly Report (Recommendations and Reports Series)*. Detailed scientific information about each systematic review is published in the *American Journal of Preventive Medicine* (*AJPM*). Accompanying the *AJPM* articles are editorial commentaries from a variety of experts describing how different audiences can use the *Community Guide* (e.g., managed care, public health, or voluntary organizations). Finally, various articles about the *Community Guide*, specific recommendations, and other aspects of the initiative occasionally appear in other journals.

The Website

The website www.thecommunityguide.org is the most comprehensive and up-to-date collection of *Community Guide* information. It includes access to all *Community Guide* reviews, short (one- or two-page) summaries of chapters and interventions, additional intervention reviews and updates completed after the publication of this book, and slide sets for use in presentations or training. For each review, details on each study included are provided in tables. Finally, links from the home page provide access to resources that link the *Community Guide* interventions to related *Healthy People 2010*[6] objectives, to related *Guide to Clinical Preventive Services*[2] interventions, and to some helpful information about how to implement interventions recommended in the *Community Guide*.

HOW DIFFERENT AUDIENCES CAN USE THE *COMMUNITY GUIDE*

The *Community Guide* can be used by decision makers in a variety of settings. Public health professionals can use the *Community Guide* for program planning and to encourage the use of effective interventions through grant guidance and planning criteria. They can also focus research on the knowledge gaps identified through the *Community Guide* systematic review process or seek resources for additional studies. Healthcare service providers can implement effective healthcare system interventions (e.g., provider reminder systems) to improve the delivery of effective clinical preventive services (e.g., advising patients to quit using tobacco products). Purchasers of health care (e.g., employers or state Medicaid officials) can use the *Community Guide* to construct and select benefit plans (e.g., reducing patients' out-of-pocket costs for vaccines or tobacco cessation therapies). In addition, employers can use the *Community Guide* to implement workplace interventions and to participate in community planning efforts. Legislators and other elected officials can support population health by enacting effective legislation (e.g., smoking bans, child safety seat laws, vaccination requirements for school admission, water fluoridation). Table I–1 provides an example of how a *Community Guide* recommendation influenced lifesaving legislation. Community-based organi-

Table I–1. Evidence-Based Recommendations at Work

An example of successful implementation of recommended interventions from the *Community Guide* illustrates the power and importance of evidence-based information. In 2001, the *Community Guide* recommendation for reducing the legal blood alcohol concentration (BAC) limit for adult drivers from 0.10% to 0.08% was influential in the decision of the U.S. Congress to include a requirement that all states pass such legislation or risk losing some federal highway construction funds. At the time the law was passed, 17 states had 0.08% BAC laws on their books. By the end of 2004, all 50 states, the District of Columbia, and Puerto Rico had enacted 0.08% BAC laws. Although most states had multiple laws aimed at reducing alcohol-impaired driving, this change should save at least 400–600 lives each year.

zations can select effective interventions for their populations and advocate for adoption of effective interventions by their local governments. Researchers can use the *Community Guide* to identify research gaps and advocate for funding to conduct research to fill those gaps. In addition, researchers can implement the *Community Guide* evaluation criteria (see Chapter 10) to ensure that their studies and reports are of the highest quality and eligible for inclusion in subsequent *Community Guide* reviews. Educators and students in all of these arenas can use the *Community Guide* as part of comprehensive training in evidence-based public health and prevention decision making.

THE *COMMUNITY GUIDE* IS PART OF COMPREHENSIVE PREVENTION PLANNING

Comprehensive program planning involves a series of activities: assessment, priority setting, objective setting, intervention selection, implementation, and evaluation.[7,8] The *Community Guide* primarily assists with intervention se-

---

Table I–2. Selected Resources for Comprehensive Prevention Planning

---

Assessment

- National Public Health Performance Standards (www.naccho.org/project48.cfm)
- MAPP: Mobilizing for Action through Planning and Partnerships (www.naccho .org/ project77.cfm)
- APEX-PH: Assessment Protocol for Excellence in Public Health (www.naccho.org/ project47.cfm)

Objective Setting

- *Healthy People 2010* objectives (www.healthypeople.gov)
- *In most states, Healthy People objectives have been tailored for state-level priorities. Your state health department will be able to provide you with state-specific objectives.*
- *Healthy People 2010* Leading Health Indicators (www.healthypeople.gov/LHI/)
- HEDIS: Health Plan Employer Data Set performance measures (www.ncqa.org/ Programs/HEDIS/)

Intervention Selection

- *Guide to Clinical Preventive Services* (www.ahrq.gov/clinic/uspstfix.htm)
- *Guide to Community Preventive Services* (www.thecommunityguide.org)
- National Guideline Clearinghouse (www.guideline.gov)

Intervention Implementation and Evaluation

- www.PreventionInfo.org has links to resources for intervention implementation
- Framework for Program Evaluation in Public Health can be found at www.cdc.gov/ mmwr/PDF/RR/RR4811.pdf
- Resources for implementing interventions are available in the Community Tool Box, http://ctb.ku.edu
- Approaches to help you plan, link, act, and network with evidence-based tools are available at Cancer Control PLANET (http://cancercontrolplanet.cancer.gov)

---

lection. Other resources assist planners and decision makers with the other steps (see Table I–2). Together, these resources can help you develop a comprehensive prevention plan for your patients, workers, students, or community members. Four key steps are briefly described below. At each step, involvement of stakeholders, recognition of intermediate objectives, monitoring of the process, and feedback of results are critical.

Assess the Primary Health Issues within Your State, Community, Workplace, School, or Health System

Evidence-based decision making requires data at each step in the process. For this first step, it is important to know which health problems and risk factors are prevalent in the community or population of interest and which health outcomes are frequent, severe, or costly. Understanding which health issues are a priority for the population, the local human and financial resources, and the political acceptability of addressing certain topics in a community is also important.

Identifying stakeholders and soliciting and incorporating their input at this and all steps in the prevention process is crucial for successfully identifying and addressing health issues. Planning tools are available to help in identifying and addressing priority health areas, and to work effectively with stakeholders (see Table I–2).

Develop Measurable Objectives to Assess Progress in Addressing Primary Health Issues

Once you identify which health issues are priorities to address, it is helpful to set specific objectives. Objectives should be reasonably attainable and must be measurable. Again, stakeholder input is important in selecting objectives so that measuring progress toward objectives will be enthusiastically endorsed by community members. Objective-setting resources for public and private entities are available (see Table I–2).

Select Effective Interventions to Help Achieve Objectives

The *Community Guide* is a primary resource for this step. Most chapters in this book include a *logic framework* or conceptual model for the topic covered in that chapter (for an example, see Figure I–1). The logic framework helps to identify the different ways in which the problem might be addressed and is essential for selecting appropriate interventions. For example, a health problem may be caused or complicated by a lack of knowledge on the part of the community members (e.g., not knowing when to get flu shots). It might be caused by the inaccessibility of health care or other resources (e.g., the ex-

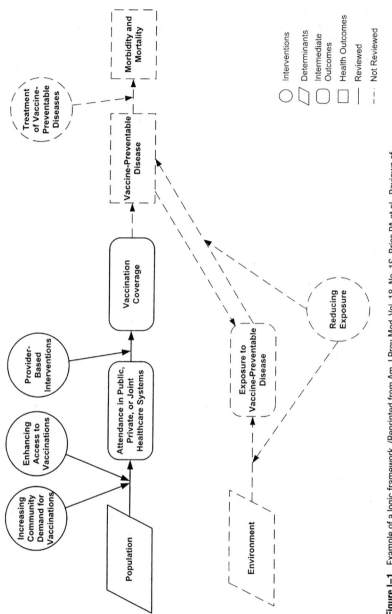

Figure I-1. Example of a logic framework. (Reprinted from Am J Prev Med, Vol. 18, No. 1S, Briss PA et al., Reviews of evidence regarding interventions to improve vaccination coverage in children, adolescents, and adults, p. 99, Copyright 2000, with permission from American Journal of Preventive Medicine.)

pense of buying a child safety seat). Or it might be aggravated by missed opportunities within the healthcare system (e.g., failure to identify a patient
who smokes and to provide appropriate counseling and therapy). To select
an intervention, it's important to know what problems are occurring or in
what proportion they are occurring. Note that the *Community Guide* does not
address all of the possible interventions that could be or have been used for
a particular health issue. Inclusion in the *Community Guide* is not a prereq-
uisite for implementing an intervention, particularly if it is a new intervention being tested for its effectiveness. Some *Community Guide* chapters include lengthy lists of intervention strategies that are applicable to the topic
but have not been reviewed. However, you should take into account whether
or not sufficient human and financial resources exist to develop, implement,
and evaluate new or untested interventions.

Once you've determined the nature of the problem you're trying to address, the remainder of the *Community Guide* chapter can be used to identify
interventions designed to address these specific areas. You'll find out whether
the intervention has been shown to be effective, ineffective, or if there's not
enough information yet to make a decision about effectiveness. And, for most
interventions, you'll find the effect size and variability that might be expected
from implementing the intervention.

With the list of intervention options narrowed, the *Community Guide* also
helps you assess several other issues that should be taken into account. For
example, you might be interested in the applicability of various interventions
to different settings and populations. Where has the intervention been implemented successfully? In which populations has the intervention worked?
For all interventions for which effectiveness has been established, our applicability information addresses both questions. In addition, citations for the
studies included in the review allow you to refer back to the original studies
or study authors.

Whenever sufficient information is available, a systematic review of the
costs, cost effectiveness, or cost–benefit of each effective intervention is provided to help you determine if you can afford to implement the intervention
and what can be achieved through your investment (see Chapter 11, Understanding and Using the Economic Evidence Provided in the *Community
Guide*). Each review also includes information on other possible benefits and
harms of the intervention. Finally, each review includes information on barriers you might encounter in implementing the intervention.

Implement and Evaluate the Selected Interventions

Careful action planning is key to successful implementation of an intervention. Although a comprehensive treatment of action planning is beyond the

scope of the *Community Guide,* excellent resources for this step exist.[7] Briefly, the intervention must be well constructed, well implemented, and evaluated.

Successful intervention implementation rests first with careful construction of the intervention. Be advised that *Community Guide* recommendations are based on summaries of numerous individual interventions that had similar components and were trying to achieve the same outcomes. Thus, the recommendations are for conceptual categories rather than particular intervention programs that have been implemented elsewhere. Therefore, when developing your local intervention, consider including all the components included in the studies summarized in the *Community Guide* intervention review. Because it is rarely possible to determine how each component contributed to intervention effectiveness, *Community Guide* recommendations are for the entire constellation of components. Next, consider local needs, culture, language, and political or social norms to help you adapt the intervention. Finally, consider how the intervention processes will be managed to make it sustainable over time.

Related to intervention construction is the implementation itself. Resources for implementing interventions well are available elsewhere (e.g., the Community Tool Box, http://ctb.ku.edu). Interventions must be implemented well to be effective. Timing, attention to detail, training of personnel, and buy-in from stakeholders are all important in ensuring success. Finally, every intervention should be evaluated over time (using formal or informal methods) to ensure that it is being implemented as intended and is achieving its desired ends. Excellent program evaluation resources are also available.[7,9-12]

The *Community Guide* can help with objective setting (by identifying the types of outcomes and effect size that can reasonably be expected from the interventions) and with evaluation (by identifying the important outcomes to measure after an intervention is implemented). It is, however, primarily designed to provide a menu of effective population-based interventions (i.e., what to choose). The *Community Guide* itself is not a cookbook that shows you how to implement the recommended interventions, although some implementation advice is provided in each chapter and additional information is provided at www.thecommunityguide.org (see Table I-2). An example of how the *Community Guide* can be used as part of comprehensive prevention planning is provided in Table I-3.

USING THE RESEARCH GAPS

The systematic review process has three possible results: we learn that an intervention is effective, that it is ineffective or harmful, or that evidence is insufficient to determine its effectiveness. Any of these findings is important information for decision making. Thus, the knowledge gaps identified through

Table I–3. Using the *Community Guide* for Strategic Intervention
Selection and Implementation: Improving Influenza Vaccination Rates

Imagine that your goal is to increase influenza vaccination rates among adults aged 65 years and older. In *Community Guide* Chapter 6, "Vaccine-Preventable Diseases," you learn that vaccine rates might be low in your population because:

1. People lack knowledge about or have attitudinal barriers to being vaccinated against a particular disease.
2. People know that they need to be vaccinated but do not have access to vaccination services.
3. People know that they need to be vaccinated and have access to services, but providers or healthcare systems are missing opportunities to vaccinate.

To select an intervention, it's important to know which of these three problems are occurring or in what combinations they are occurring. You conduct a survey and find that vaccination rates are lower than the national average and that 80% of unvaccinated adults were seen in healthcare settings during the last vaccination year but that influenza vaccine wasn't offered. Thus, you decide to start with an intervention to help providers and healthcare systems offer the vaccine more consistently.

Armed with this information, you turn to the *Community Guide* section on Provider- and System-Based Interventions for increasing coverage with universally recommended vaccines (vaccines, like influenza vaccine, recommended for all people in a particular age group). This section identifies standing orders programs as an effective strategy that can be implemented in clinics or managed care organizations. Together with your partners from local health plans, you collect more information about implementing such programs,[13] and you determine that there are no local legal, regulatory, or other barriers to implementing these programs in your area. You then decide to implement a standing orders program that identifies clients needing the vaccine and allows nurses to provide the vaccine without direct physician involvement at the time of the vaccination.

The *Community Guide* recommendation for standing orders means that these programs, which allow identification of people needing vaccination and allow them to be vaccinated without direct physician involvement at the time of the visit, generally have been shown to be effective in a variety of settings. As already noted, the implementation of such a program will vary based on characteristics of the local clinical setting (e.g., inpatient or outpatient, staff model HMO versus health department clinic) and on characteristics of the local legal and regulatory environment. However, looking at the applicability of the intervention review, you find that reasonably consistent results occurred across a broad range of populations, settings, and intervention characteristics, increasing your confidence that the intervention's effectiveness will be robust when it is adapted in your local context.

the systematic review process are an important *Community Guide* product. Chapter 12, Continuing Research Needs, can guide the organizations and government agencies that fund research to important but understudied areas. In addition, that chapter can guide researchers to important areas for developing research programs and requests for research funding.

Community Guide reviews identify promising but understudied areas with important public health implications. They can also reduce excessive repetition of research beyond that needed for appropriate replication and help allocate limited research resources more efficiently.

The *Community Guide* is an important resource for identifying research gaps, but the Task Force has purposely not established an order of priority for addressing the questions identified through their systematic review process. Research agenda setting is largely driven by the priorities and resources of the various organizations and government agencies that fund and conduct research. Thus, it is left to those groups to determine how to set priorities among the various research questions identified here.

SUMMARY

The *Community Guide* is a resource for selecting interventions to improve health and prevent disease. Systematic reviews of published literature in three key areas—changing risk behaviors; reducing specific diseases, injuries, and impairments; and addressing environmental and ecosystem challenges—provide evidence-based answers to three basic questions: What has worked for others and how well? How can I select among interventions of proven effectiveness? What might this intervention cost, and what am I likely to achieve through my investment? The *Community Guide* is also a resource for identifying areas where additional research is needed.

The *Community Guide* is really a family of products, of which this book is one part. The other parts are a website, www.thecommunityguide.org, and articles published in peer-reviewed journals. Many different audiences will find the *Community Guide* useful, including public health professionals, healthcare service providers, purchasers of health care, employers, legislators, community-based organizations, and researchers. The *Community Guide* is part of comprehensive planning for prevention activities, which includes (*1*) assessing needs; (*2*) setting objectives to measure progress; (*3*) selecting effective interventions (this is where the *Community Guide* is most helpful); and (*4*) implementing the selected interventions.

The *Community Guide* can be a valuable tool in helping you decide how to allocate limited resources and achieve desired outcomes.

Acknowledgments

This chapter was written by Stephanie Zaza, MD, MPH, Office of the Director, National Center for Chronic Disease Prevention and Health Promotion, Centers for Disease Control and Prevention (CDC), Atlanta, Georgia; Peter A. Briss, MD, MPH, Community Guide Branch, Division of Prevention Research and Analytic Methods (DPRAM), Epidemiology Program Office (EPO), CDC, Atlanta; Jonathan E. Fielding, MD, MPH, MBA, Los Angeles Department of Health Services, University of California School of Public

Health, Los Angeles, and the Task Force on Community Preventive Services; Bradford A. Myers, MPH, Community Guide Branch, DPRAM/EPO/CDC, Atlanta; and Steven M. Teutsch, MD, MPH, Outcomes Research and Management, Merck & Co., Inc., West Point, Pennsylvania.

References

1. Zaza S, Lawrence RS, Mahan CS, et al. Scope and organization of the Guide to community preventive services. Am J Prev Med 2000;18(1S):27–34.

2. U.S. Preventive Services Task Force. Guide to clinical preventive services: report of the U.S. Preventive Services Task Force. 2nd ed. Baltimore: Williams & Wilkins, 1996.

3. Glass GV. Primary, secondary, and meta-analysis. Educ Res 1976;5:3–8.

4. The Cochrane Collaboration. The Cochrane Library. Available at www.cochrane.org. Accessed March 26, 2004.

5. McGinnis JM, Foege W. Guide to community preventive services: harnessing the science [commentary]. Am J Prev Med 2000;18(1S):1–2.

6. U.S. Department of Health and Human Services. Healthy people 2010. 2nd ed. Washington, DC: U.S. Government Printing Office, 2000.

7. Brownson RC, Baker EA, Leet TL, Gillespie KN. Evidence-based public health. New York: Oxford University Press, 2003.

8. Green LW, Kreuter MW. Health promotion planning: an educational and ecological approach. 3rd ed. Mountain View, CA: Mayfield, 1999.

9. Goodman RM. Principals and tools for evaluating community-based prevention and health promotion programs. J Public Health Manag Pract 1998;4(2):37–47.

10. Israel BA, Cummings KM, Dignan MB, et al. Evaluation of health education programs: current assessment and future directions. Health Educ Q 1995;22(3):364–89.

11. Rossi PH, Freeman HE, Lipsey MW. Evaluation: a systematic approach. 6th ed. Thousand Oaks, CA: Sage, 1999.

12. Center for Disease Control and Prevention. Framework for program evaluation in public health. MMWR 1999;48(RR-11):1–40.

Part I

Changing Risk Behaviors and Addressing Environmental Challenges

Chapter 1

Tobacco

*Insufficient evidence means that we were not able to determine whether or not the intervention works.

The Task Force approved the recommendations in this chapter in 1999–2000. The research on which the findings are based was conducted between 1976 and May 2000. This information—with the exception of reviews of approaches to reduce tobacco use through interventions to restrict minors' access to tobacco products—has been previously published in the American Journal of Preventive Medicine [2001; 20(2S): 10–15 and 16–66] and the MMWR Recommendations and Reports series [2000; 49(No. RR-12):1–11]. The information on restricting minors' access to tobacco products is being prepared for publication.

Tobacco use is the leading cause of preventable illness and death in the United States.[1] Recognized as a cause of multiple cancers, heart disease, stroke, complications of pregnancy, and chronic obstructive pulmonary disease,[2] tobacco use is responsible for 430,000 deaths per year among adults, and direct medical costs are in the range of $50–$73 billion per year.[3]

Despite nearly four decades of policies, regulations, educational efforts, and increasing information on the negative health effects of tobacco use and the positive health benefits of cessation, tobacco use remains unacceptably high. In 2002, an estimated 45.8 million adults in the United States (nearly one in four adults) smoked.[4] Tobacco use and disparities in tobacco-related morbidity and mortality vary by region, level of education, socioeconomic status, race, gender, and ethnicity.[2,5] Individuals below the poverty line, for example, are more likely to smoke than individuals at or above the poverty line (32.9% compared with 22.2%).[4] By level of education, adults who had earned a General Educational Development (GED) diploma had the highest prevalence (42.3%) of smoking; people with masters, professional, and doctoral degrees had the lowest prevalence (7.2%).[4] The prevalence of smoking among American Indians and Alaska Natives (40.8%) is higher than that of other racial and ethnic groups.[4]

Regular tobacco use results in true drug dependence in most users, making attempts to quit difficult and relapses common.[6] Many users make multiple attempts to quit.[7] In 2002, an estimated 15.4 million current smokers (41.2%) had stopped smoking for at least one day during the preceding 12 months because they were trying to stop smoking entirely.[4] Although cessation significantly reduces the immediate and subsequent risks of tobacco-related morbidity and mortality,[8,9] most tobacco users do not receive assistance in quitting.[6]

Preventing the acquisition of this costly, chronic dependence is clearly desirable. However, tobacco use initiation and the transition from experimentation to addiction are not easy to prevent because they occur primarily in adolescence, when individuals are more susceptible to influences from family, friends, peers, society, and the tobacco industry that encourage tobacco use.[10] Smoking among 8th, 10th, and 12th graders increased dramatically from 1991 to 1997 and then declined just as dramatically from 1997 to 2003. For example, prevalence of current smoking among high school seniors was 28.3% in 1991, increased to 36.5% by 1997, and declined to 24.4% by 2003.[11] The high rates of smoking prevalence among young adults aged 18–24 years (28.5% in 2002), in addition to reflecting those who started smoking in high school, may also indicate an increase in tobacco use initiation among this group.[4]

Exposure to environmental tobacco smoke (ETS) is a recognized cause of heart disease and accounts for an estimated 3000 lung cancer deaths per year among adults.[12] Among infants and children, exposure to ETS causes middle ear infections and effusions, exacerbates 400,000–1,000,000 cases of asthma annually, and causes 150,000–300,000 cases of lower respiratory tract infections each year.[13] The health effects of exposure to ETS have prompted the increasing implementation of public and private policies that restrict smoking.[2] The median level of cotinine (a marker for exposure to tobacco smoke) among nonsmokers declined 70% from 1988–1991 to 1999–2000, suggesting a dramatic reduction in exposure of the general U.S. population to ETS over this time period. However, substantial gender, racial, and age disparities in exposure are evident, with children, men, and African Americans having higher exposure levels.[14] Exposure to ETS continues to occur in workplaces and public areas without smoking bans or effective restrictions and in households in which smoking indoors is allowed.

OBJECTIVES AND RECOMMENDATIONS FROM OTHER ADVISORY GROUPS

The interventions reviewed in this chapter can be useful in reaching many of the tobacco control objectives in *Healthy People 2010*[15] (Table 1–1). In the field of tobacco control, many groups have published useful guidelines. To help summarize this information, we published an article in 2001[16] comparing the *Community Guide* population-based recommendations with reviews and recommendations produced by other groups, including the Surgeon General's office, the United States Preventive Services Task Force (which publishes the *Guide to Clinical Preventive Services*[17]), and the Cochrane Collaboration. Another good source for readers interested in information on various clinical guidelines is *Treating Tobacco Use and Dependence: Clinical Practice Guideline*[6]; some information from that report is also summarized in our article.

Table 1–1. Selected *Healthy People 2010*[15] Objectives Related to Tobacco Use and Environmental Tobacco Smoke Exposure

Objective	Population	Baseline	2010 Objective
Tobacco Use in Population Groups			
Reduce cigarette smoking by adults (Objective 27–1a)	Adults	24% (1998)	12%
Reduce use of tobacco products by adolescents (in the past month)(27–2a)	Adolescents	40% (1999)	21%
Reduce the initiation of tobacco use among children and adolescents (27–3)	Children/ adolescents	Developmental	
Increase (delay) the average age of first tobacco use by adolescents (aged 12–17 years) (27–4a)	Adolescents	12 years old (1997)	14 years old
Cessation and Treatment			
Increase the percentage of smokers stopping smoking for a day or longer (27–5)	Adults	41% (1998[a])	75%
Among females aged 18–49 years, increase smoking cessation in pregnant women in the first trimester of pregnancy (27–6)	Pregnant women	14% (1998)	30%
Among adolescents in grades 9–12, increase the percentage of ever-daily smokers who try to quit (27–7)	Adolescents	76% (1999)	84%
Increase in insurance coverage of evidence-based treatment for nicotine dependency:			
• in managed care organizations: (27–8a)	All	75% (1997–98)	100%
• in Medicaid programs in states and the District of Columbia (27–8b)		24 states (1998)	51 states
Exposure to Secondhand Smoke (ETS)			
Among children aged ≤6 years, reduce the proportion of children who live in homes in which someone smokes inside the house ≥4 days per week (27–9)	Young children	27% (1994)	10%
Reduce the proportion of nonsmokers aged ≥4 years with a serum cotinine level >0.10 ng/mL (27–10)	Nonsmokers	65% (1988–94[a])	45%

Table 1-1. *Continued*

Objective	Population	Baseline	2010 Objective
Exposure to Secondhand Smoke (ETS) (continued)			
Increase the proportion of smoke-free and tobacco-free middle, junior high, and senior high schools (27–11)	Schools	37% (1994)	100%
Increase the proportion of worksites (with ≥50 workers) with formal smoking policies that prohibit smoking or limit it to separately ventilated areas (27–12)	Employees	79% (1998–99)	100%
Increase the number of states plus the District of Columbia with laws on smoke-free air:		(All 1998)	(For all)
• in private workplaces (27–13a)	All	1 state	51 states
• in public workplaces (27–13b)		13 states	
• in restaurants (27–13c)		3 states	
• on public transportation (27–13d)		16 states	
• in day-care centers (27–13e)		22 states	
• in retail stores (27–13f)		4 states	
Social and Environmental Changes			
Increase the number of states (including the District of Columbia) with a ≤5% sales rate of tobacco products to minors (27–14a)	Minors	0 states (1998)	51 states
Increase the number of states (including the District of Columbia) that can suspend or revoke state licenses for violation of laws prohibiting the sale of tobacco to minors (27–15)	Minors	34 states (1998)	51 states
Eliminate tobacco advertising and promotions that influence adolescents and young adults (27–16)	Adolescents/ young adults	Developmental	
Increase the proportion of adolescents who disapprove of smoking:		(All 1998)	
• among 8th graders (27–17a)	Adolescents	80%	95% for all

continued next page

Table 1–1. *Continued*

Objective	Population	Baseline	2010 Objective
Social and Environmental Changes (continued)			
• among 10th graders (27–17b)		75%	
• among 12th graders (27–17c)		69%	
Increase the number of tribes, territories, and states and the District of Columbia with comprehensive, evidence-based tobacco control programs (27–18)	All	Developmental	
Reduce the number of states that have laws preempting stronger tobacco control (in the areas of clean indoor air, minors' access laws, or marketing) (27–19)	All	30 states (1998)	0 states
Reduce the toxicity of tobacco products by establishing a regulatory structure to monitor toxicity (27–20)	All	Developmental	
• Increase the combined federal and average state tax (per pack) on cigarettes (27–21a)	All	$0.63 (1998)	$2
• Increase the combined federal and average state tax on spit tobacco (27–21b)		Developmental	

[a]Age adjusted for the year 2000 standard population.

METHODS

Methods used for the reviews are summarized in Chapter 10. Specific methods used in the systematic reviews of tobacco use prevention and control have been described elsewhere[16,18–20] and are available at www.thecommunityguide.org/tobacco. The logic framework depicting the conceptual approach used in these reviews is presented in Figure 1–1.

ECONOMIC EFFICIENCY

A systematic review of available economic evaluations was conducted for each recommended intervention, and a summary of each review is presented with the related intervention. The methods used to conduct these economics reviews are summarized in Chapter 11.

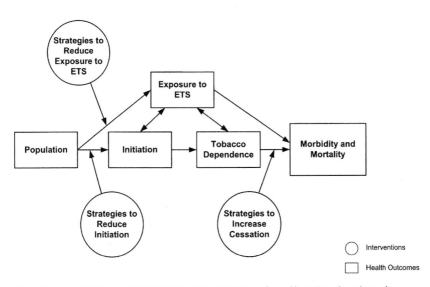

Figure 1–1. Logic framework illustrating the conceptual approach used in systematic reviews of tobacco use. (ETS = environmental tobacco smoke.) (Reprinted from Am J Prev Med, Vol. 20, No. 2S, Hopkins DP et al., Reviews of evidence regarding interventions to reduce tobacco use and exposure to environmental tobacco smoke, p. 18, Copyright 2001, with permission from American Journal of Preventive Medicine.)

RECOMMENDATIONS AND FINDINGS

This section presents a summary of the findings of the systematic reviews conducted to determine the effectiveness of the selected interventions in this topic area. We evaluated interventions to address three goals essential to tobacco prevention and control efforts: decreasing the number of people who start using tobacco products (tobacco use initiation), increasing the number of tobacco users who quit (tobacco use cessation), and reducing exposures among nonsmokers to environmental tobacco smoke (ETS).

Reducing Tobacco Use Initiation

The interventions in our reviews are designed to change knowledge, attitudes, and tobacco use among children, adolescents, and young adults. Most adults who use tobacco products began in adolescence, and nicotine addiction develops during the first few years of use.[21] Children and adolescents may perceive tobacco use to be a normal peer and adult behavior, and can often act on this belief because tobacco products are readily available and accessible.[10] Preventing or delaying experimentation with tobacco or preventing the transition from experimentation to regular use are the major goals of the interventions we reviewed: increasing the unit price for tobacco products, mass media campaigns when combined with additional efforts, and interventions to restrict minors' access to tobacco products.

Increasing the Unit Price for Tobacco Products:
Recommended (Strong Evidence of Effectiveness)

Interventions to increase the unit price for tobacco products primarily include legislation at the municipal, state, or federal level that raises the excise tax on tobacco products. In several states, excise tax increases have resulted from successful state ballot initiatives. Although other factors affect tobacco product pricing, excise tax increases have historically resulted in an equivalent or larger increase in tobacco product prices.[22]

Excise taxes on tobacco products increase the overall product cost and therefore make the use of tobacco products less attractive to young people with limited income and a variety of ways to spend their money.

Effectiveness

- Higher prices for tobacco products are associated with reduced consumption of tobacco products (a 10% price increase results in approximately a 4% decrease).
- Higher prices for tobacco products are associated with lower levels of tobacco use by adolescents and young adults who use tobacco (a 10% price increase results in approximately a 2% decrease in the amount smoked).

Applicability

- These findings should be applicable to most adolescents and young adults in the United States.

Other Effects

- Price increases also reduce tobacco use among adults.

Barriers

- Increasing the excise tax on tobacco products requires passage of legislation or a statewide referendum.

The findings of our systematic review are based on eight studies that evaluated the effectiveness of increasing the price of tobacco products on changing the tobacco use behaviors of adolescents or young adults.[23-30] Three additional articles provided information on a study already included in the review.[31-33] All studies were conducted in the United States. Studies examined the effect of product price on tobacco use by adolescents (13–18 years old) and by young adults (18–24 years or under 25 years old).

All eight studies used econometric methods to analyze surveys of students or young adults. Price elasticity of demand (the percentage change in consumption that results from a 1% change in price) estimates were calculated by combining information on local tobacco product prices, price changes, or differences over the period of study with responses to surveys on tobacco use and consumption. The price elasticity of demand estimates in these studies included participation (i.e., tobacco use prevalence), number of cigarettes smoked per day among those who smoke, and overall estimates of tobacco consumption (which includes both changes in participation and amount smoked by those who continue to smoke). All of the studies attempted to control for concurrent tobacco prevention and control efforts, including differences in smoking restrictions, youth tobacco access laws, school tobacco education programs, and exposure to anti-tobacco media. Five studies evaluated the effect of price on tobacco use for study periods that included the 1990s, and three studies reported the effect of price on tobacco use for periods before 1990.

Price elasticity of demand estimates from seven studies demonstrated that higher tobacco product prices are associated with lower levels of tobacco use by adolescents and young adults. Based on the median estimate of price elasticity from the studies in this review, for example, tobacco use prevalence among adolescents (13–18 years old) would decrease 3.7% with a 10% increase in product price (range, "no statistically significant effect" to 11.9%). The effects are at least as strong for young adults (18–24 years old). For estimates of amount smoked, the median estimate from six studies suggests that a 10% increase in product price would result in a 2.3% decrease in the amount of tobacco used by adolescents who smoke.

These findings show that increasing the unit price for tobacco products is effective in reducing both tobacco use prevalence and tobacco consumption among adolescents and young adults.

These results should be applicable to most adolescents and young adults in the United States. All studies were conducted in the United States, and most of the studies used national datasets to compare tobacco use and product price across jurisdictions (e.g., states). The study samples are representative of populations of adolescents and young adults. Studies evaluated the effect of product price on use and consumption of both cigarettes and smokeless tobacco products.

Overall, the studies showed that tobacco product price increases had a greater effect among males than among females; price affected tobacco use and consumption among whites, African Americans, and Hispanics; and African-American adolescents and young adults were more responsive to differences in product price than were white adolescents and young adults, respectively.

Increasing the price of tobacco products also reduces tobacco use among adults (for additional information see the review of Increasing the Unit Price for Tobacco Products in the next section, Increasing Tobacco Use Cessation). We found no other additional positive or negative effects of tobacco product price increases on adolescent tobacco use initiation.

Econometric analyses were included in the studies qualifying for the review of effectiveness. A separate economic evaluation was not conducted for this intervention review.

Passage of legislation or a statewide referendum is required for an excise tax increase on tobacco products and may, therefore, present a significant barrier to implementation. Political opposition has historically been well organized and funded at both the federal and state levels. Reports on both successful and unsuccessful state initiatives that proposed an increase on tobacco product excise taxes have been published.[34-36]

In conclusion, the Task Force recommends increasing the unit price for tobacco on the basis of strong evidence of effectiveness in reducing tobacco use initiation among adolescents and young adults. Raising the unit price for tobacco products (through increases in the excise tax) is effective in reducing both the number of adolescents and young adults who use tobacco products and the amount of tobacco they use. Increasing the unit price for tobacco products also reduces tobacco use among adults. The need for passage by a state legislature or a referendum can present a barrier to increasing excise taxes.

Mass Media Education Campaigns When Combined with Other Interventions: Recommended (Strong Evidence of Effectiveness)

These campaigns use mass media for an extended duration (months to years) to disseminate brief, recurring messages with the goal of providing information that will motivate people, primarily children and adolescents, to remain tobacco-free. The messages, developed through formative research, are disseminated through paid broadcast time and print space, donated time and space (as public service announcements), or a combination of the two. Mass media campaigns can be combined or coordinated with additional interventions, such as increases in tobacco product excise taxes, school-based education, and other community-wide educational activities.

Mass media techniques primarily include broadcast messages on television and radio, although other formats such as billboards, print, and movies have been used. Campaigns can focus on messages targeting children and adolescents or can include such messages as part of an overall anti-tobacco effort (e.g., including messages targeting tobacco users to increase cessation and messages about reducing exposure to secondhand tobacco smoke). The content of mass media campaigns designed to educate and motivate children and adolescents to remain tobacco-free can vary, but a recent review identified two primary strategies: agenda setting and demand reduction education.[37] Agenda-setting messages increase awareness of strategies used by the tobacco industry to promote tobacco use, and attempt to facilitate changes in both tobacco use behaviors and public tobacco policies. Demand reduction education messages provide information and support to young people to help them decide to remain tobacco-free.

Effectiveness

- Mass media education campaigns, combined with other interventions, are effective in decreasing the number of young people who use tobacco by approximately 2.4 percentage points.
- Effectiveness was increased in campaigns lasting two years or longer.

Applicability

- These findings should be applicable to most adolescents in the United States.

Other Effects

- Mass media education campaigns can also include messages that contribute to reductions in tobacco use among adults.

The findings of our systematic review are based on 12 studies that evaluated the effectiveness of mass media campaigns in reducing tobacco use among adolescents.[38-49] Two additional studies were identified but did not meet our quality criteria and were excluded from the review.[50,51] Another 28 papers provided information on studies already included in the review.[52-79] In nine studies, the mass media efforts focused on youth; in three other studies, youth-targeted messages were part of a larger anti-tobacco campaign. Only one study used mass media alone (through a variety of outlets). In 11 studies, the mass media campaign was conducted in coordination or concurrently with contests, school-based education programs, or community education programs. Two studies were conducted in settings where excise taxes on tobacco products had been increased. Two of the mass media campaigns were less than two weeks long, three were less than two years long, and seven campaigns were more than two years long.

The qualifying studies provided 12 diverse measures of tobacco use and generally showed reductions among youth (students) in the intervention communities relative to youth in the comparison communities. For example, five studies reported absolute differences in self-reported tobacco use and observed a median reduction of 2.4 percentage points (range, 0.02 increase to

9.5 decrease). In six studies, comparisons in self-reported tobacco use were expressed as odds ratios. Two of these studies reported no intervention effect on tobacco use, whereas four studies observed lower rates among people exposed to the intervention (median odds ratio of 0.60, range 0.49 to 0.74).

All seven studies evaluating campaigns of two or more years' duration observed reductions in tobacco use among youth in favor of the intervention communities. In studies reporting absolute percentage differences the median reduction in tobacco use was 8.0 percentage points (range, 2.4 to 11), and in studies calculating odds ratios the median was 0.74 (range, 0.49 to 0.74).

We could not assess the effects of the separate components of these combined intervention efforts.

These findings show that mass media education campaigns, when combined with other intervention activities, are effective in decreasing tobacco use among youth.

These results should be applicable to most adolescents in the United States. Statewide campaigns were conducted in Florida, Massachusetts, and Minnesota. Community and regional interventions were conducted in the Southeast, Northeast, and Midwest, and in Montana and Southern California. Campaigns began in the 1990s, the 1980s, and the 1970s. Both representative samples of adolescents in the general population and representative or selected samples of schools were used. Student populations were recruited or surveyed before grade 6, in grades 6–7, or after grade 7. The two most recent studies showed a greater benefit among younger adolescents. Evaluation of the Florida campaign provides evidence of effectiveness of mass media campaigns among girls, boys, whites, African Americans, and Hispanics.

Mass media campaigns, when combined with additional interventions, can also reduce tobacco use among adults (for additional information see Mass Media Education Campaigns in the next section, Increasing Tobacco Use Cessation), although the message content, broadcast times, and settings that reduce youth tobacco use may not be effective in reducing adult tobacco use. No other positive or negative effects were identified.

The findings of our systematic review of economic evaluations are based on one four-year economic study conducted in Montana, New York, and Vermont.[71] This cost-effectiveness analysis compared the effect on students of a mass media campaign combined with a school smoking prevention program to the effect of a school smoking prevention program alone. Students (from grades 5–7 through grades 8–10) were followed for two years after the intervention. Costs included personnel, travel, data entry, message research and development, and television and radio advertising. At follow-up, smoking prevalence among students exposed to the media intervention plus the school smoking prevention program was 20.4%, compared with 25.9% among students exposed only to the school program. Adjusted program cost per smoker averted was $6069, and the adjusted program cost per quality-adjusted life year (QALY) was $333.

The main barrier to implementation of mass media campaigns is the cost of purchasing advertising time. Costs of developing and test marketing messages can be offset by cooperation between tobacco control programs.

In conclusion, the Task Force recommends mass media campaigns, when combined with additional interventions, on the basis of strong evidence of effectiveness in reducing tobacco use among adolescents. These interventions were effective in decreasing the number of young people who use tobacco products. The findings of this review should be applicable to most adolescents in the United States. Mass media campaigns can produce the additional benefit of a reduction in adult tobacco use.

Restricting Minors' Access to Tobacco Products: Interventions to Reduce Tobacco Use

Access to tobacco products by minors (people under 18 years of age in most states) contributes to the initiation and regular use of tobacco by children and adolescents.[2,10] Retailers who sell tobacco products to minors (including vending machines in accessible settings) constitute one avenue of access for minors.[2,10,80] Social sources provide another route of access for many, but not all, minors. Although social sources include adults (parents, family, friends) who may purchase tobacco products legally,[81–83] illegal retailer sales to minors provide tobacco products for distribution to other minors, contributing to social access.[81]

Minors obtain tobacco from commercial sources through face-to-face purchases from retailers (from self-service displays or requests for products held behind the counter), purchases from vending machines, purchases through the mail or over the Internet, access to free product samples, and theft from retail sources. Overall, minors' access reflects the availability of tobacco products within the community, the willingness of retailers to sell them, and the efforts of minors to obtain them. Interventions to reduce access attempt to modify or to change one or more of these factors.

This section includes a review of a variety of interventions to restrict and reduce the supply of tobacco products that minors can obtain from commercial sources. Some of the intervention combinations reviewed included components intended, in whole or in part, to reduce the demand for tobacco products by minors through efforts to educate and mobilize the community and to change social norms about the acceptability of tobacco use.[84] In these efforts, minors' access to commercial sources of tobacco provided a focus for the community to address the problem of tobacco use among youth.

In conducting this review of interventions to reduce minors' access to tobacco products, we considered as evidence of effectiveness (1) measurements of differences or changes in self-reported tobacco use in the study population and (2) measurements of differences or changes in self-reported purchases of tobacco products or use of tobacco obtained from commercial sources. Because it is not clear how the compliance of any particular retailer contributes to the overall availability of tobacco to youth, differences or changes in retailer sales of tobacco products to minors were evaluated and summarized but did not by themselves provide the basis for our assessments of effectiveness.

In this section, we review studies that combined two or more interventions in a coordinated effort to restrict minors' access to tobacco products. We identified a total of 28 multicomponent studies. The 13 studies (with 14 arms) that qualified for our assessment of effectiveness evaluated a total of 10 different combinations of interventions. However, only five of these studies conducted measurements of differences or changes in tobacco use among youth, the focus of our assessment of effectiveness. The remaining studies measured differences or changes in retailer sales rates on "youth test purchase attempts" (in which recruited, trained, and supervised minors make standardized attempts to purchase tobacco products from retailers and vending machines). Overall, the body of evidence included evaluations of effectiveness for a variety of overlapping combinations of interventions. The information presented here summarizes only one of our reviews on effectiveness across the qualifying multicomponent studies.

Community Mobilization When Combined with Additional Interventions: Recommended (Sufficient Evidence of Effectiveness)

These interventions are implemented community-wide to focus public attention on the issue of youth access to tobacco products and to generate and mobilize community support for additional efforts to reduce that access. The community mobilization efforts evaluated here either fostered or were coordinated with additional interventions, such as stronger restrictions on retailer sales of tobacco products; restrictions directed at youth purchase, possession, or use; active enforcement of tobacco sales laws; and retailer education interventions (with or without reinforcement).

Educational components of the interventions included community-wide assessments of compliance by tobacco retailers—with dissemination of the results through mass media events and news coverage—and presentations to civic groups and local governments. Community and school meetings and activities, as well as direct contact with local governments through testimony, petitions, letters, and phone calls, also occurred.

We included studies in the review regardless of the order in which components were added. For example, in some studies, community mobilization was the initial intervention and contributed to the adoption of additional interventions. In other studies, community mobilization followed other interventions (such as stronger laws directed at retailers) in efforts to generate and maintain community support for reducing minors' access to tobacco products.

Effectiveness

- Community mobilization, when combined with other interventions, was effective in reducing tobacco use among youth (students) by approximately 5.8 percentage points.
- The intervention reduced the sale of tobacco products by retailers to youth making test purchase attempts by approximately 34 percentage points.

Applicability

- These findings should be applicable to most communities in the United States where not precluded by preemption legislation.

Barriers to Implementation

- The adoption or existence of a law at the state level that supersedes or precludes stronger local laws (preemption) is a significant barrier to the effective combination of community mobilization and coordinated interventions.

We identified a total of nine qualifying studies (10 intervention arms) that provided evidence on the effectiveness of community mobilization when combined with additional interventions.[85-93] Seven additional papers provided information on studies already included in our review.[94-100] Seven studies did not meet our quality criteria and were excluded from the review.[101-107]

As noted above, most of the qualifying studies did not attempt to measure differences or changes in tobacco use among youth, the focus of our assessment of effectiveness. The nine qualifying studies provided 10 measurements of changes in the percentage of retailers willing to sell tobacco products to youth in test purchase attempts. Overall, the studies observed a 33.5 percentage point reduction in retailers willing to sell tobacco to youth (range, 4.5 to 68). In the intervention communities at follow-up, the median sales rate among retailers on youth test purchase attempts was 27.5% (range, 0% to 65%).

The findings of this systematic review are based on the subset of five multicomponent intervention studies that measured differences or changes in tobacco use among youth in the study communities.[86,87,90,91,108] Four of these studies evaluated a combined intervention including community mobilization.[86,87,90,91] In these studies, the interventions coordinated with community mobilization included retailer education with reinforcement,[86,87,91] stronger local ordinances directed at retailers,[90,91] active enforcement of retailer sales laws,[90,91] local ordinances directed at youth tobacco purchase, possession, or use,[90,91] and school-based education.[87]

All four studies evaluating interventions combined with community mobilization observed decreases in self-reported tobacco use by students, with a median decrease of 5.8 percentage points (range, 3.8 to 11) over follow-up periods of 24–48 months. In addition, all four studies observed both reductions in the sale of tobacco products on youth test purchase attempts (median –44 percentage points) and low post-intervention sales rates by retailers on youth test purchase attempts (median 7.9%; range, 0% to 24%) in the intervention communities.

The fifth qualifying study that measured youth tobacco use as an intervention outcome evaluated the combination of sustained, active enforcement of sales laws directed at retailers following a brief retailer education effort (notification of existing sales laws).[108] Despite a significant reduction of 30 percentage points in retailer sale of tobacco products on youth test purchase attempts (the post-intervention sales rate was 18% in the intervention community), self-reported tobacco use by surveyed high school students was not significantly different at two-year follow-up.

Overall, these results indicate that the combination of community mobilization and additional activities is effective in reducing youth access to tobacco.

These results should be applicable to some communities in the United States (barriers are described below). The multicomponent interventions evaluated in this body of evidence were implemented in a variety of settings and populations, including urban, suburban, and rural communities in the United States and Australia. Interventions were implemented in U.S. communities that included predominantly African-American, Hispanic, or white populations.

We found no information on other positive or negative effects of community mobilization. One report observed that youth who took part in test purchase attempts had not increased smoking or intentions to smoke at a two-year follow-up.[109]

The findings of our systematic review of economic evaluations are based on one study of a component of community mobilization.[110] This one-year study modeled the cost effectiveness of active enforcement of tobacco sales to minors on a national level. The intervention included employing minors to attempt tobacco purchases, licensing tobacco vendors, and civil penalties for vendors who illegally sold tobacco products to minors. Program costs included personnel, salary, and benefits for minors and for adult inspectors; liability insurance; money to purchase tobacco; transportation; and overhead (analyses were based on enforcement costs of $50, $150, $250, and $350, where marginal expense is lowest at the community level and highest at the federal level). Primary outcome measures consisted of four levels of reduction in youth tobacco use ranging from 5% to 50%, with subsequent cost-effectiveness ratios ranging from $44 to $3100 per year of life saved.

Barriers to implementation are well described in the published literature. Preemption, the adoption or existence of a law at the state level that supersedes or precludes stronger local laws, is the subject of a *Healthy People 2010*[15] objective (see Table 1–1). Preemption is a significant barrier to the effective combination of community mobilization and coordinated interventions, such as laws directed at retailers and the conduct of active enforcement.[2,90,106,111,112] Preemption statutes in many states hinder or prevent implementation of the effective combinations of interventions described in this review.[2,106] In addition, some preemption laws hinder or obstruct compliance checks of retailers, making it more difficult for communities to recognize and address minors' access to commercial sources of tobacco products.

Opposition by retailers, retail associations, and the tobacco industry can be a significant barrier to the implementation and conduct of sustained, active enforcement of sales laws.[2,90] Lack of resources or interest in conducting active enforcement can affect the impact and duration of enforcement efforts.[113]

Judicial nullification of penalties directed at retailers was noted as a potential barrier in achieving and maintaining retailer compliance through active enforcement.[89,114] Other reviews have suggested that replacing criminal offense statutes with specified civil penalties (e.g., graduated fines or license suspension) would improve enforcement efforts and minimize court appearances.[2,84,114]

Another barrier to implementation can come from legislative efforts to weaken, replace, or prevent the implementation and conduct of interventions to reduce minors' access. Several reports identified in this review summarized these efforts.[2,80,115,116]

In conclusion, the Task Force recommends community mobilization combined with additional interventions—such as stronger local laws directed at retailers, active enforcement of retailer sales laws, and retailer education with reinforcement—on the basis of sufficient evidence of effectiveness in reducing youth tobacco use and access to tobacco products from commercial sources. Preemption is a significant barrier to the implementation of the intervention combinations evaluated in this report. The published literature describes a number of legislative efforts to weaken, replace, or prevent the implementation and conduct of these interventions.

We also evaluated the effectiveness of several interventions implemented alone in reducing minors' access to and use of tobacco products. The evidence was insufficient to determine the effectiveness of any of these interventions by itself.

Sales Laws Directed at Tobacco Retailers to Reduce Illegal Sales to Minors When Implemented Alone: Insufficient Evidence to Determine Effectiveness

In addition to general laws governing the sale of tobacco, laws directed at retailers provide specific regulation or restriction of the sale of tobacco products to minors. These laws include licensing requirements for tobacco retailers and bans or restrictions on tobacco product vending machines and self-service displays. The laws may include additional conditions, such as requiring proof of the purchaser's age before selling tobacco, displaying sales laws (such as warning signs at the point of purchase), banning the sale of single cigarettes, and restricting the age of the seller.

These laws may designate the method of enforcement and establish the penalties and the responsible parties for each violation (for example, civil penalties directed at the retail owner or license holder). The interventions described in the studies we reviewed were implemented by local governments and were not limited by state preemption legislation. (The effectiveness of active enforcement of these laws is reviewed separately in this chapter.)

Effectiveness

- We found insufficient evidence to determine the effectiveness of sales laws directed at retailers, when implemented alone, in reducing minors' access to and use of tobacco products.
- Only one study qualified for review; it had limitations in study execution and lacked measurements of youth tobacco use or purchase behaviors.
- Insufficient evidence means that we were not able to determine whether or not the intervention works.

The findings of our systematic review are based on a single qualifying study.[117] Four additional reports[24,32,118,119] (on three studies) were identified but did not meet our quality criteria and were excluded from the review. The single qualifying study evaluated the effect of a local county ban of self-service displays on sales of tobacco products to youth. No measurements of differences in tobacco use among youth were attempted. A slight reduction (3.2 percentage points from a baseline of 17.5%) in the number of retailers willing to sell tobacco to youth was observed. Results from this single qualifying study provided insufficient evidence to determine the effectiveness of sales laws directed at retailers when implemented alone in reducing youth access to tobacco.

Because we could not establish the effectiveness of these laws, we did not examine situations in which these laws would be applicable, information about economic efficiency, or possible barriers to implementation.

A potential benefit of these laws is that license requirements for the sale of tobacco products enable communities to identify commercial sources of tobacco. These laws also provide support for additional interventions, such as active enforcement of sales laws. Finally, self-service display bans reduce or eliminate minors' ability to obtain cigarettes by stealing them. No harms were identified.

In conclusion, the Task Force found insufficient evidence to determine the effectiveness of laws directed at retailers when implemented alone in reducing youth access to tobacco, because only one study qualified for our review, and that study had limitations in execution and lacked measurements of youth tobacco use or purchase behaviors.

Laws Directed at Minors' Purchase, Possession, or Use of Tobacco Products When Implemented Alone: Insufficient Evidence to Determine Effectiveness

These laws prohibit the purchase, possession, or use of tobacco products by minors. Communities have implemented laws directed at minors, and state governments are increasingly doing so. The laws may designate which agency is responsible for enforcement as well as the penalty for violations. Some laws require minors who have received citations to participate in educational programs that provide assistance in quitting smoking.

Effectiveness

- We found insufficient evidence to determine the effectiveness of laws directed at minors' purchase, possession, or use of tobacco products when implemented alone in reducing minors' access to and use of tobacco products.
- The evidence was insufficient because we identified no studies that met the quality criteria for our review.
- Insufficient evidence means that we were not able to determine whether or not the intervention works.

Our search identified no studies that evaluated the effectiveness of laws directed at minors' purchase, possession, or use of tobacco products when implemented alone. We therefore found insufficient evidence to determine whether or not these laws are effective in reducing minors' access to tobacco.

Because we could not establish the effectiveness of these laws, we did not examine situations in which they would be applicable, information about economic efficiency, or possible barriers to implementation.

Although we could not determine whether these laws are effective, we did note other published effects of the laws. Preemption legislation and policies in some states have directed resources and priority of enforcement away from laws directed at retailers in favor of laws directed at youth.[114,120] Some laws establish or mandate participation in programs providing education and cessation assistance to cited youth.[121]

In conclusion, the Task Force found insufficient evidence to determine the effectiveness of laws directed at minors' purchase, possession, or use of tobacco products when implemented alone, because no studies qualified for the review.

Active Enforcement of Sales Laws Directed at Retailers When Implemented Alone: Insufficient Evidence to Determine Effectiveness

Active enforcement is used to achieve and maintain retailer compliance with sales laws. This enforcement consists of periodic unannounced compliance checks, which employ recruited, trained, and supervised minors to make standardized attempts to purchase tobacco products from retailers and vending machines. Retailers who violate sales laws receive citations from law enforcement officers or officers in designated government agencies (e.g., health department inspectors).

Local enforcement operations identified in this review were not limited by state preemption legislation.

Effectiveness

- We found insufficient evidence to determine the effectiveness of active enforcement of sales laws when implemented alone in reducing minors' access to and use of tobacco products.
- Evidence was insufficient because only one qualifying study was identified, which did not measure differences or changes in youth tobacco use or purchase behaviors.
- Insufficient evidence means that we were not able to determine whether or not the intervention works.

The findings of our systematic review are based on one study.[122] An additional study was identified but did not meet our quality criteria and was excluded from the review.[123]

The single qualifying study evaluated the effect of an enforcement campaign on the sale of single cigarettes by tobacco retailers in New York City. Starting from a 100% baseline, the percentage of retailers willing to sell cigarettes in the intervention (enforcement) group decreased by 47.7 percentage points (singles or packs) on youth test purchases (the post-intervention sales rate was 46.9%). This study did not measure differences or changes in youth tobacco use or purchase behaviors. We therefore found insufficient evidence to determine if active enforcement of existing laws against sale of tobacco products to minors, when implemented alone, is effective in reducing such sales.

Because we could not establish the effectiveness of these laws, we did not examine situations in which they would be applicable, information about economic efficiency, or possible barriers to implementation.

In conclusion, the Task Force found insufficient evidence to determine the effectiveness of active enforcement of sales laws when implemented alone in reducing youth access to tobacco, because only one qualifying study was identified and it did not provide measurements of youth tobacco use or purchase behaviors.

Our review identified two types of education interventions directed to tobacco retailers. In both interventions, the messages emphasized the importance of refusing to sell tobacco products to minors. These education interventions differed in the intensity and content of the educational messages, and in whether or not they provided reinforcement to retailers (in the form of follow-up and feedback).

Retailer Education with Reinforcement and Information on Health Consequences When Implemented Alone: Insufficient Evidence to Determine Effectiveness

These interventions aim to increase retailer compliance with prohibitions on tobacco sales to minors through repeated educational messages and feedback on retailer performance. Reviewed interventions involved face-to-face delivery of education messages by concerned citizens, health department workers, or law enforcement officers. The educational component included follow-up that provided either positive or negative reinforcement of retailer or clerk compliance with sales laws based on periodic unannounced compliance checks. In most cases, these interventions included information on the health consequences of tobacco use.

Effectiveness

- We found insufficient evidence to determine the effectiveness of retailer education providing reinforcement and information on health consequences when implemented alone in reducing minors' access to and use of tobacco products.
- The evidence was insufficient because we found no studies that met our quality criteria for review.

- Insufficient evidence means that we were not able to determine whether or not the intervention works.

Our search identified two studies in which retailer education with reinforcement was implemented alone.[124,125] Both studies were excluded from the review, however, because one had limitations in the quality of execution and the other had a least suitable study design. Additionally, neither study evaluated differences or changes in youth tobacco use or purchase behaviors. Therefore, we found insufficient evidence to determine whether or not retailer education with reinforcement and information on health consequences, by itself, is effective in increasing retailer compliance with laws prohibiting the sale of tobacco products to minors.

Because we could not establish the effectiveness of this intervention, we did not examine situations in which such programs would be applicable, information about economic efficiency, or possible barriers to implementation.

In conclusion, the Task Force found insufficient evidence to determine the effectiveness of retailer education providing reinforcement and information on health consequences when implemented alone in reducing minors' access to tobacco, because no studies met our quality criteria for inclusion in the review.

Retailer Education without Reinforcement When Implemented Alone: Insufficient Evidence to Determine Effectiveness

These education interventions deliver messages to retailers about tobacco sales to minors without providing follow-up and feedback on retailer performance. Education interventions, which aim to increase retailer compliance with prohibitions on the sale of tobacco to minors, include distribution of information about current or recent changes in local or state laws governing sales to minors as well as distribution of materials such as display signs or training manuals for clerks. In the studies evaluated in this review, education was carried out by mail; in face-to-face encounters; or through training sessions conducted by concerned citizens, health department workers, or law enforcement officers. The educational messages did not address the health consequences of tobacco use. Our review did not identify any studies evaluating mandatory training sessions for retailers or clerks or provisions to reduce or eliminate penalties for retailers who participated in education programs.

Effectiveness

- We found insufficient evidence to determine the effectiveness of retailer education without reinforcement when implemented alone in reducing minors' access to and use of tobacco products.

- Only three studies qualified for our review, and none of these measured youth tobacco use or purchase behaviors.
- Insufficient evidence means that we were not able to determine whether or not the intervention works.

The findings of our systematic review are based on three studies.[122,126,127] Three additional studies were identified but did not meet our quality criteria and were excluded from the review.[128-130] The three reviewed studies evaluated mailed educational messages or a combination of mailed messages and face-to-face encounters. Although one study observed an increase (+21.3 percentage points) in the number of retailers requiring proof of age from youth making test purchase attempts and two studies observed absolute reductions in retailer sales rates of 9 and 27.5 percentage points, respectively, none of the studies provided measurements of differences or changes in youth tobacco use or purchase behaviors. Therefore, we were unable to determine the effectiveness of retailer education without reinforcement, by itself, in increasing retailer compliance with laws prohibiting the sale of tobacco products to minors.

Because we could not establish the effectiveness of the intervention, we did not examine situations in which it would be applicable, information about economic efficiency, or possible barriers to implementation.

In conclusion, the Task Force found insufficient evidence to determine the effectiveness of this intervention because of the small number of qualifying studies and lack of measurement of youth tobacco use or purchase behaviors.

Community Education about Minors' Access to Tobacco Products When Implemented Alone: Insufficient Evidence to Determine Effectiveness

These interventions attempt to disseminate information community-wide to focus public attention on the issue of youth access to tobacco products. The educational components include community-wide assessments of compliance by tobacco retailers, with results disseminated through mass media events, news coverage, and presentations to civic groups and local governments. The interventions can also include community and school meetings and activities as well as direct contact with local governments through testimony, petitions, letters, and phone calls.

In this review, we distinguished between community education efforts (reviewed here) and community mobilization, in which the education efforts fostered or were coordinated with additional interventions directed at minors' access to tobacco products (see Reducing Tobacco Use Initiation—Community Mobilization Combined with Additional Interventions).

Effectiveness

- We found insufficient evidence to determine the effectiveness of community education when implemented alone in reducing minors' access to and use of tobacco products.
- We identified no studies that evaluated this intervention.
- Insufficient evidence means that we were not able to determine whether or not the intervention works.

Our search identified no studies in which community education interventions were implemented and evaluated alone. We therefore had insufficient evidence to determine whether community education, by itself, is effective in increasing community awareness of the issue of youth access to tobacco products.

Because we could not establish the effectiveness of this intervention, we did not examine situations in which it would be applicable, information about economic efficiency, or possible barriers to implementation.

In conclusion, the Task Force found insufficient evidence to determine the effectiveness of this intervention in reducing minors' access to tobacco, because no qualifying studies of community education alone were identified.

Increasing Tobacco Use Cessation

Interventions to increase the number of tobacco users who successfully quit include efforts to increase the number of people who attempt to quit, efforts to improve the success rate for quit attempts, and efforts that support both of these goals. We reviewed two approaches appropriate for communities (increasing the unit price for tobacco products and mass media education); five approaches that can be implemented in healthcare systems (provider reminder systems alone; provider education programs alone; provider reminder systems and provider education programs together, with or without client education materials; provider feedback systems; and reducing client out-of-pocket costs for effective cessation therapies); and one intervention appropriate for both communities and healthcare systems (telephone cessation support).

In conducting this review of the evidence, the Task Force noted that spontaneous and unassisted rates of tobacco use cessation among tobacco users are low (3%–10%).[6,131] Although the interventions reviewed in this section showed relatively small effects (increases of 2.2 to 4.1 percentage points), they represent relatively large improvements in the success rates for tobacco use cessation. Task Force assessments and conclusions of the evidence on effectiveness reflect these aspects of tobacco use cessation.

Increasing the Unit Price for Tobacco Products: Recommended (Strong Evidence of Effectiveness)

Excise tax increases at the municipal, state, or federal level can raise the unit price for tobacco products. In several states, excise tax increases on tobacco products resulted from successful state ballot initiatives. Although other factors affect tobacco product pricing, excise tax increases have historically resulted in an equivalent or larger increase in tobacco product prices.[22]

Effectiveness

- Increases in tobacco product price are consistently effective in reducing tobacco use (a 10% price increase results in approximately a 4% decrease).

Applicability

- These findings should be applicable to most adults in the United States.

Other Effects

- Price increases also reduce tobacco use among adolescents and young adults.

Barriers

- Increasing the excise tax on tobacco products requires passage of legislation or a statewide referendum.

The findings of our systematic review are based on 17 aggregate studies, which were consolidated from 51 papers that evaluated the effectiveness of price increases for tobacco products in reducing tobacco use.[23,29,30,33,132–178] Because many of these papers analyzed the same data during similar, identical, or overlapping periods of time, we decided to consolidate papers into aggregate studies on the basis of similarities in location, the period of study, and the dataset employed. Five additional studies were identified but did not meet our quality criteria and were excluded from the review.[179–183]

The 17 aggregate studies reviewed evaluated the effect of tobacco product price on tobacco use in California; Massachusetts; Oregon; 11 Western states; national evaluations conducted in the 1990s, 1980s, and 1970s; and three studies conducted in Canada, three in the United Kingdom, and one each in Austria, Finland, Switzerland, and New Zealand.

Price elasticity of demand (the percentage change in consumption that results from a 1% change in price) was the most common measure used in these studies to estimate the effect of tobacco product price increases. Of the 17 aggregate studies, 13 included measurements of price elasticity of demand, which generally showed decreases in consumption. For example, in 10 aggregate studies that measured cigarette sales data, a 10% increase in product price would result in a 4.1% decrease in population consumption (range,

2.7% to 7.6%). Similar effects were seen in all measures of changes in tobacco prevalence and amount smoked.

Overall, this body of evidence documented consistent effectiveness of increases in tobacco product price in reducing tobacco use, regardless of the measurements reported or calculated, the setting or period of time evaluated, or differences in the control of potential confounders.

Four studies using measures other than price elasticity of demand (for example, measurements of tobacco product sales or consumption) showed that tobacco use declined in response to price increases, whereas excise tax decreases significantly slowed this decline.

These results should be applicable to most adults in the United States. All of the reviewed studies evaluated the effect of price on the consumption of cigarettes. Some also evaluated the effect of price increases on consumption of smokeless tobacco, cigars, and pipe tobacco. Studies demonstrated the effectiveness of state excise tax increases and federal excise tax increases in reducing tobacco consumption; effectiveness was also shown for whites, African Americans, Hispanics, men and women, across most social classes, and among people with incomes below median or with less than a high school education.

A positive effect of increasing the unit price for tobacco products is a decrease in tobacco use among adolescents and young adults (discussed under Reducing Tobacco Use Initiation). One potential negative effect of increases in tobacco product excise taxes is an increase in smuggling (illegal cross-border transport and sale of untaxed tobacco products). No recent studies of the effects of organized smuggling in the United States were identified in this review, however, and an analysis in 1985 reported a significant reduction in activity following federal legislation in 1978.[184]

Effects of tobacco product price increases that might reduce (but would not eliminate) the potential health benefits of more cessation and less consumption include legal individual cross-border purchases of tobacco products; substitution of tobacco products (e.g., smokeless tobacco for cigarettes) created by unequal taxation on different kinds of tobacco products; and modification of individual tobacco use patterns, such as smoking cigarettes longer or changing to a higher-tar, higher-nicotine brand.[148]

Econometric analyses were included in the studies qualifying for review of effectiveness. A separate economic evaluation was not conducted for this intervention review.

Passage of legislation or a statewide referendum is needed to increase the excise tax and may therefore present a barrier to implementation. Political opposition has historically been well organized and funded at the municipal, state, and federal levels. Reports on both successful and unsuccessful state initiatives that proposed an increase on tobacco product excise taxes have been published.[34-36]

In conclusion, the Task Force recommends increasing the unit price for tobacco products on the basis of strong evidence of effectiveness in increasing the number of people who stop using tobacco. Raising the unit price for tobacco products, through increases in excise taxes for tobacco products, is consistently effective in reducing tobacco use, regardless of the measure used. The findings of this review should be applicable to most adults in the United States. Tobacco product price increases also reduce tobacco use among adolescents and young adults. The need for passage by a state legislature or a referendum can be a significant barrier to efforts to raise excise taxes on tobacco products.

Mass Media Education

Mass media messages (broadcast and print) are disseminated to provide cessation information, motivation to assist tobacco users in their efforts to quit, or both. In our review, we distinguished among three subtypes of mass media interventions—campaigns, cessation series, and cessation contests—which differ in the duration, intent, and intensity of the media messages. Each is addressed separately below.

Mass Media Education Campaigns Combined with Other Interventions: Recommended (Strong Evidence of Effectiveness)

Mass media campaigns employ brief, recurring messages over time (weeks to years) to provide information or motivation to tobacco users and others (family members, households, peers) with the goal of increasing or improving efforts to quit using tobacco products. The messages, developed through formative research, are disseminated through paid broadcast time and print space, donated time and space (as public service announcements), or a combination of the two. Campaigns can focus on cessation or can include cessation themes within a broader range of tobacco messages (including messages directed at reducing tobacco use among youth, reducing secondhand smoke exposure, or both). Mass media campaigns can be combined with other interventions, such as an excise tax increase or additional community-wide education efforts.

Effectiveness

- Mass media education campaigns, when combined with other activities, were effective in increasing tobacco use cessation by approximately 2 additional quitters per 100.
- These interventions were also effective in reducing tobacco use in the population, as measured in states and in communities. Changes in tobacco use include reductions in consumption (by approximately 12.8%) and reductions in the prevalence of tobacco use (by approximately 3 people per 100 tobacco users).

Applicability

- These findings should be applicable to most people in the United States.

Other Effects

- Mass media education campaigns can increase the number of people who seek help from telephone "quit" lines.

The findings of our systematic review are based on 15 studies that evaluated the effectiveness of mass media campaigns in reducing tobacco use.[138–140,185–196] Another 14 papers provided information on studies already included in the review.[75,135,197–208] Three studies measured the effect of a mass media campaign in increasing use of a telephone cessation information service: these results are described below (see Multicomponent Interventions that Include Client Telephone Support).[209–211] Six studies did not meet our quality criteria and were excluded from the review.[212–217] All of the reviewed studies evaluated the combination of a mass media education campaign coordinated or concurrent with at least one other intervention: an excise tax increase (6 studies), community education programs such as the distribution of self-help cessation information (12 studies), individual or group cardiovascular disease risk factor reduction or smoking cessation counseling (7 studies), and other mass media efforts (2 studies).

The reviewed studies measured changes in tobacco use in terms of changes in individual tobacco use cessation, changes in population consumption (measured by statewide sales of cigarettes), and changes in the prevalence of tobacco use in the study population. In general, the studies observed increases in tobacco use cessation and decreases in population consumption and prevalence.

Five studies evaluated the effect of combined interventions including mass media campaigns on tobacco use cessation among groups of recruited tobacco users. In study periods of one to five years' duration, the median difference in cessation between intervention group participants and comparison group participants (who were potentially exposed to the media component in three studies) was an increase of 2.2 percentage points (representing approximately 2 additional people per 100 who quit using tobacco; range, 2 to 35).

Three studies, with follow-up periods of two to eight years, evaluated the effect of statewide mass media campaigns when combined with additional interventions (excise tax increase, community and school education activities) on consumption of cigarettes as determined by sales of taxed cigarette packs. In all three states, overall tobacco consumption declined at a greater rate than in the rest of the United States (median 12.8% decrease).

Finally, seven studies measured changes in tobacco use prevalence in communities exposed to a mass media campaign combined with additional interventions. Six studies observed decreases in tobacco use prevalence over study periods of 6 months to 20 years, and five of these studies included a concurrent comparison population. In these studies, tobacco use prevalence decreased in the intervention population by a median of 3.4 percentage points (range, −7 to +0.2) when compared with the unexposed community.

The results of these studies provide strong evidence of the effectiveness of mass media education campaigns, when combined with other activities, in increasing tobacco use cessation and reducing tobacco consumption.

These findings should be applicable to people throughout the United States. All of the reviewed studies focused on cigarette use. These studies included statewide and regional campaigns in the United States, national campaigns in Scotland, and regional campaigns in Finland. Studies were conducted in large cities as well as in smaller communities. In the United States, studies were also conducted specifically among Hispanics and among Vietnamese men.

Mass media campaigns, when combined with additional interventions, can also be effective in reducing tobacco use among youth (see Reducing Tobacco Use Initiation), especially when the campaign includes a variety of targeted messages and broadcast times. In California, Oregon, and Massachusetts, for example, campaigns included messages for children and adolescents as well as messages about the health effects of exposure to environmental tobacco smoke. Several studies noted significant increases in the use of telephone cessation information or support services ("quit" lines) when the media messages told audiences about these services.

The findings of our systematic review of economic evaluations of community-wide interventions to increase cessation among adult tobacco users are based on two cost-effectiveness studies (one conducted in the Netherlands[218] and the other in Scotland[219]). Both studies reported program costs per quitter. In addition, the study in Scotland reported program cost per life-years saved, which was converted to dollars per QALY based on preference weights provided by Fiscella and Franks (a standard economic approach used to adjust health-related quality-of-life measures on a continuum from 0.0 [death] to 1.0 [optimal health]).[220]

The intervention conducted in the Netherlands evaluated the effect of a mass media campaign, a self-help manual, a hotline, and a nine-session group cessation program. Self-reported seven-day abstinence was determined at six-month follow-up. Costs included were wages, overhead, calls to the hot-line, participant time, transportation, and charges for the group session. The effect size was estimated as the difference in smoking prevalence before and after the intervention. The self-reported cessation rate was 11% for partici-pants using the self-help manual alone and 22% for participants using the self-help manual combined with the cessation program. Based on this effect size, adjusted program cost per quitter ranged from $796 to $1593.

The study conducted in Scotland consisted of a mass media campaign, telephone help line, and information booklet. At the 12-month follow-up, 9.8% of program participants reported having quit smoking for at least six months. Costs included research, production, design fees, printing, dissemi-nation, staff salaries, and overhead. The adjusted program cost per quitter in this study ranged from $298 to $655. Adjusted program cost per QALY ranged from $151 to $328. The range was based on lower and upper bound estimates of adult participants.

The primary barrier to the implementation of mass media campaigns is the funding needed to develop and maintain an extended-duration, high-intensity campaign using paid and targeted broadcast times to deliver messages that resonate with target audiences. Cooperation between tobacco control pro-grams can reduce program development costs. The barriers encountered by the tobacco control program in the state of California provide important les-sons on the need for both public and political support and vigilance in main-taining an effective campaign.[221,222]

In conclusion, the Task Force recommends mass media education campaigns combined with additional interventions on the basis of strong evidence of ef-fectiveness in increasing tobacco use cessation and in reducing tobacco con-sumption. The findings of this review should be applicable to most people in the United States. An additional benefit of these campaigns can be an in-crease in the number of people who call in to dedicated telephone cessation support services' quit lines.

Mass Media Education—Cessation Series: Insufficient Evidence to Determine Effectiveness

Cessation series consist of broadcasted instructional segments designed to re-cruit, inform, and motivate users of tobacco products to try quitting and to succeed. Cessation series can be coordinated with pre-series broadcast or print promotion, community education (e.g., distribution of self-help cessation materials), and organization of cessation groups in the community. The series can extend for a period of several weeks to several months. Techniques include nightly or weekly segments on news or informational programs giving expert advice or sharing peer group experiences on cessation issues (e.g., dealing with the symptoms of withdrawal). The series can encourage tobacco users to join a community-wide quit effort. Over the course of the broadcasts, viewers can receive ongoing support and assistance from cessation experts and recruited peers.

Effectiveness

- We found insufficient evidence to determine the effectiveness of mass media education cessation series in increasing the number of people who quit using tobacco products.
- Evidence was insufficient because of inconsistent results and inadequate comparison groups.
- Insufficient evidence means that we were not able to determine whether or not the intervention works.

The findings of our systematic review are based on nine studies that evaluated the effectiveness of cessation series in increasing tobacco use cessation.[223–231] Eleven additional studies were identified but did not meet our quality criteria and were excluded from the review.[208,232–241] Ten other reports provided information on studies already included in the review.[242–251]

All of the reviewed studies evaluated the effectiveness of cessation series combined with other interventions, such as community education (typically, access to or distribution of self-help cessation manuals), organized cessation groups or programs, or telephone cessation support (quit lines). Eight studies evaluated televised cessation series broadcast over periods of 20 days to three months, and one study evaluated a week-long newspaper cessation series. Five of the nine studies in the review evaluated broadcast cessation series conducted in the Chicago metropolitan area (in one of three waves) between 1985 and 1987. These studies were evaluated separately because of differences in the study populations or settings.

The reviewed studies provided insufficient evidence to determine the effectiveness of mass media eduction cessation series in increasing tobacco use cessation. The differences in cessation observed in these studies might be the result of (1) baseline differences in motivation to quit between intervention and comparison smokers and (2) the small group cessation sessions provided to the intervention group participants.

Because we could not establish the effectiveness of mass media cessation series in increasing the number of people who successfully quit using tobacco products, we did not examine situations in which they would be applicable, information about economic efficiency, or possible barriers to implementation.

No harms or benefits of mass media cessation series were identified.

In conclusion, the Task Force found insufficient evidence to determine the effectiveness of mass media cessation series in increasing the number of people who successfully quit using tobacco products because of inconsistent results and inadequate comparison groups.

Mass Media Education—Cessation Contests: Insufficient Evidence to Determine Effectiveness

Cessation contests are community-wide events of short duration that use mass media to recruit and motivate users of tobacco products to participate in a program to quit by a certain date or during a specified time period. Cessation contests use both mass media and such small media as posters and flyers as the primary tool for promotion and to recruit tobacco product users in the community. Contests can increase cessation in the community by changing tobacco product users' attitudes about cessation, recruiting users to initiate a quit attempt, and motivating those who attempt to quit to remain abstinent through incentives or by mobilizing support from family, friends, and other participants. We evaluated contests that offered additional incentives for participation and successful cessation, as well as targeted quit events conducted without additional incentives.

Effectiveness

- We found insufficient evidence to determine the effectiveness of mass media education cessation contests in increasing the number of people who quit using tobacco products.
- Evidence was insufficient because only one study met the quality criteria for this review, and that study lacked sufficient evidence on which to base a recommendation.
- Insufficient evidence means that we were not able to determine whether or not the intervention works.

The findings of our systematic review are based on one study.[252] We identified another 16 studies that did not meet our quality criteria and were excluded from the review.[234,253-267] Three other papers provided information on the study already included in the review.[268-270]

The single reviewed study evaluated a multicomponent smoking cessation program in New York City. Interventions included a cessation manual and video, telephone cessation support, and the opportunity to participate in smoking cessation contests.

Although the single reviewed study showed some improvements in self-reported cessation at a six-month follow-up, the evidence was insufficient to determine the effectiveness of mass media cessation series in increasing the number of people who successfully quit using tobacco products because the evidence in this single study was not sufficient to support a recommendation.

Because we could not establish the effectiveness of mass media cessation contests in increasing the number of people who successfully quit using tobacco products, we did not examine situations in which the programs would be applicable, information about economic efficiency, or possible barriers to implementation.

No harms or benefits of mass media cessation contests were identified.

In conclusion, evidence was insufficient to determine the effectiveness of mass media education cessation contests in increasing the number of people who successfully quit using tobacco products because only a single study, showing only moderate improvement, qualified for review.

Provider- and System-Based Interventions

We reviewed six interventions that can be implemented by healthcare systems and providers to increase cessation of tobacco use by clients. We did not evaluate the effectiveness of provider counseling to tobacco-using clients or the effectiveness of specific clinical therapies, which have been thoroughly reviewed by others.[2,6,7,17]

Healthcare Provider Reminder Systems: Recommended (Sufficient Evidence of Effectiveness)

Provider reminder systems can identify clients who use tobacco products and prompt providers to discuss cessation with their clients or advise clients to quit at every encounter. Because even brief provider advice has a demonstrated effect on getting clients to quit,[6,17] increasing the delivery of advice by providers should increase the number of clients who quit.

Reminders can be delivered by a variety of methods, including chart stickers, vital sign stamps, medical record flowsheets, and checklists, and the content of the reminders can vary. Provider reminder systems are often combined with other interventions, such as provider education and client education. Here we review provider reminder systems used alone; multicomponent interventions including provider reminders are considered below (see Healthcare Provider Reminder Systems with Provider Education, with or without Client Education).

Effectiveness

- Provider reminder systems were effective in increasing the number of clients who quit smoking by approximately 4 additional clients per 100.
- Provider reminder systems were also effective in increasing the number of clients whom providers advise to quit smoking by approximately 13 additional clients per 100.
- These systems were also effective in increasing the determination of client smoking status by providers by approximately 32 additional clients per 100.

Applicability

- These findings should be applicable to most clinical setting in the United States.

Other Effects

- The use of provider reminder systems may also increase delivery of other preventive services.

The findings of our systematic review are based on seven studies evaluating the effectiveness of provider reminder systems when used alone.[271-277] One additional paper was identified but did not meet our quality criteria and was excluded from the review.[278] The reviewed studies prompted providers with chart prompts or stickers, "expanded vital signs" that indicate whether or not a client uses tobacco, and flowsheets. In one study, analysis was based on receipt of a consultation that encouraged implementation of a provider reminder system, not on actual implementation of the reminder system.

The seven reviewed studies used diverse measures to document changes in client smoking status, provider delivery of advice to quit, and client smoking cessation. The median improvement in determining client smoking status was 32.5 percentage points (range, 26 to 57.6; four studies); that is, the intervention resulted in determining the smoking status of approximately 32 additional clients per 100, with results ranging from 26 to 58 additional clients per 100. These results were measured 8 to 24 months after implementation (median, 15 months). For provider delivery of advice to quit, a median change of 13 percentage points was observed (range, 7 to 31; five studies) in assessments extending 2 to 24 months after implementation (median 8 months). One study reported a difference in biochemically confirmed smoking cessation of 4 percentage points six months after a clinic visit. These findings provide sufficient evidence that healthcare provider reminder systems are effective in increasing the number of tobacco-using clients who receive advice to quit from their providers.

These findings should be applicable in most clinical settings in the United States. Studies were conducted in primary care clinics, family practice clinics, and pulmonary clinics. Most studies did not provide demographic information about client populations.

Two studies[274,276] evaluated provider reminder systems that included preventive services in addition to delivering advice to quit to tobacco-using clients. Improvements were observed in some or all of the prompted activities. No other positive or negative effects were identified in this review.

We did not find any economic evaluations of provider reminder systems.

Although one potential barrier to the implementation of a provider reminder system could be the administrative burden, this was not identified as a problem in any of the reviewed studies, and most of the reminder systems (e.g., "expanded vital signs") were easily implemented.

In conclusion, the Task Force recommends provider reminder systems on the basis of sufficient evidence of effectiveness in increasing the number of tobacco-using clients whom providers advise to quit (because this outcome has been previously shown to increase subsequent tobacco use cessation[17]). These findings should be applicable to most clinical settings in the United States. An additional benefit of provider reminder systems can be increased delivery of other preventive services.

Healthcare Provider Reminder Systems with Provider Education, with or without Client Education: Recommended (Strong Evidence of Effectiveness)

These multicomponent interventions to increase tobacco use cessation include efforts to educate and to prompt providers to identify and to intervene with tobacco-using clients, as well as to provide supplementary educational materials when appropriate. The interventions consist of a provider reminder system and a provider education program, and may or may not include client education materials (e.g., self-help cessation manuals).

A multicomponent intervention can provide an integrated approach to increasing and improving tobacco use cessation by clients. Goals of the interventions include educating, motivating, and prompting providers to increase and improve their interaction with tobacco-using clients, as well as improving client cessation by increasing knowledge and motivation to quit and to remain abstinent. The multicomponent interventions evaluated in this section include at least one provider-directed component.

Effectiveness

- These interventions were effective in increasing the number of clients who quit smoking by approximately 5 additional clients per 100.
- The interventions were also effective in increasing the number of tobacco-

using clients who received advice to quit from their healthcare provider by approximately 20 additional clients per 100.

Applicability

- These findings should be applicable to most clinical settings in the United States and to a variety of provider specialties.

Other Effects

- The use of provider reminder systems plus provider education, with or without client education, may also increase delivery of other preventive services.

The findings of our systematic review are based on 31 studies that evaluated the effectiveness of these interventions in reducing tobacco use among clients.[272,275,279-307] One study measured changes in adolescent tobacco use initiation and is not considered further in this section.[290] Fifteen additional papers provided information on studies already included in the review.[308-322] Six additional studies were identified but did not meet our quality criteria and were excluded from the review.[323-328]

Overall, studies that measured providers' delivery of advice to quit using tobacco and the number of clients who quit showed significant improvements. For example, the 20 studies that evaluated the effectiveness of a multi-component intervention combining at least a provider reminder system and a provider education program found a median change of 20 percentage points (range, 5 to 60) in the number of clients receiving advice to quit from their providers and a median change of 5 percentage points (range, −1 to +26) in the number of clients who quit using tobacco (in follow-up periods of five weeks to 12 months). Similar results were found in the subsets of studies that evaluated interventions using only a provider reminder system and a provider education program (seven studies); interventions that also included client education materials (13 studies); and interventions that included provider reminders and client education but not provider education (three studies). Interventions that included only provider education are discussed below (see Healthcare Provider Education Alone).

These results show that healthcare provider reminder systems plus provider education programs, whether or not combined with client education, are effective in increasing the number of tobacco-using clients who receive advice to quit from their healthcare providers.

These findings should be applicable to a variety of healthcare settings and provider specialties. Studies were conducted in health maintenance organizations (HMOs), private practices, academic health care centers, physician training programs, and public health clinics, among providers in primary care, internal medicine, family medicine, obstetrics, pediatrics, and dentistry. One study focused on reducing use of smokeless tobacco.

Provider reminder systems can include prompts for additional preventive services. No other positive or negative effects were identified in the review.

We did not find any economic evaluations of these interventions.

The burden of administering provider reminder systems is a potential barrier to their implementation.

In conclusion, the Task Force recommends multicomponent interventions including provider reminder systems and provider education, with or without client education, on the basis of strong evidence of effectiveness in increasing the number of providers who advise their clients to quit smoking and in increasing the number of clients who quit. These findings should be applicable to most clinical settings in the United States and to relevant clinical specialties. Reminder systems can include prompts for additional preventive services.

Healthcare Provider Education Alone: Insufficient Evidence to Determine Effectiveness

The goal of provider education is to increase providers' knowledge about tobacco use and cessation, to change their attitudes and practices, and increase or improve their interactions with clients who use tobacco. These interactions can include identifying more tobacco-using clients, increasing delivery of advice to quit, improving the quality of advice to quit, and both increasing and improving providers' efforts to assist clients in their attempts to quit and to remain tobacco-free.

Information can be delivered in a variety of ways, including lectures, written materials, videos, and continuing medical education seminars. Physicians, nurses, physician assistants, students, and office staff can receive this education.

Provider education efforts are frequently combined with other interventions, such as provider reminders and client education efforts. Multicomponent interventions that include provider reminders are considered above (see Healthcare Provider Reminder Systems with Provider Education, with or without Client Education).

Effectiveness

- We found insufficient evidence to determine the effectiveness of provider education alone in increasing the number of people who quit using tobacco products.
- Evidence was insufficient because (1) few studies measured the effect of the intervention on tobacco use cessation and (2) the results of studies that

measured changes in the number of clients whom providers advise to quit smoking were inconsistent.
- Insufficient evidence means that we were not able to determine whether or not the intervention works.

The findings of our systematic review are based on 16 studies that evaluated the effectiveness of provider education interventions when implemented alone.[272,275,285,294,301,302,329-338] Two additional papers provided information on studies already included in the review.[339,340] Nine other studies were identified but did not meet our quality criteria and were excluded from the review.[327,341-348]

Provider education techniques evaluated in the reviewed studies included day-long seminars, lectures for practitioners and for resident physicians, lectures and office visits or contacts, small group tutorial sessions, mock interviews with feedback, and education materials. The provider education sessions ranged from two hours to three days (median, two and a half hours) in the 11 studies that provided this information.

The 16 qualifying studies reported a total of 19 measures of change in provider counseling skills or behaviors and 2 measures of client tobacco use. Of the 10 studies that measured differences in provider delivery of advice to quit, 4 observed either no effect or a negative effect (median change 2.2 percentage points; range, −5 to 73). Only two studies reported differences in client tobacco use cessation, showing small increases (1.7 and 5.2 percentage points, respectively). Five studies measured differences in provider determination of client smoking status, with percentage differences ranging from 0.1 to 35 percentage points (median, 8).

These results provide insufficient evidence to determine whether healthcare provider education alone is effective in changing providers' knowledge, attitudes, and practices about tobacco use or in increasing the number of people who stop using tobacco products.

Because we could not establish the effectiveness of these interventions, we did not examine situations in which they would be applicable, information about economic efficiency, or possible barriers to implementation.

No harms or benefits of provider education alone were identified.

In conclusion, the Task Force found insufficient evidence to determine the effectiveness of provider education interventions when implemented alone in increasing the number of people who quit using tobacco products. Evidence was insufficient because (1) few studies evaluated the effect on client tobacco use cessation and (2) studies that evaluated provider delivery of advice to quit had inconsistent results.

Healthcare Provider Feedback and Assessment: Insufficient Evidence to Determine Effectiveness

Feedback interventions inform and motivate providers by assessing their performance in identifying client tobacco use status, delivering advice to quit, or both. Assessment techniques include chart reviews and the use of computerized records. These interventions can be combined with other activities, such as provider reminders and provider education, and these combinations were considered in our review.

Provider assessment and feedback can motivate providers to increase and improve their interactions with clients in such areas as advising clients to stop using tobacco. Evaluation of provider assessment and feedback is timely because (1) clinical information systems are improving and are increasingly common; (2) effective cessation therapies are available, and an increase in provider interactions with tobacco-using clients could increase the use of these therapies; and (3) quality assurance approaches such as the Healthplan Employer Data and Information Set (HEDIS) are being used more often.

Effectiveness

- We found insufficient evidence to determine the effectiveness of provider assessment and feedback in increasing either provider advice to clients to quit using tobacco or the number of clients who quit using tobacco products.
- Evidence was insufficient because the small number of available studies did not measure these outcomes.
- Insufficient evidence means that we were not able to determine whether or not the intervention works.

The findings of our systematic review of the effectiveness of provider assessment and feedback interventions in changing provider behaviors toward tobacco-using clients are based on three studies.[349–351] Two additional studies were identified but did not meet our quality criteria and were excluded from the review.[352,353]

A provider assessment and feedback program was evaluated alone in one study, and in combination with other components in two studies that included a provider education program and a provider reminder flowsheet. In all three studies, provider documentation or recognition of a client's tobacco use status was only 1 of up to 26 preventive care practices for which assessment and feedback were provided. Only one study used a computer system to collect information and enable providers to obtain feedback information.

None of the qualifying studies attempted to measure changes in provider delivery of advice to quit or whether clients quit using tobacco. The three studies did, however, provide measures of effectiveness in increasing provider recognition of client tobacco use status, showing a median increase of

21 percentage points (range, 13 to 39) in study periods that ranged from three months to six years. This improvement, however, provides insufficient evidence to determine the effectiveness of healthcare provider feedback alone in changing providers' knowledge, attitudes, and practices about tobacco use or in increasing the number of people who stop using tobacco products.

Because we could not establish the effectiveness of these interventions, we did not examine situations in which the programs would be applicable, information about economic efficiency, or possible barriers to implementation.

An additional benefit of increased provider delivery of other preventive care practices was found in two studies. No other positive or negative effects were identified in this review.

In conclusion, the Task Force found insufficient evidence to determine the effectiveness of provider assessment and feedback interventions, when implemented alone, in increasing either provider advice to clients to quit using tobacco or the number of clients who quit using tobacco products. Evidence was insufficient because the small number of available studies did not provide measurements of provider advice to clients to quit using tobacco or the number of clients who quit using tobacco products.

Reducing Client Out-of-Pocket Costs for Effective Cessation Therapies: Recommended (Sufficient Evidence of Effectiveness)

Reducing the financial barriers that may prevent clients from using effective cessation therapies such as nicotine replacement,[6] other pharmacologic therapy,[6] behavioral therapies such as cessation groups,[6] or a combination of these approaches is intended to increase the use of effective therapies, increase the number of people who try to quit, and increase the number of people who succeed in quitting.

Effectiveness

- Reducing client out-of-pocket costs is effective in increasing the number of people who successfully quit using tobacco by approximately 8 clients per 100.
- The intervention is also effective in increasing the number of people who use cessation therapies by approximately 7 clients per 100.

Applicability

- These findings should be applicable in a variety of clinical settings in the United States, in rural and mixed rural-urban settings.

Other Effects

- Clients may use nicotine gum beyond the recommended length of time.

Barriers

- Insurance requirements to combine pharmaceutical therapies with behavioral programs may discourage some clients from trying to quit.

The findings of our systematic review are based on five studies that evaluated the effectiveness of reducing clients' out-of-pocket costs for nicotine gum or nicotine replacements.[354-358] In two studies, nicotine gum or a nicotine replacement were provided as part of, or in addition to, a behavioral program. Access to a behavioral program was provided but rarely used in a third study. In three studies, nicotine gum or nicotine replacement was provided free of charge to participants in the intervention group. In one study, the out-of-pocket costs of the combination of behavioral program and nicotine replacement were $10 for intervention group clients and $52.50 for comparison group clients.

Overall, studies showed improvement in both the use of cessation therapies and the number of clients who quit using tobacco. For example, three studies reported a median difference in use of cessation therapies of 7 percentage points (range, 6.5 to 28). Four studies that measured changes in the number of people who stopped using tobacco showed a median increase of 7.8 percentage points (range, 2.1 to 11) in follow-up periods that ranged from 6 to 12 months (median, 9 months). These findings show that reducing client out-of-pocket costs for tobacco cessation therapies is effective in increasing both the use of these therapies and the number of tobacco users who quit.

These findings should be applicable to different settings and populations. Studies were conducted in the United States; in HMOs, private practices, and a Department of Defense hospital; in rural and mixed rural-urban settings; and among a low-income population.

A potential harm of nicotine replacement therapy was found in the extended use of nicotine gum beyond the recommended duration (four months) in one study. No other potential benefits or harms were identified in this review

The findings of our systematic review of economic evaluations are based on two studies.[355,356] One study,[355] a cost-effectiveness analysis that reported program cost per quitter, was conducted in a healthcare setting in Washington State for employees enrolled in a health plan. The intervention consisted of insurance coverage for clients in a behavioral program that included nicotine replacement, with a 12-month follow-up. Four types of insurance coverage, with different out-of-pocket costs to users, were available: (*1*) standard coverage: a 50% co-payment for the behavioral program and the usual $5 co-payment per prescription for nicotine replacement therapy; (2) reduced coverage: a 50% co-payment for both the behavioral program and nicotine-replacement therapy; (3) flipped coverage: no co-payment for the behavioral program but a 50% co-payment for nicotine-replacement therapy, and; (4) full coverage: no co-payment for the behavioral program and the usual $5 co-payment per prescription for nicotine replacement therapy. Costs measured included drugs, personnel, and cost of the behavioral program. Development, marketing, and implementation of the coverage plan were not included in the analysis. The adjusted program costs per quitter were $135, $141, $149, and $195 for standard, reduced, flipped, and full coverage, respectively.

The second study[356] was a cost–benefit analysis conducted in Vermont, reporting net benefit. The intervention, conducted at a rural family practice clinic with low-income clients, consisted of brief physician advice and a prescription for free nicotine gum, with a six-month follow-up. Costs measured included physician time, nicotine gum, smoking cessation booklets, and client time. Development, promotion, and evaluation costs were not included. The adjusted quit rate for the intervention group was 9.4%. When costs and benefits from averted illness were compared, the intervention was shown to be cost-saving.

Potential barriers to increased use of effective cessation therapies are created by coverage requirements that tie pharmacotherapy to behavioral therapy interventions. Recent reviews have identified each strategy as effective alone.[6] The combinations demonstrate higher cost-effectiveness[359] but also limit the use of effective therapies for smokers who are unwilling to participate in the behavioral program. Including proactive telephone counseling as a behavioral therapy option might reduce these barriers.[360]

In conclusion, the Task Force recommends reducing out-of-pocket costs on the basis of sufficient evidence of effectiveness in increasing the number of people who use cessation therapies and in increasing the number of people who successfully quit using tobacco. This approach has been tried successfully in a variety of clinical settings in both rural and rural-urban settings. A potential harm is that clients may continue to use nicotine gum beyond the recommended length of time. Healthcare coverage requirements for behavioral programs along with pharmaceutical therapies may discourage clients who do not wish to be part of the behavioral programs.

Multicomponent Interventions That Include Client Telephone Support:
Recommended (Strong Evidence of Effectiveness)

Telephone support for people trying to stop using tobacco provides counseling or assistance in quitting and in staying tobacco-free. Depending on the program, tobacco users or healthcare providers can initiate contact. Telephone support can include trained counselors, healthcare providers, or taped messages in single or multiple sessions that usually follow a standardized protocol for providing advice and counseling. Telephone support is usually combined with other interventions, such as client education materials, individual or group cessation counseling, or nicotine replacement therapies.

Telephone contact is intended to increase the motivation of tobacco users to attempt to quit, and can help to reduce relapses by providing support and assistance to recent quitters. In community settings, telephone support typically provides access to self-help cessation materials and available local resources (such as group sessions), and may provide counseling and motivation sessions. In clinical settings, telephone follow-up calls usually support other clinical cessation interventions such as provider counseling, group cessation sessions, or nicotine replacement or other therapies.

Effectiveness

- These multicomponent interventions were effective in increasing the number of people who stop using tobacco by approximately 3 people per 100.

Applicability

- These findings should be applicable to most adults in a variety of clinical and community-wide settings in the United States.

The findings of our systematic review are based on 32 studies that evaluated the effectiveness of telephone cessation support.[248,285,288,289,293,297,300,304,361–384] Sixteen additional papers provided information on studies already included in the review.[309,310,312,315–319,321,385–391] Seven additional studies were identified but did not meet our quality criteria and were excluded from the review.[216,328,392–396]

In all of the reviewed studies, telephone support was coordinated with additional interventions including client education (29 studies), provider-delivered counseling (17 studies), nicotine replacement (4 studies), a smoking cessation clinic (1 study), and a televised cessation series (1 study). Telephone support was reactive (the caller initiated all contact) in 5 studies and proactive (the provider initiated contact or the caller initiated contact, with provider follow-up) in 27 studies.

Thirty studies compared differences in tobacco use cessation based on use of or exposure to telephone support. In follow-up periods of 5 weeks to 34 months (median, 12 months) the median difference was an increase in tobacco use cessation of 2.6 percentage points (range, −3.4 to +23). Studies that compared telephone support plus client education to client education alone found similar increases in cessation. These findings show that multicomponent interventions that include client telephone support are effective in increasing tobacco use cessation.

These findings should be applicable in many settings and to many populations throughout the United States. Studies were conducted in HMOs, private practices, public health clinics, medical centers and hospitals, and resident training programs. Provider specialties included dentistry, obstetrics, gynecology and family planning, primary care, family practice, and internal medicine. Clients included hospitalized smokers, veterans, pregnant women, African Americans, and smokers over 60 years of age. One study focused on reducing the use of smokeless tobacco.

We found no other positive or negative effects of telephone cessation support.

The findings of our systematic review of economic evaluations are based on five cost-effectiveness studies.[389,397–400] Two studies reported program costs per quitter,[398,400] and three studies[389,397,399] reported program costs per life-year saved ratios, which were converted to cost per QALY using preference weights reported by Fiscella and Franks (a standard economic approach used to adjust health-related quality-of-life measures on a continuum from 0.0 [death] to 1.0 [optimal health]).[220]

Both studies reporting program costs per quitter evaluated interventions to increase tobacco use cessation among pregnant women. The first study was conducted in Southern California in an HMO setting.[398] The intervention consisted of a combined prenatal nutrition counseling and smoking cessation program aimed at reducing the incidence of low-birthweight infants. The smoking cessation program consisted of an eight-week home correspondence program that included weekly telephone calls to an automated answering service. Smoking cessation increased by 12 percentage points over the comparison group cessation rate of 38%. Costs included salaries, overhead, supplies, printing, phone, and postage. Adjusted program cost per quitter was $677. The second study was a nationwide modeled intervention in the United States.[400] It consisted of a single 15-minute counseling session conducted by a nonmedical counselor, instructional material, and two follow-up telephone calls. The change in cessation was an increase of 15 percentage points modeled from earlier randomized trials of smoking cessation among pregnant women. Costs included instructional materials, staff time, overhead, and training. The adjusted program cost per quitter was $292. The difference in program cost between the two studies can be explained by the fact that the first study looked at a comprehensive intervention using more resources.

Of the three studies reporting program costs in terms of life-years saved, two studies looked at interventions conducted in hospital settings with adult clients who smoked. One study was conducted at the Mayo Clinic in Minnesota,[397] and the other was conducted at HMO hospitals in Oregon and Washington.[389] The comparison group quit rates for the studies were 10.7% and 9.2%, respectively; the intervention group showed cessation increases of 12 percentage points and 4 percentage points above the comparison quit rates, respectively. The Mayo Clinic intervention consisted of two programs: an individual nicotine-dependency treatment program and a relapse prevention program. The relapse prevention program included telephone follow-up calls, letters, and a mailed survey. The comparison group consisted of clients who received no program. Costs included personnel, supplies, telephone, drugs, and capital equipment. The adjusted program cost per QALY was $2532. The HMO hospital intervention consisted of a 20-minute bedside counseling session, a video, self-help materials, and follow-up calls. Costs included program development, personnel, communications, and overhead. The adjusted program cost per QALY of this intervention was $1248. The Mayo Clinic intervention had a higher program cost per QALY in spite of showing a higher net effect size, because programs costs of this intervention included letters, surveys, and treatment for nicotine dependency in addition to counseling and telephone calls. The third study,[399] conducted at a Boston hospital with clients who had had an acute myocardial infarction, modeled an intervention consisting of nurse-managed smoking-cessation counseling including telephone support after discharge. The comparison group—clients exposed to standard smoking cessation counseling designed for survivors of acute myocardial infarction—had a quit rate of 45%. Cessation increased by 26 percentage points in the intervention group. Costs included were personnel and instructional materials. Time spent on the phone, follow-up time, program development, and training costs were not included. The adjusted program cost per QALY was $73.

Lack of client awareness of, or interest in, support lines can limit the effectiveness of this intervention. Making clients aware of this available support (e.g., though media messages) is one way to increase use of support (quit) lines.

In conclusion, the Task Force Recommends telephone cessation support on the basis of strong evidence of effectiveness in increasing tobacco use cessation when implemented with other interventions (e.g., other educational approaches or clinical therapies) in both clinical and community settings. Effective interventions combined at least proactive telephone support and client cessation materials.

Reducing Exposure to Environmental Tobacco Smoke

Interventions to reduce exposure to environmental tobacco smoke (ETS) require or encourage the establishment of smoke-free areas in workplaces, in public areas, and in the home in an effort to reduce tobacco-related morbidity and mortality. Having smoke-free areas can reduce exposure to ETS and ETS-related illness and death.[12,13,401] Smoke-free policies can change the attitudes and behaviors of smokers and increase both the number of people who try to quit and the number of attempts made by each person. Smoke-free policies may also improve the success rate for each quit attempt by reducing opportunities for relapse.[402] Smoke-free policies also challenge the perception of smoking as a normal adult behavior.[403] By changing this perception, these policies can change the attitudes and behaviors of adolescents, resulting in a reduction in tobacco use initiation.[404]

The interventions reviewed here are smoking bans and restrictions to address exposure in the workplace and in public areas and community education to reduce exposure to ETS, especially among children, in the home environment.

Smoking Bans and Restrictions: Recommended (Strong Evidence of Effectiveness)

Smoking bans and restrictions are policies, regulations, and laws established by private, nongovernment, and government groups and agencies. Smoking bans entirely prohibit smoking in geographically defined areas, whereas smoking restrictions limit smoking to designated areas. Smoking bans and restrictions can be implemented with additional interventions, such as education and tobacco use treatment programs.

Businesses establish smoking policies to protect employees and customers from exposure to ETS in the workplace. Accrediting agencies (e.g., the Joint Commission on Accreditation of Healthcare Organizations) set regulations to protect employees and patrons within their organizations. Federal, state, or local laws are implemented to protect people from ETS exposure in public areas, and to establish minimum standards for both public and private workplaces. Standards for regulations and laws establishing smoking restrictions often include the size, location, and ventilation requirements for designated smoking areas.

Effectiveness

- Smoking bans and restrictions were effective in decreasing the amount of ETS by approximately 72%.
- Bans and restrictions were also effective in reducing exposure to ETS by approximately 60%.

Applicability

- These findings should be applicable to most indoor workers in the United States.

Other Effects

- Smoking bans and restrictions also helped to reduce cigarette consumption and to increase the number of people who quit smoking.
- We found no adverse economic impacts on business or tourism as a result of these policies.

Barriers

- Preemption, the adoption or existence of a law at the state level that supersedes or precludes stronger local laws, can prevent implementation of smoking bans or restrictions.

The findings of our systematic review are based on 10 studies that evaluated the effect of smoking bans and restrictions on exposure to ETS.[405-414] Seven additional studies were identified but did not meet our quality criteria and were excluded from the review.[415-421]

The 10 studies provided a total of 12 measures of the effect of smoking bans and restrictions on exposure to ETS. Overall, 9 of the 10 studies observed reductions or differences in ETS exposure in workplaces that had smoking bans or restrictions. In four studies that measured environmental components of ETS (such as nicotine vapor) before and after implementation of the smoking ban or restriction, the median change, assessed 6 to 12 months after implementation of the ban or restriction, was a decrease of 72% (range, 44% to 97%). Six studies provided a total of eight measures of differences in self-reported exposure to ETS. In assessments conducted 4 to 18 months after implementation, the median change in self-reported ETS exposure was a decrease of 60% (range, 4% increase to 94% decrease).

Four studies evaluated the effect of smoking restrictions, four studies measured the effect of smoking bans, and two studies measured differences in workplace ETS exposure for both. In general, reductions in ETS exposure were greater in workplaces that had smoking bans than in those with only smoking restrictions.

These results show that smoking bans and restrictions are effective in decreasing both the amount of and exposure to ETS.

These results should be applicable to most indoor workers in the United States. Smoking bans and restrictions were evaluated in a variety of settings including hospitals and medical centers, healthcare provider offices, government or public sector workplaces, and a university. Studied bans and restrictions were created through a government law, private-sector policies, workplace policies, and local ordinance. Studies on representative samples of indoor workers in the states of California and Missouri, and on large, diverse samples of government employees in Texas and HMO employees in Oregon showed that smoking bans and restrictions reduced self-reported ETS exposure in workplaces community-wide. No studies evaluated the effect of smoking bans or restrictions in public settings outside of the workplace, such as public transportation systems or sports and entertainment venues.

A number of additional benefits of smoking bans and restrictions were described in the studies in this review. Workers exposed to a workplace smoking ban or restriction reported a greater reduction in daily consumption of cigarettes (median, −1.2 cigarettes per day, nine qualifying studies[409,410,412,422 − 427]) than did workers not exposed to a workplace smoking policy. Four studies of workplace smoking bans[423,425 − 427] found that tobacco users exposed to the ban quit at a greater rate than did tobacco users who were not exposed to a ban in the workplace. Six studies[428 − 434] (in seven reports) identified in this review evaluated the economic impact of smoking ordinances and found no adverse economic effects on businesses (including bars and restaurants) or on tourism.

The findings of our systematic review of economic evaluations are based on one study conducted in the United States, which modeled the costs and benefits of a proposed national smoke-free environment act to restrict or ban smoking inside all nonresidential buildings regularly entered by 10 or more people per week.[435] Costs included implementation of the restriction or ban by the establishment, construction and maintenance of smoking lounges, and enforcement. Benefits included savings on medical costs by averting heart disease, the value of lives saved, costs averted by reduced smoking-related fires, and productivity improvements. The net present benefit to society (benefits minus costs) was in the range of $42 to $78 billion. This range was based on high and low estimates of benefits and costs.

A major barrier to efforts by local governments to adopt smoking bans is preemption, which is the passage or presence of a state law with weaker restrictions that prevents implementation and enforcement of stronger local laws. (Eliminating preemption statutes is one of the tobacco objectives of *Healthy People 2010*[15] [Table 1–1].) Political opposition to legislative efforts to reduce ETS exposures in all workplaces and in a variety of public areas can be significant, and may include organizations representing tobacco users, businesses concerned about potential changes in revenue, and groups sponsored by the tobacco industry.

In conclusion, the Task Force recommends smoking bans and restrictions on the basis of strong evidence of effectiveness in decreasing both the amount of, and exposure to, environmental tobacco smoke. The findings of this review should be applicable to most indoor workers in the United States. Additional benefits of these interventions include reductions in daily consumption of cigarettes among workers exposed to bans or restrictions and increases in tobacco use cessation by smokers exposed to workplace smoking bans.

Community Education to Reduce Exposure to Environmental Tobacco Smoke in the Home: Insufficient Evidence to Determine Effectiveness

Community education includes all efforts to increase knowledge and to change attitudes about the health effects of exposure to environmental tobacco smoke (ETS). Techniques may include mass media messages, small media messages (including educational materials), and counseling provided outside of healthcare settings.

Community education provides information to parents, other occupants, and visitors about the health risks for nonsmoking adults and for children caused by smoking in the home (infants and children get most of their ETS exposure in the home[436]). Information is disseminated to households to motivate (1) tobacco users to reduce exposures to ETS in the household by quitting or by smoking outdoors, (2) nonsmokers in the household to assist smokers in their efforts to quit, and (3) members of the household to establish home smoking bans or restrictions. The combination of reduced indoor smoking and increased cessation will result in a reduction in indoor ETS exposure and, therefore, a reduction in tobacco-related illness and death.

Effectiveness

- We found insufficient evidence to determine the effectiveness of community education to reduce exposure to ETS in the home.
- Evidence was insufficient because of the small number of available studies and limitations in their design and execution.
- Insufficient evidence means that we were not able to determine whether or not the intervention works.

The findings of our systematic review are based on one study.[437] Two additional studies were identified but did not meet our quality criteria and were excluded from the review.[438,439] The reviewed study evaluated the effect on infant exposure to ETS of education provided by nurses during home visits. At one-year follow-up, the difference in ETS exposure between intervention and comparison households was a reduction of 4 percentage points; overall exposure, however, increased in both study arms. The inconsistency of these findings provides insufficient evidence to determine the effectiveness of community education in reducing home exposure to ETS.

Because we could not establish the effectiveness of this intervention, we did not examine situations in which it would be applicable, information about economic efficiency, or possible barriers to implementation.

Potential benefits of education to reduce ETS exposure in the home include motivating tobacco users in the household to try to quit. No harms were identified.

In conclusion, the Task Force found insufficient evidence to determine the effectiveness of community education in reducing exposure to ETS in the home because of the small number of available studies and limitations in their design and execution.

USE OF THESE RECOMMENDATIONS

The evidence reviews and recommendations presented in this chapter provide a list of effective options to support efforts by states, communities, and healthcare systems to reduce tobacco use and exposures to environmental tobacco smoke. Prevention programs and planners can compare their current prevention activities with these recommendations, take steps to ensure that existing interventions are adequately implemented and funded, and consider additional interventions in the ongoing effort to build and maintain comprehensive tobacco prevention programs.

Based on evidence of effectiveness documented in the scientific literature, recommendations from the Task Force support the following population-based tobacco prevention and control efforts:

- Clean indoor air legislation prohibiting tobacco use in indoor public and private workplaces.
- Federal, state, and local efforts to increase tobacco product excise taxes as an effective public health intervention to promote tobacco use cessation and to reduce the initiation of tobacco use among youth.
- The funding and implementation of long-term, high-intensity mass media campaigns using paid broadcast times and media messages developed through formative research.
- Proactive telephone cessation support services (quit lines).
- Reduced or eliminated co-payments for effective cessation therapies.
- Reminder systems for healthcare providers.
- Combinations of efforts to mobilize communities to identify and reduce the commercial availability of tobacco products to youth.

In reflecting the available evidence on effectiveness, recommendations from the Task Force confirm the importance of coordinated or combined intervention efforts in tobacco prevention. Evidence of effectiveness in efforts to reduce tobacco use among youth through access restrictions, to disseminate anti-tobacco messages through mass media, and to assist tobacco users in their efforts to quit via telephone comes predominantly from studies that implemented these interventions in combination with other strategies.

The contribution to our available evidence on the effectiveness of multi-component intervention efforts should be fully appreciated by program planners. The available evidence on effectiveness for any single-component intervention is small and is concentrated in evaluations of policy interventions. In this review, only one single-component program intervention—healthcare provider reminder systems—had a sufficient body of evidence on effectiveness to support a Task Force recommendation for use. For the multicomponent reviews described in this chapter, readers are encouraged to go beyond the short recommendation summaries and to learn more about the intervention combinations described in the studies contributing to the recommendation from the Task Force.

A comprehensive tobacco prevention program is often interpreted to represent concurrent intervention efforts to promote or assist tobacco use cessation, to reduce tobacco use initiation, and to implement clean indoor air policies. The *Community Guide* reviews suggest that effectiveness within each of these strategic directions (cessation, initiation, reducing secondhand smoke) demands a similar comprehensive approach in the combination and coordination of interventions.

Recommendations from the Task Force also confirm the effectiveness (and the importance) of laws and policies in tobacco prevention. State and community clean indoor air laws are effective in reducing exposure to secondhand tobacco smoke. Excise taxes on tobacco products are effective in reducing tobacco use among both adults and youth. Healthcare system policies reducing out-of-pocket costs for effective cessation therapies increase and improve client cessation efforts. Although public policies have political implications and opposition, these effective intervention options should not be prematurely "taken off the table" for consideration by prevention programs and planners.

Although these reviews include summary measurements of the magnitude of effect, readers are strongly advised to also consider the size and scope of their target population for the intervention when drawing comparisons. Mass media campaigns and policies (excise tax increases, clean indoor air legislation) deliver an intervention impact across a very broad (and potentially very large) population. Interventions with effects of relatively small magnitude, when applied across an entire community, can contribute to significant change within the population.

In many states, preemption is a major barrier to the implementation of effective tobacco prevention policies and programs. It is a direct obstacle to the adoption of local clean indoor air ordinances and to local efforts to restrict youth access to tobacco products from commercial sources. In settings where effective options are blocked, programs should determine whether or not effective intervention combinations are still feasible to address the prevention objective. In some cases, program resources may be better spent on implementing effective interventions to address other prevention goals. Programs must also remain vigilant for the introduction of new preemption legislation.

The work of the Task Force on Community Preventive Services complements an array of useful evidence reviews and guidelines[2,3,6,17,84,440,441] available to tobacco prevention and control programs. These reviews, employing different methods to select, appraise, and summarize the available evidence, report similar findings and evidence-based conclusions.

In summary, *Community Guide* reviews provide programs and planners with a (1) concise summary on effectiveness of interventions and recommendations for use; (2) convenient guide to specific studies contributing to the evidence-based conclusions on effectiveness; and (3) complementary review to support similar conclusions across the available guidelines. The reviews and the recommendations provided in this chapter, therefore, can contribute in different ways to tobacco prevention and control efforts across a range of audiences, settings, and situations.

CONCLUSION

This chapter summarizes conclusions and recommendations to date from the Task Force on interventions to reduce the initiation of tobacco use, to increase tobacco use cessation, and to reduce exposure to ETS. To reduce the initiation of tobacco use, the Task Force recommends increasing the unit price for tobacco products; mass media education campaigns combined with other interventions; and community mobilization combined with additional interventions to restrict minors' access to tobacco products. Evidence was insufficient to determine the effectiveness of restricting minors' access to tobacco through the following interventions when implemented alone: sales laws directed at retailers; laws directed at minors' purchase, possession, or use of tobacco products; active enforcement of sales laws; retailer education with reinforcement; retailer education without reinforcement; and community education.

To increase cessation of tobacco use, the Task Force recommends increasing the unit price for tobacco products; mass media campaigns combined with other interventions; healthcare provider reminder systems; provider reminders combined with provider education; reducing client out-of-pocket costs for effective cessation therapies; and multicomponent interventions that include client telephone support (quit lines). Evidence was insufficient to determine the effectiveness of mass media cessation series; mass media cessation contests; healthcare provider education alone; and healthcare provider feedback and assessment.

To reduce exposure to ETS, the Task Force recommends smoking bans and restrictions. Evidence was insufficient to determine the effectiveness of community education to reduce exposure to ETS in the home.

Details of these reviews have been published[18-19] and these articles, along with additional information about the reviews, are available at www.the communityguide.org/tobacco.

Acknowledgments

This chapter was written by the members of the systematic review development team: Jonathan E. Fielding, MD, MPH, MBA, Los Angeles Department of Health Services, University of California Los Angeles School of Public Health, University of California Los Angeles School of Medicine, Los Angeles, California, and the Task Force on Community Preventive Services; Peter A. Briss, MD, Division of Prevention Research and Analytic Methods (DPRAM), Epidemiology Program Office (EPO), Centers for Disease Control and Prevention (CDC), Atlanta; Vilma G. Carande-Kulis, MS, PhD, DPRAM/EPO/CDC; David P. Hopkins, DPRAM/EPO/CDC; Corinne G. Husten, MD, MPH; Terry F. Pechacek, PhD, Office on Smoking and Health (OSH), National Centers for Chronic Disease Prevention and Health Promotion (NCCDPHP), Centers for Disease Control and Prevention, Atlanta; Tom J. Glynn, PhD, American Cancer Society, Washington, DC.

Consultants for all reviews were: Dileep G. Bal, MD, California Department of Health Services, Sacramento; Anthony Biglan, PhD, Oregon Research Institute, Eugene; Patricia A. Buffler, PhD, MPH, University of California, Berkeley and the Task Force on Community Preventive Services; Gregory Connolly, DMD, MPH, Massachusetts Tobacco Control Program, Boston; K. Michael Cummings, PhD, MPH, Roswell Park Institute, Buffalo, New York; Michael C. Fiore, MD, MPH, University of Wisconsin Medical School, Madison; David W. Fleming, MD, Centers for Disease Control and Prevention, Atlanta; Sally Malek, MPH, North Carolina Department of Health, Raleigh; Patricia A, Mullen, DrPH, University of Texas Health Sciences Center, Houston and the Task Force on Community Preventive Services; Cheryl L. Perry, PhD, University of Minnesota, Minneapolis; John P. Pierce, PhD, University of California, San Diego; Helen H. Schauffler, PhD, University of California, Berkeley; Randy H. Schwartz, MSPH, Maine Bureau of Health, Augusta; Mitchell Zeller, American Legacy Foundation, Washington, DC.

Consultants who worked on specific intervention reviews were: Namita Sharma MA, MPA; Trevor A. Woollery, PhD; Don J. Sharp, MD, DTMH; Jeff W. McKenna, MS; Corinne G. Husten, MD, MPH, OSH/NCCDPHP/CDC, Atlanta; Connie J. Ricard, MPH; Jeffrey R. Harris, MD, MPH, DPRAM/EPO/CDC, Atlanta.

Articles included in the reviews were abstracted by: J.F. Bond, MS; C.D. Archbald, MD, MPH; B.M. Morissette, MPH, PhD; J.A. Dake, MPH; C. Herrington, MPH; N.L. Lee, BS; L.M. Tomich, MS, RD; Y. Yousey, MS, RN.

References

1. McGinnis JM, Foege WH. Actual causes of death in the United States. JAMA 1993;270:2207–12.
2. U.S. Department of Health and Human Services. Reducing tobacco use: a report of

the Surgeon General. Atlanta, GA: U.S. Department of Health and Human Services, Centers for Disease Control and Prevention, Office on Smoking and Health, 2000.

3. Centers for Disease Control and Prevention. Best practices for comprehensive tobacco control programs—August 1999. Atlanta, GA: U.S. Department of Health and Human Services, Centers for Disease Control and Prevention, National Center for Chronic Disease Prevention and Health Promotion, Office on Smoking and Health, 1999.

4. Centers for Disease Control and Prevention. Cigarette smoking among adults— United States, 2002. MMWR 2004;53(20): 427–31.

5. U.S. Department of Health and Human Services. Tobacco use among U.S. racial/ethnic minority groups—African Americans, American Indians and Alaska Natives, Asian Americans and Pacific Islanders, and Hispanics: a report of the Surgeon General. Atlanta, GA: U.S. Department of Health and Human Services, Centers for Disease Control and Prevention, National Center for Chronic Disease Prevention and Health Promotion, Office on Smoking and Health, 1998.

6. Fiore MC, Bailey WC, Cohen SJ, et al. Treating tobacco use and dependence. Clinical practice guideline. Rockville, MD: U.S. Department of Health and Human Services, Public Health Service, 2000. Available at: http://www.surgeongeneral.gov/tobacco. Accessed July 13, 2000.

7. National Institutes of Health. Tobacco and the clinician: interventions for medical and dental practice. Washington, DC: U.S. Department of Health and Human Services, Public Health Service, National Institutes of Health, 1994. NIH Pub No 94–3693.

8. U.S. Department of Health and Human Services. Reducing the health consequences of smoking: 25 years of progress. A report of the Surgeon General. Rockville, MD: U.S. Department of Health and Human Services, Public Health Service, Centers for Disease Control and Prevention, 1989. DHHS Pub No (CDC) 89–8411.

9. U.S. Department of Health and Human Services. The health benefits of smoking cessation. A report of the Surgeon General. Rockville, MD: U.S. Department of Health and Human Services, Public Health Service, Centers for Disease Control, Center for Chronic Disease Prevention and Health Promotion, Office on Smoking and Health, 1990. DHHS Pub No (CDC) 90–8416.

10. U.S. Department of Health and Human Services. Preventing tobacco use among young people: a report of the Surgeon General. Atlanta, GA: U.S. Department of Health and Human Services, Centers for Disease Control and Prevention, National Center for Chronic Disease Prevention and Health Promotion, Office on Smoking and Health, 1994.

11. University of Michigan, Institute for Social Research. Monitoring the Future Survey. Available at: http://www.monitoringthefuture.org/data/03data.html#2003data-cigs. Accessed March 16, 2004.

12. U.S. Environmental Protection Agency. Respiratory health effects of passive smoking: lung cancer and other disorders. Washington, DC: U.S. Environmental Protection Agency, Office of Research and Development, Office of Health and Environmental Assessment, 1992. EPA/600/6–90/006F.

13. California Environmental Protection Agency. Health effects of exposure to environmental tobacco smoke—final report and appendices. Sacramento: California Environmental Protection Agency, Office of Environmental Health Hazard Assessment, 1997.

14. Centers for Disease Control and Prevention. Second national report on human exposure to environmental chemicals. Available at: http://www.cdc.gov/exposurereport/tobacco/pdf/tobaccosmoke.pdf. Accessed March 16, 2004.

15. U.S. Department of Health and Human Services. Healthy people 2010. 2nd ed. Washington, DC: U.S. Government Printing Office, 2000.

16. Hopkins DP, Husten CG, Fielding JE, Rosenquist JN, Westphal LL. Evidence reviews and recommendations on interventions to reduce tobacco use and exposure to environmental tobacco smoke. A summary of selected guidelines. Am J Prev Med 2001; 20(2S):67–87.

17. U.S. Preventive Services Task Force. Guide to clinical preventive services: report of the U.S. Preventive Services Task Force. 2nd ed. Baltimore: Williams & Wilkins, 1996.

18. Centers for Disease Control and Prevention. Strategies for reducing exposure to environmental tobacco smoke, increasing tobacco-use cessation, and reducing initiation in communities and health-care systems. A report on recommendations of the Task Force on Community Preventive Services. MMWR 2000;49(No. RR-12):1–11.

19. Task Force on Community Preventive Services. Recommendations regarding interventions to reduce tobacco use and exposure to environmental tobacco smoke. Am J Prev Med 2001;20(2S):10–5.

20. Hopkins DP, Briss PA, Ricard CJ, et al. Reviews of evidence regarding interventions to reduce tobacco use and exposure to environmental tobacco smoke. Am J Prev Med 2001;20(2S):16–66.

21. Lynch BS, Bonnie RJ, Institute of Medicine: Committee on Preventing Nicotine Addiction in Children and Youths. Overview: growing up tobacco free. Preventing nicotine addiction in children and youths. Washington, DC: National Academy Press, 1994.

22. Chaloupka F, Warner K. The economics of smoking. In: Culyer AJ, Newhouse JP, eds. Handbook of health economics. Vol. 1B. Amsterdam: Elsevier Science, 2000: 1539–627.

23. Centers for Disease Control and Prevention. Response to increases in cigarette prices by race/ethnicity, income, and age groups—United States, 1976–1993. MMWR 1998;47(29):605–9.

24. Chaloupka FJ, Pacula RL. Sex and race differences in young people's responsiveness to price and tobacco control policies. Tob Control 1999;8(4):373–7.

25. Chaloupka FJ, Wechsler H. Price, tobacco control policies and smoking among young adults. J Health Econ 1997;16:359–73.

26. Gruber J. Youth smoking in the U.S.: prices and policies. Available at: http://papers .nber.org/papers/w7506. Accessed April 12, 2004.

27. Lewit EM, Coate D, Grossman M. The effects of government regulation on teenage smoking. J Polit Econ 1981;24:545–70.

28. Lewit EM, Hyland A, Kerrebrock N, Cummings KM. Price, public policy, and smoking in young people. Tob Control 1997;6(suppl 2):S17-S24.

29. Ohsfeldt RL, Boyle RG, Capilouto E. Effects of tobacco excise taxes on the use of smokeless tobacco products in the USA. Health Educ 1997;6:525–31.

30. Wasserman J, Manning WG, Newhouse JP, Winkler JD. The effects of excise taxes and regulations on cigarette smoking. J Health Econ 1991;10:43–64.

31. Chaloupka FJ, Grossman M. Price, tobacco control policies and youth smoking. National Bureau of Economic Research 1996;Working Paper 5740:1–39.

32. Chaloupka FJ, Tauras JA, Grossman M. Public policy and youth smokeless tobacco use. South Econ J 1997;64(2):503–16.

33. Ohsfeldt RL, Boyle RG. Tobacco excise taxes and rates of smokeless tobacco use in the U.S.: an exploratory ecological analysis. Tob Control 1994;3:316–23.

34. Koh HK. An analysis of the successful 1992 Massachusetts tobacco tax initiative. Tob Control 1996;5(3):220–5.

35. Nicholl J. Tobacco tax initiatives to prevent tobacco use. Cancer 1998;83:2666–79.

36. Traynor MP, Glantz SA. California's tobacco tax initiative: the development and passage of Proposition 99. J Health Polit Policy Law 1996;21(3):543–85.

37. Worden JK, Flynn BS. Effective use of mass media to prevent cigarette smoking. J Public Health Manag Pract 2000;6(3):vii–viii.

38. Bauman KE, LaPrelle J, Brown JD, Koch GG, Padgett CA. The influence of three mass media campaigns on variables related to adolescent cigarette smoking: results of a field experiment. Am J Public Health 1991;81(5):597–604.

39. Centers for Disease Control and Prevention. Tobacco use among middle and high school students—Florida, 1998 and 1999. MMWR 1999;48(12):248–53.

40. Flay BR, Hansen WB, Johnson CA, et al. Implementation effectiveness trial of a social influences smoking prevention program using schools and television. Health Educ Res 1987;2(4):385–400.

41. Flay BR, Miller TQ, Hedeker D, et al. The television, school, and family smoking prevention and cessation project. VIII. Student outcomes and mediating variables. Prev Med 1995;24(1):29–40.

42. Flynn BS, Worden JK, Secker-Walker RH, Pirie PL, Badger GJ, Carpenter JH. Long-term responses of higher and lower risk youths to smoking prevention interventions. Prev Med 1997;26(3):389–94.

43. Hafstad A, Straypedersen B, Langmark F. Use of provocative emotional appeals in a mass media campaign designed to prevent smoking among adolescents. Eur J Public Health 1997;7(2):122–7.

44. Johnson CA, Pentz MA, Weber MD, et al. Relative effectiveness of comprehensive community programming for drug abuse prevention with high-risk and low-risk adolescents. J Consult Clin Psychol 1990;58(4):447–56.

45. Kaufman JS, Jason LA, Sawlski LM, Halpert JA. A comprehensive multi-media program to prevent smoking among black students. J Drug Educ 1994;24(2):95–108.

46. Murray DM, Prokhorov AV, Harty KC. Effects of a statewide antismoking campaign on mass media messages and smoking beliefs. Prev Med 1994;23(1):54–60.

47. Perry CL, Kelder SH, Murray DM, Klepp KI. Communitywide smoking prevention: long-term outcomes of the Minnesota Heart Health Program and the Class of 1989 Study. Am J Public Health 1992;82(9):1210–6.

48. Siegel M, Biener L. The impact of an antismoking media campaign on progressions to established smoking: results of a longitudinal youth study. Am J Public Health 2000;90(3):1–7.

49. Vartiainen E, Paavola M, McAlister A, Puska P. Fifteen-year follow-up of smoking prevention effects in the North Karelia Youth Project. Am J Public Health 1998;88(1):81–5.

50. Meister JS. Designing an effective statewide tobacco control program—Arizona. Cancer 1998;83(12 suppl rep):2728–32.

51. Seghers T, Foland S. Anti-tobacco media campaign for young people. Tob Control 1998;7(suppl):S29–S30 (discussion).

52. Bauman KE, Brown JD, Bryan ES, Fisher LA, Padgett CA, Sweeney JM. Three mass media campaigns to prevent adolescent cigarette smoking. Prev Med 1988;17(5):510–30.

53. Bauman KE, Padgett CA, Koch GG. A media-based campaign to encourage personal communication among adolescents about not smoking cigarettes: participation, selection and consequences. Special issue: smoking. Health Educ Res 1989;4(1):35–44.

54. Brannon BR, Dent CW, Flay BR, et al. The television, school, and family project. V. The impact of curriculum delivery format on program acceptance. Prev Med 1989; 18:492–502.

55. Flay BR, Brannon BR, Johnson CA, et al. The television school and family smoking prevention and cessation project. 1. Theoretical basis and program development. Prev Med 1988;17(5):585–607.

56. Florida Department of Health. Florida Tobacco Youth Survey. Available at: http://www.doh.state.fl.us/disease_ctrl/epi/FYTS/index.htm. Accessed March 18, 2004.

57. Flynn BS, Worden JK, Secker-Walker RH, Badger GJ, Geller BM, Costanza MC. Prevention of cigarette smoking through mass media intervention and school programs. Am J Public Health 1992;82(6):827–34.

58. Flynn BS, Worden JK, Secker-Walker RH, et al. Mass media and school interventions for cigarette smoking prevention: effects 2 years after completion. Am J Public Health 1994;84(7):1148–50.

59. Hafstad A, Aaro LE, Langmark F. Evaluation of an anti-smoking mass media campaign targeting adolescents: the role of affective responses and interpersonal communication. Health Educ Res 1996;11(1):29–38.

60. Hafstad A, Aaro LE. Activating interpersonal influence through provocative appeals—evaluation of a mass media-based antismoking campaign targeting adolescents. Health Commun 1997;9(3):253–72.

61. Hafstad A, Aaro LE, Engeland A, Andersen A, Langmark F, Straypedersen B. Provocative appeals in anti-smoking mass media campaigns targeting adolescents—the accumulated effect of multiple exposures. Health Educ Res 1997;12(2):227–36.

62. MacKinnon DP, Johnson CA, Pentz MA, et al. Mediating mechanisms in a school-based drug prevention program: first-year effects of the Midwestern Prevention Project. Health Psychol 1991;10(3):164–72.

63. Murray DM, Perry CL, Griffin G, et al. Results from a statewide approach to adolescent tobacco use prevention. Prev Med 1992;21(4):449–72.

64. Pentz MA, MacKinnon DP, Flay BR, Hansen WB, Johnson CA, Dwyer JH. Primary prevention of chronic diseases in adolescence: effects of the Midwestern Prevention Project on tobacco use. Am J Epidemiol 1989;130(4):713–24.

65. Pentz MA, MacKinnon DP, Dwyer JH, et al. Longitudinal effects of the Midwestern Prevention Project on regular and experimental smoking in adolescents. Prev Med 1989;18(2):304–21.

66. Pentz MA, Johnson A, Dwyer JH, MacKinnon DM, Hansen WB, Flay BR. A comprehensive community approach to adolescent drug abuse prevention: effects on cardiovascular disease risk behaviors. Ann Med 1989;21(3):219–22.

67. Pentz MA, Trebow EA, Hansen WB, et al. Effects of program implementation on adolescent drug use behavior: the Midwestern Prevention Project (MPP). Eval Rev 1990; 14(3):264–89.

68. Perry CL, Klepp KI, Sillers C. Community-wide strategies for cardiovascular health: the Minnesota Heart Health Program youth program. Special issue: smoking. Health Educ Res 1989;4(1):87–101.

69. Puska P, Vartiainen E, Pallonen U, et al. The North Karelia Youth Project. A

community-based intervention study on CVD risk factors among 13- to 15-year-old children: study design and preliminary findings. Prev Med 1981;10(2):133–48.

70. Puska P, Vartiainen E, Pallonen U, et al. The North Karelia Youth Project: evaluation of two years of intervention on health behavior and CVD risk factors among 13- to 15-year old children. Prev Med 1982;11(5):550–70.

71. Secker-Walker RH, Worden JK, Holland RR, Flynn BS, Detsky AS. A mass media programme to prevent smoking among adolescents: costs and cost effectiveness. Tob Control 1997;6:207–12.

72. Sussman S, Brannon BR, Flay BR, et al. The television, school, and family smoking prevention/cessation project. II. Formative evaluation of television segments by teenagers and parents—implications for parental involvement in drug education. Health Educ Res 1986;1(3):185–94.

73. Sussman S, Dent CW, Brannon BR, et al. The television, school and family smoking prevention/cessation project. IV. Controlling for program success expectancies across experimental and control conditions. Addict Behav 1989;14(6):601–10.

74. Vartiainen E, Pallonen U, McAlister A, Koskela K, Puska P. Effect of two years of educational intervention on adolescent smoking (the North Karelia Youth Project). Bull World Health Organ 1983;61(3):529–32.

75. Vartiainen E, Pallonen U, McAlister A, Koskela K, Puska P. Four-year follow-up results of the smoking prevention program in the North Karelia Youth Project. Prev Med 1986;15(6):692–8.

76. Vartiainen E, Fallonen U, McAlister AL, Puska P. Eight-year follow-up results of an adolescent smoking prevention program: the North Karelia Youth Project. Am J Public Health 1990;80(1):78–9.

77. Vartiainen E, Tossavainen K, Viri L, Niskanen E, Puska P. The North Karelia Youth Programs. Ann N Y Acad Sci 1991;623:332–49.

78. Worden JK, Flynn BS, Geller BM, et al. Development of a smoking prevention mass media program using diagnostic and formative research. Prev Med 1988;17(5): 531–58.

79. Worden JK, Flynn BS, Solomon LJ, Secker-Walker RH, Badger GJ, Carpenter JH. Using mass media to prevent cigarette smoking among adolescent girls. Health Educ Q 1996;23(4):453–68.

80. Forster JL, Wolfson M. Youth access to tobacco: policies and politics. Annu Rev Public Health 1998;19:203–35.

81. Forster JL, Wolfson M, Murray DM, Wagenaar AC, Claxton AJ. Perceived and measured availability of tobacco to youths in 14 Minnesota communities: the TPOP Study. Tobacco Policy Options for Prevention. Am J Prev Med 1997;13(3):167–74.

82. Harrison PA, Fulkerson JA, Park E. The relative importance of social versus commercial sources in youth access to tobacco, alcohol, and other drugs. Prev Med 2000; 31(1):39–48.

83. Hinds MW. Impact of a local ordinance banning tobacco sales to minors. Public Health Rep 1992;107(3):355–8.

84. Institute of Medicine. Growing up tobacco free: preventing nicotine addiction in children and youths. Lynch BS, Bonnie RJ, eds. Washington, DC: National Academy Press, 1994.

85. Altman DG, Rasenick-Douss L, Foster V, Tye JB. Sustained effects of an educational program to reduce sales of cigarettes to minors. Am J Public Health 1991;81(7):891–3.

86. Altman DG, Wheelis AY, McFarlane M, Lee H, Fortmann SP. The relationship between tobacco access and use among adolescents: a four community study. Soc Sci Med 1999;48(6):759–75.

87. Biglan A, Ary DV, Smolkowski K, Duncan T, Black C. A randomised controlled trial of a community intervention to prevent adolescent tobacco use. Tob Control 2000; 9(1):24–32.

88. Chapman S, King M, Andrews B, McKay E, Markham P, Woodward S. Effects of publicity and a warning letter on illegal cigarette sales to minors. Aust J Public Health 1994;18(1):39–42.

89. Feighery E, Altman DG, Shaffer G. The effects of combining education and enforcement to reduce tobacco sales to minors. A study of four northern California communities. JAMA 1991;266(22):3168–71.

90. Forster JL, Murray DM, Wolfson M, Blaine TM, Wagenaar AC, Hennrikus DJ. The effects of community policies to reduce youth access to tobacco. Am J Public Health 1998;88(8):1193–8.

91. Jason LA, Billows WD, Schnopp-Wyatt DL, King C. Long term findings from Woodridge in reducing illegal cigarette sale to older minors. Eval Health Prof 1996;19(1):3–13.

92. Wildey MB, Woodruff SI, Pampalone SZ, Conway TL. Self-service sale of tobacco: how it contributes to youth access. Tob Control 1995;4:355–61.

93. Junck E, Humphries J, Rissel C. Reducing tobacco sales to minors in Manly: 10 months follow-up. Health Promot J Aust 1997;70:29–34.

94. Altman DG, Foster V, Rasenick-Douss L, Tye JB. Reducing the illegal sale of cigarettes to minors. JAMA 1989;261(1):80–3.

95. Biglan A, Ary DV, Koehn V, et al. Mobilizing positive reinforcement in communities to reduce youth access to tobacco. Am J Community Psychol 1996;24(5):625–38.

96. Jason LA, Ji PY, Anes MD, Birkhead SH. Active enforcement of cigarette control laws in the prevention of cigarette sales to minors [see comments]. JAMA 1991;266(22): 3159–61.

97. Keay KD, Woodruff SI, Wildey MB, Kenney EM. Effect of retailer intervention on cigarette sales to minors in San Diego County, California. Tob Control 1993;2:145–51.

98. Biglan A, Henderson J, Humphrey D. Mobilising positive reinforcement to reduce youth access to tobacco. Tob Control 1995;4:42–8.

99. Erickson AD, Woodruff SI, Wildey MB, Kenney E. A baseline assessment of cigarette sales to minors in San Diego, California. J Community Health 1993;18(4):213–24.

100. Jason LA, Katz R, Vavra J, Schnopp-Wyatt DL, Talbot B. Long-term follow-up of youth access to tobacco laws' impact on smoking prevalence. J Hum Behav Soc Environ 1999;2(3):1–13.

101. Cummings KM, Coogan K. Organizing communities to prevent the sale of tobacco products to minors. Int Q Community Health Educ 1992;13(1):77–86.

102. Dovell RA, Mowat DL, Dorland J, Lam M. Changes among retailers selling cigarettes to minors. Can J Public Health 1996;87(1):66–8.

103. Lewis RK, Paine-Andrews A, Fawcett SB, et al. Evaluating the effects of a community coalition's efforts to reduce illegal sales of alcohol and tobacco products to minors. J Community Health 1996;21(6):429–36.

104. Schensky AE, Smith SS, Icenogle DL, Fiore MC. Youth tobacco sale compliance checks: impact on vendor practices and community policy. Wis Med J 1996;95(11): 775–8.

105. Staff M, March L, Brnabic A, et al. Can non-prosecutory enforcement of public health legislation reduce smoking among high school students? [see comments]. Aust N Z J Public Health 1998;22(3 suppl):332–5.

106. Centers for Disease Control and Prevention. Illegal sales of cigarettes to minors—Ciudad Juarez, Mexico; El Paso, Texas; and Las Cruces, New Mexico, 1999. MMWR 1999;48:394–8.

107. Naidoo J, Platts C. Smoking prevention in Bristol: getting maximum results using minimum resources. Health Educ J 1985;44:39–42.

108. Rigotti NA, DiFranza JR, Chang Y, Tisdale T, Kemp B, Singer DE. The effect of enforcing tobacco-sales laws on adolescents' access to tobacco and smoking behavior. N Engl J Med 1997;337(15):1044–51.

109. Alcaraz R, Klonoff EA, Landrine H. The effects on children of participating in studies of minors' access to tobacco. Prev Med 1997;26(2):236–40.

110. DiFranza JR, Peck RM, Radecki TE, Savageau JA. What is the potential cost-effectiveness of enforcing a prohibition on the sale of tobacco to minors? Prev Med 2001; 32(2):168–74.

111. Siegel M, Carol J, Jordan J, et al. Preemption in tobacco control: review of an emerging public health problem. JAMA 1997;278:858–63.

112. Gorovitz E, Mosher J, Pertschuk M. Preemption or prevention?: Lessons learned from efforts to control firearms, alcohol, and tobacco. J Public Health Policy 1998; 19(1):36–50.

113. Jacobson PD, Wasserman J. The implementation and enforcement of tobacco control laws: policy implications for the activists and the industry. J Health Polit Policy Law 1999;24(3):567–98.

114. Mosher JF. The merchants, not the customers: resisting the alcohol and tobacco industries' strategy to blame young people for illegal alcohol and tobacco sales. J Public Health Policy 1995;16(4):412–32.

115. DiFranza JR. The empire strikes back. Tob Access Law News 1994;25:1–8.

116. DiFranza JR, Godshall B. Tobacco industry lobbies to sabotage Synar law. Tobacco-Free Youth Rep 1994;6(3):7–10.

117. Bidell MP, Furlong MJ, Dunn DM, Koegler JE. Case study of attempts to enact self service tobacco display ordinances: a tale of three communities. Tob Control 2000;9:71–7.

118. Forster JL, Hourigan ME, Kelder S. Locking devices on cigarette vending machines: evaluation of a city ordinance. Am J Public Health 1992;82(9):1217–9.

119. Siegel M, Biener L, Rigotti NA. The effect of local tobacco sales laws on adolescent smoking initiation. Prev Med 1999;29(5):334–42.

120. Cismoski J. Blinded by the light: the folly of tobacco possession laws against minors. Wis Med J 1994;93(11):591–8.

121. Lazovich D, Ford J, Forster J, Riley B. A pilot study to evaluate a tobacco diversion program. Am J Public Health 2001;91(11):1790–1.

122. Gemson DH, Moats HL, Watkins BX, Ganz ML, Robinson S, Healton E. Laying down the law: reducing illegal tobacco sales to minors in Central Harlem. Am J Public Health 1998;88(6):936–9.

123. Bagott M, Jordan C, Wright C, Jarvis S. How easy is it for young people to obtain cigarettes, and do test sales by trading standards have any effect? A survey of two schools in Gateshead. Child Care Health Dev 1998;24(3):207–16.

124. McDermott SR, Scott KL, Frintner MP. Accessibility of cigarettes to minors in suburban Cook County, Illinois. J Community Health 1998;23(2):153–60.

125. Woodruff SI, Wildey MB, Conway TL, Clapp EJ. Effect of a brief retailer intervention to reduce the sale of single cigarettes. Am J Health Promot 1995;9(3):172–4.

126. Skretny MT, Cummings KM, Sciandra R, Marshall J. An intervention to reduce the sale of cigarettes to minors. N Y State J Med 1990;90(2):54–5.

127. Schofield MJ, Sanson-Fisher RW, Gulliver S. Interventions with retailers to reduce cigarette sales to minors: a randomised controlled trial. Aust N Z J Public Health 1997;21(6):590–6.

128. Voorhees CC, Yanek LR, Stillman FA, Becker DM. Reducing cigarette sales to minors in an urban setting: issues and opportunities for merchant intervention. Am J Prev Med 1998;14(2):138–42.

129. Abernathy TJ. Compliance for Kids: a community-based tobacco prevention project. Can J Public Health 1994;85(2):82–4.

130. DiFranza JR, Brown LJ. The Tobacco Institute's "It's the Law" campaign: has it halted illegal sales of tobacco to children? Am J Public Health 1992;82(9):1271–3.

131. National Cancer Institute. Population-based smoking cessation: proceedings of a conference on what works to influence cessation in the general population. Smoking and tobacco control monograph No. 12. Bethesda, MD: U.S. Department of Health and Human Services, National Institutes of Health, National Cancer Institute, 2000. NIH Pub. No 00–4892.

132. Flewelling RL, Kenney E, Elder JP, Pierce J, Johnson M, Bal DG. First-year impact of the 1989 California cigarette tax increase on cigarette consumption. Am J Public Health 1992;82(6):867–9.

133. Glantz S. Changes in cigarette consumption, prices, and tobacco industry revenues associated with California's Proposition 99. Tob Control 1993;2:311–4.

134. Hu TW, Bai J, Keeler TE, Barnett PG, Sung HY. The impact of California Proposition 99, a major anti-smoking law, on cigarette consumption. J Public Health Policy 1994;15(1):26–36.

135. Hu TW, Sung HY, Keeler TE. Reducing cigarette consumption in California: tobacco taxes vs an anti-smoking media campaign. Am J Public Health 1995;85(9):1218–22.

136. Hu TW, Ren QF, Keeler TE, Bartlett J. The demand for cigarettes in California and behavioural risk factors. Health Econ 1995;4(1):7–14.

137. Keeler TE, Hu T, Barnett PG, Manning WG. Taxation, regulation, and addiction: a demand function for cigarettes based on time-series evidence. J Health Econ 1993; 12:1–18.

138. Pierce JP, Gilpin E, Emery SL, White MM, Rosbrook B, Berry C. Has the California Tobacco Control Program reduced smoking? JAMA 1998;280(10):893–9.

139. Centers for Disease Control and Prevention. Cigarette smoking before and after an excise tax increase and an antismoking campaign—Massachusetts, 1990–1996. MMWR 1996;45(44):966–70.

140. Centers for Disease Control and Prevention. Decline in cigarette consumption following implementation of a comprehensive tobacco prevention and education program—Oregon, 1996–1998. MMWR 1999;48(7):140–3.

141. Sung H, Hu T, Keeler TE. Cigarette taxation and demand: an empirical model. Contemp Econ Policy 1994;12:91–100.

142. Meier KJ, Licari MJ. The effect of cigarette taxes on cigarette consumption, 1955 through 1994. Am J Public Health 1997;87(7):1126–30.

143. Evans WN, Ringel JS, Stech D. Tobacco taxes and public policy to discourage smoking. In:Tax policy and the economy—Vol. 13. Poterba JM, ed. Cambridge, MA: MIT Press, 1999:1–56.

144. Baltagi BH, Goel RK. Quasi-experimental price elasticities of cigarette demand and the bootlegging effect. Am Agric Econ Assoc 1987;69(4):750–4.

145. Barnett PG, Keeler TE, Hu T. Oligopoly structure and the incidence of cigarette excise taxes. J Public Econ 1995;57:457–70.

146. Becker GS, Grossman M, Murphy KM. An empirical analysis of cigarette addiction. Am Econ Rev 1994;84(3):396–418.

147. Chaloupka F, Saffer H. Clean indoor air laws and the demand for cigarettes. Contemp Policy Issues 1992;10:72–83.

148. Evans WN, Farrelly MC. The compensating behavior of smokers: taxes, tar, and nicotine. Rand J Econ 1998;29(3):578–95.

149. Jackson JD, Saba RP. Some limits on taxing sin: cigarette taxation and health care finance. South Econ J 1997;63:761–75.

150. Moore MJ. Death and tobacco taxes. Rand J Econ 1996;27(2):415–28.

151. Peterson DE, Zeger SL, Remington PL, Anderson HA. The effect of state cigarette tax increases on cigarette sales, 1955 to 1988. Am J Public Health 1992;82(1):94–6.

152. Saba RP, Beard TR, Ekelund RB, Ressler RW. The demand for cigarette smuggling. Econ Inq 1995;23:189–202.

153. Seldon BJ, Doroodian K. A simultaneous model of cigarette advertising: effects on demand and industry response to public policy. Rev Econ Stat 1989;71(4):673–7.

154. Seldon BJ, Boyd R. The stability of cigarette demand. Appl Econ 1991;23(2):319–26.

155. Tegene A. Kalman filter and the demand for cigarettes. Appl Econ 1991;23(7):1175–82.

156. Thursby JG, Thursby MC. Interstate cigarette bootlegging: extent, revenue losses, and effects of federal intervention. National Tax J 2000;53(1):59–77.

157. Tremblay CH, Tremblay VJ. The impact of cigarette advertising on consumer surplus, profit, and social welfare. Contemp Econ Policy 1995;13:113–24.

158. Goel RK, Morey MJ. The interdependence of cigarette and liquor demand. South Econ J 1995;62(2):451–9.

159. Baltagi BH, Levin D. Estimating dynamic demand for cigarettes using panel data: the effects of bootlegging, taxation and advertising reconsidered. Rev Econ Stat 1986;68(1):148–55.

160. Bishop JA, Yoo JH. Health scare, excise taxes and advertising ban in the cigarette demand and supply. South Econ J 1985;52(2):402–11.

161. Chaloupka FJ. Clean indoor air laws, addiction, and cigarette smoking. Appl Econ 1992;24:193–205.

162. Chaloupka FJ. Rational addictive behavior and cigarette smoking. J Polit Econ 1991;99(41):722–42.

163. Douglas S, Hariharan G. The hazard of starting smoking: estimates from a split population duration model. J Health Econ 1994;13:213–30.

164. Fujii ET. The demand for cigarettes: further empirical evidence and its implications for public policy. Appl Econ 1980;12:479–89.

165. Lewit EM, Coate D. The potential for using excise taxes to reduce smoking. J Health Econ 1982;1(2):121–45.

166. Schneider L, Klein B, Murphy KM. Governmental regulation of cigarette health information. J Law Econ 1981;24:575–612.

167. Young T. The demand for cigarettes: alternative specifications of Fujii's model. Appl Econ 1983;15:203–11.

168. Galbraith JW, Kaiserman M. Taxation, smuggling and demand for cigarettes in Canada: evidence from time-series data. J Health Econ 1997;16:287–301.

169. Hamilton VH, Levinton C, St-Pierre Y, Grimard F. The effect of tobacco tax cuts on cigarette smoking in Canada. Can Med Assoc J 1997;156(2):187–91.

170. Mummery WK, Hagen LC. Tobacco pricing, taxation, consumption and revenue: Alberta 1985–1995. Can J Public Health 1996;87(5):314–6.

171. Jones A. UK demand for cigarettes 1954–1986, a double-hurdle approach. J Health Econ 1989;8(1):133–41.

172. Townsend J, Roderick P, Cooper J. Cigarette smoking by socioeconomic group, sex, and age: effects of price, income, and health publicity. BMJ 1994;309(6959):923–7.

173. Townsend JL. Cigarette tax, economic welfare, and social class patterns of smoking. Appl Econ 1987;19:355–65.

174. Worgotter GF, Kunze M. Cigarette prices and cigarette consumption in Austria, 1955–1983. N Y State J Med 1986;86(9):478–9.

175. Pekurinen M. The demand for tobacco products in Finland. Brit J Addict 1989; 84(10):1183–92.

176. Leu R. The effects of cigarette price and anti-smoking publicity on cigarette consumption in Switzerland. Rev Epidemiol Sante Publique 1979;27(4):359–62.

177. Leu R. Anti-smoking publicity, taxation, and the demand for cigarettes. J Health Econ 1984;3:101–16.

178. Laugesen M, Meads C. Advertising, price, income and publicity effects on weekly cigarette sales in New Zealand supermarkets. Brit J Addict 1991;86(1):83–9.

179. Kaiserman MJ, Rogers B. Tobacco consumption declining faster in Canada than in the U.S. Am J Public Health 1991;81(7):902–4.

180. Labeaga JM. Individual behaviour and tobacco consumption: a panel data approach. Health Econ 1993;2(2):103–12.

181. Laugesen M, Meads C. Tobacco advertising restrictions, price, income and tobacco consumption in OECD countries, 1960–1986. Brit J Addict 1991;86(10):1343–54.

182. Miller E. Taxes, cigarettes and the health of Maine citizens. J Maine Med Assoc 1977;68(2):58–62.

183. Reekie WD. Consumers' surplus and the demand for cigarettes. Manage Decis Econ 1994;15:223–34.

184. Advisory Commission on Intergovernmental Relations. Cigarette tax evasion: a second look. Washington, DC: Advisory Commission on Intergovernmental Relations, 1985.

185. Cummings KM, Sciandra R, Davis S, Rimer BK. Results of an antismoking media campaign utilizing the Cancer Information Service. J Natl Cancer Inst Monogr 1993; (14):113–8.

186. Fortmann SP, Taylor CB, Flora JA, Jatulis DE. Changes in adult cigarette smoking prevalence after 5 years of community health education: the Stanford Five-City Project. Am J Epidemiol 1993;137(1):82–96.

187. Jenkins CN, McPhee SJ, Le A, Pham GQ, Ha NT, Stewart S. The effectiveness of a media-led intervention to reduce smoking among Vietnamese-American men. Am J Public Health 1997;87(6):1031–4.

188. Ledwith F. Immediate and delayed effects of postal advice on stopping smoking. Health Bull 1984;42(6):332–44.

189. Luepker RV, Murray DM, Jacobs DJ, et al. Community education for cardiovascular disease prevention: risk factor changes in the Minnesota Heart Health Program. Am J Public Health 1994;84(9):1383–93.

190. Marin G, Perez-Stable EJ. Effectiveness of disseminating culturally appropriate smoking-cessation information: Programa Latino para Dejar de Fumar. J Natl Cancer Inst Monogr 1995;(18):155–63.

191. McAlister AL, Ramirez AG, Amezcua C, Pulley L, Stern MP, Mercado S. Smoking cessation in Texas-Mexico border communities: a quasi-experimental panel study. Am J Health Promot 1992;6(4):274–9.

192. McPhee SJ, Jenkins CN, Wong C, et al. Smoking cessation intervention among Vietnamese Americans: a controlled trial. Tob Control 1997;4(suppl 1):S16–S24.

193. Meyer AJ. Skills training in a cardiovascular health education campaign. J Consult Clin Psychol 1980;48(2):129–42.

194. Mudde AN, de Vries H, Dolders MG. Evaluation of a Dutch community-based smoking cessation intervention. Prev Med 1995;24(1):61–70.

195. Pierce JP, Macaskill P, Hill D. Long-term effectiveness of mass media led anti-smoking campaigns in Australia. Am J Public Health 1990;80(5):565–9.

196. Vartiainen E, Puska P, Jousilahti P, Korhonen HJ, Tuomilehto J, Nissinen A. Twenty-year trends in coronary risk factors in north Karelia and in other areas of Finland. Int J Epidemiol 1994;23(3):495–504.

197. Dwyer T, Pierce JP, Hannam CD, Burke N. Evaluation of the Sydney "Quit For Life" anti-smoking campaign. Part 2. Changes in smoking prevalence. Med J Aust 1986;144(7):344–7.

198. Farquhar JW, Maccoby N, Wood PD, et al. Community education for cardiovascular health. Lancet 1977;1(8023):1192–5.

199. Farquhar JW, Fortmann SP, Maccoby N, et al. The Stanford Five-City Project: design and methods. Am J Epidemiol 1985;122(2):323–34.

200. Farquhar JW, Fortmann SP, Flora JA, et al. Effects of communitywide education on cardiovascular disease risk factors. The Stanford Five-City Project. JAMA 1990;264(3):359–65.

201. Jacobs DR Jr, Luepker RV, Mittelmark MB, et al. Community-wide prevention strategies: evaluation design of the Minnesota Heart Health Program. J Chronic Dis 1986;39(10):775–88.

202. Marin BV, Perez-Stable EJ, Marin G, Hauck WW. Effects of a community intervention to change smoking behavior among Hispanics. Am J Prev Med 1994;10(6):340–7.

203. Marin G, Marin BV, Perez-Stable EJ, Sabogal F, Otero-Sabogal R. Changes in information as a function of a culturally appropriate smoking cessation community intervention for Hispanics. Am J Community Psychol 1990;18(6):847–64.

204. Perez-Stable EJ, Marin BV, Marin G. A comprehensive smoking cessation program for the San Francisco Bay area Latino community: Programa Latino para Dejar de Fumar. Am J Health Promot 1993;7(6):430–42.

205. Pierce JP, Dwyer T, Frape G, Chapman S, Chamberlain A, Burke N. Evaluation of the Sydney "Quit For Life" anti-smoking campaign. Part 1. Achievement of intermediate goals. Med J Aust 1986;144(7):341–4.

206. Pierce JP, Burns DM, Berry C, et al. Reducing tobacco consumption in California: Proposition 99 seems to work [letter]. JAMA 1991;265(10):1257–8.

207. Popham WJ, Potter LD, Hetrick MA, Muthen LK, Duerr JM, Johnson MD. Effectiveness of the California 1990–1991 tobacco education media campaign. Am J Prev Med 1994;10(6):319–26.

208. Puska P, Wiio J, McAlister A, et al. Planned use of mass media in national health promotion: the "Keys to Health" TV program in 1982 in Finland. Can J Public Health 1985;76(5):336–42.

209. Boyd NR, Sutton C, Orleans CT, et al. Quit Today: a targeted communications campaign to increase use of the cancer information service by African American smokers. Prev Med 1998;27(5 (Pt 2)):S50–S60.

210. Ossip-Klein DJ, Shapiro RM, Stiggins J. Freedom line: increasing utilization of a telephone support service for ex-smokers. Addict Behav 1984;9(2):227–30.

211. Pierce JP, Anderson DM, Romano RM, Meissner HI, Odenkirchen JC. Promoting smoking cessation in the United States: effect of public service announcements on the Cancer Information Service telephone line. J Natl Cancer Inst 1992;84(9):677–83.

212. Barber JJ, Grichting WL. Australia's media campaign against drug abuse. Int J Addict 1990;25(6):693–708.

213. Campion P, Owen L, McNeill A, McGuire C. Evaluation of a mass media campaign on smoking and pregnancy. Addiction 1994;89(10):1245–54.

214. Gredler B, Kunze M. Impact of a national campaign on smoking attitudes and patterns in Austria. Int J Health Educ 1981;24(4):271–9.

215. Mogielnicki RP, Neslin S, Dulac J, Balestra D, Gillie E, Corson J. Tailored media can enhance the success of smoking cessation clinics. J Behav Med 1986;9(2):141–61.

216. Platt S, Tannahill A, Watson J, Fraser E. Effectiveness of antismoking telephone helpline: follow up survey. BMJ 1997;314(7091):1371–5.

217. Shuster GF, Utz SW, Merwin E. Implementation and outcomes of a community-based self-help smoking cessation program. J Community Health Nurs 1996;13(3): 187–98.

218. Mudde AN, de Vries H, Strecher VJ. Cost-effectiveness of smoking cessation modalities: comparing apples with oranges? Prev Med 1996;25(6):708–16.

219. Ratcliffe J, Cairns J, Platt S. Cost effectiveness of a mass media-led anti-smoking campaign in Scotland. Tob Control 1997;6(2):104–10.

220. Fiscella K, Franks P. Cost-effectiveness of the transdermal nicotine patch as an adjunct to physicians' smoking cessation counseling. JAMA 1996;275(16):1247–51.

221. Novotny TE, Siegel MB. California's tobacco control saga. Health Aff 1996; 15(1):58–72.

222. Begay ME, Traynor M, Glantz SA. The tobacco industry, state politics, and tobacco education in California. Am J Public Health 1993;83(9):1214–21.

223. Cummings KM, Sciandra R, Markello S. Impact of a newspaper mediated quit smoking program. Am J Public Health 1987;77(11):1452–3.

224. Flay BR, Gruder CL, Warnecke RB, Jason LA, Peterson P. One year follow-up of the Chicago televised smoking cessation program. Am J Public Health 1989;79(10): 1377–80.

225. Jason LA, Gruder CL, Martino S, Flay BR, Warnecke R, Thomas N. Work site group meetings and the effectiveness of a televised smoking cessation intervention. Am J Community Psychol 1987;15(1):57–72.

226. Jason LA, Tait E, Goodman D, Buckenberger L, Gruder CL. Effects of a televised smoking cessation intervention among low-income and minority smokers. Am J Community Psychol 1988;16(6):863–76.

227. Millar WJ, Naegele BE. Time to quit: community involvement in smoking cessation. Can J Public Health 1987;78(2):109–14.

228. Mudde AN, de Vries H. The reach and effectiveness of a national mass media-led smoking cessation campaign in The Netherlands. Am J Public Health 1999;89(3): 346–50.

229. Salina D, Jason LA, Hedeker D, et al. A follow-up of a media-based, worksite smoking cessation program. Am J Community Psychol 1994;22(2):257–71.

230. Sutton S, Hallett R. Randomized trial of brief individual treatment for smoking using nicotine chewing gum in a workplace setting. Am J Public Health 1987;77(9): 1210–1.

231. Warnecke RB, Langenberg P, Wong SC, Flay BR, Cook TD. The second Chicago televised smoking cessation program: a 24-month follow-up. Am J Public Health 1992; 82(6):835–40.

232. Ben-Sira Z. The health promoting function of mass media and reference groups: motivating or reinforcing of behavior change. Soc Sci Med 1982;16(7):825–34.

233. Danaher BG, Berkanovic E, Gerber B. Mass media based health behavior change: televised smoking cessation program. Addict Behav 1984;9(3):245–53.

234. Korhonen HJ, Niemensivu H, Piha T, et al. National TV smoking cessation program and contest in Finland. Prev Med 1992;21(1):74–87.

235. Leroux RS, Miller ME. Electronic media-based smoking cessation clinic in the USA. Hygie 1983;2(1):23–37.

236. Ryan B, Coffin K, Smillie C, Porter K. Smoking cessation in Nova Scotia: results of the Time to Quit program. Can J Public Health 1990;81(2):166–7.

237. Sallis JF, Flora JA, Fortmann SP, Taylor CB, Maccoby N. Mediated smoking cessation programs in the Stanford Five-City Project. Addict Behav 1985;10(4):441–3.

238. Thompson B, Curry SJ. Characteristics and predictors of participation and success in a televised smoking cessation activity. Am J Health Promot 1994;8(3):175–7.

239. Valois RF, Adams KG, Kammermann SK. One-year evaluation results from Cable-Quit: a community cable television smoking cessation pilot program. J Behav Med 1996; 19(5):479–99.

240. Wewers ME, Ahijevych K, Page JA. Evaluation of a mass media community smoking cessation campaign. Addict Behav 1991;16(5):289–94.

241. Harvey M, Tuffin A, Tuffin K. An evaluation of a community based antismoking campaign. N Z Med J 1990;103(890):243–5.

242. Gruder CL, Warnecke RB, Jason LA, Flay BR, Peterson P. A televised, self-help, cigarette smoking cessation intervention. Addict Behav 1990;15(6):505–16.

243. Gruder CL, Mermelstein RJ, Kirkendol S, et al. Effects of social support and relapse prevention training as adjuncts to a televised smoking-cessation intervention. J Consult Clin Psychol 1993;61(1):113–20.

244. Jason L, Gruder CL, Buckenberger L, et al. A 12-month follow-up of a worksite smoking cessation intervention. Health Educ Res 1987;2(3):185–94.

245. Jason LA, Lesowitz T, Michaels M, et al. A worksite smoking cessation intervention involving the media and incentives. Am J Community Psychol 1989;17(6): 785–99.

246. Kviz FJ, Crittenden KS, Belzer LJ, Warnecke RB. Psychosocial factors and enrollment in a televised smoking cessation program. Health Educ Q 1991;18(4):445–61.

247. Kviz FJ, Crittenden KS, Clark MA, Madura KJ, Warnecke RB. Buddy support among older smokers in a smoking cessation program. J Aging Health 1994;6(2):229–54.

248. McFall SL, Michener A, Rubin D, et al. The effects and use of maintenance newsletters in a smoking cessation intervention. Addict Behav 1993;18(2):151–8.

249. Smillie C, Coffin K, Porter K, Ryan B. Primary health care through a community based smoking-cessation program. J Community Health 1988;13(3):156–70.

250. Warnecke RB, Langenberg P, Gruder CL, Flay BR, Jason LA. Factors in smoking cessation among participants in a televised intervention. Prev Med 1989;18(6):833–46.

251. Warnecke RB, Flay BR, Kviz FJ, et al. Characteristics of participants in a televised smoking cessation intervention. Prev Med 1991;20(3):389–403.

252. Resnicow K, Vaughan R, Futterman R, et al. A self-help smoking cessation program for inner-city African Americans: results from the Harlem Health Connection Project. Health Educ Behav 1997;24(2):201–17.

253. Centers for Disease Control and Prevention. Impact of promotion of the Great American Smokeout and availability of over-the-counter nicotine medications, 1996. MMWR 1997;46(37):867–71.

254. Chapman S, Smith W, Mowbray G, Hugo C, Egger G. Quit and win smoking cessation contests: how should effectiveness be evaluated? Prev Med 1993;22(3):423–32.

255. Chapman S, Smith W. Deception in quit smoking lottery entrants. Am J Health Promot 1994;8:328–30.

256. Donovan RJ, Fisher DA, Armstrong BK. "Give it away for a day": an evaluation of Western Australia's first smoke free day. Community Health Stud 1984;8(3):301–6.

257. Elder JP, McGraw SA, Rodrigues A, et al. Evaluation of two community-wide smoking cessation contests. Prev Med 1987;16(2):221–34.

258. Elder JP, Campbell NR, Mielchen SD, Hovell MF, Litrownik AJ. Implementation and evaluation of a community-sponsored smoking cessation contest. Am J Health Promot 1991;5(3):200–7.

259. Glasgow RE, Klesges RC, Mizes JS, Pechacek TF. Quitting smoking: strategies used and variables associated with success in a stop-smoking contest. J Consult Clin Psychol 1985;53(6):905–12.

260. Gritz ER, Carr CR, Marcus AC. Unaided smoking cessation: Great American Smokeout and New Year's Day quitters. Special Issue: Clinical research issues in psychosocial oncology. J Psychosoc Oncol 1988;6(3–4):217–34.

261. Hantula D, Stillman FA, Waranch HR. Can a mass media campaign modify tobacco smoking in a large organization? Evaluation of the Great American Smokeout in an urban hospital. J Organ Behav Manage 1992;13(1):33–47.

262. King AC, Flora JA, Fortmann SP, Taylor CB. Smokers' challenge: immediate and long-term findings of a community smoking cessation contest. Am J Public Health 1987; 77(10):1340–1.

263. Korhonen T, Urjanheimo E, Mannonen P, Korhonen HJ, Uutela A, Puska P. Quit and Win campaigns as a long-term anit-smoking intervention in North Karelia and other parts of Finland. Tob Control 1999;8:175–81.

264. Lando HA, Loken B, Howard-Pitney B, Pechacek T. Community impact of a localized smoking cessation contest. Am J Public Health 1990;80(5):601–3.

265. Lando HA, Pirie PL, Dusich KH, Elsen C, Bernards J. Community incorporation of quit and win contests in Bloomington, Minnesota. Am J Public Health 1995;85(2): 263–4.

266. Leinweber CE, Macdonald JM, Campbell HS. Community smoking cessation contests: an effective public health strategy. Can J Public Health 1994;85(2):95–8.

267. Tillgren P, Haglund BJ, Ainetdin T, Holm LE. Who is a successful quitter? One-year follow-up of a National Tobacco Quit and Win Contest in Sweden. Scand J Soc Med 1995;23(3):193–201.

268. Resnicow K, Futterman R, Weston RE, et al. Smoking prevalence in Harlem, New York. Am J Health Promot 1996;10(5):343–6.

269. Resnicow K, Royce J, Vaughan R, Orlandi MA, Smith M. Analysis of a multi-component smoking cessation project: what worked and why. Prev Med 1997;26(3): 373–81.

270. Tillgren P, Haglund BJ, Gilljam H, Holm LE. A tobacco quit and win model in the Stockholm cancer prevention programme. Eur J Cancer Prev 1992;1(5):361–6.

271. Chang HC, Zimmerman LH, Beck JM. Impact of chart reminders on smoking cessation practices of pulmonary physicians. Am J Respir Crit Care Med 1995;152(3): 984–7.

272. Dietrich AJ, O'Conner GT, Keller A, Carney PA, Levy D, Whaley FS. Cancer: improving early detection and prevention. A community practice randomised trial. BMJ 1992;304:687–91.

273. Robinson MD, Laurent SL, Little JJ. Including smoking status as a new vital sign: it works. J Fam Pract 1995;40(6):556–61.

274. Hahn DL, Berger MG. Implementation of a systematic health maintenance protocol in a private practice. J Fam Pract 1990;31(5):492–502.

275. Strecher VJ, O'Malley MS, Villagra VG, et al. Can residents be trained to counsel patients about quitting smoking? Results from a randomized trial. J Gen Intern Med 1991;6(1):9–17.

276. Rosser WW, McDowell I, Newell C. Use of reminders for preventive procedures in family medicine. Can Med Assoc J 1991;145(7):807–13.

277. Spencer E, Swanson T, Hueston WJ, Edberg DL. Tools to improve documentation of smoking status. Continuous quality improvement and electronic medical records. Arch Fam Med 1999;8(1):18–22.

278. Fiore MC, Jorenby DE, Schensky AE, Smith SS, Bauer RR, Baker TB. Smoking status as the new vital sign: effect on assessment and intervention in patients who smoke. Mayo Clin Proc 1995;70(3):209–13.

279. Cohen SJ, Stookey GK, Katz BP, Drook CA, Smith DM. Encouraging primary care physicians to help smokers quit. A randomized, controlled trial. Ann Intern Med 1989; 110(8):648–52.

280. Cohen SJ, Stookey GK, Katz BP, Drook CA, Christen AG. Helping smokers quit: a randomized controlled trial with private practice dentists. J Am Dent Assoc 1989;118: 41–5.

281. Conger B, Nelson EC, Dietrich AJ, et al. Effectiveness of physician antismoking advice. Am J Prev Med 1987;3(4):223–6.

282. Cummings SR, Richard RJ, Duncan CL, et al. Training physicians about smoking cessation: a controlled trial in private practice. J Gen Intern Med 1989;4(6):482–9.

283. Cummings SR, Coates TJ, Richard RJ, et al. Training physicians in counseling about smoking cessation. A randomized trial of the "Quit for Life" program. Ann Intern Med 1989;110(8):640–7.

284. Davies BL, Matte-Lewis L, O'Connor AM, Dulberg CS, Drake ER. Evaluation of the "Time to Quit" self-help smoking cessation program. Can J Public Health 1992; 83(1):19–23.

285. Duncan C, Stein MJ, Cummings SR. Staff involvement and special follow-up time increase physicians' counseling about smoking cessation: a controlled trial. Am J Public Health 1991;81(7):899–901.

286. Gilbert JR, Wilson DM, Singer J, et al. A family physician smoking cessation program: an evaluation of the role of follow-up visits. Am J Prev Med 1992;8(2):91–5.

287. Goldberg DN, Hoffman AM, Farinha MF, et al. Physician delivery of smoking-cessation advice based on the stages-of-change model. Am J Prev Med 1994;10(5): 267–74.

288. Hartmann KE, Thorp JMJ, Pahel-Short L, Koch MA. A randomized controlled trial of smoking cessation intervention in pregnancy in an academic clinic. Obstet Gynecol 1996;87(4):621–6.

289. Hollis JF, Lichtenstein E, Vogt TM, Stevens VJ, Biglan A. Nurse-assisted counseling for smokers in primary care. Ann Intern Med 1993;118:521–5.

290. Hovell MF, Slymen DJ, Jones JA, et al. An adolescent tobacco-use prevention trial in orthodontic offices. Am J Public Health 1996;86(12):1760–6.

291. Kottke TE, Brekke ML, Solberg LI, Hughes JR. A randomized trial to increase smoking intervention by physicians: Doctors Helping Smokers, Round I. JAMA 1989; 261(14):2101–6.

292. Kottke TE, Solberg LI, Brekke ML, Conn SA, Maxwell P, Brekke MJ. A controlled trial to integrate smoking cessation advice into primary care practice: Doctors Helping Smokers, Round III. J Fam Pract 1992;34(6):701–8.

293. Manfredi C, Crittenden KS, Warnecke RB, Engler J, Cho YI, Shaligram C. Evaluation of a motivational smoking cessation intervention for women in public health clinics. Prev Med 1999;28:51–60.

294. McIlvain HE, Susman JL, Manners MA, Davis CM, Gilbert CS. Improving smoking cessation counseling by family practice residents. J Fam Pract 1992;34(6):745–9.

295. McPhee S, Bird J, Fordham D, Rodnick J. Promoting cancer prevention activities by primary care physicians: results of a randomized, controlled trial. JAMA 1991;266: 538–44.

296. Morgan GD, Noll EL, Orleans CT, Rimer BK, Amfoh K, Bonney G. Reaching midlife and older smokers: tailored interventions for routine medical care. Prev Med 1996;25(3):346–54.

297. Ockene JK, Kristeller J, Pbert L, et al. The physician-delivered smoking intervention project: can short-term interventions produce long-term effects for a general outpatient population? Health Psychol 1994;13(3):278–81.

298. Petersen L, Handel J, Kotch J, Podedworny T, Rosen A. Smoking reduction during pregnancy by a program of self-help and clinical support. Obstet Gynecol 1992; 79(6):924–30.

299. Richmond R, Mendelsohn C, Kehoe L. Family physicians' utilization of a brief smoking cessation program following reinforcement contact after training: a randomized trial. Prev Med 1998;27(1):77–83.

300. Rigotti NA, Arnsten JH, McKool KM, Wood-Reid KM, Pasternak RC, Singer DE. Efficacy of a smoking cessation program for hospital patients. Arch Intern Med 1997; 157(22):2653–60.

301. Rodney WM, Nutter D, Widoff B. Recording patients' consumption of social drugs in a family medicine residency: a longitudinal study. Fam Pract 1985;2(2):86–90.

302. Secker-Walker RH, Solomon LJ, Flynn BS, Skelly JM, Mead PB. Reducing smoking during pregnancy and postpartum: physician's advice supported by individual counseling. Prev Med 1998;27:422–30.

303. Sinclair HK, Bond CM, Lennox AS, Silcock J, Windfield AJ, Donnan PT. Training pharmacists and pharmacy assistants in the stage-of-change model of smoking cessation: a randomised controlled trial in Scotland. Tob Control 1998;7:253–61.

304. Stevens VJ, Severson H, Lichtenstein E, Little SJ, Leben J. Making the most of a teachable moment: a smokeless-tobacco cessation intervention in the dental office. Am J Public Health 1995;85(2):231–5.

305. Wall MA, Severson HH, Andrews JA, Lichtenstein E, Zoref L. Pediatric office-based smoking intervention: impact on maternal smoking and relapse. Pediatrics 1995; 96(4 pt 1):622–8.

306. Wilson DM, Taylor DW, Gilbert JR, et al. A randomized trial of a family physician intervention for smoking cessation. JAMA 1988;260(11):1570–4.

307. Windsor RA, Lowe JB, Perkins LL, et al. Health education for pregnant smokers: its behavioral impact and cost benefit. Am J Public Health 1993;83(2):201–6.

308. Cohen SJ, Christen AG, Katz BP, et al. Counseling medical and dental patients about cigarette smoking: the impact of nicotine gum and chart reminders. Am J Public Health 1987;77(3):313–6.

309. Hebert JR, Kristeller J, Ockene JK, et al. Patient characteristics and the effect of three physician-delivered smoking interventions. Prev Med 1992;21(5):557–73.

310. Hollis JF, Lichtenstein E, Mount K, Vogt TM, Stevens VJ. Nurse-assisted smoking counseling in medical settings: minimizing demands on physicians. Prev Med 1991; 20(4):497–507.

311. Kottke TE, Solberg LI, Conn S, et al. A comparison of two methods to recruit physicians to deliver smoking cessation interventions. Arch Intern Med 1990;150(7): 1477–81.

312. Lichtenstein E, Hollis J. Patient referral to a smoking cessation program: who follows through? J Fam Pract 1992;34(6):739–44.

313. Lindsay-McIntyre E, Wilson D, Best JA, et al. The impact of a continuing education package for smoking cessation on physicians' clinical behavior and patient smoking. Proc Annu Conf Res Med Educ 1987;26:14–9.

314. Lindsay EA, Wilson D, Best JA, Singer J, Gilbert JR, Taylor DW. A randomized trial of physician training for smoking cessation. Am J Health Promot 1989;3(3):11–8.

315. Little SJ, Stevens VJ, Severson HH, Lichtenstein E. Effective smokeless tobacco intervention for dental hygiene patients. J Dent Hyg 1992;66(4):185–90.

316. Manfredi C, Crittenden KS, Cho YI, Engler J, Warnecke RB. Minimal smoking cessation interventions in prenatal, family planing, and well-child public health clinics. Am J Public Health 2000;90:423–7.

317. Manfredi C, Crittenden KS, Cho YI, Engler J, Warnecke RB. The effect of a structured smoking cesation program, independent of exposure to existing interventions. Am J Public Health 2000;90:751–6.

318. Ockene JK, Kristeller J, Goldberg R, et al. Increasing the efficacy of physician-delivered smoking interventions: a randomized clinical trial. J Gen Intern Med 1991; 6(1):1–8.

319. Rosal MC, Ockene JK, Hurley TG, Kalan K, Hebert JR. Effectiveness of nicotine-containing gum in the Physician-Delivered Smoking Intervention Study. Prev Med 1998; 27(2):262–7.

320. Secker-Walker RH, Solomon LJ, Flynn BS, et al. Training obstetric and family practice residents to give smoking cessation advice during prenatal care. Am J Obstet Gynecol 1992;166(5):1356–63.

321. Whitlock EP, Vogt TM, Hollis JF, Lichtenstein E. Does gender affect response to a brief clinic-based smoking intervention? Am J Med 1997;13(3):159–66.

322. Windsor RA, Lowe JB, Artz L, Contreras L. Smoking cessation and pregnancy intervention trial: preliminary mid-trial results. Prog Clin Biol Res 1990;339:107–17.

323. Allen B, Pederson LL, Leonard EH. Effectiveness of physicians-in-training counseling for smoking cessation in African Americans. J Natl Med Assoc 1998;90(10): 597–604.

324. Kosower E, Ernst A, Taub B, Berman N, Andrews J, Seidel J. Tobacco prevention education in a pediatric residency program. Arch Pediatr Adolesc Med 1995;149(4): 430–5.

325. Leshan LA, Fitzsimmons M, Marbella A, Gottlieb M. Increasing clinical prevention efforts in a family practice residency program through CQI methods. J Qual Improv 1997;23(7):391–400.

326. Narce-Valente S, Kligman EW. Increasing physician screening and counseling for passive smoking. J Fam Pract 1992;34(6):722–8.

327. Russell MA, Stapleton JA, Jackson PH, Hajek P, Belcher M. District programme to reduce smoking: effect of clinic supported brief intervention by general practitioners. BMJ (Clinical Research Ed) 1987;295:1240–4.

328. Solberg LI, Maxwell PL, Kottke TE, Gepner GJ, Brekke ML. A systematic primary care office-based smoking cessation program. J Fam Pract 1990;30(6):647–54.

329. Allen SS, Bland CJ, Dawson SJ. A mini-workshop to train medical students to use a patient-centered approach to smoking cessation. Am J Prev Med 1990;6(1): 28–33.

330. Carney PA, Dietrich AJ, Freeman DJ, Mott LA. A standardized-patient assessment of a continuing medical education program to improve physicians' cancer-control clinical skills. Acad Med 1995;70(1):52–8.

331. Cockburn J, Ruth D, Silagy C, et al. Randomised trial of three approaches for marketing smoking cessation programmes to Australian general practitioners. BMJ 1992; 304(6828):691–4.

332. Giovino GA, Cummings KM, Koenigsberg MR, Sciandra RC. An evaluation of a physician training program on patient smoking cessation. Prog Clin Biol Res 1990;339: 27–48.

333. Klein JD, Portilla M, Goldstein A, Leininger L. Training pediatric residents to prevent tobacco use. Pediatrics 1995;96(2 pt 1):326–30.

334. Ockene JK, Lindsay EA, Hymowitz N, et al. Tobacco control activities of primary-

care physicians in the Community Intervention Trial for Smoking Cessation. COMMIT Research Group. Tob Control 1997;6(suppl 2):S49–S56.

335. Quirk M, Ockene J, Kristeller J, et al. Training family practice and internal medicine residents to counsel patients who smoke: improvement and retention of counseling skills. Fam Med 1991;23(2):108–11.

336. Roche AM, Eccleston P, Sanson-Fisher R. Teaching smoking cessation skills to senior medical students: a block-randomized controlled trial of four different approaches. Prev Med 1996;25(3):251–8.

337. Royce JM, Gorin SS, Edelman B, Rendino-Perrone R, Orlandi MA. Student nurses and smoking cessation. Prog Clin Biol Res 1990;339:49–71.

338. Ward J, Sanson-Fisher R. Does a 3-day workshop for family medicine trainees improve preventive care? A randomized control trial. Prev Med 1996;25(6):741–7.

339. Dietrich AJ, Barrett J, Levy D, Carney-Gersten P. Impact of an educational program on physician cancer control knowledge and activities. Am J Prev Med 1990;6(6):346–52.

340. Ockene JK, Quirk ME, Goldberg RJ, et al. A residents' training program for the development of smoking intervention skills. Arch Intern Med 1988;148(5):1039–45.

341. Anonymous. The impact of providing physicians with quit-smoking materials for smoking patients. CA Cancer J Clin 1981;31(2):75–8.

342. Chu F, Day R. Smoking recognition by family physicians. J Fam Pract 1981;12(4):657–60.

343. Dunkley J. Training midwives to help pregnant women stop smoking. Nurs Times 1997;93(5):64–6.

344. Hall MN, Pettice YJ, Robinson MD, Alexander M. Teaching smoking cessation to family practice residents: an experiential approach. Fam Med 1996;28(5):331–6.

345. Leininger LS, Earp JA. The effect of training staff in office-based smoking cessation counseling. Patient Educ Couns 1993;20(1):17–25.

346. Montner P, Bennett G, Brown C. An evaluation of a smoking cessation training program for medical residents in an inner-city hospital. J Natl Med Assoc 1994;86(9):671–5.

347. Patterson J, Fried RA, Nagle JP. Impact of a comprehensive health promotion curriculum on physician behavior and attitudes. Am J Prev Med 1989;5(1):44–9.

348. Wood GJ, Cecchini JJ, Nathason N, Hiroshige K. Office-based training in tobacco cessation for dental professionals. J Am Dent Assoc 1997;128(2):216–24.

349. Bonevski B, Sanson-Fisher RW, Campbell E, Carruthers A, Reid AL, Ireland M. Randomized controlled trial of a computer strategy to increase general practitioner preventive care. Prev Med 1999;29(6 pt 1):478–86.

350. Kern D, Harris W. Use of an outpatient medical record audit to achieve educational objectives. J Gen Intern Med 1990;5:218–24.

351. Shank JC, Powell T, Llewelyn J. A five-year demonstration project association with improvement in physician health maintenance behavior. Fam Med 1989;21(4):273–8.

352. Ewart CK, Li VC, Coates TJ. Increasing physicians' antismoking influence by applying an inexpensive feedback technique. J Med Educ 1983;58(6):468–73.

353. Frame P, Kowulich B, Llewellyn A. Improving physician compliance with a health maintenance protocol. J Fam Pract 1984;19:341–4.

354. Cox JL, McKenna JP. Nicotine gum: does providing it free in a smoking cessation program alter success rates? J Fam Pract 1990;31(3):278–80.

355. Curry SJ, Grothaus LC, McAfee T, Pabiniak C. Use and cost effectiveness of smoking-cessation services under four insurance plans in a health maintenance organization. N Engl J Med 1998;339(10):673–9.

356. Hughes JR, Wadland WC, Fenwick JW, Lewis J, Bickel WK. Effect of cost on the self-administration and efficacy of nicotine gum: a preliminary study. Prev Med 1991; 20(4):486–96.

357. Johnson RE, Hollis JF, Stevens VJ, Woodson GT. Patterns of nicotine gum use in a health maintenance organization. DICP 1991;25:730–5.

358. Schauffler HH, McMenamin S, Olson K, Boyce-Smith G, Rideout JA, Kamil J. Variations in treatment benefits influence smoking cessation: results of a randomized controlled trial. Tob Control 2001;10(2):175–80.

359. Cromwell J, Bartosch WJ, Fiore MC, Hasselblad V, Baker T. Cost-effectiveness of the clinical practice recommendations in the AHCPR guideline for smoking cessation. Agency for Health Care Policy and Research. JAMA 1997;278(21):1759–66.

360. Sofian NS, McAfee T, Wilson J, Levan S. Telephone smoking cessation intervention: the Free and Clear Program. HMO Pract 1995;9(3):144–6.

361. Curry SJ, McBride C, Grothaus LC, Louie D, Wagner EH. A randomized trial of self-help materials, personalized feedback, and telephone counseling with nonvolunteer smokers. J Consult Clin Psychol 1995;63(6):1005–14.

362. Decker BD, Evans RG. Efficacy of a minimal contact version of a multimodal smoking cessation program. Addict Behav 1989;14(5):487–91.

363. Gebauer C, Kwo CY, Haynes EF, Wewers ME. A nurse-managed smoking cessation intervention during pregnancy. J Obstet Gynecol Neonatal Nurs 1998;27(1):47–53.

364. Glasgow RE, Whitlock EP, Eakin EG, Lichtenstein E. A brief smoking cessation intervention for women in low-income planned parenthood clinics. Am J Public Health 2000;90(5):786–9.

365. Johnson JL, Budz B, Mackay M, Miller C. Evaluation of a nurse-delivered smoking cessation intervention for hospitalized patients with cardiac disease. Heart Lung 1999;28(1):55–64.

366. Lando HA, Hellerstedt WL, Pirie PL, McGovern PG. Brief supportive telephone outreach as a recruitment and intervention strategy for smoking cessation. Am J Public Health 1992;82(1):41–6.

367. Lando HA, Pirie PL, Roski J, McGovern PG, Schmid LA. Promoting abstinence among relapsed chronic smokers: the effect of telephone support. Am J Public Health 1996;86(12):1786–90.

368. Lando HA, Rolnick S, Klevan D, Roski J, Cherney L, Lauger G. Telephone support as an adjunct to transdermal nicotine in smoking cessation. Am J Public Health 1997;87(10):1670–4.

369. Lewis SF, Piasecki TM, Fiore MC, Anderson JE, Baker TB. Transdermal nicotine replacement for hospitalized patients: a randomized clinical trial. Prev Med 1998;27(2): 296–303.

370. McBride CM, Curry SJ, Lando HA, Pirie PL, Grothaus LC, Nelson JC. Prevention of relapse in women who quit smoking during pregnancy. Am J Public Health 1999; 89(5):706–11.

371. McBride CM, Scholes D, Grothaus LC, Curry SJ, Ludman E, Albright J. Evaluation of a minimal self-help smoking cessation intervention following cervical cancer screening. Prev Med 1999;29(2):133–8.

372. Miller N, Smith P, DeBusk RF, Sobel DS, Taylor CB. Smoking cessation in hospitalized patients: results of a randomized trial. Arch Fam Med 1997;157:409–15.

373. Orleans CT, Schoenbach VJ, Wagner EH, et al. Self-help quit smoking interventions: effects of self-help materials, social support instructions, and telephone counseling. J Consult Clin Psychol 1991;59(3):439–48.

374. Orleans CT, Boyd NR, Bingler R, et al. A self-help intervention for African American smokers: tailoring cancer information service counseling for a special population. Prev Med 1998;27(5 (pt 2)):S61–S70.

375. Ossip-Klein DJ, Giovino GA, Megahed N, et al. Effects of a smoker's hotline: results of a 10-county self-help trial. J Consult Clin Psychol 1991;59(2):325–32.

376. Ossip-Klein DJ, Carosella AM, Krusch DA. Self-help interventions for older smokers. Tob Control 1997;6(3):188–93.

377. Prochaska JO, DiClemente CC, Velicer WF, Rossi JS. Standardized, individualized, interactive, and personalized self-help programs for smoking cessation. Health Psychol 1993;12(5):399–405.

378. Sexton M, Hebel JR. A clinical trial of change in maternal smoking and its effect on birth weight. JAMA 1984;251(7):911–5.

379. Simon JA, Solkowitz SN, Carmody TP, Browner WS. Smoking cessation after surgery, a ramdomized trial. Arch Fam Med 1997;157:1371–6.

380. Stevens VJ, Glasgow RE, Hollis JF, Lichtenstein E, Vogt TM. A smoking-cessation intervention for hospital patients. Med Care 1993;31(1):65–72.

381. Thompson B, Kinne S, Lewis FM, Woolridge JA. Randomized telephone smoking-intervention trial initially directed at blue-collar workers. J Natl Cancer Inst Monogr 1993; 14:105–12.

382. Weissfeld JL, Holloway JL. Treatment for cigarette smoking in a Department of Veterans Affairs outpatient clinic. Arch Intern Med 1991;151(5):973–7.

383. Westman EC, Levin ED, Rose JE. The nicotine patch in smoking cessation. A randomized trial with telephone counseling. Arch Intern Med 1993;153(16):1917–23.

384. Zhu SH, Stretch V, Balabanis M, Rosbrook B, Sadler G, Pierce JP. Telephone counseling for smoking cessation: effects of single-session and multiple-session interventions. J Consult Clin Psychol 1996;64(1):202–11.

385. Britt J, Curry SJ, McBride C, Grothaus L, Louie D. Implementation and acceptance of outreach telephone counseling for smoking cessation with nonvolunteer smokers. Health Educ Q 1994;21(1):55–68.

386. Glasgow RE, Lando H, Hollis J, McRae SG, La Chance PA. A stop-smoking telephone help line that nobody called. Am J Public Health 1993;83(2):252–3.

387. Hebel JR, Nowicki P, Sexton M. The effect of antismoking intervention during pregnancy: an assessment of interactions with maternal characteristics. Am J Epidemiol 1985;122(1):135–48.

388. Kinne S, Thompson B, Wooldridge JA. Response to a telephone smoking information line. Am J Health Promot 1991;5(6):410–3.

389. Meenan RT, Stevens VJ, Hornbrook MC, et al. Cost-effectiveness of a hospital-based smoking cessation intervention. Med Care 1998;36(5):670–8.

390. Taylor CB, Miller N, Herman S, et al. A nurse-managed smoking cessation program for hospitalized smokers. Am J Public Health 1996;86(11):1557–60.

391. Vogt TM, Lichtenstein E, Ary D, et al. Integrating tobacco intervention into a

health maintenance organization: the TRACC program. Special Issue: Smoking. Health Educ Res 1989;4(1):125–35.

392. Amos A, White DA, Elton RA. Is a telephone helpline of value to the workplace smoker? Occup Med 1995;45(5):234–8.

393. Bachman DS. Smoking cessation via telephone counseling and tools for helping your patients quit smoking once and for all. J Ark Med Soc 1997;94(4):147–8.

394. Dubren R. Self-reinforcement by recorded telephone messages to maintain non-smoking behavior. J Consult Clin Psychol 1977;45(3):358–60.

395. Glasgow RE, Hollis JF, McRae SG, Lando HA, LaChance P. Providing an integrated program of low intensity tobacco cessation services in a health maintenance organization. Health Educ Res 1991;6(1):87–9.

396. Racelis MC, Lombardo K, Verdin J. Impact of telephone reinforcement of risk reduction education on patient compliance. J Vasc Nurs 1998;16(1):16–20.

397. Croghan IT, Offord KP, Evans RW, et al. Cost-effectiveness of treating nicotine dependence: the Mayo Clinic experience. Mayo Clin Proc 1997;72(10):917–24.

398. Ershoff DH, Aaronson NK, Danaher BG, Wasserman FW. Behavioral, health, and cost outcomes of an HMO-based prenatal health education program. Public Health Rep 1983;98(6):536–47.

399. Krumholz HM, Cohen BJ, Tsevat J, Pasternak RC, Weinstein MC. Cost-effectiveness of a smoking cessation program after myocardial infarction. J Am Coll Cardiol 1993;22(6):1697–702.

400. Marks JS, Koplan JP, Hogue CJ, Dalmat ME. A cost-benefit/cost-effectiveness analysis of smoking cessation for pregnant women. Am J Prev Med 1990;6(5):282–9.

401. U.S. Office on Smoking and Health. The health consequences of involuntary smoking. A report of the Surgeon General. Rockville, MD: U.S. Department of Health and Human Services, Public Health Service, Centers for Disease Control, Center for Health Promotion and Education, Office on Smoking and Health, 1986. DHHS Pub No (CDC) 87–8398.

402. Burns DM, Axelrad R, Bal D, et al. Report of the Tobacco Policy Research Study Group on Smoke-Free Indoor Air Policies. Tob Control 1992;1(suppl):S14–S18.

403. Fielding JE. Banning worksite smoking. Am J Public Health 1986;76(8):957–9.

404. Pierce JP, Naquin M, Gilpin E, Giovino G, Mills S, Marcus S. Smoking initiation in the United States: a role for worksite and college smoking bans. J Natl Cancer Inst 1991;83(14):1009–13.

405. Becker DM, Conner HF, Waranch HR, et al. The impact of a total ban on smoking in the Johns Hopkins Children's Center. JAMA 1989;262(6):799–802.

406. Borland R, Pierce JP, Burns DM, Gilpin E, Johnson M, Bal D. Protection from environmental tobacco smoke in California: the case for a smoke-free workplace. JAMA 1992;268(6):749–52.

407. Broder I, Pilger C, Corey P. Environment and well-being before and following smoking ban in office building. Can J Public Health 1993;84(4):254–8.

408. Brownson RC, Davis J, Jackson-Thompson J, Wilkerson J. Environmental tobacco smoke awareness and exposure: impact of a statewide clean indoor air law and the report of the U.S. Environmental Protection Agency. Tob Control 1995;4:132–8.

409. Etter J, Ronchi A, Perneger TV. Short-term impact of a university based smoke free campaign. J Epidemiol Community Health 1999;53:710–5.

410. Gottlieb NH, Eriksen MP, Lovato CY, Weinstein RP, Green LW. Impact of a restrictive work site smoking policy on smoking behavior, attitudes, and norms. J Occup Med 1990;32(1):16–23.

411. Millar WJ. Evaluation of the impact of smoking restrictions in a government work setting. Can J Public Health 1988;79(5):379–82.

412. Mullooly JP, Schuman KL, Stevens VJ, Glasgow RE, Vogt TM. Smoking behavior and attitudes of employees of a large HMO before and after a work site ban on cigarette smoking. Public Health Rep 1990;105(6):623–8.

413. Patten CA, Pierce JP, Cavin SW, Berry C, Kaplan R. Progress in protecting nonsmokers from environmental tobacco smoke in California workplaces. Tob Control 1995;4:139–44.

414. Stillman FA, Becker DM, Swank RT, et al. Ending smoking at the Johns Hopkins Medical Institutions. An evaluation of smoking prevalence and indoor air pollution. JAMA 1990;264(12):1565–9.

415. Abernathy T, O'Grady B, Dukeshire S. Changes in ETS following anti-smoking legislation. Can J Public Health 1998;89(1):33–4.

416. Batlle E, Boixet M, Agudo A, Almirall J, Salvador T. Tobacco prevention in hospitals: long-term follow-up of a smoking control programme. Brit J Addict 1991;86(6): 709–17.

417. Borland R, Owen N, Hocking B. Changes in smoking behaviour after a total workplace smoking ban. Aust J Public Health 1991;15(2):130–4.

418. Centers for Disease Control. Evaluation of an employee smoking policy—Pueblo, Colorado, 1989–90. MMWR 1990;39(38):673–6.

419. Eisner MD, Smith AK, Blanc PD. Bartenders' respiratory health after establishment of smoke-free bars and taverns. JAMA 1998;280(22):1909–14.

420. Hammond SK, Sorensen G, Youngstrom R, Ockene JK. Occupational exposure to environmental tobacco smoke. JAMA 1995;274(12):956–60.

421. Marcus BH, Emmons K, Abrams DB, et al. Restrictive workplace smoking policies: impact on nonsmokers' tobacco exposure. J Public Health Policy 1992;13:42–51.

422. Biener L, Abrams DB, Follick MJ, Dean L. A comparative evaluation of a restrictive smoking policy in a general hospital. Am J Public Health 1989;79(2):192–5.

423. Brigham J, Gross J, Stitzer ML, Felch LJ. Effects of a restricted work-site smoking policy on employees who smoke. Am J Public Health 1994;84(5):773–8.

424. Jeffery RW, Kelder SH, Forster JL, French SA, Lando HA, Baxter JE. Restrictive smoking policies in the workplace: effects on smoking prevalence and cigarette consumption. Prev Med 1994;23(1):78–82.

425. Longo DR, Brownson RC, Johnson JC, et al. Hospital smoking bans and employee smoking behavior: results of a national survey. JAMA 1996;275(16):1252–7.

426. Patten CA, Gilpin E, Cavin SW, Pierce JP. Workplace smoking policy and changes in smoking behavior in California: a suggested association. Tob Control 1995;4:36–41.

427. Stave GM, Jackson GW. Effect of a total work-site smoking ban on employee smoking and attitudes. J Occup Med 1991;33(8):884–90.

428. Bartosch W, Pope G. The economic effect of smoke-free restaurant policies on restaurant business in Massachusetts. J Public Health Manag Pract 1999;5:53–62.

429. Centers for Disease Control and Prevention. Assessment of the impact of a 100% smoke-free ordinance on restaurant sales—West Lake Hills, Texas, 1992–1994. MMWR 1995;44(19):370–2.

430. Glantz S, Smith L. The effect of ordinances requiring smoke-free restraunts and bars on revenues: a follow-up. Am J Public Health 1997;87(10):1687–93.

431. Glantz SA, Smith LR. The effect of ordinances requiring smoke-free restaurants on restaurant sales. Am J Public Health 1994;84(7):1081–5.

432. Glantz SA, Charlesworth A. Tourism and hotel revenues before and after passage of smoke-free restaurant ordinances. JAMA 1999;281(20):1911–8.

433. Hyland A, Cummings KM, Nauenberg E. Analysis of taxable sales receipts: was New York City's smoke-free air bad for restaurant business? J Public Health Manag Pract 1999;5:14–21.

434. Sciacca J, Eckrem M. Effects of a city ordinance regulating smoking in restaurants and retail stores. J Community Health 1993;18(3):175–82.

435. Mudarri DH. The costs and benefits of smoking restrictions: an assessment of the Smoke-Free Environment Act of 1993 (H.R. 3434). Government Document 1994; H.R. 3434, April 1994.

436. Ashley MJ, Ferrence R. Reducing children's exposure to environmental tobacco smoke in homes: issues and strategies. Tob Control 1998;7:61–5.

437. Greenberg RA, Strecher VJ, Bauman KE, et al. Evaluation of a home-based intervention program to reduce infant passive smoking and lower respiratory illness. J Behav Med 1994;17(3):273–90.

438. Farkas AJ, Gilpin E, Distefan JM, Pierce JP. The effects of household and workplace smoking restrictions on quitting behaviors. Tob Control 1999;8:261–5.

439. Borland R, Mullins R, Trotter L, White V. Trends in environmental tobacco smoke restrictions in the home in Victoria, Australia. Tob Control 1999;8:266–71.

440. Cochrane Collaboration. The Cochrane Library, Issue 4. Available at: www.cochrane.org. Accessed January 6, 2003.

441. National Cancer Policy Board—Institute of Medicine and Commission on Life Sciences—National Research Council. Taking action to reduce tobacco use. Washington, DC: National Academy Press, 1998.

Chapter 2

Physical Activity

There is no doubt that Americans are not physically active enough. Only 45% of adults get the recommended 30 minutes of physical activity on five or more days per week, and adolescents are similarly inactive.[1,2] Regular physical activity improves aerobic capacity, muscular strength, body agility and coordination, and metabolic functioning.[3] Those who are physically active have a reduced risk of cardiovascular disease,[4–9] ischemic stroke,[10,11] type 2 (non-

*Insufficient evidence means that we were not able to determine whether or not the intervention works.

The Task Force approved the recommendations in this chapter in 2001. The research on which the findings are based was conducted between 1980 and 2000. This information has been previously published in the American Journal of Preventive Medicine [2002; 22(4S):67–72 and 73–107] and the MMWR Recommendations and Reports [2001; 50(No. RR-18):1–14].

insulin-dependent) diabetes,[12-18] colon cancers,[19-22] osteoporosis,[23-25] depression,[26-29] and fall-related injuries.[30-33]

Recommendations for increasing physical activity have been made for individuals and for clinical settings. In this chapter we present recommendations for increasing physical activity through interventions in community settings. Because increasing physical activity involves behavioral, social, and environmental factors (both physical and social), interventions in community settings to promote physical activity have emerged as a critical piece of an overall strategy to increase physical activity in the United States. The interventions we reviewed used several approaches to increasing physical activity: informational, behavioral and social, and environmental and policy changes.

RECOMMENDATIONS FROM OTHER ADVISORY GROUPS

Healthy People 2010[1] ranks physical activity as 1 of 10 leading health indicators. The *Healthy People* objectives aim to (1) increase the amount of moderate or vigorous physical activity performed by all people and (2) increase opportunities for physical activity through creating and enhancing access to places and facilities where people can be physically active. The *Healthy People* objectives to improve levels of physical activity for adults, adolescents, and children, and to reduce sedentary behavior among adolescents, are shown in Table 2–1.

In 2002, the U.S. Preventive Services Task Force concluded that the evidence is insufficient to recommend for or against behavioral counseling in primary care settings to promote physical activity.[34] They noted that the effectiveness of physical activity in reducing morbidity or mortality related to chronic diseases has been well documented, so it was not the focus of their review. The review also did not focus on counseling in other settings.

A consensus statement developed by a panel of the American College of Sports Medicine and the Centers for Disease Control and Prevention[35] recommends that every adult accumulate 30 minutes or more of moderate-intensity physical activity on most, preferably all, days of the week. This recommendation was modified to emphasize that even activity that is not strenuous or continuous (e.g., three 10-minute exercise sessions per day instead of one 30-minute session) can produce health results. The recommendation is supported by the Surgeon General[3] and the National Institutes of Health.[36]

METHODS

Methods used for the reviews are summarized in Chapter 10. Specific methods used in the systematic reviews of physical activity have been described

Table 2–1. Selected *Healthy People 2010*[1,2] Objectives for Increasing Physical Activity

Objective	Population	Baseline	2010 Objective
Reduce the proportion of adults ≥18 years engaged in no leisure-time physical activity (Objective 22–1)	Adults	40% (1997[a])	20%
Increase the proportion of adults ≥18 years who either engage regularly, preferably daily, in moderate physical activity for ≥30 minutes or engage in vigorous physical activity ≥3 days per week for ≥20 minutes per occasion (22–2, updated 2004)	Adults	32% (1997[a])	50%
Increase the proportion of adults ≥18 years engaged in vigorous physical activity ≥3 days per week for ≥20 minutes per occasion (22–3)	Adults	23% (1997[a])	30%
Increase the proportion of adolescents (students in grades 9–12) who engage in moderate physical activity for ≥30 minutes on ≥5 of the previous 7 days (22–6)	Adolescents	27% (1999)	35%
Increase the proportion of adolescents (students in grades 9–12) engaged in vigorous physical activity ≥3 days per week for ≥20 minutes per occasion (22–7)	Adolescents	65% (1999)	85%
Increase the proportion of adolescents (students in grades 9–12) who participate in daily school physical education (22–9)	Adolescents	29% (1999)	50%
Increase the proportion of adolescents (students in grades 9–12) who view television ≤2 hours on a school day (22–11)	Adolescents	57% (1999)	75%
Increase the proportion of trips of ≤1 mile made by walking by adults ≥18 years (22–14a)	Adults	17% (1995[a])	25%
Increase the proportion of trips to school of ≤1 mile made by children and adolescents[b] walking (22–14b)	Children/ adolescents	31% (1995[a])	50%
Increase the proportion of trips of ≤5 miles made by bicycle by adults ≥18 years (22–15a)	Adults	0.6% (1995[a])	2.0%
Increase the proportion of trips to school of ≤2 miles made by bicycle by children and adolescents[b] (22–14b)	Children/ adolescents	2.4% (1995[a])	5.0%

[a]Age adjusted to the year 2000 standard population.

[b]*Children and adolescents* defined as aged 5–15 years.

Reprinted from Am J Prev Med, Vol. 22, No. 4S, Kahn EB et al., The effectiveness of interventions to increase physical activity: a systematic review, p. 74, Copyright 2002, with permission from American Journal of Preventive Medicine.

in detail elsewhere[37] and are available at www.thecommunityguide.org/pa. The logic framework depicting the conceptual approach used in these reviews is presented in Figure 2–1.

ECONOMIC EFFICIENCY

A systematic review of available economic evaluations was conducted for all recommended interventions, and a summary of each review is presented with the related intervention. The methods used to conduct these economics reviews are summarized in Chapter 11.

RECOMMENDATIONS AND FINDINGS

This section presents a summary of the findings of the systematic reviews conducted to determine the effectiveness of the selected interventions in this topic area. We evaluated three kinds of approaches to increasing physical activity: informational, behavioral and social, and environmental and policy approaches.

Informational Approaches to Increasing Physical Activity

Informational approaches focus on increasing physical activity by providing information to motivate and enable people to change their behavior and to maintain that change over time. The interventions primarily use educational approaches to present both specific information about physical activity and exercise and general information (e.g., ways to reduce the risk of cardio-vascular disease). The information is intended to change people's knowledge about the benefits of physical activity, increase their awareness of opportunities for increasing physical activity, explain methods for overcoming barriers and negative attitudes about physical activity, and ultimately increase physical activity.

Community-Wide Campaigns: Recommended (Strong Evidence of Effectiveness)

Community-wide campaigns involve many community sectors in highly visible, broad-based, multicomponent approaches to increasing physical activity. In addition to considering sedentary behavior, most of the campaigns reviewed also addressed other cardiovascular disease risk factors, particularly diet and smoking.

These campaigns are effective in increasing the level of physical activity and the fitness of both adults and children. They also increase knowledge

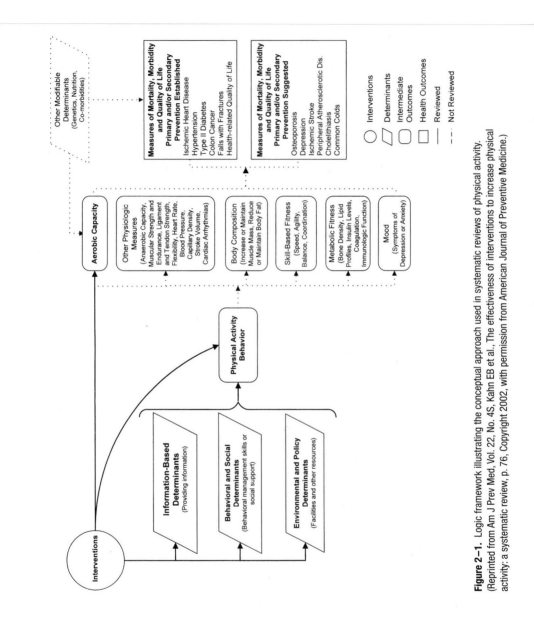

Figure 2–1. Logic framework illustrating the conceptual approach used in systematic reviews of physical activity. (Reprinted from Am J Prev Med, Vol. 22, No. 4S, Kahn EB et al., The effectiveness of interventions to increase physical activity: a systematic review, p. 76, Copyright 2002, with permission from American Journal of Preventive Medicine.)

about exercise and physical activity, as well as intentions to be more physically active.

Effectiveness

- Community-wide campaigns are effective in increasing the percentage of active people by approximately 4%.
- These campaigns are also effective in increasing energy expenditure by approximately 16%.

Applicability

- The findings of this review should be applicable to most communities in the United States if the campaign is adapted to the target population.

The findings of our systematic review are based on 10 studies of the effectiveness of large-scale, community-wide campaigns in increasing physical activity and improving physical fitness.[38-47] Some programs sought to decrease levels of cardiovascular disease by increasing physical activity and improving diet over a period of years; others lasted from six weeks to six months. We studied only multicomponent campaigns and evaluated them as such because we could not separate the effects of each component.

Campaign messages were directed to large audiences through a variety of channels, including television, radio, newspapers, direct mail, billboards, posters at bus stops and train stations, and trailers in movie theaters. Messages were delivered through paid advertisements, donated public service announcements, news releases, the creation of feature items in newspapers, or any combination of these approaches. The campaigns reviewed also included such components as support and self-help groups; physical activity counseling; risk factor screening and education at worksites, schools, and community health fairs; community events; and creation of walking trails.

Many of the interventions were designed to decrease levels of cardiovascular disease in a community over a period of several years by increasing levels of physical activity and improving dietary behaviors. These interventions included activities supported by media efforts but conducted independently. The remaining studies were six weeks to six months long and activities, although more limited, were still presented community-wide.

The percentage of people engaging in physical activity increased by a median of 4.2% (range, -2.9% to 9.4%; six arms of five studies). Energy expenditure also increased by a median of 16.3% (range, 7.6% to 21.4%; three arms of two studies). Four out of five other measures of physical activity also showed increases. These results show that large-scale, community-wide campaigns are effective in increasing physical activity and improving physical fitness.

These results should be applicable to diverse communities—rural, urban, and suburban—and to populations of any race, ethnicity, or socioeconomic status, if the program is adapted to the target population. For example, bilingual campaign materials and leaders can be used, materials can be written at a reading level appropriate for the target population, or campaigns can be adapted to the physical setting (e.g., emphasizing skiing in northern states during the winter or walking on the beach in warmer coastal climates).

Community-wide campaigns produced some additional benefits, including increases in knowledge about exercise as well as intentions to increase physical activity. Studies that measured change in weight, however, had mixed results. Some showed losses, others showed no change, and still others showed slight gains.

These campaigns can also produce a decrease in risk factors for cardiovascular disease. Communities themselves can benefit, too, by developing a greater sense of cohesion and a collective motivation to exercise, developing or strengthening social networks to achieve program goals, and even becoming involved in local government or civic organizations, thereby increasing social capital.

We did not find any economic evaluations of community-wide campaigns.

Poor planning and coordination of the campaigns, inadequately trained staff, and insufficient resources to implement a campaign of sufficient scope are all barriers to the success of community-wide campaigns. To change people's knowledge, attitudes, or behaviors, especially in high-risk populations, considerable exposure to campaign messages is required. Community buy-in (the involvement and acceptance of any targeted community) is also needed, and achieving it usually requires considerable effort.

In conclusion, the Task Force recommends community-wide campaigns on the basis of strong evidence of effectiveness in increasing both the number of people who are active and the energy expended by active individuals. The findings of this review should be applicable to most communities in the United States, provided that the campaigns are adapted to the specific needs and interests of the target population.

Point-of-Decision Prompts: Recommended (Sufficient Evidence of Effectiveness)

Point-of-decision prompts are signs placed by elevators and escalators to motivate people to use nearby stairs for health benefits or weight loss. These signs appear to motivate both people who want to be more active and those interested in the general health benefits of using the stairs. All interventions evaluated were single component, in which placement of signs was the only activity.

Effectiveness

- Point-of-decision prompts are effective in increasing the percentage of people taking the stairs (rather than escalators or elevators) by approximately 54%.
- These prompts are also effective in increasing levels of physical activity.
- Prompts are more effective among obese than non-obese people, especially when signs link use of stairs to weight loss rather than general health benefits.

Applicability

- These findings should be generally applicable in diverse populations and settings, provided that the intervention is adapted to the target population.

The findings of our systematic review of the effectiveness of point-of-decision prompts are based on six studies (two studies in one report) conducted between 1980 and 2000.[48-52] These studies were conducted in shopping malls, train and bus stations, and a university library.

Stair use was quite low at baseline: under 12% in all but one study (range, 4.8% to 39.6%). Five studies showed a median increase in stair-climbing of 53.9% (range, 5.5% to 128.6%). The remaining study showed an unspecified increase in stair-climbing and also found that the signs were effective in getting those who were less active (as measured by responses to a brief survey) to take the stairs. Both obese and non-obese people increased their stair use in response to the signs, although obese people seemed more likely to use the stairs than did non-obese people. Among obese people, a sign that linked stair use to the potential for weight loss produced a higher increase in stair use than a sign linking stair use to general health benefits.

These results show that point-of-decision prompts are effective in increasing the percentage of people who use the stairs, as well as in increasing physical activity.

These results should be applicable across diverse settings and population groups, provided that appropriate care is taken to adapt the messages to the target groups. As noted above, a study that reported results separately for obese people found that a message linking stair use to weight loss was more effective in increasing the percentage of stair users than a message emphasizing general health benefits. Another way to adapt the message can be to use culturally appropriate language on the signs.

We did not find any economic evaluations of point-of-decision prompts.

Several potential barriers to increased stair use are all related to the condition and accessibility of the stairs themselves. Stairways in many buildings and facilities are difficult to find and are poorly lit, maintained, or secured, making them apparently or actually unsafe. Additionally, some stairwells are locked, preventing access to them.

In conclusion, the Task Force recommends point-of-decision prompts on the basis of sufficient evidence of effectiveness in increasing levels of physical activity, as measured by the number of people who choose to use the stairs instead of riding escalators or elevators. Signs linking stair climbing to weight loss may be more effective among obese people than generic signs.

Mass Media Campaigns: Insufficient Evidence to Determine Effectiveness

These single-component campaigns are designed to increase knowledge about physical activity, influence attitudes and beliefs, and change behavior by transmitting messages through newspapers, radio, television, and billboards, singly or in combination. Paid advertisements, donated time and space for promotions, and news or lifestyle features are used. Unlike the community-wide campaigns discussed above, these interventions do not include other components such as support groups, risk factor screening and education, or community events.

Effectiveness

- We found insufficient evidence to determine the effectiveness of mass media campaigns alone in increasing physical activity or improving fitness.
- Evidence was insufficient because of the small number of available studies, limitations in their design and execution, and inconsistent findings.
- Insufficient evidence means that we were not able to determine whether or not the intervention works.

The findings of our systematic review are based on three studies[40,45,53] that measured the effectiveness of mass media campaigns in changing (1) the percentage of people achieving a specified level of activity (i.e., walking, moderate- or vigorous-intensity physical activity, aerobic or non-aerobic activity), (2) the percentage of people categorized as sedentary, and (3) energy expenditure. Some—but not all—measures suggested a modest trend toward increasing physical activity, especially among people who were less physically active at the start of the programs. Because of the small number of available studies and limitations in their design and execution, the evidence was insufficient to determine the effectiveness of mass media campaigns, when used alone, in increasing physical activity or improving fitness.

Because we could not establish the effectiveness of these programs, we did not examine situations in which the programs would be applicable, information about economic efficiency, or possible barriers to implementation.

Even in the absence of sufficient evidence to determine effectiveness, some positive effects of mass media campaigns are apparent. Significant and substantial improvements in knowledge and beliefs were seen in two of the studies. Mass media campaigns might also play important roles in changing awareness of opportunities for and benefits of physical activity, helping to build support for environmental and policy changes that improve physical activity behavior, fitness, or both. We did not, however, assess the effect of mass media campaigns on these outcomes.

In conclusion, the Task Force found insufficient evidence to determine the effectiveness of mass media campaigns, when used alone, in increasing physical activity or improving fitness. (When combined with other activities, such as support groups, risk factor screening and education, and community events, these are regarded as community-wide campaigns, which are recommended and discussed in this chapter.) At the time of our systematic review, only three studies were available, which had limitations in their design and execution and showed inconsistent evidence of effectiveness in increasing physical activity.

Classroom-Based Health Education Focused on Providing Information: Insufficient Evidence to Determine Effectiveness

These programs consist of health education classes in elementary, middle, or high schools whose goal is to help students develop the skills they need to make rational decisions about adopting healthier behaviors. Class content is usually multicomponent, with teachers educating students about aspects of physical inactivity, nutrition, smoking, and alcohol and drug misuse. Behavioral skills components (e.g., role-play, goal-setting, contingency planning) can also be part of the classes. Spending additional time in physical activity is not usually part of the curriculum.

Effectiveness

- We found insufficient evidence to determine the effectiveness of classroom-based health education focused on providing information in increasing physical activity levels and physical fitness.
- Evidence was insufficient because of inconsistent results in the available studies.
- Insufficient evidence means that we were not able to determine whether or not the intervention works.

The findings of our systematic review are based on 10 studies, most of which sought to reduce students' risk of developing chronic disease.[54-63] An additional three studies were identified but did not meet our quality criteria and were excluded from the review.[64-66] Four programs were based on the Know Your Body curriculum,[67] designed to provide children with the skills needed to adopt behaviors that reduce the risk of developing cardiovascular disease. These classes focused on nutrition, physical fitness, and preventing cigarette smoking. One program focused on preventing type 2 diabetes by encouraging students to eat low-fat foods and exercise regularly. Programs lasted from three months to five years.

There was no clear trend in the effects of these classes. Some of the studies showed increases in time spent in physical activity outside the school setting, while others showed decreases. Changes in self-reported physical activity behavior also varied: some programs produced positive changes in self-reported behavior, while others showed no effect or reported negative changes. Aerobic capacity was not measured in any of these studies. These findings provided insufficient evidence to determine if classroom-based health education focused on providing information is effective in increasing levels of physical activity or physical fitness.

Because we could not establish the effectiveness of these programs, we did not examine situations in which the programs would be applicable, information about economic efficiency, or possible barriers to implementation.

Although these studies did not show clear changes in activity, many showed other benefits, including increases in general health knowledge, exercise-related knowledge, and personal motivation to exercise. The programs may also provide additional benefits, such as more supportive attitudes for physical activity initiatives or changes in other health-related behaviors.

In conclusion, the Task Force found insufficient evidence to determine the effectiveness of classroom-based health education focused on providing information in increasing physical activity levels and physical fitness because of inconsistent results in the available studies.

Behavioral and Social Approaches to Increasing Physical Activity

Behavioral and social approaches focus on increasing physical activity by teaching behavior management skills that can be used in many settings and by structuring the social environment to provide support for people trying to change their health and activity habits. These interventions often involve group behavioral counseling and may also involve an individual's friends or family members. Skills focus on recognizing cues and opportunities for physical activity, ways to manage high-risk situations, and ways to maintain desired behaviors and prevent relapse. These interventions also involve making changes in the home, family, school, and work environments.

School-Based Physical Education: Recommended (Strong Evidence of Effectiveness)

These programs modify school-based physical education (PE) classes by increasing the amount of time students spend in PE class, the amount of time they are active during PE classes, or the amount of moderate or vigorous physical activity (MVPA) they engage in during PE classes. Most studies reviewed increased the amount of physical activity during already-scheduled PE classes by changing the activities taught (e.g., substituting soccer for softball) or modifying the rules of the game so that students are more active (e.g., the entire team runs the bases together if the batter makes a base hit). Health education was often part of the program as well.

Effectiveness

- School-based PE is effective in increasing levels of physical activity and improving physical fitness.
- Time spent in PE classes increased by approximately 10%, and time spent in MVPA in PE classes increased by approximately 50%.
- Aerobic capacity increased by approximately 8%.

Applicability

- These programs should be generally applicable to elementary and high school students if the program is adapted to the students receiving it.

Other Effects

- School-based PE produced small improvements in flexibility and muscular endurance as well as increases in knowledge about exercise, fitness, nutrition, general health, and personal motivation to exercise.
- We found no evidence to support the perception that time spent in PE classes harms academic performance.

The findings of our systematic review are based on 14 studies in 13 reports.[68-80] An additional four studies were identified but did not meet our quality criteria and were excluded from the review.[81-84] Studies evaluated the effectiveness of modifying school-based PE curricula and policies by increasing the amount of time students spend in PE class, the amount of time they are active during PE class, or the amount of MVPA they engage in during PE classes (the last can be accomplished by adding new PE classes or increasing the number of existing classes, lengthening existing PE class sessions, or increasing the MVPA of students during PE classes without necessarily lengthening class time). Studies looked at a variety of measures of improved fitness and increased activity, including energy expenditure, percent of class time spent in MVPA, minutes spent in MVPA, observed activity score, physical activities outside of school, aerobic capacity results from timed runs, and endurance testing. The amount and percent of time spent in MVPA at school showed consistent increases in five arms from four studies: the median increase in the amount of PE class time spent in MVPA was 50.3% (range, 6.0% to 125.3%), and the increase in percent of time spent in MVPA in PE classes was 10% (range, 3.3% to 15.7%). Studies also showed an increase in energy expenditure, and 14 arms from 11 studies showed a median increase in aerobic capacity of 8.4% (interquartile range, 3.1% to 18.9%). These results show that school-based PE is effective in increasing levels of physical activity and in improving physical fitness.

These findings should be applicable to elementary, middle, and high school students, provided that the program is adapted to the students receiving it.

Other benefits of these programs included small improvements in flexibility and muscular endurance; decreases in skinfold measurements; and increases in knowledge about exercise, fitness, nutrition, general health, and personal motivation to exercise. We searched for, but did not find, any evidence that time spent in PE classes harms academic performance.

We did not find any economic evaluations of modifying school-based PE classes.

School systems present the primary barriers to implementing these programs. Although PE is mandated in almost every state, requirements for the amount of PE instruction are generally low. Few middle and high schools require daily PE, and schools face increasing pressure to eliminate PE to make more time available for academic subjects.

In conclusion, the Task Force recommends modifying school-based PE classes on the basis of strong evidence of effectiveness in increasing students' activity levels and aerobic capacity. Adapting the program to the students who receive it should make this intervention applicable to all elementary, middle, and high school students. No evidence was found to support the belief that time spent in physical education harms academic performance.

Individually-Adapted Health Behavior Change Programs:
Recommended (Strong Evidence of Effectiveness)

Individually-adapted health behavior change programs are tailored to participants' specific interests, preferences, and readiness to change, teaching specific behavioral skills that enable participants to make moderate-intensity physical activity part of their daily routines. The behavioral skills taught include setting goals for physical activity and monitoring one's progress toward those goals, building social support for new behavioral patterns, reinforcing new behaviors through self-reward and positive self-talk, structured problem solving to help maintain behavior change, and preventing relapse into sedentary behaviors. Participants can engage in activities that are planned (e.g., a daily scheduled walk) or unplanned (e.g., taking the stairs when the opportunity arises). Established health behavior change models (e.g., Social Cognitive Theory,[85] the Health Belief Model,[86] or the Transtheoretical Model of Change[87]) are the basis for many individually adapted programs.

Effectiveness

- These programs are effective in increasing levels of physical activity.
- Energy expenditure increased by approximately 64%, and time spent in physical activity increased by approximately 35%.
- Increases were also seen in attendance at exercise sessions, number of sessions completed, percentage of people starting exercise programs, and frequency of physical activity.
- The programs decreased body weight and body fat and increased strength and flexibility.

Applicability

- These programs should be generally applicable in diverse populations and settings, if the programs are adapted to the people receiving them.

The findings of our systematic review are based on 18 studies that evaluated the effectiveness of individually-adapted health behavior change programs in changing physical activity patterns.[46,88-104] An additional two studies were identified but did not meet our quality criteria and were excluded from the review.[105,106] All of the interventions were delivered either in person to groups or by mail, telephone, or directed media. Programs typically involved recruiting volunteers who selected physical activity goals and worked in groups to achieve those goals. Group members provided companionship and support for one another. Study staff also provided encouragement in the form of phone calls to check on participants' progress and to encourage them to continue, and by leading formal group discussions about negative views of exercise and other barriers to change.

Studies used various measures of progress, including how often and how long people exercised in terms of blocks walked daily; flights of stairs climbed daily; number of minutes spent in activity; and how often they attended exercise sessions, ran, or participated in exercise and organized sports.

Participants increased time spent in physical activity (median 35.4%; interquartile range, 16.7% to 83.3%; 20 arms of 10 studies), energy expenditure (median 64.3%; interquartile range, 31.2% to 85.5%; 15 arms of 4 studies), and maximal oxygen uptake (VO_2 max) (median 6.3%; interquartile range, 5.1% to 9.8%; 13 arms of 4 studies). Increases were also seen in frequency of attendance at exercise sessions, the number of prescribed exercise sessions completed, the percentage of people starting exercise programs, and the frequency of physical activity. These findings show that individually-adapted health behavior change programs are effective in increasing levels of physical activity, time spent in physical activity, and energy expenditure.

These results should be applicable to diverse settings and populations, provided that the program is adapted to the people participating in it.

Other benefits of these programs included decreases in body weight and percentage of body fat and increases in strength and flexibility.

The findings of our systematic review of economic evaluations of individually-adapted health behavior change programs are based on one report.[107] This two-year study, conducted at a fitness facility in Dallas, Texas, evaluated the cost-effectiveness of two physical activity interventions—lifestyle and structured—for adults 35–60 years of age. The lifestyle intervention provided behavioral skills training to integrate moderate to intense physical activity into the lives of participants. The structured intervention consisted of supervised center-based exercise sessions. The adjusted cost-effectiveness ratio range was $0.05–$3.94 per person for the lifestyle intervention and $0.07–$5.39 for the structured intervention.

Inadequate resources, lack of planning and coordination, and lack of professionally trained staff may present barriers to thorough implementation and evaluation of these programs.

In conclusion, the Task Force recommends individually-adapted health behavior change programs on the basis of strong evidence that they increase levels of physical activity, time spent in physical activity, and energy expenditure and decrease body weight and fat. These programs, when tailored to their intended recipients, should be applicable to diverse populations and settings. The need for adequate resources and trained staff presents a potential barrier to implementation of these programs.

Social Support Interventions in Community Settings:
Recommended (Strong Evidence of Effectiveness)

These interventions build, strengthen, and maintain social networks that support increases in physical activity. New social networks can be created or existing networks in social settings outside the family, such as the workplace, can be used. Typically, participants set up a *buddy* system and make *contracts* to guarantee that both buddies will be active, or they form walking groups or other groups to provide companionship and support while being physically active.

Effectiveness

- Social support increased time spent in activity by approximately 44%.
- Frequency of exercise increased by approximately 20%.
- Aerobic capacity increased by approximately 5%.
- Participation in these programs improved fitness levels, lowered percentage of body fat, increased knowledge about exercise, and improved confidence in the ability to exercise.

Applicability

- These findings should be generally applicable for people of all ages and levels of activity, and in diverse settings, if the programs are adapted to the people participating in them.

The findings of our systematic review are based on nine reports that evaluated the effectiveness of social support interventions in community settings (e.g., walking programs in the neighborhood, exercising at home).[45,108–115] Programs typically involved recruiting volunteers who selected physical activity goals and worked in groups to achieve those goals. Group members provided companionship and support for one another. Study staff also provided encouragement in the form of phone calls to check on participants' progress and to encourage them to continue, and by leading formal group discussions about negative views of exercise and other barriers to change.

Studies used various measures of progress, including how often and how long people exercised in terms of blocks walked daily; flights of stairs climbed daily; number of minutes spent in activity; and how often they attended exercise sessions, ran, or participated in exercise and organized sports.

Participants spent more time in physical activity (44.2% median increase; interquartile range, 19.9% to 45.6%; five arms from four studies); exercised more often (19.6% median increase; interquartile range, 14.6% to 57.6%; six arms from three studies); and improved their aerobic capacity (4.7% median increase; interquartile range, 3.3% to 6.1%; five arms from three studies). One study showed that more frequent support, whether structured or informal, effectively encouraged people to be more active.

These results show that social support interventions in community settings are effective in increasing physical activity.

These results should be applicable to men and women; young and old; initially sedentary or at any level of activity; and in settings including communities, worksites, and universities, provided that the program is adapted to the people participating in it.

The studies also showed other benefits: participants reduced body fat (−7.3% median; interquartile range, −6.8% to −8.1%) and increased their knowledge of, confidence about, and social support for exercise.

We did not find any economic evaluations of social support interventions in community settings.

We found no barriers to implementing social support in community settings to promote physical activity.

In conclusion, the Task Force recommends social support to increase physical activity on the basis of strong evidence that such support increases time spent in and frequency of physical activity, increases physical fitness and aerobic capacity, and improves participants' confidence in their ability to exercise. Programs fostering this support should be applicable to people of all ages and levels of activity, and in diverse settings, if the programs are adapted to the people participating in them.

College-Based Health Education and Physical Education:
Insufficient Evidence to Determine Effectiveness

These interventions use didactic and behavioral education to increase and retain physical activity levels among college students and to help students develop lifelong exercise habits. The physical education (PE) classes may or may not be offered by PE or wellness departments at colleges and universities but must include supervised activity in the class. Classes include both lectures and laboratory-type activities. Students engage in supervised physical activity, develop goals and activity plans, and write term papers based on their experiences. Social support is also built into these programs.

Effectiveness

- We found insufficient evidence to determine the effectiveness of college-based health education and PE in increasing physical activity levels.
- Evidence was insufficient because of the small number of studies and limitations in their design and execution.
- Insufficient evidence means that we were not able to determine whether or not the intervention works.

The findings of our systematic review are based on two studies in three reports.[116-118] An additional three studies were identified but did not meet our quality criteria and were excluded from the review.[119-121] In both reviewed studies, participants showed short-term improvements in physical activity levels and aerobic capacity, but in one study, which followed up over two years, these gains were generally lost. Because of the small number of available studies and limitations in design and execution, the evidence was insufficient to determine the effectiveness of college-based health education and PE programs to help participants become more physically active and stay active after the end of the program.

Because we could not establish the effectiveness of these programs, we did not examine situations in which the programs would be applicable, information about economic efficiency, or possible barriers to implementation.

Although we found insufficient evidence to determine whether or not these programs are effective, the studies did indicate some benefits, especially in behaviors that can support increased physical activity. Men, in particular, showed some increase in giving social support to others and in resisting falling back into inactivity. Participants' perception of potential barriers to exercising may also be reduced. Women showed an increased enjoyment of physical activity as well as changes in their perception of benefits and barriers, their social support for fellow exercisers, and their ability to begin or maintain an exercise program.

In conclusion, the Task Force found insufficient evidence to determine the effectiveness of college-based health education and PE interventions in increasing physical activity because of the small number of studies and limitations in their design and execution.

Classroom-Based Health Education Focused on Reducing Television Viewing and Video Game Playing: Insufficient Evidence to Determine Effectiveness

These health education classes, based in elementary school classrooms, encourage students to spend less time watching television and playing video games. Students are taught techniques or strategies to help achieve these goals, such as limiting access to TV and video games and self-monitoring and budgeting of the time spent watching TV and playing video games. All classes include a "TV turnoff challenge" encouraging students not to watch TV for a specified number of days. Classes do not specifically encourage physical activity as an alternative to watching TV and playing video games. Parental involvement is prominent, and all households are given automatic TV use monitors.

Effectiveness

- We found insufficient evidence to determine the effectiveness of health education classes focused on reducing television viewing and video game playing in increasing physical activity.

- Evidence was insufficient because of inconsistent results in the available studies.
- Insufficient evidence means that we were not able to determine whether or not the intervention works.

The findings of our systematic review are based on three studies, one[122] lasting six months, the other two[123,124] lasting two years. Each study measured the amount of time students spent playing video games and watching TV; one study also measured time spent in other sedentary behaviors. All studies used the amount of sedentary time in some form, usually time spent watching TV or playing video games, as the primary measure of effectiveness.

The programs produced consistent reductions in the time spent watching TV, playing video games, and other sedentary behaviors, according to both the children and their parents. Studies reported inconsistent results, however, for corresponding increases in physical activity among participants, with two measures showing increases and four showing decreases. These inconsistent results provide insufficient evidence to determine the effectiveness of these interventions in increasing physical activity.

Because we could not establish the effectiveness of these programs, we did not examine situations in which the programs would be applicable, information about economic efficiency, or possible barriers to implementation.

The studies suggest some benefits even though the evidence was insufficient to determine effectiveness. Body fat (measured by body mass index scores and skinfold tests) and rates of obesity decreased among participants according to some measures, despite inconsistent measures of increased physical activity. This may be because reduced TV viewing time also meant reduced time for snacking or because participants engaged in physical activity not recorded by the studies.

In conclusion, the Task Force found insufficient evidence to determine the effectiveness of health education classes focused on reducing television viewing and video game playing in increasing physical activity because of inconsistent results in the reviewed studies.

Family-Based Social Support: Insufficient Evidence to Determine Effectiveness

These interventions help families of those trying to increase physical activity (parents, siblings, or partners) to encourage this effort by modeling healthy behavior and by being supportive of exercise. Intervention components—which may include goal setting, problem solving, contracts to exercise among family members, and other techniques for promoting physical activity—are often delivered in conjunction with other school-based activities, such as physical education (PE) or health education. Family involvement may be promoted through take-home packets, reward systems, and family record keeping. Some programs, such as CATCH (Child and Adolescent Trial for Cardiovascular Health), also included family-oriented special events (e.g., a "mini" health fair).

Effectiveness

- We found insufficient evidence to determine the effectiveness of family-based social support in increasing physical activity.
- Evidence was insufficient because of inconsistent results in the available studies.
- Insufficient evidence means that we were not able to determine whether or not the intervention works.

The findings of our systematic review are based on 11 studies (in 12 reports).[56,73-78,125-129] One additional study was identified but did not meet our quality criteria and was excluded from the review.[130] Studies showed inconsistent results: most showed no change, and others showed increases in activity, and others showed decreases. These disparities occurred both between and within studies. These inconsistent results provided insufficient evidence to determine whether or not family-based social support is an effective approach to increasing physical activity.

Because we could not establish the effectiveness of these programs, we did not examine situations in which the programs would be applicable, information about economic efficiency, or possible barriers to implementation.

The studies indicate some benefits even though the evidence was insufficient to determine effectiveness. Among both children and adults, several studies showed increases in knowledge of disease risk factors, fitness, exercise, or health. Participants in one study were more self-motivated to exercise, and in another study they reported being more satisfied with the amount of family activity.

In conclusion, the Task Force found insufficient evidence to determine the effectiveness of family-based social support in increasing physical activity because of inconsistent results.

Environmental and Policy Approaches to Increasing Physical Activity

The goal of these interventions is to help people adopt healthier behaviors by changing the physical environment, social networks, organizational norms and policies, and laws through environmental and policy approaches. Physical activity levels are affected by a wide variety of factors beyond individual motivation and knowledge; these include being physically active close to home as well as environmental and neighborhood factors such as weather, air pollution, and lighting. Public policy that supports healthy lifestyles, creating environments to support these lifestyles, and strengthening the involvement of communities will result in healthier physical and organizational environments for all.

Interventions in this category affect entire populations by targeting physical and organizational structures. They are implemented and evaluated over a longer period of time than interventions directed to individuals. Although these interventions are conducted by traditional health professionals, they may also include others not previously involved with public health directly, such as community agencies and organizations; legislators; departments of parks, recreation, transportation, and planning; and the media.

In addition to the intervention reviewed here, we are investigating two additional approaches: urban form (design) and land-use planning strategies that lead to increased physical activity, and changes to transportation and travel policy and infrastructure that reduce dependence on motorized transport and increase physical activity. When published, the results of these reviews will be available at www.thecommunityguide.org/pa.

Creation of or Enhanced Access to Places for Physical Activity Combined with Informational Outreach Activities: Recommended (Strong Evidence of Effectiveness)

These multicomponent interventions involve the efforts of businesses, coalitions, agencies, and communities to create or provide access to places where people can be physically active. Creating walking trails or providing access to fitness equipment in nearby fitness or community centers can increase the opportunities for people to be more active.

In addition to promoting access, many of the studies in our review included training people to use weight and aerobic fitness equipment; teaching about healthy behaviors; creating health and fitness programs and support or buddy systems; and providing seminars, counseling, risk screening, health forums and workshops, and referrals to physicians or additional services.

Effectiveness

- These programs are effective in getting people to exercise more.
- Participants usually report loss of weight or body fat.
- Frequency of physical activity increased by approximately 48% among participants.
- Aerobic capacity increased by approximately 5% and energy expenditure by approximately 8%.

- These programs should be applicable to both men and women in various settings if appropriately adapted to participants.

The findings of our systematic review are based on 10 studies.[131–140] An additional two studies were identified but did not meet our quality criteria and were excluded from the review.[141,142] Reviewed studies showed improvements in many measures of physical fitness. For example, the median increase in aerobic capacity was 5.1% (interquartile range, 2.8% to 9.6%; 8 arms from 5 studies). Changes were also noted in energy expenditure, people reporting some leisure time physical activity, and exercise score. In five studies that measured how often people exercised and how many people exercised three or more times per week, the median increase was an impressive 48.4% (interquartile range, 21.0% to 83.8%). Although measured in a variety of ways, the results indicate that these interventions are effective in increasing physical activity.

All studies were conducted in the United States, including eight at worksites (industrial locations such as automotive, brewing, and printing plants, plus universities and federal agencies). Two studies were conducted in low-income communities. One study included only men and one included only African Americans. Two studies stratified their results for men and women, and one study reported effects specific to African Americans. The reviewed interventions should therefore be applicable to diverse populations and settings.

Other benefits of these programs included weight reduction or loss of body fat, increases in perceived energy and confidence in the ability to exercise regularly, improved flexibility, and improved strength and better composite scores on the Physical Readiness Test. Information addressing cardiovascular disease risk factors, particularly diet and smoking, may have provided other health benefits for participants.

The findings of our systematic review of economic evaluations of interventions to create or enhance access to places for physical activity are based on two studies, both conducted in worksites.[143,144] In a four-year study at an employee fitness facility in a Houston, Texas, insurance company, a cost–benefit analysis of a structured physical fitness program was conducted. The program included regularly scheduled exercise classes and health seminars. Adjusted benefits were estimated at $1106 per participant and adjusted costs at $451 per participant.

A 5-year study with projections for an additional 10 years was conducted in a workplace setting among 36,000 employees and retirees of an insurance company. The researchers conducted a cost–benefit analysis of a company-sponsored health and fitness program that used health promotion centers, newsletters, medical reference texts, videotapes, and quarterly media blitzes. Adjusted benefits were estimated at $139 million and adjusted costs at $43 million over the 15-year life of the program.

In both studies, the adjusted benefits substantially exceeded the adjusted costs of creating or enhancing access to places for physical activity.

The amount of time and money required to build or enhance facilities promoting physical activity may present barriers to implementation. Getting the community to support such projects, and finding the expertise to plan and coordinate them, may also be difficult.

In conclusion, the Task Force recommends interventions to create or enhance access to places for physical activity combined with informational outreach activities on the basis of strong evidence of effectiveness in increasing frequency of physical activity, aerobic capacity, energy expenditure, and other indicators of fitness. When adapted to recipients, these interventions should be applicable to both men and women in a variety of settings.

Point-of-Decision Prompts: Recommended (Sufficient Evidence of Effectiveness)

See the discussion of point-of-decision prompts under Informational Approaches to Increasing Physical Activity in this chapter.

INCREASING PHYSICAL ACTIVITY THROUGH USE OF THESE RECOMMENDATIONS

In the United States, physical inactivity is a leading contributor to disability and premature death, accounting for 22% of coronary heart disease, 22% of colon cancer, 18% of osteoporosis-related fractures, 12% of diabetes and hypertension, and 5% of breast cancer.[145] Physical inactivity accounts for about 2.4% of the cost of U.S. health care or approximately $24 billion a year.[145] The recommendations in this chapter provide a variety of ways to meet the need to increase physical activity, be it at work, at school, at home, or in the community.

Those interested in increasing physical activity (e.g., employers and employees; school administrators, teachers, and students; families; and community groups) can begin by assessing several factors: current levels of activity; the presence of particularly inactive groups (who will benefit more from becoming active than will active people who increase their levels of activity); and local barriers to implementation (e.g., access barriers; deficits in individual knowledge, attitudes, or skills; or lack of resources including funding and physical locations for physical activity) and current activities to improve them. The results should be compared with the recommendations in this chapter to determine whether existing efforts are recommended, appropriately implemented, and adequately funded. The choice of new interventions should rely in part on the interventions described by the *Community Guide*, including those that are recommended, but should also take into account local goals, characteristics, and resources.

Next, setting measurable goals, both for existing and for new interventions, can help you assess whether or not the desired results are being achieved. These goals can be as simple or as complex as your time and resources allow. *Healthy People 2010* provides national objectives (Table 2–1), which can also be measured at the local level. You may find additional goals that are relevant to the particular interventions you choose to implement or to your ability to measure them. For example, some programs might measure access to and use of services. Keeping in mind the goal of increasing physical activity can help you determine what kinds of measurements are appropriate for your program(s).

Information about applicability, which describes the settings and populations involved in the recommended interventions, can help you assess the extent to which the intervention might be useful in a particular setting or population. Economic information, provided wherever available for recommended interventions, can be useful both in identifying what resources are needed and in choosing interventions that are more economically efficient in meeting public health goals than other available options.

In choosing recommended interventions, remember that the reviewed interventions were conducted among populations, not individuals. Although only small improvements were noted in some interventions, these small changes in populations can add up to significant public health improvements. Furthermore, the largest public health benefit of interventions to increase physical activity comes from getting sedentary people to be active rather than getting already active people to be more active.[146] Therefore, implementation of the recommendations in a variety of settings, involving many kinds of people, can produce significant public health benefits.

We examined a variety of settings for improving physical activity, which should be relevant to most communities. Schools can choose to increase the length or number of physical education classes or simply to increase students' activity levels during existing classes. In workplaces, many possibilities exist, depending on available space and resources. Point-of-decision prompts can be posted to encourage people to use the stairs as an alternate to elevators or escalators. Social support interventions can form the basis for exercise teams or groups, and individually-adapted health behavior change programs can augment these groups or involve individuals who prefer to work toward their activity goals alone. Access to places to exercise can be increased (e.g., extending gym hours beyond working hours) and creating walking trails or other areas for physical activity (e.g., a health center or gym) may be possible.

Community centers and faith-based groups may also choose to implement social support interventions and individually-adapted health behavior change programs. Depending on the structure of their facilities, the opportunity may exist to use point-of-decision prompts. These groups may also help members get to nearby exercise facilities (e.g., by providing transportation or child care).

Community-wide campaigns involve many community sectors. Increasingly, practitioners who conduct interventions in community settings to increase physical activity are recognizing that involvement of sectors outside of traditional public health is essential. These partnerships often involve urban and transportation planners, officials in parks and recreation, economists, and elected officials concerned about urban sprawl. Each community can decide for itself which groups to involve in the planning and implementing of these programs and the specific approaches to be used (e.g., where and how often to advertise). Even communities with limited resources may find that simple campaigns (e.g., supported by donated time and services from local media outlets, charitable groups, print shops, or delivery services) can help raise awareness of the need to increase physical activity and provide suggestions for doing so.

CONCLUSION

This chapter summarizes conclusions and recommendations to date from the Task Force on interventions to increase physical activity using three types of approaches: informational, behavioral and social, and environmental and policy. To increase physical activity using informational approaches, the Task Force recommends community-wide campaigns and point-of-decision prompts. Evidence was insufficient to determine the effectiveness in increasing physical activity of mass media campaigns or classroom-based health education focused on providing information.

To increase physical activity using behavioral or social approaches, the Task Force recommends school-based physical education, individually-adapted health behavior change programs, and social support interventions in community settings. Evidence was insufficient to determine the effectiveness in increasing physical activity of college-based health education and physical education; classroom-based health education focusing on reducing television viewing and video game playing; or family-based social support.

To increase physical activity using environmental or policy approaches, the Task Force recommends creation of or enhanced access to places for physical activity combined with informational outreach activities, and point-of-decision prompts.

Details of these reviews have been published[37,147,148] and these articles, along with additional information about the reviews, are available at www .thecommunityguide.org/pa.

Acknowledgments

This chapter was written by the members of the systematic review development team: Emily B. Kahn, PhD, MPH and Leigh T. Ramsey, PhD, Division of Prevention Research and Analytic Methods (DPRAM), Epidemiology Program Office (EPO), Centers for Disease Control and Prevention (CDC), Atlanta, Georgia; Ross C. Brownson, PhD, St. Louis University School of Public Health, St. Louis, Missouri, and the Task Force on Community Preventive Services; Gregory W. Heath, DHSc, MPH, Division of Nutrition and Physical Activity (DNPA), National Center for Chronic Disease Prevention and Health Promotion (NCCDPHP), CDC, Atlanta; Elizabeth H. Howze, ScD, Division of Health Education and Promotion, Agency for Toxic Substances and Disease Registry, Atlanta; Kenneth E. Powell, MD, MPH, Epidemiology and Prevention Branch, Georgia Department of Human Resources, Atlanta; and Elaine J. Stone, PhD, MPH, National Heart, Lung, and Blood Institute (NHLBI), National Institutes of Health (NIH), Bethesda, Maryland.

Consultants for the reviews were: Terry Bazzarre, PhD, Robert Wood Johnson Foundation, Princeton, New Jersey; Carl J. Caspersen, PhD, NCCDPHP/CDC, Atlanta; Diana Cassady, DrPH, California Department of Health Services, Sacramento; Carlos J. Crespo, DrPH, State University of New York School of Medicine and Biomedical Sciences, Buffalo; Steve Hooker, PhD, California Department of Health Services, Sacramento; Jonathan E. Fielding, MD, MPH, MBA, Los Angeles Department of Health Services, University of California School of Public Health, Los Angeles, and the Task Force on Community Preventive Services; Barbara Fraser, RD, MS, Nebraska Department of Health and Human Services, Lincoln; George J. Isham, MD, HealthPartners, Minneapolis, Minnesota, and the Task Force on Community Preventive Services; Abby C. King, PhD, Stanford University School of Medicine, Stanford, California; I-Min Lee, MD, ScD, Harvard Medical School/Brigham and Women's Hospital, Boston, Massachusetts; Denise G. Simons-Morton, MD, PhD, NHLBI/NIH, Bethesda, Maryland; Reba A. Norman, MLM, NCCDPHP/CDC, Atlanta; Cindy Porteous, MA, Indianapolis Park Foundation, Indianapolis, Indiana; Michael Pratt, MD, MPH, NCCDPHP/CDC, Atlanta; Thomas Schmid, PhD, NCCDPHP/ CDC, Atlanta; Christine G. Spain, MA, The President's Council on Physical Fitness and Sports, Washington, DC; Wendell C. Taylor, PhD, MPH, University of Texas Health Science Center at Houston.

Articles included in the reviews were abstracted by: Modupe AinaAkinpelu, MBBS, MPH; Amy Eyler, MS; Kristi Heesch, MPH; Hoang C. Le, BS; Ann MacIntyre, MHS; Pam Overberger, MS; Amar Pandya, BS; Jacqueline Pesa, PhD; Melissa Stigler, MPH; and Sarah Levin, MS, PhD.

References

1. U.S. Department of Health and Human Services. Healthy people 2010. 2nd edition. Washington, DC: U.S. Government Printing Office, 2000.

2. Centers for Disease Control and Prevention. DATA2010: The Healthy People 2010 database. Available at: http://wonder.cdc.gov/DATA2010. Accessed March 23, 2004.

3. U.S. Department of Health and Human Services. Physical activity and health: a report of the Surgeon General. Atlanta, GA: U.S. Department of Health and Human Services, Centers for Disease Control and Prevention, National Center for Chronic Disease Prevention and Health Promotion, 1996.

4. Paffenbarger RS Jr, Hyde RT, Wing AL, Steinmetz CH. A natural history of athleticism and cardiovascular health. JAMA 1984;252(4):491–5.

5. Wannamethee SG, Shaper AG. Physical activity in the prevention of cardiovascular disease: an epidemiological perspective. Sports Med 2001;31(2):101–14.

6. Sesso HD, Paffenbarger RS Jr, Lee IM. Physical activity and coronary heart disease in men: The Harvard Alumni Health Study. Circulation 2000;102(9):975–80.

7. Kannel WB, Sorlie P. Some health benefits of physical activity. The Framingham Study. Arch Intern Med 1979;139(8):857–61.

8. LaCroix AZ, Leveille SG, Hecht JA, Grothaus LC, Wagner EH. Does walking decrease the risk of cardiovascular disease hospitalizations and death in older adults? J Am Geriatr Soc 1996;44(2):113–20.

9. Kannel WB, Belanger A, D'Agostino R, Israel I. Physical activity and physical demand on the job and risk of cardiovascular disease and death: the Framingham Study. Am Heart J 1986;112(4):820–5.

10. Hu FB, Stampfer MJ, Colditz GA, et al. Physical activity and risk of stroke in women. JAMA 2000;283(22):2961–7.

11. Gorelick PB, Sacco RL, Smith DB, et al. Prevention of a first stroke: a review of guidelines and a multidisciplinary consensus statement from the National Stroke Association. JAMA 1999;281(12):1112–20.

12. Hu FB, Manson JE, Stampfer MJ, et al. Diet, lifestyle, and the risk of type 2 diabetes mellitus in women. N Engl J Med 2001;345(11):790–7.

13. Hu FB, Leitzmann MF, Stampfer MJ, Colditz GA, Willett WC, Rimm EB. Physical activity and television watching in relation to risk for type 2 diabetes mellitus in men. Arch Intern Med 2001;161(12):1542–8.

14. Pfohl M, Schatz H. Strategies for the prevention of type 2 diabetes. Exp Clin Endocrinol Diabetes 2001;109(suppl 2):S240–S249.

15. Fulton-Kehoe D, Hamman RF, Baxter J, Marshall J. A case-control study of physical activity and non-insulin-dependent diabetes mellitus (NIDDM). The San Luis Valley Diabetes Study. Ann Epidemiol 2001;11(5):320–7.

16. Helmrich SP, Ragland DR, Leung RW, Paffenbarger RS Jr. Physical activity and reduced occurrence of non-insulin-dependent diabetes mellitus. N Engl J Med 1991;325(3): 147–52.

17. Kaye SA, Folsom AR, Sprafka JM, Prineas RJ, Wallace RB. Increased incidence of diabetes mellitus in relation to abdominal adiposity in older women. J Clin Epidemiol 1991;44(3):329–34.

18. Uusitupa M, Siitonen O, Pyorala K, et al. The relationship of cardiovascular risk factors to the prevalence of coronary heart disease in newly diagnosed type 2 (non-insulin-dependent) diabetes. Diabetologia 1985;28(9):653–9.

19. Brownson RC, Zahm SH, Chang JC, Blair A. Occupational risk of colon cancer. An analysis by anatomic subsite. Am J Epidemiol 1989;130(4):675–87.

20. Brownson RC, Chang JC, Davis JR, Smith CA. Physical activity on the job and cancer in Missouri. Am J Public Health 1991;81(5):639–42.

21. Dosemeci M, Hayes RB, Vetter R, et al. Occupational physical activity, socioeconomic status, and risks of 15 cancer sites in Turkey. Cancer Causes Control 1993;4(4): 313–21.

22. Giovannucci E, Ascherio A, Rimm EB, Colditz GA, Stampfer MJ, Willett WC. Physical activity, obesity, and risk for colon cancer and adenoma in men. Ann Intern Med 1995;122(5):327–34.

23. Nichols DL, Sanborn CF, Bonnick SL, Ben Ezra V, Gench B, DiMarco NM. The effects of gymnastics training on bone mineral density. Med Sci Sports Exerc 1994;26(10): 1220–5.

24. Rubin K, Schirduan V, Gendreau P, Sarfarazi M, Mendola R, Dalsky G. Predictors of axial and peripheral bone mineral density in healthy children and adolescents, with special attention to the role of puberty. J Pediatr 1993;123(6):863–70.

25. Kohrt WM, Snead DB, Slatopolsky E, Birge SJ Jr. Additive effects of weight-bearing exercise and estrogen on bone mineral density in older women. J Bone Miner Res 1995;10(9):1303–11.

26. Fox KR. The influence of physical activity on mental well-being. Public Health Nutr 1999;2(3A):411–8.

27. Ross CE, Hayes D. Exercise and psychologic well-being in the community. Am J Epidemiol 1988;127(4):762–71.

28. Camacho TC, Roberts RE, Lazarus NB, Kaplan GA, Cohen RD. Physical activity and depression: evidence from the Alameda County Study. Am J Epidemiol 1991;134(2): 220–31.

29. Weyerer S. Physical inactivity and depression in the community. Evidence from the Upper Bavarian Field Study. Int J Sports Med 1992;13(6):492–6.

30. Farmer ME, Harris T, Madans JH, Wallace RB, Cornoni-Huntley J, White LR. Anthropometric indicators and hip fracture. The NHANES I epidemiologic follow-up study. J Am Geriatr Soc 1989;37(1):9–16.

31. Meyer HE, Tverdal A, Falch JA. Risk factors for hip fracture in middle-aged Norwegian women and men. Am J Epidemiol 1993;137(11):1203–11.

32. Cummings SR, Nevitt MC, Browner WS, et al. Risk factors for hip fracture in white women. Study of Osteoporotic Fractures Research Group. N Engl J Med 1995; 332(12):767–73.

33. Jaglal SB, Kreiger N, Darlington G. Past and recent physical activity and risk of hip fracture. Am J Epidemiol 1993;138(2):107–18.

34. U.S. Preventive Services Task Force. Physical activity—counseling. Available at: www.ahrq.gov/clinic/uspstf/uspsphys.htm. Accessed January 9, 2004.

35. Pate RR, Pratt M, Blair SN, et al. Physical activity and public health. A recommendation from the Centers for Disease Control and Prevention and the American College of Sports Medicine. JAMA 1995;273(5):402–7.

36. Physical activity and cardiovascular health. NIH Consens Statement 1995;13:1–33.

37. Kahn E, Ramsey LT, Brownson RC, et al. The effectiveness of interventions to increase physical activity: a systematic review. Am J Prev Med 2002;22(4S):73–107.

38. Luepker RV, Murray DM, Jacobs DJ, et al. Community education for cardiovascular disease prevention: risk factor changes in the Minnesota Heart Health Program. Am J Public Health 1994;84(9):1383–93.

39. Tudor-Smith C, Nutbeam D, Moore L, Catford J. Effects of the Heartbeat Wales programme over five years on behavioural risks for cardiovascular disease: quasi-

experimental comparison of results from Wales and a matched reference area. BMJ 1998;316(7134):818–22.

40. Meyer AJ. Skills training in a cardiovascular health education campaign. J Consult Clin Psychol 1980;48(2):129–42.

41. Osler M, Jespersen NB. The effect of a community-based cardiovascular disease prevention project in a Danish municipality. Dan Med Bull 1993;40:485–9.

42. Goodman RM, Wheeler FC, Lee PR. Evaluation of the Heart To Heart Project: lessons from a community- based chronic disease prevention project. Am J Health Promot 1995;9(6):443–55.

43. Malmgren S, Andersson G. Who were reached by and participated in a one year newspaper health information campaign? Scand J Soc Med 1986;14(3):133–40.

44. Young DR, Haskell WL, Taylor CB, Fortmann SP. Effect of community health education on physical activity knowledge, attitudes, and behavior. The Stanford Five-City Project. Am J Epidemiol 1996;144(3):264–74.

45. Jason LA, Greiner BJ, Naylor K, Johnson SP, Van Egeren L. A large-scale, short-term, media-based weight loss program. Am J Health Promot 1991;5(6):432–7.

46. Owen N, Lee C, Naccarella L, Haag K. Exercise by mail: a mediated behavior-change program for aerobic exercise. J Sport Psychol 1987;9(4):346–57.

47. Wimbush E, MacGregor A, Fraser E. Impacts of a national mass media campaign on walking in Scotland. Health Promot Int 1998;13(1):45–53.

48. Andersen RE, Franckowiak SC, Snyder J, Bartlett SJ, Fontaine KR. Can inexpensive signs encourage the use of stairs? Results from a community intervention. Ann Intern Med 1998;129(5):363–9.

49. Blamey A, Mutrie N, Aitchison T. Health promotion by encouraged use of stairs. BMJ 1995;311:289–90.

50. Brownell KD, Stunkard AJ, Albaum JM. Evaluation and modification of exercise patterns in the natural environment. Am J Psychiatry 1980;137:1540–5.

51. Kerr J, Eves F, Carroll D. Posters can prompt less active people to use the stairs. J Epidemiol Community Health 2000;54(12):942.

52. Russell W, Dzewaltowski D, Ryan G. The effectiveness of a point-of-decision prompt in deterring sedentary behavior. Am J Health Promot 1999;13(5):257–9.

53. Booth M, Bauman A, Oldenburg B, Owen N, Magnus P. Effects of a national mass-media campaign on physical activity participation. Health Promot Int 1992;7(4):241–7.

54. Bush PJ, Zuckerman AE, Theiss PK, et al. Cardiovascular risk factor prevention in black schoolchildren: two-year results of the "Know Your Body" program. Am J Epidemiol 1989;129(3):466–82.

55. Dale D, Corbin CB. Physical activity participation of high school graduates following exposure to conceptual or traditional physical education. Res Q Exerc Sport 2000; 71(1):61–8.

56. Davis SM, Lambert LC, Gomez Y, Skipper B. Southwest cardiovascular curriculum project: study findings for American Indian elementary students. J Health Educ 1995; 26:S72–S81.

57. Holcomb JD, Lira J, Kingery PM, Smith DW, Lane D, Goodway J. Evaluation of Jump Into Action: a program to reduce the risk of non-insulin-dependent diabetes mellitus in school children on the Texas-Mexico border. J School Health 1998;68(7):282–8.

58. Killen JD, Robinson TN, Telch MJ, et al. The Stanford Adolescent Heart Health Program. Health Educ Q 1989;16(2):263–83.

59. Marcus AC, Wheeler RC, Cullen JW, Crane LA. Quasi-experimental evaluation of the Los Angeles Know Your Body Program: knowledge, beliefs, and self-reported behaviors. Prev Med 1987;16:803–15.

60. Perry CL, Klepp KI, Dudovitz B, Golden D, Griffin, Smyth M. Promoting healthy eating and physical activity patterns among adolescents: a pilot study of "Slice of Life." Health Educ Q 1987;2:93–103.

61. Petchers MK, Hirsch EZ, Bloch BA. A longitudinal study of the impact of a school heart health curriculum. J Community Health 1988;13(2):85–94.

62. Walter HJ, Hofman A, Connelly PA, Barrett LT, Kost KL. Primary prevention of chronic disease in childhood: changes in risk factors after one year of intervention. Am J Epidemiol 1985;122(5):772–81.

63. Walter HJ, Hofman A, Connelly PA, Barrett LT, Kost KL. Coronary heart disease prevention in childhood: one-year results of a randomized intervention study. Am J Prev Med 1986;2(4):239–45.

64. Coates TJ, Jeffery RW, Slinkard LA. Heart healthy eating and exercise: introducing and maintaining changes in health behaviors. Am J Public Health 1981;71(1):15–23.

65. Homel PJ, Daniels P, Reid TR, Lawson JS. Results of an experimental school-based health development programme in Australia. Int J Health Educ 1981;263–70.

66. Moon AM, Mullee MA, Rogers L, Thompson RL, Speller V, Roderick P. Helping schools to become health-promoting environments—an evaluation of the Wessex Healthy Schools award. Health Promot Int 1999;14(2):111–22.

67. American Health Foundation. Know Your Body (KYB) school health promotion program. Available at: http://www.ed.gov/pubs/EPTW/eptw9/eptw9d.html. Accessed January 28, 2003.

68. Donnelly JE, Jacobsen DJ, Whatley JE, et al. Nutrition and physical activity program to attenuate obesity and promote physical and metabolic fitness in elementary school children. Obes Res 1996;4:229–43.

69. Dwyer T, Coonan WE, Leitch DR, Hetzel BS, Baghurst RA. An investigation of the effects of daily physical activity on the health of primary school students in South Australia. Int J Epidemiol 1983;12(3):308–13.

70. Ewart CK, Young DR, Hagberg JM. Effects of school-based aerobic exercise on blood pressure in adolescent girls at risk for hypertension. Am J Public Health 1998; 88:949–51.

71. Fardy PS, White RE, Haltiwanger-Schmitz K, et al. Coronary disease risk factor reduction and behavior modification in minority adolescents: the PATH program. J Adolesc Health 1996;18(4):247–53.

72. Harrell JS, McMurray RG, Gansky SA, Bangdiwala SI, Bradley CB. A public health vs a risk-based intervention to improve cardiovascular health in elementary school children: the Cardiovascular Health in Children Study. Am J Public Health 1999;89(10): 1529–35.

73. Hopper CA, Gruber MB, Munoz KD, Herb RA. Effect of including parents in a school-based exercise and nutrition program for children. Res Q Exerc Sport 1992;63(3): 315–21.

74. Hopper CA, Munoz KD, Gruber MB, MacConnie S. A school-based cardiovascular exercise and nutrition program with parent participation: An evaluation study. Child Health Care 1996;25(3):221–35.

75. Luepker RV, Perry CL, McKinlay SM, et al. Outcomes of a field trial to improve

children's dietary patterns and physical activity. The Child and Adolescent Trial for Cardiovascular Health. CATCH collaborative group . JAMA 1996;275(10):768–76.

76. Manios Y, Moschandreas J, Hatzis C, Kafatos A. Evaluation of a health and nutrition education program in primary school children of Crete over a three-year period. Prev Med 1999;28(2):149–59.

77. McKenzie TL, Nader PR, Strikmiller PK, et al. School physical education: effect of the Child and Adolescent Trial for Cardiovascular Health. Prev Med 1996;25(4):423–31.

78. Sallis JF, McKenzie TL, Alcaraz JE, Kolody B, Faucette N, Hovell MF. The effects of a 2-year physical education program (SPARK) on physical activity and fitness in elementary school students. Sports, Play and Active Recreation for Kids. Am J Public Health 1997;87(8):1328–34.

79. Simons-Morton BG, Parcel GS, Baranowski T, Forthofer R, O'Hara NM. Promoting physical activity and a healthful diet among children: results of a school-based intervention study. Am J Public Health 1991;81:986–91.

80. Vandongen R, Jenner DA, Thompson C, et al. A controlled evaluation of a fitness and nutrition intervention program on cardiovascular health in 10- to 12-year-old children. Prev Med 1995;24(1):9–22.

81. Duncan B, Boyce WT, Itami R, Puffenbarger N. A controlled trial of a physical fitness program for fifth grade students. J School Health 1983;(8):467–71.

82. Flores R. Dance for health: improving fitness in African American and Hispanic adolescents. Public Health Rep 1995;110(2):189–93.

83. Halfon ST, Bronner S. The influence of a physical ability intervention program on improved running time and increased sport motivation among Jerusalem schoolchildren. Adolescence 1988;23(90):405–16.

84. Tell GS, Vellar OD. Noncommunicable disease risk factor intervention in Norwegian adolescents: the Oslo Youth Study. In: Hetzel B, Berenson GS, eds. Cardiovascular risk factors in childhood: epidemiology and prevention. Amsterdam: Elsevier Science Publishers B.V., 1987:203–17.

85. Bandura A. Social foundations of thought and action: a social-cognitive theory. Englewood Cliffs, NJ: Prentice-Hall, 1986.

86. Rosenstock IM. The health belief model: explaining health behavior through expectancies. In: Health behavior and health education. Theory, research, and practice. Glanz K, Lewis FM, Rimer BK, eds. San Francisco: Jossey-Bass Publishers, 1990:39–62.

87. Prochaska JO, DiClemente CC. The transtheoretical approach: crossing traditional boundaries of change. Homewood, IL: Dorsey Press, 1984.

88. Blair SN, Smith M, Collingwood TR, Reynolds R, Prentice MC, Sterling CL. Health promotion for educators: impact on absenteeism. Prev Med 1986;15(2):166–75.

89. Cardinal BJ, Sachs ML. Prospective analysis of stage-of-exercise movement following mail-delivered, self-instructional exercise packets. Am J Health Promot 1995;9:430–2.

90. Chen A. A home-based behavioral intervention to promote walking in sedentary ethnic minority women: project WALK. Womens Health 1998;4(1):19–39.

91. Coleman KJ, Raynor HR, Mueller DM, Cerny FJ, Dorn JM, Epstein LH. Providing sedentary adults with choices for meeting their walking goals. Prev Med 1999;28(5):510–9.

92. Dunn AL, Marcus BH, Kampert JB, Garcia ME, Kohl HWI, Blair SN. Comparison

of lifestyle and structured interventions to increase physical activity and cardiovascular fitness: a randomized trial. JAMA 1999;281(4):327–34.

93. Foreyt JP, Goodrick GK, Reeves RS, Raynaud AS. Response of free-living adults to behavioral treatment of obesity: attrition and compliance to exercise. Behav Ther 1993; 24(4):659–69.

94. Jarvis KL, Friedman RH, Heeren T, Cullinane PM. Older women and physical activity: using the telephone to walk. Womens Health Issues 1997;7(1):24–9.

95. Jeffery RW, Wing RR, Thorson C, Burton LR. Use of personal trainers and financial incentives to increase exercise in a behavioral weight-loss program. J Consult Clin Psychol 1998;66(5):777–83.

96. Jette A, Lachman M, Giorgetti M, et al. Exercise—it's never too late: the Strong-for-Life program. Am J Public Health 1999;89(1):66–72.

97. Kanders BS, Ullmann-Joy P, Foreyt JP, et al. The black American lifestyle intervention (BALI): the design of a weight loss program for working-class African-American women. J Am Diet Assoc 1994;94(3):310–2.

98. King A, Haskell WL, Taylor CB, Kraemer HC, DeBusk RF. Group vs home based exercise training in healthy older men and women. JAMA 1991;266(11):1535–42.

99. Marcus B, Emmons KM, Simkin-Silverman LR, et al. Evaluation of motivationally tailored vs. standard self-help physical activity interventions at the workplace. Am J Health Promot 1998;12:246–53.

100. Mayer JA, Jermanovich A, Wright BL, Elder JP, Drew JA, Williams SJ. Changes in health behaviors of older adults: the San Diego Medicare Preventive Health Project. Prev Med 1994;23(2):127–33.

101. McAuley E, Courneya KS, Rudolph DL, Lox CL. Enhancing exercise adherence in middle-aged males and females. Prev Med 1994;23(4):498–506.

102. Noland MP. The effects of self-monitoring and reinforcement on exercise adherence. Res Q Exerc Sport 1989;60(3):216–24.

103. Peterson TR, Aldana SG. Improving exercise behavior: an application of the stages of change model in a worksite setting. Am J Health Promot 1999;13(4):229–32.

104. Wing RR, Jeffery RW, Pronk N, Hellerstedt WL. Effects of a personal trainer and financial incentives on exercise adherence in overweight women in a behavioral weight loss program. Obes Res 1996;4(5):457–62.

105. Robison JI, Rogers MA, Carlson JJ, et al. Effects of a 6-month incentive-based exercise program on adherence and work capacity. Med Sci Sports Exerc 1992;24(1):85–93.

106. Taggart AC, Taggart J, Siedentop D. Effects of a home-based activity program. A study with low fitness elementary school children. Behav Modif 1986;10(4):487–507.

107. Sevick MA, Dunn AL, Morrow MS, Marcus BH, Chen GJ, Blair SN. Cost-effectiveness of lifestyle and structured exercise interventions in sedentary adults. Results of project ACTIVE. Am J Prev Med 2000;19(1):1–8.

108. Avila P, Hovell MF. Physical activity training for weight loss in Latinas: a controlled trial. Int J Obes Relat Metab Disord 1994;18(7):476–82.

109. Gill AA, Veigl VL, Shuster JJ, Notelovitz M. A well woman's health maintenance study comparing physical fitness and group support programs. Occup Ther J Res 1984; 4(4):286–308.

110. King AC, Taylor CB, Haskell WL, DeBusk RF. Strategies for increasing early ad-

herence to and long-term maintenance of home-base exercise training in health middle-aged men and women. Am J Cardiol 1988;61(8):628–32.

111. King AC, Frederiksen LW. Low-cost strategies for increasing exercise behavior: relapse preparation training and social support. Behav Modif 1984;8(1):3–21.

112. Kriska AM, Bayles C, Cauley JA, LaPorte RE, Sandler RB, Pambianco G. A randomized exercise trial in older women: increased activity over two years and the factors associated with compliance. Med Sci Sports Exerc 1986;18(5):557–62.

113. Lombard DN, Lombard TN, Winett RA. Walking to meet health guidelines: the effect of prompting frequency and prompt structure. Health Psychol 1995;14(2):164–70.

114. Simmons D, Fleming C, Voyle J, Fou F, Feo S, Gatland B. A pilot urban church-based programme to reduce risk factors for diabetes among Western Samoans in New Zealand. Diabet Med 1998;15(2):136–42.

115. Wankel LM, Yardley JK, Graham J. The effects of motivational interventions upon the exercise adherence of high and low self-motivated adults. Can J Appl Sport Sci 1985;10(3):147–56.

116. Calfas KJ, Sallis JF, Nichols JF, et al. Project GRAD: two-year outcomes of a randomized controlled physical activity intervention among young adults. Graduate Ready for Activity Daily. Am J Prev Med 2000;18(1):28–37.

117. Epstein LH, Wing RR, Thompson JK, Griffin W. Attendance and fitness in aerobics exercise: the effects of contract and lottery procedures. Behav Modif 1980;4(4):465–79.

118. Sallis JF, Calfas KJ, Nichols JF, et al. Evaluation of a university course to promote physical activity: project GRAD. Res Q Exerc Sport 1999;70(1):1–10.

119. Brynteson P, Adams TM. The effects of conceptually based physical education programs on attitudes and exercise habits of college alumni. Res Q Exerc Sport 1993; 64(2):208–12.

120. Lock RS. College women's decision-making skills relating to voluntary participation in physical activity during leisure time. Percept Mot Skills 1990;71(1):141–6.

121. Slava S, Laurie DR, Corbin CB. Long-term effects of a conceptual physical education program. Res Q Exerc Sport 1984;55(2):161–8.

122. Robinson TN. Reducing children's television viewing to prevent obesity: a randomized controlled trial. JAMA 1999;282(16):1561–7.

123. Gortmaker SL, Peterson K, Wiecha J, et al. Reducing obesity via a school-based interdisciplinary intervention among youth: Planet Health. Arch Pediatr Adolesc Med 1999;153(4):409–18.

124. Gortmaker SL, Cheung LW, Peterson KE, et al. Impact of a school-based interdisciplinary intervention on diet and physical activity among urban primary school children: eat well and keep moving. Arch Pediatr Adolesc Med 1999;153(9):975–83.

125. Baranowski T, Simons-Morton B, Hooks P, et al. A center-based program for exercise change among black-American families. Health Educ Q 1990;17(2):179–96.

126. Bishop P, Donnelly JE. Home based activity program for obese children. Am Correct Ther 1987;41(1):12–9.

127. Johnson CC, Nicklas TA, Arbeit ML, et al. Cardiovascular intervention for high-risk families: the Heart Smart Program. South Med J 1991;84(11):1305–12.

128. Nader PR, Baranowski T, Vanderpool NA, Dunn K, Dworkin R, Ray L. The family health project: cardiovascular risk reduction education for children and parents. J Devel Behav Pediatr 1983;4(1):3–10.

129. Nader PR, Sallis JF, Patterson TL, et al. A family approach to cardiovascular risk

reduction: results from the San Diego Family Health Project. Health Educ Q 1989;16(2): 229–44.

130. Zimmerman RS, Gerace TA, Smith JC, Benezra J. The effects of a worksite health promotion program on the wives of fire fighters. Soc Sci Med 1988;26(5):537–43.

131. Bertera RL. Behavioral risk factor and illness day changes with workplace health promotion: two-year results. Am J Health Promot 1993;7(5):365–73.

132. Blair SN, Piserchia PV, Wilbur CS, Crowder JH. A public health intervention model for work-site health promotion. Impact on exercise and physical fitness in a health promotion plan after 24 months. JAMA 1986;255(7):921–6.

133. Brownson RC, Smith CA, Pratt M, et al. Preventing cardiovascular disease through community-based risk reduction: the Bootheel Heart Health Project. Am J Public Health 1996;86(2):206–13.

134. Heirich MA, Foote A, Erfurt JC, Konopka B. Work-site physical fitness programs: comparing the impact of different program designs on cardiovascular risks. J Occup Med 1993;35:510–7.

135. Henritze J, Brammell HL, McGloin J. LIFECHECK: a successful, low touch, low tech, in-plant, cardiovascular disease risk identification and modification program. Am J Health Promot 1992;7(2):129–36.

136. King AC, Carl F, Birkel L, Haskell WL. Increasing exercise among blue-collar employees: the tailoring of worksite programs to meet specific needs. Prev Med 1988;17(3):357–65.

137. Larsen P, Simons N. Evaluating a federal health and fitness program: indicators of improving health. AAOHN J 1993;41(3):143–8.

138. Lewis CE, Raczynski JM, Heath GW, Levinson R, Hilyer JJ, Cutter GR. Promoting physical activity in low-income African-American communities: the PARR project. Ethn Dis 1993;3(2):106–18.

139. Linenger JM, Chesson CV, Nice DS. Physical fitness gains following simple environmental change. Am J Prev Med 1991;7(5):298–310.

140. Ostwald SK. Changing employees' dietary and exercise practices: an experimental study in a small company. J Occup Med 1989;31(2):90–7.

141. Cady LD Jr, Thomas PC, Karwasky RJ. Program for increasing health and physical fitness of fire fighters. J Occup Med 1985;27(2):110–4.

142. Eddy JM, Eynon D, Nagy S, Paradossi PJ. Impact of a physical fitness program in a blue-collar workforce. Health Values 1990;14(6):14–23.

143. Golaszewski T, Snow D, Lynch W, Yen L, Solomita D. A benefit-to-cost analysis of a work-site health promotion program. J Occup Med 1992;34(12):1164–72.

144. Bowne DW, Russell ML, Morgan JL, Optenberg SA, Clarke AE. Reduced disability and health care costs in an industrial fitness program. J Occup Med 1984;26(11):809–16.

145. Colditz GA. Economic costs of obesity and inactivity. Med Sci Sports Exerc 1999; 31(11 suppl):S663–S667.

146. Blair SN, Kohl HW III, Barlow CE, Paffenbarger RS Jr, Gibbons LW, Macera CA. Changes in physical fitness and all-cause mortality. A prospective study of healthy and unhealthy men. JAMA 1995;273(14):1093–8.

147. Centers for Disease Control and Prevention. Increasing physical activity. A report on recommendations of the Task Force on Community Preventive Services. MMWR 2001;50(No. RR-18):1–14.

148. Task Force on Community Preventive Services. Recommendations to increase physical activity in communities. Am J Prev Med 2002;22(4S):67–72.

Chapter 3

The Social Environment

Social environments lacking basic resources—healthy food, safe housing, living-wage jobs, decent schools, supportive social networks, access to health care and other public and private goods and services—present the highest public health risk for serious illness and premature death.[1,2] Understanding why this happens requires an ecologic approach to population health, one that recognizes that individuals and communities interact with their physical and social environments.[3] Conceptualizing health as a product, in part, of social conditions facilitates the identification of relationships between social determinants and health outcomes that may be amenable to community interventions.[4]

*Insufficient evidence means that we were not able to determine whether or not the intervention works.

The Task Force approved the recommendations in this chapter in 2000–2001. The research on which the findings are based was conducted from 1966 to 2000. This information has been previously published in the American Journal of Preventive Medicine [2003; 24(suppl 3):12–79] and the MMWR Recommendations and Reports series [2002; 51(no. RR-1):1–8].

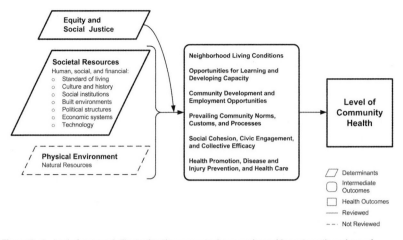

Figure 3-1. Logic framework illustrating the conceptual approach used in systematic reviews of interventions in the social environment to improve community health. (Reprinted from Am J Prev Med, Vol. 24, No. 3S, Anderson LM et al., Methods for conducting systematic reviews of the evidence of effectiveness and economic efficiency of interventions to promote healthy social environments, p. 26, Copyright 2003, with permission from American Journal of Preventive Medicine.)

The fundamental premise of the *Community Guide*'s social environment and health model (Figure 3-1) is that access to societal resources determines community health outcomes.[5] Standard of living, culture and history, social institutions, built environments, political structures, economic systems, and technology are all societal resources that a population draws upon to sustain health. Patterns of exposure to risk vary among socioeconomic groups and are associated with a fundamental access to resources.[5] Prosperity, whether at the community, family, or personal level, provides such resources as knowledge, money, power, and prestige, which can be used to avoid or buffer exposure to health risks. Poverty, on the other hand, with all of its attendant burdens, also powerfully influences health status. An impoverished social environment is a potential source of stressors (e.g., high-crime neighborhood or job scarcity) as well as resources (e.g., after-school programs or homeless shelters).[6-8]

In this chapter, we focus on three broad areas of the social environment that affect health: early childhood development, affordable housing, and culturally competent health care. These three topics, covering broad and essential areas, represent just a small beginning of the review of evidence that interventions can effectively address the social conditions that influence health.

OBJECTIVES AND RECOMMENDATIONS FROM OTHER ADVISORY GROUPS

Table 3-1 shows the goals and objectives outlined in *Healthy People 2010*[9] for all three topics covered in this chapter: early childhood education, housing,

Table 3–1. Selected Healthy People 2010[9] Goals and Objectives
Directly Relevant to the Social Environment

Objective	Population	Baseline	2010 Objective
Early Childhood Development: Maternal and Child Health			
Increase the proportion of pregnant women who receive early and adequate prenatal care (Objective 16–6b)	Pregnant women	74% (1998)	90%
Reduce:		(Both 1998)	
• low birthweight (LBW) (16–10a)	Infants	7.6%	5.0%
• very low birthweight (VLBW) (16–10b)		1.4%	0.9%
Reduce the occurrence of developmental disabilities per 10,000 people:		(Both 1991–94)	
• Mental retardation (16–14a)	All	131[a]	124
• Cerebral palsy (16–14b)		32.2[b]	31.5
• Autism spectrum disorder (16–14c)		Developmental	
• Epilepsy (16–14d)		Developmental	
Early Childhood Development: Educational and Community-Based Programs			
Increase high school completion among 18- to 24-year-olds (7–1)	Adolescents/ young adults	85% (1998)	90%
Housing: Educational and Community-Based Programs			
Increase the proportion of Tribal and local health service areas or jurisdictions that have established a community health promotion program that addresses multiple Healthy People 2010 focus areas (7–10)	American Indian communities	Developmental	
Culturally Competent Health Care: Educational and Community-Based Programs			
Increase the proportion of patients who report that they are satisfied with the patient education they receive from their healthcare organization (7–8)	All	Developmental	
Increase the proportion of local health departments that have established culturally appropriate and linguistically competent community health promotion and disease prevention programs (7–11)	Health departments	Vary by condition	

Table 3–1. *Continued*

Objective	Population	Baseline	2010 Objective
Culturally Competent Health Care: Programs Using Communication to Improve Health			
Increase the proportion of persons who report that their healthcare providers have satisfactory communication skills (11–6)	All	Developmental	
Culturally Competent Health Care: Programs to Improve Access to Appropriate, Quality Mental Health Services			
Increase the number of States, Territories, and the District of Columbia with an operational mental health plan that addresses cultural competence (18–13)	All	Developmental	

[a]Children aged 8 years in metropolitan Atlanta having an IQ of 70 or less.

[b]Children aged 8 years in metropolitan Atlanta.

and culturally competent health care. Objectives and recommendations specific to each topic are listed below.

Early Childhood Development

The National Education Goals panel (created in 1994 by the Goals 2000: Educate America Act) established a national priority for research in education: improve learning and development in early childhood so that all children can enter kindergarten prepared to learn and succeed in elementary and secondary school. Two goals of this panel are directly relevant here.

Goal 1 states that "By the year 2000, all children in America will start school ready to learn."[10] Two objectives toward achieving that goal are: (*1*) Children will receive the nutrition, physical activity experiences, and health care needed to arrive at school with healthy minds and bodies, and to maintain the mental alertness necessary to be prepared to learn, and the number of low-birthweight babies will be significantly reduced through enhanced prenatal health systems; and (*2*) All children will have access to high-quality and developmentally appropriate preschool programs that help prepare children for school. Goal 2 was to increase the high school graduation rate to at least 90% by the year 2000.

The Institute of Medicine's Committee on Capitalizing on Social Science and Behavioral Research to Improve the Public's Health issued corresponding recommendations in 2000.[11] Two of their nine recommendations apply to early childhood education interventions:

- Recommendation 2: Rather than focusing on a single or limited number of health determinants, interventions on social and behavioral factors should link multiple levels of influence (i.e., individual, interpersonal, institutional, community, and policy levels).
- Recommendation 6: High-quality, center-based early education programs should be more widely implemented. Future interventions directed at infants and young children should focus on strengthening other processes affecting child outcomes such as the home environment, school and neighborhood influences, and physical health and growth.

Housing

The FY 2000–2006 Strategic Plan of the U.S. Department of Housing and Urban Development[12] included four goals related to housing programs whose aim is to reduce residential segregation by income. These goals and their corresponding objectives are:

Goal 1: Increase the availability of decent, safe, and affordable housing in American communities.
Objective: By 2005, the number of families with children, elderly households and persons with disabilities with worst-case housing needs will decrease by 30% from 1997 levels. (*Worst-case housing needs* are defined as the needs of unassisted very-low-income renters who pay more than half of their income for housing or live in severely substandard housing.)

Goal 2: Ensure equal opportunity in housing for all Americans.
Objective: Segregation of racial and ethnic minorities and low-income households will decline.

Goal 3: Promote housing stability, self-sufficiency, and asset development of families and individuals.
Objective: The annual percentage growth in earnings of families in public and assisted housing increases.

Goal 4: Improve community quality of life and economic vitality.
Objective: The share of households located in neighborhoods with extreme poverty decreases.
Among low- and moderate-income residents, the share with a good opinion of their neighborhood increases.
Residents of public housing are more satisfied with their safety. (Note: For the purposes of this measure, a "good opinion" of the neighbor-

hood is defined as a response of 7–10 on a 10-point scale assessing "overall opinion of neighborhood.")

Culturally Competent Health Care

In March 2001, the Department of Health and Human Services' Office of Minority Health published National Standards for Culturally and Linguistically Appropriate Services in Health Care (CLAS).[13] The CLAS standards were developed to provide a common understanding and a consistent definition of culturally and linguistically appropriate healthcare services. Additionally, they were proposed as one means of correcting inequities in the provision of health services and making healthcare systems more responsive to the needs of all clients. Ultimately, the standards aim to eliminate racial and ethnic disparities in health status and improve the health of the entire population.

The interventions selected for this review complement the recommended CLAS standards for linguistic and cultural competency by examining the extent to which meeting some of these standards results in improved processes and outcomes of care.

METHODS

Methods used for the reviews are summarized in Chapter 10. Specific methods used in the systematic reviews of the social environment have been described elsewhere[14] and are available at www.thecommunityguide.org/social. The logic framework depicting the conceptual approach used in reviews of interventions in the social environment to improve community health is presented in Figure 3–1.

ECONOMIC EFFICIENCY

A systematic review of economic evaluations was conducted for all recommended interventions (i.e., those shown to be effective), and a summary of each economic review is presented with the related intervention. The methods used to conduct these economics reviews are summarized in Chapter 11.

RECOMMENDATIONS AND FINDINGS

This section presents a summary of the findings of the systematic reviews conducted to determine the effectiveness of the selected interventions in this topic area. Three areas were reviewed: early childhood development, housing, and culturally competent health care.

Early Childhood Development

Infancy and early childhood are periods of opportunity for growth as well as vulnerability to harm.[15] Living in poverty can affect a child's cognitive and behavioral development, which, in turn, affects readiness for school.[16,17] A child's readiness when starting school is related to motivation and intellectual performance in subsequent years and is therefore critical to establishing a trajectory for successful educational attainment. Educational attainment, in turn, is related to a wide range of adult disease outcomes.[18,19]

Early childhood development programs are designed to promote social competence and school readiness among children three to five years old. Publicly funded programs such as Head Start target preschool children disadvantaged by poverty. These programs address cognitive, social, emotional, and physical development, as well as the ability of the child's family to provide a home environment appropriate for healthy development.

Comprehensive, Center-Based, Early Childhood Development Programs for Low-Income Children: Recommended (Strong Evidence of Effectiveness)

Comprehensive early childhood development programs are designed to improve the cognitive, social, and emotional functioning of preschool children, which, in turn, influence readiness to learn in the school setting. School readiness, particularly among poor children, may help prevent the cascade of consequences of early academic failure and school behavioral problems: dropping out of high school, delinquency, unemployment, and psychological and physical problems in young adulthood.

Effectiveness

- These programs are effective in improving children's cognitive and social development.

Applicability

- Our findings should be applicable to all preschool children in the United States, especially those disadvantaged by poverty.

The findings of our systematic review are based on assessment of four different aspects of early childhood development: cognitive, social, health, and family. We identified a total of 90 effect measures for the four outcomes, with over 70% of the reported effects measuring cognitive outcomes.

In terms of cognitive change, consistent improvements were found in measures of intellectual ability (IQ), standardized academic achievement tests, standardized tests of school readiness, promotion to the next grade level, and decreased placement in special education classes because of learning problems. These results came from 12 studies (in 17 reports).[20-36] The median effect size for improvement in academic achievement tests was 0.35 (the effect size is the difference between the means of the intervention and control groups divided by the standard deviation of the control group); for standardized tests to determine school readiness, 0.38; and for standardized tests measuring IQ, 0.43. The median reduction in students held back to repeat a grade was 13 percentage points; placement in special education programs because of various sources of learning difficulty showed a median reduction of 14 percentage points. Use of comprehensive, center-based early childhood development programs for low-income children is recommended on the basis of these improvements in cognitive outcomes.

Of the five studies (in six reports)[22,31,33,34,37,38] reporting on social outcomes as measures of early childhood development, one year after the program two studies showed improved behavior and motivation in the classroom and one study showed a decline. Long-term social outcomes (e.g., increased employment, home ownership, decreased teen pregnancy, arrest) showed improvement in two studies, although no numbers were provided in the reports.

We found only one qualifying study that examined whether more children in early childhood development programs were being screened for general health and dental health than those not in programs.[39] This study found a 44% increase in health screenings and a 61% increase in dental screenings.

Two studies examined whether enrollment of a child in an early childhood development program corresponded to an improvement in measures of education, employment, poverty, and public assistance among the household.[39,40] One of these studies showed an increase in health screenings for siblings of children enrolled in early childhood development programs.

These results should apply to most preschool children from disadvantaged backgrounds. Study settings ranged from urban to rural, and the populations of different studies included people of African-American, Latino, Asian, Native American, and other ethnic or cultural backgrounds.

No additional harms or benefits from these programs were identified during the review.

The findings of our systematic review of economic evaluations are based on one study,[41] conducted in a low-income area in Ypsilanti, Michigan, which modeled the costs and benefits of the Perry Preschool program.[34] The study was conducted in preschool facilities and homes throughout the community. The population consisted of 128 African-American three-year-olds of low socioeconomic status from a single school attendance area. The study had a follow-up of 24 years, but lifetime benefits were factored in. The net benefit of the program (in 1997 US$) was $108,516 for males and $110,333 for females.

The Perry Preschool program differs from other programs, however, in terms of the degree of support and quality of implementation. Its results, therefore, cannot necessarily be generalized to less intensive programs, such as Head Start. Nevertheless, careful consideration of the program is valuable because of the importance of the outcomes, long-term effects, consistency of findings across numerous measures, and the strong quality of the research design.

Our systematic review identified no barriers to implementing these programs.

In conclusion, the Task Force recommends early childhood development programs on the basis of strong evidence that they improve intermediate cognitive and social outcomes, which in some cases are markers of improved long-term health outcomes. Specifically, participants scored higher on cognitive skills tests, were less likely to be retained in grade in school, and were less likely to require placement in special education classes. Long-term follow-up of the Perry Preschool program, in particular, indicates that the benefits of an early childhood development program may extend to adulthood. That study showed a correlation between participation in early childhood development programs and improved educational and economic outcomes.

Housing

Among the most prevalent community health concerns related to family housing are the inadequate supply of affordable housing for low-income families and the increasing segregation of households into unsafe neighborhoods based on income, race, ethnicity, or social class. When affordable housing is not available to low-income households, family resources needed for food, medical or dental care, and other necessities are diverted to housing costs. We reviewed two housing programs intended to provide affordable housing and, concurrently, reduce the residential segregation of low-income families into unsafe neighborhoods of concentrated poverty: tenant-based rental assistance programs and the creation of mixed-income housing developments.

Tenant-Based Rental Assistance Programs: Recommended (Sufficient Evidence of Effectiveness)

Tenant-based rental assistance programs subsidize the cost of housing secured by low-income households within the private rental market through the use of vouchers or direct cash subsidies. The Section 8 program of the U.S. Department of Housing and Urban Development (HUD) is administered by local and state housing agencies under contract to the federal government. The Section 8 program subsidizes rental costs for families with incomes

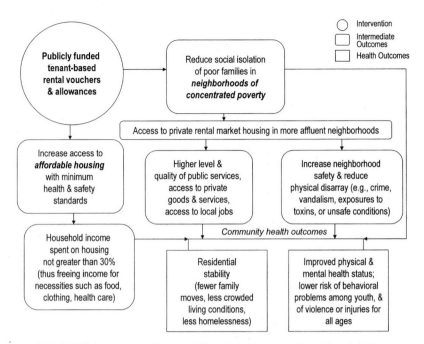

Figure 3–2. Analytic framework used to conduct the systematic reviews of tenant-based rental assistance programs. (Reprinted from Am J Prev Med, Vol. 24, No. 3S, Anderson LM et al., Providing affordable family housing and reducing residential segregation by income: a systematic review, p. 52, Copyright 2003, with permission from American Journal of Preventive Medicine.)

below 50% of area median income. Families contribute 30% of their monthly income to housing costs, and the Section 8 subsidy provides the remainder for rental costs up to a locally defined standard. Figure 3–2 is the conceptual model (analytic framework) we used to conduct this review.

The success of Section 8 vouchers and certificates in moving assisted families to less impoverished or less racially segregated areas is dependent on several factors, including housing market discrimination, the inexperience of program participants as housing "consumers," the desire of many to remain near established social ties and the conveniences of the urban core, the time and transportation constraints that hinder such households in conducting housing searches in suburban locations, and administrative and programmatic shortcomings of local housing authorities.[42,43] In light of this, some rental voucher programs are augmented with housing search counseling, employment and transportation assistance, community networking, landlord outreach, or post-placement services.[44]

Effectiveness

- These programs are effective in reducing individuals' likelihood of being a victim of crime; in reducing neighborhood social disorder (e.g., trash, graffiti, abandoned buildings, public drinking); in improving the quality of housing; in decreasing behavioral problems among youth, both at home and in school; and in improving the physical and psychological health of heads of household.

Applicability

- The findings of our review should be applicable to most low-income families in urban areas, regardless of race or ethnic origin.

The findings of our systematic review are based on 12 studies (in 23 papers) on the effectiveness of tenant-based rental assistance (or voucher) programs in improving community health outcomes.[45-67] These 12 studies represent four broad groups of federal housing evaluation efforts: (1) the Housing Allowance Experiment; (2) HUD's Section 8 Rental Certificate and Voucher program; (3) the Gautreaux program, in which rental vouchers were provided to African-American families in racially segregated public housing in Chicago; and (4) Moving to Opportunity for Fair Housing research, implemented in five large cities, which combines rental vouchers with household counseling to help low-income families move from public housing to nonpoverty neighborhoods.

Five studies reported measures of neighborhood safety and found that household victimization, measured, on average, six months after the intervention took place, decreased by a median of 6 percentage points. Four studies examined changes in neighborhood social disorder and found a median decrease of 15.5 percentage points. One study compared murder rates in the neighborhood to which households relocated with rates in their neighborhood of origin and reported a decrease. One study reported decreases in health and safety risks including peeling paint, inadequate plumbing, rodent infestation, and broken or missing locks on housing unit doors.

Three studies reported on youth risk behaviors, measured between 1 and 5 years (mean, 2.9 years) after the intervention took place. The median difference was a decrease in behavioral problems of 7.8 percentage points. Two studies examined self-reported symptoms of depression and anxiety by heads of households and found a median decrease of 8 percentage points. The same two studies reported self-rated health status and found a median increase of 11.5 percentage points among people rating their health as "good" or "excellent" compared with "fair" or "poor." One study reported on diverse child health outcomes. A median decrease of 4.5% was observed in the need for acute medical care for injuries or asthma episodes, although a median decrease of 5.5% was also observed for use of child preventive services for children (e.g., well-child check-ups and vaccinations).

Overall, these results provide sufficient evidence of the effectiveness of tenant-based rental assistance programs in improving household safety through reducing exposure to crimes against person and property and decreasing neighborhood social disorder.

These findings should be applicable to most low-income families in urban areas. Studies were conducted among white, Latino, and African-American populations, and effects were similar for all of these groups. We did not examine housing programs that targeted the elderly or people with special health needs.

Two unintended effects of these programs are common. When families move from one neighborhood to another, social ties and supports are disrupted. And, if families move to weak or declining neighborhoods because that is where they can find affordable housing, new areas of concentrated poverty can be created. A third postulated effect might be found in the Moving to Opportunity program. The very name implies that residents must move to find opportunities, and could make those who stay in the old neighborhoods feel that the neighborhoods are undesirable.

We did not find any economic evaluations of tenant-based rental assistance programs.

Barriers to implementing tenant-based rental assistance programs are described in the literature. Families may be limited in their search for housing in better neighborhoods if they lack transportation, lack money for apartment application fees, fear discrimination, or fear encountering landlords who refuse to accept them as tenants. Local housing market conditions may also inflate rents above what rental voucher recipients can afford to pay.

In conclusion, the Task Force recommends tenant-based rental assistance programs to improve household safety, on the basis of sufficient evidence of effectiveness in reducing exposure to crimes against person and property and decreasing neighborhood social disorder. This recommendation should be applicable to all low-income urban families. A conclusion about the effectiveness of these programs in reducing housing hazards, youth risk behaviors, and psychological and physical morbidity could not be made because only a few studies reported these outcomes.

Mixed-Income Housing Developments: Insufficient Evidence to Determine Effectiveness

In our systematic review, we defined a mixed-income housing development as a publicly subsidized multifamily rental housing development in which the deliberate mixing of income groups is a fundamental part of the development's operating and financial plans. A portion of a development's units must be reserved for, and made affordable to, households whose incomes are at least below 60% of the area median, although the income levels of all residents and the relative representation of each income group may vary among developments. These developments can be created either through new construction or conversion of existing developments, but must exist within neighborhoods where over 20% of households have income below the federal poverty level.

Effectiveness

- We found insufficient evidence to determine the effectiveness of mixed-income housing developments in improving an array of family and neighborhood conditions.
- Evidence was insufficient because no qualifying studies could be found.
- Insufficient evidence means that we were not able to determine whether or not the intervention works.

We could not determine the effectiveness of mixed-income housing developments in providing affordable housing in safe neighborhood environments, because we found no studies comparing families who had moved to such developments with families who stayed in their old neighborhoods.

Because we could not establish the effectiveness of mixed-income housing developments in improving neighborhood conditions or family safety or achievement, we did not examine situations in which such programs would be applicable, information about economic efficiency, or possible barriers to implementation.

In conclusion, the Task Force found insufficient evidence to determine the effectiveness of mixed-income housing developments because no qualifying studies were found.

Culturally Competent Health Care

When a healthcare provider speaks one language and the client speaks a different language, how is the quality of health care affected? When the provider bases his or her actions on one set of beliefs and the client on another, what kind of communication can be expected? The solution to this and other cross-cultural challenges in health care may lie in developing culturally competent health care. The goal of culturally competent care is to ensure that appropriate services are provided and to reduce medical errors resulting from misunderstandings caused by differences in language or culture. Cultural competence has the potential to improve the efficiency of care by reducing unnecessary diagnostic testing or inappropriate use of services. A culturally competent healthcare setting includes an appropriate mix of a culturally diverse staff that reflects the community(ies) served, providers or translators who speak the clients' language(s), training for providers about the culture and language of the people they serve, signage and instructional literature in the clients' language(s) and consistent with their cultural norms, and culturally specific healthcare settings.

An inability to communicate with a healthcare provider not only creates a barrier to accessing health care[68–70] but also undermines trust in the quality of medical care received and decreases the likelihood of appropriate follow-up.[71] Furthermore, lack of a common language between client and provider can result in diagnostic errors and inappropriate treatment.[70] According to the Current Population Reports,[72] in March 2000 the foreign-born population of the United States was estimated to be 28.4 million—a substantial increase from the population of 9.6 million foreign-born in 1970, reflecting the high level of immigration over the past three decades.

Differences in referral and treatment patterns of providers (after controlling for medical need) are associated with a client's racial or ethnic group.[13,73] Whether conscious or unconscious, negative social stereotypes shape behaviors and influence decisions made by providers and their clients.[74] For example, differences between African Americans and whites in referral for cardiac procedures,[75,76] analgesic prescribing patterns for ethnic minorities compared with nonminority clients,[77] racial differences in cancer treatment,[78] receipt of the best available treatments for depression and anxiety by ethnic minorities compared with nonminority clients,[79] and differences in HIV treatment modalities[80] are just a few ways in which race and ethnicity can affect care. Clients' delay or refusal to seek needed care can result from mistrust, perceived discrimination, and negative experiences in interactions with the healthcare system.[81–84] In 2002, the Institute of Medicine report[73] on unequal medical treatment noted: "The sources of these disparities are complex, are rooted in historic and contemporary inequities, and involve many participants at several levels, including health systems, their administrative and bureaucratic processes, utilization managers, healthcare professionals, and patients."

Programs to Recruit and Retain Staff Who Reflect the Cultural Diversity of the Community Served: Insufficient Evidence to Determine Effectiveness

Workforce diversity in the healthcare setting can be a means of providing relevant and effective services. Workforce diversity programs can go beyond hiring practices to include identification of barriers that prevent employees from full participation and success. Achieving diversity at all levels of healthcare organizations could influence the manner and extent to which the needs of clients of various cultural and linguistic backgrounds are met. In our systematic review, we searched for healthcare system interventions to recruit or retain diverse staff.

Effectiveness

- We found insufficient evidence to determine the effectiveness of programs to recruit and retain staff who reflect the cultural diversity of the community served in improving health care.
- Evidence was insufficient because no qualifying studies could be found.
- Insufficient evidence means that we were not able to determine whether or not the intervention works.

No comparative studies evaluated these programs. Therefore, evidence was insufficient to determine the effectiveness of healthcare system interventions to recruit and retain diverse staff.

Because we could not establish the effectiveness of these programs, we did not examine situations in which such programs would be applicable, information about economic efficiency, or possible barriers to implementation.

In conclusion, the Task Force found insufficient evidence to determine the effectiveness of programs to recruit and retain staff who reflect the cultural diversity of the community served in improving health care because no qualifying studies were found.

Use of Interpreter Services or Bilingual Providers for Clients with Limited English Proficiency: Insufficient Evidence to Determine Effectiveness

Clients should be able to understand the nature and purpose of the healthcare services they receive. Accurate, appropriate communication increases the likelihood of receiving appropriate care, both in terms of the best technical care for symptoms or conditions and in terms of client preferences. Language capacity varies: a person may understand enough English to complete an intake form, but may need considerable help to understand diagnosis and treatment options. Or an English-speaking provider may know basic vocabulary or medical terminology in the client's language, but may lack understanding of the cultural nuances that affect the meaning of words or phrases. In the healthcare setting, non-English-speaking clients can be assisted by family members, by staff with other primary duties who act as interpreters, or by professionally trained interpreters (whose training in medical terminology and confidentiality may both prevent communication errors and protect privacy). Nonverbal communication also should be considered, as it too may be culturally bound.

Effectiveness

- We found insufficient evidence to determine the effectiveness of interpreter services or bilingual providers in improving health care.
- Evidence was insufficient because only one study, with limitations in the quality of execution, was available.
- Insufficient evidence means that we were not able to determine whether or not the intervention works.

The findings of our systematic review are based on one study that examined the effectiveness of using bilingual staff or providers or professionally trained interpreters.[85] One other study did not meet our quality criteria and was excluded from the review.[86] We searched for studies that examined the effectiveness of bilingual providers, bilingual staff members who serve as interpreters (in addition to their regular duties), and professionally trained interpreters in improving client satisfaction and health status and reducing racial or ethnic differentials in the use of healthcare services.

The reviewed study, conducted in an urban hospital emergency department serving predominantly Latino clients (74%), included subjects who were predominantly female (64%), between 18 and 60 years of age (92%), and uninsured (68%). Clients presenting with overt psychiatric illness and those too ill to complete an interview were not included. The study evaluated whether or not physicians and clients could use the same language or if an interpreter (both professionally trained and untrained) was needed. The need for an interpreter was determined by the physician or nurse. A comparison group consisted of clients who reported that an interpreter was needed but not used. Most interpreters (88%) were family members or hospital staff serving as ad hoc interpreters; only 12% of interpreters were professionally trained.

Clients who reported that an interpreter was needed but not used were more likely to be discharged without a follow-up appointment than clients who were able to communicate directly with their physicians in a common language (OR = 1.79, 95% CI 1.00–3.23). Similarly, clients who communicated through interpreters were more likely to be discharged without follow-up appointments than clients with language-concordant physicians (OR = 1.92, 95% CI 1.11–3.33).

The results of this one study provide insufficient evidence to determine if interpreters or bilingual providers are effective in improving health care.

Because we could not establish the effectiveness of these programs, we did not examine situations in which such programs would be applicable, information about economic efficiency, or possible barriers to implementation.

In conclusion, the Task Force found insufficient evidence to determine the effectiveness of interpreter services or bilingual providers for clients with limited English proficiency in improving health care. Evidence was insufficient because only one comparative study, with limitations in the quality of execution, was available.

Cultural Competency Training for Healthcare Providers: Insufficient Evidence to Determine Effectiveness

A person's health is shaped by cultural beliefs and experiences that influence the identification and labeling of symptoms; beliefs about causality, prognosis, and prevention; and choices among treatment options. Family, social, and cultural networks reinforce these processes. Cultural competence includes the capacity to identify, understand, and respect the values and beliefs of others.

Cultural competency training is designed to (1) enhance self-awareness of attitudes towards people of different racial and ethnic groups; (2) improve care by increasing knowledge about the cultural beliefs and practices, attitudes toward health care, healthcare-seeking behaviors, and burden of various diseases in different populations served; and (3) improve skills such as communication. We searched for studies that examined the effectiveness of cultural competency training programs for healthcare providers in improving the outcomes of client satisfaction, racial or ethnic differentials in use and treatment, and health status measures.

Effectiveness

- We found insufficient evidence to determine the effectiveness of cultural competency training for healthcare providers in improving health care.
- Evidence was insufficient because only one study, with limitations in the quality of execution, was available.
- Insufficient evidence means that we were not able to determine whether or not the intervention works.

The findings of our systematic review are based on one study that examined the effectiveness of cultural competency training for healthcare professionals in improving at least one of these outcomes: client satisfaction, racial or ethnic differentials in use and treatment, or health status measures.[87] Eighty women, all lower-income African Americans who resided in the community, sought help at a counseling clinic (in a metropolitan college mental health center) or were referred by area social services agencies. Counseling staff (two white and two African-American counselors) had either received four hours of cultural sensitivity training or had received only usual training. Those clients who met with counselors who had cultural sensitivity training reported greater satisfaction with counseling than those who met with counselors in the "usual training" group (standard effect size 1.6, $p < .001$), inde-

pendent of the counselor's race. Further, those clients who met with culturally sensitive counselors returned for more sessions than did those assigned
to the other counselors (difference of 33%, $p < .001$).

Although this study's results were promising, one study with limitations in
the quality of execution is insufficient to determine the effectiveness of cultural competency training in improving client satisfaction or health status, or
in reducing racial and ethnic differences.

Because we could not establish the effectiveness of cultural competency training, we did not examine situations in which such programs would be applicable, information about economic efficiency, or possible barriers to implementation.

In conclusion, the Task Force found insufficient evidence to determine the effectiveness of cultural competency training programs for healthcare providers in improving health care because only one qualifying study, with limitations in the quality of execution, was available.

Use of Linguistically and Culturally Appropriate Health Education Materials: Insufficient Evidence to Determine Effectiveness

Culture defines how health information is received, understood, and acted
upon. Language is a powerful transmitter of culture. Nonverbal expression differs among ethnic groups. Health information messages (i.e., print materials,
videos, television or radio messages) developed for the majority population
may be inaccessible by or unsuitable for other cultural or ethnic groups.

Culturally and linguistically appropriate health education materials are designed to take into account differences in language and nonverbal communication patterns, and to be sensitive to cultural beliefs and practices.

Effectiveness

- We found insufficient evidence to determine the effectiveness of linguistically and culturally appropriate health education materials in improving
  health care.
- Evidence was insufficient because only a small number of studies, with
  limitations in the quality of execution, was available.
- Insufficient evidence means that we were not able to determine whether or
  not the intervention works.

The findings of our systematic review are based on four studies that evaluated the effectiveness of linguistically and culturally appropriate health education materials in improving client satisfaction, racial or ethnic differentials
in use of services or treatment, or health status measures.[88–91] Two other studies did not meet our quality criteria and were excluded from the review.[92,93]

All four reviewed studies examined the effectiveness of culturally sensitive health education videos among African-American or mixed African-American and Latino populations. Three studies examined HIV knowledge, attitudes, or behaviors—two among adults and one among adolescents. The remaining study examined tobacco use knowledge and behavior among adolescents.

The cultural communication techniques used in the videos included race or ethnic concordance between actors and the target audience, multicultural messages versus those targeted specifically to African Americans, and similarity in contemporary music and dress between actors and audience. Of the four studies reviewed, one reported a change in health behavior: African-American women exposed to a video specifically designed to emphasize culturally relevant values had an 18% increase ($p < .01$) in self-reported HIV testing in a two-week period after the intervention. The remaining studies included measures of satisfaction with the cultural relevance of the videos. Significant positive differences in satisfaction with the educational video and credibility of content and attractiveness of the announcer were reported. One study reported no difference in preference for a "rap" format video targeted to African-American youth over a standard video.

Although these studies showed promising results, the Task Force found that they did not provide sufficient evidence to determine whether or not linguistically and culturally appropriate health education materials are effective in improving client satisfaction or health status or in reducing racial or ethnic differences in health care.

Because we could not establish the effectiveness of these materials, we did not examine situations in which their use would be applicable, information about economic efficiency, or possible barriers to implementation.

In conclusion, the Task Force found insufficient evidence to determine the effectiveness of interventions to provide linguistically and culturally appropriate health education materials in improving health care, because only a small number of comparative studies, with limitations in the quality of execution, were available.

Culturally Specific Healthcare Settings: Insufficient Evidence to Determine Effectiveness

Healthcare settings may raise both linguistic and cultural barriers for ethnic subgroups, particularly recent immigrants with limited acculturation. People with limited English language proficiency or who are of a different ethnic group from local healthcare providers may delay seeking health care. Ethnic or culturally specific clinics for immigrant populations provide a welcoming healthcare environment for clients.

Effectiveness

- We found insufficient evidence to determine the effectiveness of culturally specific healthcare settings in improving health care.
- Evidence was insufficient because no qualifying studies could be found.
- Insufficient evidence means that we were not able to determine whether or not the intervention works.

For our systematic review, we searched for studies that evaluated the effectiveness of culturally or ethnically specific clinics and services located within the community served. No comparative studies evaluated these programs. Therefore, evidence was insufficient to determine whether or not interventions to deliver services in culturally or ethnically specific settings are effective in increasing client satisfaction or health status, or in decreasing racial or ethnic differences in health care.

Because we could not establish the effectiveness of culturally specific healthcare settings, we did not examine situations in which such programs would be applicable, information about economic efficiency, or possible barriers to implementation.

In conclusion, the Task Force found insufficient evidence to determine the effectiveness of culturally specific healthcare settings in improving health care because no qualifying studies were found.

IMPROVING HEALTH FACTORS IN THE SOCIAL ENVIRONMENT THROUGH USE OF THESE RECOMMENDATIONS

In this chapter, the Task Force recommends early childhood development programs and tenant-based rental assistance programs as ways to improve community health.

Interventions that improve children's opportunities to learn and develop capacity are particularly important for children in communities disadvantaged by high rates of poverty, violence, substance abuse, and physical and social disorder. Communities can assess the quality and availability of early childhood development programs in terms of local needs and resources, and can use the Task Force recommendation to advocate for continued or expanded funding of early childhood development programs. Current levels of federal and state funding are not adequate to support accessible quality services for the number of at-risk children who would benefit from participation.[94] Child health advocates from all disciplines can use this recommendation to develop testimony for those making policy and funding decisions about the effectiveness of these programs. Healthcare providers can use the recommendation to promote participation in an early childhood development program as part of well-child care. Public health agencies can use the recommendation to inform communities about the importance of early childhood development opportunities and their long-lasting effects on children's well-being and ability to learn.

The Task Force recommendation for use of tenant-based rental assistance programs can be used by public health agencies in conjunction with local housing authorities to inform policy makers of the effectiveness of such programs for increasing family safety in the neighborhood environment.

The Task Force made no recommendations on mixed-income housing developments or culturally competent health care.

CONCLUSION

This chapter summarizes Task Force conclusions and recommendations on interventions in the social environment to improve community health. To improve children's readiness for school and to reduce retention in grade and placement in special education, the Task Force recommends comprehensive, center-based, early childhood development programs for low-income children. To improve family safety, the Task Force recommends tenant-based rental assistance programs (voucher programs), which are effective in reducing individuals' experience of victimization and neighborhood social disorder.

Details of these reviews have been published[14,95-100] and these articles, along with additional information about the reviews, are available at www .thecommunityguide.org/social.

Acknowledgments

This chapter was written by the members of the systematic review development teams: Laurie M. Anderson, PhD, MPH, Division of Prevention Research and Analytic Methods (DPRAM), Epidemiology Program Office (EPO), Centers for Disease Control and Prevention (CDC), Olympia, Washington; Mindy T. Fullilove, MD, Columbia University, New York, New York and the Task Force on Community Preventive Services; Susan C. Scrimshaw, PhD, University of Illinois School of Public Health, Chicago and the Task Force on Community Preventive Services; Jonathan E. Fielding, MD, MPH, MBA, Los Angeles Department of Health Services, University of California School of Public Health, Los Angeles, and the Task Force on Community Preventive Services; Jacques Normand, PhD, National Institute on Drug Abuse, National Institutes of Health, Bethesda, Maryland; Carolynne Shinn, MS, DPRAM/EPO/CDC, Olympia; Joseph St. Charles, MPA, DPRAM/ EPO/CDC, Olympia.

Consultants for all topics were: Regina M. Benjamin, MD, MBA, Bayou La Batre Rural Health Clinic, Bayou La Batre, Alabama; David Chavis, PhD, Association for the Study and Development of Community, Gaithersburg, Maryland; Shelly Cooper-Ashford, Center for Multicultural Health, Seattle, Washington; Leonard J. Duhl, MD, School of Public Health, University of California, Berkeley; Ruth Enid-Zambrana, PhD, Department of Women's Studies, University of Maryland, College Park; Stephen B. Fawcette, PhD, Work Group on Health Promotion and Community Development, University of Kansas, Lawrence; Nicholas Freudenberg, DrPH, Urban Public Health, Hunter College, City University of New York, New York; Douglas Greenwell, PhD, The Atlanta Project, Atlanta, Georgia; Robert A. Hahn, PhD, MPH, DPRAM/EPO/CDC, Atlanta, Georgia; Camara P. Jones, MD, PhD, MPH, National Center for Chronic Disease Prevention and Health Promotion (NCCDPHP), CDC, Atlanta; Joan Kraft, PhD, NCCDPHP/CDC, Atlanta; Nancy Krieger, PhD, School of Public Health, Harvard University, Cambridge, Massachusetts; Robert S. Lawrence, MD, Bloomberg School of Public Health, Johns Hopkins University, Baltimore, Maryland; David V. McQueen, NCCDPHP/CDC, Atlanta; Jesus Ramirez-Valles, PhD, MPH, School of Public Health, University of Illinois, Chicago; Robert Sampson, PhD, Social Sciences Division, University of Chicago, Chicago, Illinois; Leonard S. Syme, PhD, School of Public Health, University of California, Berkeley; David R. Williams, PhD, Institute for Social Research, University of Michigan, Ann Arbor.

Articles included in the reviews were abstracted by: Kim Danforth, MPH; Maya Tholandi, MPH; Carolynne Shinn, MS; Garth Kruger, MA; Michelle Weiner, PhD; Jessie Satia, PhD; and Kathy O'Connor, MD, MPH.

References

1. Daniels N, Kennedy B, Kawachi I. Is inequality bad for our health? Boston: Beacon Press, 2000.

2. Evans RG, Barer ML, Marmor TR. Why are some people healthy and others not? The determinants of health of populations. New York: A. de Gruyter, 1994.

3. Institute of Medicine (U.S.), Committee on Health and Behavior: Research Practice and Policy. Health and behavior: the interplay of biological, behavioral, and societal influences. Smedley BD, Syme SL, eds. Washington, DC: National Academy Press, 2001.

4. Anderson L, Fullilove M, Scrimshaw S, et al. A framework for evidence-based reviews of interventions for supportive social environments. Ann N Y Acad Sci 1999;896: 487–9.

5. Link BG, Phelan J. Social conditions as fundamental causes of disease. J Health Soc Behav 1995;Spec No:80–94.

6. Elliot M. The stress process in neighborhood context. Health Place 2000;6:287–99.

7. Singer B, Ryff CD. Hierarchies of life histories and associated health risks. Ann N Y Acad Sci 1999;896:96–115.

8. McEwen BS. From molecules to mind. Stress, individual differences, and the social environment. Ann N Y Acad Sci 2001;935:42–9.

9. U.S. Department of Health and Human Services. Healthy people 2010. 2nd edition. Washington, DC: U.S. Government Printing Office, 2000.

10. U.S. Department of Education. National education goals. Available at: http://www.ed.gov/legislation/GOALS2000/TheAct/sec102.html. Accessed July 19, 2002.

11. Institute of Medicine (U.S.), Committee on Capitalizing on Social Science and Behavioral Research to Improve the Public's Health, Division of Health Promotion and Disease Prevention. Promoting health: intervention strategies from social and behavioral research. Smedley BD, Syme SL, eds. Washington, DC: National Academy Press, 2001.

12. U.S. Department of Housing and Urban Development. FY 2000-FY 2006 strategic plan. Available at: http://www.hud.gov/reform/strategicplan.pdf. Accessed June 20, 2002.

13. U.S. Department of Health and Human Services, Office of Minority Health. National standards for culturally and linguistically appropriate services in health care: final report. Available at: http://www.omhrc.gov/clas/. Accessed August 20, 2002.

14. Anderson LM, Fielding JE, Fullilove M, Scrimshaw SC, Carande-Kulis VG, Task Force on Community Preventive Services. Methods for conducting systematic reviews of the evidence of effectiveness and economic efficiency of interventions to promote healthy social environments. Am J Prev Med 2003;24(3S):25–31.

15. Levine MD. Neurodevelopmental dysfunction in the school-aged child. In: Nelson WE, Behrman RE, Kliegman RM, Arvin AM, eds. Nelson textbook of pediatrics. Philadelphia, PA: W.B. Saunders, 1996:100–7.

16. Income, socioeconomic status and health. Auerbach JA, Krimgold BK, eds. Washington, DC: National Policy Association, 2001.

17. Yeung WJ, Linver MR, Brooks-Gunn J. How money matters for young children's development: parental investment and family processes. Child Dev 2002;73(6):1861–79.

18. Power C, Hertzman C. Health, wellbeing and coping skills. In: Keating DP, Hertzman C, eds. Developmental health and the wealth of nations: social, biological, and educational dynamics. New York: Guilford Press, 1999:41–54.

19. Board on Children, Youth, and Families, Committee on Integrating the Science of Early Childhood Development. From neurons to neighborhoods: the science of early child development. Shonkoff JP, Phillips D, eds. Washington, DC: National Academy Press, 2000.

20. Barnett WS, Frede EC, Mobasher H, Mohr P. The efficacy of public preschool programs and the relationship of program quality to efficacy. Educ Eval Policy Anal 1987; 10(1):37–49.

21. Bee CK. A longitudinal study to determine if Head Start has lasting effects on school achievement. Unpublished doctoral dissertation: University of South Dakota, 1981.

22. Berrueta-Clement JR, Schweinhart LJ, Barnett WS, Epstein AS, Weikart DP. Changed lives: The effects of the Perry Preschool Program on youths through age 19. Ypsilanti, MI: High/Scope Press, 1984.

23. Bryant D, Bernier K, Taylor K, Maxwell K. The effects of Smart Start child care on kindergarten entry skills. North Carolina University, 1998. ERIC Document # ED 423 068.

24. Campbell FA, Ramey CT. Effects of early intervention on intellectual and academic achievement: a follow-up study of children from low-income families. Child Dev 1994;65:684–98.

25. Campbell FA, Ramey CT. Cognitive and school outcomes for high-risk African-American students at middle adolescence: positive effects of early intervention. Am Educ Res J 1995;32(4):743–72.

26. Copple CE, Cline MG, Smith AN. Path to the future: long-term effects of Head Start in the Philadelphia school district. Washington, DC: U.S. Department of Health and Human Services, Office of Human Development Services, Administration for Children, Youth and Families, Head Start Bureau, 1987.

27. Eisenberg L, Conners C. The effect of Headstart on developmental processes. Washington, DC: Department of Health, Education and Welfare, Office of Economic Opportunity, 1966. OEO-510.

28. Howard JL, Plant WT. Psychometric evaluation of an Operation Headstart program. J Genet Psychol 1967;111:281–8.

29. Lazar I, Darlington R. Lasting effects of early education: a report from the Consortium for Longitudinal Studies. Horowitz F, ed. Chicago: University of Chicago Press, Monographs of the Society for Research in Child Development, 1982: Serial No. 195, Vol. 47, Nos. 2–3.

30. Lee VE, Brooks-Gunn J, Schnur E. Does Head Start work? A 1-year follow-up comparison of disadvantaged children attending Head Start, no preschool, and other preschool programs. Dev Psychol 1988;24(2):210–22.

31. Lee VE, Brooks-Gunn J, Schnur E, Liaw F. Are Head Start effects sustained? A longitudinal follow-up comparison of disadvantaged children attending Head Start, no preschool, and other preschool programs. Child Dev 1990;61(2):495–507.

32. Ramey CT, Campbell FA. Poverty, early childhood education and academic competence: the Abecedarian experiment. In: Huston A, ed. Children in poverty: child development and public policy. New York: Cambridge University Press, 1991:190–221.

33. Schweinhart LJ, Weikart DP, Larner MB. Consequences of three preschool curriculum models through age 15. Early Child Res Q 1986;1:15–45.

34. Schweinhart LJ, Barnes HV, Weikart DP. Significant benefits: the High/Scope Perry Preschool study through age 27. Ypsilanti, MI: High/Scope Press, 1993.

35. Sontag M, Sella A, Thorndike R. The effect of Head Start training on the cognitive growth of disadvantaged children. J Educ Res 1969;62(9):387–9.

36. Zigler E, Abelson W, Trickett P, Seitz V. Is an intervention program necessary in order to improve economically disadvantaged children's IQ scores? Child Dev 1982;53:340–8.

37. Malakoff ME, Underhill JM, Zigler E. Influence of inner-city environment and Head Start experience on effectance motivation. Am J Orthopsychiatry 1998;68(4):630–8.

38. Sklerov AJ. The effect of preschool experience on the cognitive style of reflectivity-impulsivity of disadvantaged children. Grad Res Educ Relat Discip 1974;7(2):77–91.

39. Hale BA, Seitz V, Zigler E. Health services and Head Start: a forgotten formula. J Appl Dev Psychol 1990;11:447–58.

40. Oyemade UJ, Washington V, Gullo DF. The relationship between Head Start parental involvement and the economic and social self-sufficiency of Head Start families. J Negro Educ 1989;58(1):5–15.

41. Barnett WS. Lives in the balance: age-27 benefit-cost analysis of the High/Scope Perry Preschool Program. Ypsilanti, MI: High/Scope Press, 1996.

42. Goering J, Stebbins H, Siewert M. Promoting housing choice in HUD's rental assistance programs. Washington, DC: U.S. Department of Housing and Urban Development, 1995.

43. Maney B, Crowley S. Scarcity and success: perspectives on assisted housing. Washington, DC: National Low Income Housing Coalition, 1999.

44. Peterson G, Williams K. Housing mobility: what has it accomplished and what is its promise? Washington, DC: The Urban Institute, 1994.

45. Abt Associates. Participation and benefits in the urban Section 8 program: new construction and existing housing (2 vols.). Cambridge, MA: Abt Associates Inc., 1981.

46. Atkinson R, Hamilton W, Myers D. Economic and racial/ethnic concentration in the housing allowance demand experiment. Cambridge, MA: Abt Associates Inc, 1980.

47. Katz LF, Kling JR, Liebman JB. Moving to Opportunity in Boston: early results of

a randomized mobility experiment. Working Paper No. 441. Available at: http://www
.wws.princeton.edu/ ~ kling/mto/. Accessed July 12, 2002.

48. Katz LF, Kling JR, Liebman JB. The early impacts of Moving to Opportunity in
Boston: final report to the U.S. Department of Housing and Urban Development. Available at: http://www.wws.princeton.edu/ ~ kling/mto/. Accessed June 20, 2002.

49. Kaufman JE. Low-income black youth in white suburbs: education and employment outcomes. PhD dissertation, Northwestern University, 1991.

50. Kennedy SD. Housing Allowance Demand Experiment: final report. Cambridge,
MA: Abt Associates Inc., 1980.

51. Kennedy SD, Finkel M. Section 8 rental voucher and rental certificate utilization
study: final report. Washington, DC: U.S. Department of Housing and Urban Development, 1994.

52. Leger ML, Kennedy SD. Final comprehensive report of the freestanding housing
voucher demonstration (2 vols). Cambridge, MA: Abt Associates Inc., 1990.

53. Leventhal T, Brooks-Gunn J. Moving to Opportunity: what about the kids? Available at: http://www.wws.princeton.edu/ ~ kling/mto/. Accessed June 20, 2002.

54. Ludwig J, Duncan GJ, Pinkston JC. Neighborhood effects on economic self-
sufficiency: evidence from a randomized housing-mobility experiment. Available at:
http://www.wws.princeton.edu/ ~ kling/mto/. Accessed July 12, 2002.

55. Ludwig J, Duncan GJ, Hirschfield P. Urban poverty and juvenile crime: evidence
from a randomized housing-mobility experiment. JCPR Working Paper 158. Available at:
http://www.jcpr.org/wp/wpprofile.cfm?id=162. Accessed July 12, 2002.

56. Meaden PM. Social integration and self-esteem outcomes among low-income
black adolescents in middle-class white suburbs. PhD dissertation, Northwestern University, 1993.

57. Peroff KA, Davis CL, Jones R, Curtin RT, Marans RW. Gautreaux housing demonstration: an evaluation of its impact on participating households. U.S. Department of
Housing and Urban Development, Office of Policy Development and Research, Division
of Policy Studies, 1979.

58. Pettit B, McLanahan S, Hanratty M. Moving to Opportunity: benefits and hidden
costs. Working Paper 98–11. Available at: http://www.wws.princeton.edu/ ~ kling/mto/.
Accessed June 20, 2002.

59. Popkin S, Rosenbaum J, Meaden P. Labor market experiences of low-income
black women in middle-class suburbs: evidence from a survey of Gautreaux program
participants. J Policy Anal Manage 1993;12(3):556–73.

60. Rosenbaum E, Harris LE. Low-income families in their new neighborhoods: the
short-term effects of moving from Chicago's public housing. Available at: http://www
.wws.princeton.edu/ ~ kling/mto/chicago.htm#Chi3. Accessed June 20, 2002.

61. Rosenbaum E, Harris LE. Residential mobility and opportunities: early impacts of
the Moving to Opportunity demonstration program in Chicago. Available at: http://www
.wws.princeton.edu/ ~ kling/mto/. Accessed June 20, 2002.

62. Rosenbaum J, Popkin SJ. Economic and social impacts of housing integration.
Evanston, IL: Northwestern University Press, 1990.

63. Rosenbaum JE, Kulieke MJ, Rubinowitz LS. Low-income black children in white
suburban schools: a study of school and student responses. J Negro Educ 1987;56(1):
35–43.

64. Rosenbaum JE, Popkin SJ. Employment and earnings of low-income blacks who

move to middle-class suburbs. In: Jencks C, Peterson PE, eds. The urban underclass. Washington, DC: The Brookings Institution, 1991:342–56.

65. Rosenbaum JE, Popkin SJ, Kaufman JE, Rusin J. Social integration of low-income black adults in middle-class white suburbs. Soc Probl 1991;38(4):448–61.

66. Rusin-White J. Self-efficacy, residential integration and attainment in Gautreaux families: a longitudinal study. PhD dissertation, Northwestern University, 1993.

67. Solomon AP, Fenton CG. The nation's first experience with housing allowances: the Kansas City demonstration. Working Paper No. 23. Cambridge, MA: Joint Center for Urban Studies of M.I.T. and Harvard University, 1973.

68. Gazmararian JA, Baker DW, Williams MV, et al. Health literacy among Medicare enrollees in a managed care organization. JAMA 1999;281(6):545–51.

69. Weinick RM, Krauss NA. Racial and ethnic differences in children's access to care. Am J Public Health 2000;90(11):1771–4.

70. Woloshin S, Bickell N, Shwartz L, Gany F, Welch G. Language barriers in medicine in the United States. JAMA 1995;273(9):724–8.

71. Brach C, Fraser I. Can cultural competency reduce racial and ethnic disparities? A review and conceptual model. Med Care Res Rev 2000;57(suppl 1):181–217.

72. Schmidley AD. Profile of the foreign-born population in the United States: 2000. U.S. Census Bureau, Current Population Reports, Series P23–206. Washington, DC: U.S. Government Printing Office, 2001.

73. Institute of Medicine Board on Health Sciences Policy. Unequal treatment: confronting racial and ethnic disparities in healthcare. Smedley BD, Stith AY, Nelson AR, eds. Washington, DC: National Academy Press, 2002.

74. Geiger JH. Racial stereotyping and medicine: the need for cultural competence. Can Med Assoc J 2001;164(12):1699–700.

75. Giles WH, Anda RF, Casper ML, Esconbedo LG, Taylor HA. Race and sex differences in rates of invasive cardiac procedures in U.S. hospitals. Data from the National Hospital Discharge Survey. Arch Intern Med 1995;155:318–24.

76. Shiefer SE, Escarce JJ, Schulman KA. Race and sex differences in the management of coronary artery disease. Am Heart J 2000;139:848–57.

77. Todd KH, Samaroo N, Hoffman JR. Ethnicity as a risk factor for inadequate emergency department analgesia. JAMA 1993;269:1537–9.

78. Bach PB, Cramer LD, Warren JL, Begg CB. Racial differences in the treatment of early-stage lung cancer. N Engl J Med 1999;341:1198–205.

79. Young AS, Klap R, Sherbourne CD, Wells KB. The quality of care for depressive and anxiety disorders in the United States. Arch Gen Psychiatry 2001;58:55–61.

80. Sambamoorthi U, Moynihan PJ, McSpiritt E, Crystal S. Use of protease inhibitors and non-nucleoside reverse transcriptase inhibitors among Medicaid beneficiaries with AIDS. Am J Public Health 2001;91:1474–81.

81. LaVeist TA, Nickerson KJ, Bowie JV. Attitudes about racism, medical mistrust and satisfaction with care among African American and white cardiac patients. Med Care Res Rev 2000;57(suppl 1):146–61.

82. Lillie-Blanton M, Brodie M, Rowland D, Altman D, McIntosh M. Race, ethnicity and the health care system: public perceptions and experiences. Med Care Res Rev 2000; 57(1):218–35.

83. O'Malley AS, Forrest CB, Mandelblatt J. Adherence of low-income women to cancer screening recommendations. J Gen Intern Med 2002;17(2):144–54.

84. Ong LM, de Haes JC, Hoos AM, Lammes FB. Doctor-patient communication: a review of the literature. Soc Sci Med 1995;40(7):903–18.

85. Sarver J, Baker D. Effect of language barriers on follow-up appointments after an emergency department visit. J Intern Med 2000;15(4):256–64.

86. Enguidanos ER, Rosen P. Language as a factor affecting follow-up compliance from an emergency department. J Emerg Med 1997;15(1):9–12.

87. Wade P, Bernstein B. Culture sensitivity training and counselor's race: effects on black female client's perceptions and attrition. J Couns Psychol 1991;38(1):9–15.

88. Herek GM, Gillis JR, Glunt EK, Lewis J, Welton D, Capitanio JP. Culturally sensitive AIDS educational videos for African American audiences: effects of source, message, receiver, and context. Am J Community Psychol 1998;26(5):705–43.

89. Kalichman SC, Kelly JA, Hunter TL, Murphy DA, Tyler R. Culturally tailored HIV-AIDS risk-reduction messages targeted to African American urban women: impact on risk sensitization and risk reduction. J Consult Clin Psychol 1993;61(2):291–5.

90. Stevenson HC, Davis G. Impact of culturally sensitive AIDS video education on the AIDS risk knowledge of African-American adolescents. AIDS Educ Prev 1994;6(1):40–52.

91. Sussman S, Parker VC, Lopes C, Crippens DL, Elder P, Scholl D. Empirical development of brief smoking prevention videotapes which target African-American adolescents. Int J Addict 1995;30(9):1141–64.

92. Stevenson HC, Gay KM, Josar L. Culturally sensitive AIDS education and perceived AIDS risk knowledge: reaching the "know-it-all" teenager. AIDS Educ Prev 1995;7(2):134–44.

93. Lavizzo-Mourey R, Smith V, Sims R, Taylor L. Hearing loss: an educational and screening program for African-American and Latino elderly. J Natl Med Assoc 1994;86(1):53–9.

94. Shumacher R, Greenberg M, Lombardi J. State initiatives to promote early learning: next steps in coordinating subsidized child care, Head Start, and state kindergarten. Policy brief. Washington, DC: Center for Law and Social Policy, 2001.

95. Centers for Disease Control and Prevention. Community interventions to promote healthy social environments: early childhood development and family housing. A report on recommendations of the Task Force on Community Preventive Services. MMWR 2002;51(RR-1):1–8.

96. Anderson LM, Scrimshaw SC, Fullilove MT, Fielding JE, Task Force on Community Preventive Services. The Community Guide's model for linking the social environment to health. Am J Prev Med 2003;24(3S):12–20.

97. Task Force on Community Preventive Services. Recommendations to promote healthy social environments. Am J Prev Med 2003;24(3S):21–4.

98. Anderson LM, Shinn C, Fullilove MT, et al. The effectiveness of early childhood development programs: a systematic review. Am J Prev Med 2003;24(3S):32–46.

99. Anderson LM, St Charles J, Fullilove MT, et al. Providing affordable family housing and reducing residential segregation by income: a systematic review. Am J Prev Med 2003;24(3S):47–67.

100. Anderson LM, Scrimshaw SC, Fullilove MT, Fielding JE, Normand J, Task Force on Community Preventive Services. Culturally competent healthcare systems: a systematic review. Am J Prev Med 2003;24(3S):68–79.

Part II

Reducing Disease, Injury, and Impairment

Chapter 4

Cancer

Cancer is a leading cause of death in the United States (second only to heart disease), accounting for more than one in four deaths nationally and more than an estimated 1500 deaths every day.[1] Many cancer deaths can be prevented: for example, all deaths related to cigarette smoking (estimated to be more than 180,000 in 2004) could be prevented.[2,3] About one-third of the half million cancer deaths expected in 2004 could be prevented by adopting a healthy

---

*Insufficient evidence means that we were not able to determine whether or not the intervention works.

The Task Force approved the recommendations in this chapter for reducing exposure to ultraviolet radiation in 2001–2002. The research on which the findings are based was conducted prior to July 2001. This information has been published in the MMWR Recommendations and Reports series [2003; 52(no. RR-15):1–12] and the American Journal of Preventive Medicine [2004; in press]. The Task Force considered the evidence on effectiveness of interventions to increase informed decision making in cancer screening in 2003, and this information has been published in the American Journal of Preventive Medicine, 2004;26(1):67–80.

diet, maintaining a healthy weight and increasing physical activity,[2-6] reducing heavy drinking, and other changes in lifestyle. Cancers related to exposure to infectious diseases, such as hepatitis B or human immunodeficiency virus (HIV), can be prevented through vaccines or behavior change.[1] Regular screening by healthcare professionals can also detect certain cancers early in their course, thereby increasing the likelihood of successful treatment.[7-13]

Systematic reviews for the *Community Guide* explore many population-based interventions that can help reduce the incidence of, reduce the consequences of, or improve decisions about cancer. This chapter includes reviews about (*1*) reducing skin cancer by limiting exposure to ultraviolet (UV) radiation and (*2*) promoting informed decision making about cancer screening. Chapter 7 (Oral Health) finds that evidence was insufficient to determine whether community approaches to detecting oral and pharyngeal cancers improve outcomes. Other chapters evaluate approaches to improving health by increasing the number of people who quit smoking and reducing the number who start (Chapter 1, Tobacco); increasing physical activity (Chapter 2, Physical Activity); and increasing coverage with vaccines including the hepatitis B vaccine (Chapter 6, Vaccine-Preventable Diseases). Systematic reviews for the *Community Guide* are also underway on population-based approaches for increasing use of effective cancer screening, reducing obesity, improving nutrition, reducing the number of HIV-infected people, and reducing abuse of alcohol.

PREVENTING SKIN CANCER BY REDUCING EXPOSURE TO ULTRAVIOLET RADIATION

Skin cancer is the most common type of cancer in the United States.[14] The two most common types of skin cancer—basal cell carcinoma and squamous cell carcinoma—both respond well to treatment. Melanoma, the third most common type of skin cancer, is much more likely to be fatal. Estimates for 2004 indicated that more than 1 million people would be diagnosed as having basal cell or squamous cell carcinoma, and approximately 2300 deaths from both cancers combined were predicted. In contrast, an estimated 55,100 diagnoses of melanoma will account for 7910 deaths—more than three-quarters of all skin cancer fatalities.[1]

Reducing the Risk of Skin Cancer

Preventable risk factors for skin cancer include excessive exposure to UV radiation, especially during childhood and adolescence. Sunlight is the primary source of UV radiation. (Sunlamps and tanning beds are other sources.) People with high levels of exposure to UV radiation are at greater risk for all three major forms of skin cancer, and approximately 65% – 90% of melanomas are caused by UV exposure.[15] Exposure to UV radiation during childhood and adolescence plays a role in the future development of both melanoma and basal cell cancer.[16-21] The risk of developing melanoma is strongly related to a history of one or more sunburns (an indicator of intense UV exposure) in childhood or adolescence.[17,22-24] Sunburns during these periods have also recently been found to increase the risk of basal cell carcinoma.[19,20]

Moles are an important risk factor for skin cancer, and most moles develop during childhood. Sun exposure in childhood may heighten the risk of melanoma by increasing the number of moles.[23] Sun protection during childhood may therefore reduce the risk of melanoma in adulthood.[25,26]

"Sun-protective" behaviors that reduce skin cancer risk include limiting or minimizing exposure to the sun during peak hours (10 A.M. to 4 P.M.), when UV rays are more intense; wearing protective clothing; and using appropriate sunscreen protection. As noted in more detail below, however, sunscreens may not protect against melanoma, should not be used as the sole method for skin cancer prevention, and should not be used as a means to extend the duration of UV exposure.

Environmental factors can also affect the amount of UV exposure. These include proximity to the equator; high altitude; low levels of cloud coverage (which can allow up to 80% of UV rays to penetrate the atmosphere); the presence of materials that reflect the sun, such as pavement, water, snow, and sand; exposure to the sun around midday; and spending time outside in the spring or summer.[27,28]

OBJECTIVES AND RECOMMENDATIONS FROM OTHER ADVISORY GROUPS

Two goals of *Healthy People 2010*[29] are to (*1*) increase to 75% the proportion of people who use at least one of the following protective measures that may reduce the risk of skin cancer: avoid the sun between 10 A.M. and 4 P.M., wear sun-protective clothing when exposed to the sun, use sunscreen with a sun protection factor (SPF) of 15 or higher, and avoid artificial sources of UV light; and (*2*) reduce melanoma deaths to less than 2.5 per 100,000 people.

Recommendations for sunscreen use, including recommended public health strategies, are available from the International Agency for Research on Cancer (IARC).[30] Specifically, because the relationship between sunscreen use and melanoma is complex, the IARC recommends that sunscreens not be used as the sole method for skin cancer prevention and not be used as a means to extend the duration of UV exposure.

The Centers for Disease Control and Prevention (CDC) recommends that schools engage in skin cancer prevention activities.[31] The U.S. Preventive

Services Task Force found insufficient evidence to determine whether clinician counseling was effective in getting patients to change their behavior and thereby reduce skin cancer risk.[32]

METHODS

Methods used for the reviews are summarized in Chapter 10. Specific methods used in the systematic reviews of interventions to prevent skin cancer through reducing exposure to UV radiation have been described elsewhere.[33] An example of the kind of conceptual model we used to guide our reviews is presented in Figure 4–1, which shows the analytic framework for the reviews of mass media campaigns to reduce UV exposure and increase sun-protective behaviors. These reviews used the key health outcomes (e.g., sunburn or nevi [moles]) and sun-protective behaviors of limiting or minimizing exposure to the sun during peak hours (10 A.M. to 4 P.M.), wearing protective clothing, and seeking shade to measure the success of programs and policies and to support recommendations. Changes in knowledge, attitudes, or intentions were not used to support recommendations.

ECONOMIC EFFICIENCY

A systematic review of available economic evaluations was conducted for each of the two recommended interventions, and no economic evaluations were found for either one. The methods used to conduct those economics reviews are summarized in Chapter 11.

RECOMMENDATIONS AND FINDINGS

Interventions in Specific Settings

Many skin cancer prevention activities are carried out in specific settings. These settings are often convenient ways of organizing intervention activities for specific interveners and target populations.

We reviewed six interventions carried out in specific settings. Four were educational and policy interventions—in child care centers, primary schools, secondary schools and colleges, and recreational and tourism settings—and two were programs—in outdoor occupational settings and in healthcare system and provider settings.

Most sun-safety programs have been evaluated in formal educational settings. Such settings facilitate integration of skin cancer education into existing learning situations as well as supporting policy and environmental interventions.

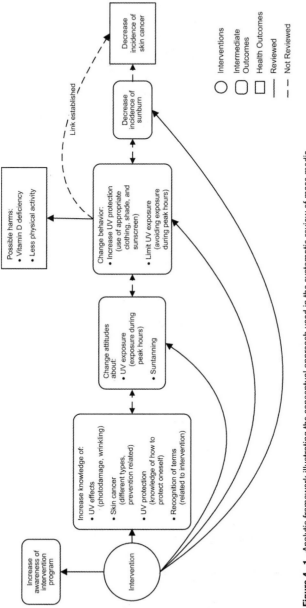

Figure 4–1. Analytic framework illustrating the conceptual approach used in the systematic review of mass media campaigns to reduce ultraviolet (UV) exposure and increase sun-protective behaviors.

Educational and Policy Interventions in Primary Schools: Recommended (Sufficient Evidence of Effectiveness) for Improving Children's "Covering-Up" Behaviors

Interventions in primary schools promote sun-protective behaviors among children in kindergarten through eighth grade. These interventions include at least one of the following activities: providing information to children (through instruction, small media education, or both); influencing children's behavior (e.g., modeling, demonstration, or role playing); attempting to change the knowledge, attitudes, or behavior of caregivers (e.g., teachers or parents); and environmental and policy approaches (e.g., providing sunscreen, increasing availability of shade, or scheduling outdoor activities to avoid hours of peak sunlight).

Effectiveness

- Educational and policy interventions in primary schools are effective in improving children's sun-protective behavior of covering up.

Applicability

- These findings should be applicable to most school-age children.

Students spend a large part of their day in school or in school-related activities during hours of peak ultraviolet (UV) light. Children are more receptive than adolescents to practicing sun-protective behaviors and are more amenable to parents' or other adults' instruction. Primary schools are therefore more likely than high schools to have success with sun-protection programs.

The findings of our systematic review are based on 20 studies.[34–53] An additional five studies[54] were identified but did not meet our quality criteria and were excluded from the review. Eight reports provided additional information on studies already included in the review.[55–62] Many of the reports included several intervention arms and multiple behavioral outcomes.

These studies examined improvements in four sun-protective behaviors: (1) covering up (wearing hats, long-sleeved clothing, or pants); (2) using sunscreen; (3) avoiding the sun (seeking shade, rescheduling activities, not going out in the sun during peak UV hours); and (4) composite behaviors (a combination of at least two of the above behaviors). We found consistent improvement in covering-up behaviors but not in any of the other three behaviors.

Intervention activities used included didactic classroom teaching, didactic teaching using sunscreen samples, interactive class and home-based activities, health fairs, an educational picture book, teaching by medical students, interactive CD-ROM multimedia programs, and peer education. Relatively few studies included environmental or policy approaches.

Study design markedly affected changes in study outcomes. For sun-avoidance behaviors, we found a median change that ranged from 4% (for concurrent comparison groups) to 16% (for before-and-after measures). For covering-up behaviors, the median change ranged from 25% (concurrent comparison) to 70% (before-and-after). For sunscreen use, the median change ranged from 17% (concurrent comparison) to 34% (before-and-after). The improvement in covering-up behaviors was consistent and large enough for the Task Force to recommend educational and policy interventions in primary schools as an effective approach for preventing skin cancer.

In general, these interventions also improved knowledge and attitudes related to sunscreen use and to skin cancer prevention. Evidence was insufficient to determine the effectiveness of interventions to improve other sun-protective behaviors because of inconsistent results. Evidence was also insufficient to determine the effectiveness of interventions in primary schools to change policies and practices or health outcomes based on small numbers of studies and limitations in their design and execution.

These findings should be applicable to most school-age children. Studies were conducted in geographically diverse areas including Arizona, North Carolina, Canada, France, and Australia. Most studies were conducted among primarily white populations.

We found no information on other potential benefits of these interventions, such as reduction in the risk of overexposure to heat. One paper reported on the potential harm of transmitting lice via hats or other clothing and found that hats were not a major factor in transmission.[63]

We did not find any economic evaluations of these interventions.

A potential barrier to implementation of educational and policy interventions in primary schools might be concerns of parents or teachers that these changes will lead to reductions in physical activity. Parents or teachers may also be concerned that covering up will lead to wearing of gang insignia, although this is perhaps less of a concern in primary schools than in secondary schools. (Until recently, California schools did not permit students to wear clothing such as hats because of concerns about gang affiliation. Now students in California can wear hats.)

In conclusion, available studies provide sufficient evidence that interventions in primary schools are effective in improving covering-up behavior. Evidence was insufficient to determine effectiveness in improving the other two sun-protective behaviors (i.e., using sunscreen, avoiding the sun) because of inconsistent evidence; evidence was also insufficient to determine effectiveness in decreasing sunburns. These findings should be applicable to most school-age children.

Educational and Policy Interventions in Recreational and Tourism Settings: Recommended (Sufficient Evidence of Effectiveness) for Improving Adults' Covering-Up Behaviors

Interventions in recreational and tourism settings involve efforts to promote the sun-protective behaviors of adults, children, and their parents. These interventions include at least one of the following: providing information to children and adults (i.e., through instruction, small media education, or both); activities intended to change the knowledge, attitudes, beliefs, or intentions of children and adults; additional activities to influence the behavior of children and adults (such as modeling, demonstration, or role playing); and environmental or policy approaches, including providing sunscreen or shade or scheduling outdoor activities to avoid hours of peak sunlight.

Effectiveness

- Educational and policy interventions in recreational and tourism settings are effective in increasing adults' sun-protective behavior of covering up.
- We found insufficient evidence to determine the effectiveness of the interventions in reducing sunburn in adults or children.

Applicability

- These findings should be widely applicable to adults in most settings.

Domestic and international travel has increased substantially over the past decade, particularly among overseas vacationers traveling from temperate climates to regions where the UV level is high.[64] Participation in outdoor leisure activities has also increased, resulting in increased exposure to sunlight, which appears to increase the risk of melanoma.[65] Recreational and tourism settings are therefore important sites for sun-protection programs. In such settings, skin cancer education can be integrated into existing recreational or tourism activities, and supportive policy and environmental interventions can also be implemented.

The findings of our systematic review are based on 11 studies[66–76] that evaluated the effectiveness of reducing UV exposure through educational and policy interventions in recreational and tourism settings. We identified two other reports[77,78] that did not meet our quality criteria and were excluded from the review. Another five reports[79–83] provided additional information on studies already included in the review.

Intervention activities for both children and adults included interactive sun-protection education activities (stories, games, puzzles, stamps, arts and crafts); activities to promote sun-safe environments; a UV-reduction curriculum at poolside; home-based activities for children and their parents; brochures to help educate participants about the prevalence and severity of skin cancer, the effects of the sun on the skin, or sun-protective measures; a sun sensitivity assessment, photographs providing examples of sun damage to skin, and suggestions on reducing unprotected UV exposure; and peer-leader modeling by lifeguards, informational posters and fliers, posters listing goals, and a "commitment raffle" to influence the sun-protective behaviors of children and adults.

The outcomes examined were similarly wide-ranging, and included changes in parent-reported sun-protective behaviors among children (using sunscreen; seeking shade; wearing a hat, shirt, or other protective clothing; and composite behaviors); incidence of children's sunburns; children's degree of tanness; adult sun-protective behaviors; incidence of adult sunburn; and adult information-seeking behaviors, follow-up study participation, knowledge, attitudes, beliefs, or intentions; as well as sun-protective measures and environmental supports reported by parents at outdoor recreational centers or swimming pools.

The adult sun-protective behavior of wearing protective clothing (hat or shirt) increased by a median of 11.2% (interquartile range, 5.1% to 12.9%) in five arms of three reports. This increase is the basis for recommending use of this intervention. Three other outcomes were evaluated, but none provided sufficient evidence to determine the effectiveness of the intervention: the evidence of effectiveness in reducing the adult incidence of sunburn and increasing children's sun-protective behaviors was inconsistent and, although children's sunburn decreased in two arms of one report by about 41.2%, the single study did not provide sufficient evidence for a recommendation.

We also measured several outcomes that would not, by themselves, form the basis for a recommendation. Five arms from four reports showed a 9.8% increase in children's sunscreen use and a 15.4% increase in composite sun-protective behaviors. We found inconsistent effects on adults' information-seeking behavior; follow-up study participation; knowledge; attitudes or beliefs; or intentions. Available reports also demonstrated inconsistent effects of the intervention on sun-protective measures and environmental supports at outdoor recreational centers or swimming pools.

These findings should be applicable to a wide variety of settings and populations. Studies were conducted in Australia, England, Hawaii, Southern California, Virginia, and New England. Study participants' ages ranged from 6.5 to 79 years (median 31.5 years). Most of the reports that identified race or ethnicity were conducted with a predominantly white population; three reports involved Hawaiian or Asian/Pacific Islander populations. Of the reports that identified gender, most studies were conducted among predominantly female populations. Annual household income of study participants ranged from $20,000 to greater than $90,000. Only one study reported educational level; in this study, 88% of the participants were high school graduates.

The studies in this review did not include information on other potential benefits or harms of these interventions. Benefits may include reaching populations not otherwise exposed to skin cancer prevention and reducing the risk of overexposure to heat and UV radiation that comes from over-reliance on sunscreen. Potential negative effects include reduction in outdoor physical activity.

We did not find any economic evaluations of educational and policy interventions in recreational and tourism settings.

Potential barriers to implementation include the limited time that recreational center staff may have to implement the special activity component of an intervention[69] and limitations imposed by swimming class schedules.[68] Additionally, some in the tourism trade might worry that sun-safety concerns could adversely affect their business and would therefore be unwilling to partner in these efforts.

In conclusion, the Task Force recommends educational and policy interventions in recreational and tourism settings on the basis of sufficient evidence of effectiveness in improving the adult sun-protective behavior of covering up. Evidence was insufficient to determine the effectiveness of the intervention in reducing sunburns in adults and children, because results were inconsistent (adults' sunburns) or too few studies were available (children's sunburns). Available reports also demonstrate evidence of effectiveness of the intervention in changing children's sun-protective behaviors, including sunscreen use and composite sun-protective behaviors; these, however, are not outcomes that form the basis for a recommendation. These findings should be applicable to a wide range of settings and populations.

Educational and Policy Interventions in Child Care Centers: Insufficient Evidence to Determine Effectiveness

Interventions in child care centers involve efforts to promote the sun-protective behaviors of children under five years of age. These interventions include at least one of the following: providing information directly or indirectly to the children (through instruction or small media education); additional activities to influence children's behavior (modeling, demonstration, or role playing); activities intended to change the knowledge, attitudes, or behavior of teachers, parents, and other caregivers; and environmental or policy approaches (such as providing sunscreen and shade or scheduling outdoor activities to avoid hours of peak sunlight).

Effectiveness

- We found insufficient evidence to determine the effectiveness of educational and policy interventions in child care centers in reducing children's adverse health effects or changing children's behavior related to sun exposure, in changing caregivers' behavior related to sun exposure, or in changing policies and practices in child care centers.
- Evidence was insufficient because of the small number of studies, lack of relevant outcomes, and inconsistent results.
- Insufficient evidence means that we were not able to determine whether or not the intervention works.

Much of lifetime sun exposure occurs in childhood.[84,85] Sun exposure varies among infants and preschool-age children and is largely dependent on the discretion of parents and other adult care providers. Studies have found that parental protective behaviors often depend on whether the child tends to sunburn and that parents most often rely on sunscreen for protection.[86–91] As children progress from infancy to childhood, increased mobility and a greater tendency to play outdoors often lead to increased UV exposure.[92]

Child care centers also represent an important, although often missed, opportunity to reduce children's UV exposure by providing shady play areas or scheduling outdoor activities during non-peak UV hours.[93]

The findings of our systematic review are based on two studies.[93,94] Two additional studies were identified but did not meet our quality criteria and were excluded from the review.[95,96] One report evaluated the "Be Sunsafe" curriculum (interactive classroom and take-home activities that promote covering up, finding shade, and asking for sunscreen) but did not evaluate behavioral or policy outcomes. The other study used a workshop for staff, an activity packet for parents, and a working session to develop skin protection plans for centers to focus on increasing application of sunscreen, scheduling activities to avoid peak sun, increasing availability of shade, and encouraging children to play in shady areas and to wear protective clothing. This study did not show statistically significant effects on policy outcomes or measures of children's behavior. Although both studies showed generally consistent and statistically significant improvements in knowledge, the small number of studies, with inconsistencies in results and few measures of key outcomes, provided insufficient evidence to determine the effectiveness of this intervention.

Because we could not establish the effectiveness of this intervention, we did not examine situations where it would be applicable, information about economic efficiency, or possible barriers to implementation.

The reviewed reports did not include information on other potential benefits of these interventions, such as reduction in the risk of overexposure to heat, or on potential harms, such as reduction in outdoor physical activity or transmission of lice via hats or other clothing.

In conclusion, the Task Force found insufficient evidence to determine the effectiveness of educational and policy interventions in child care centers in reducing children's adverse health effects or changing children's behavior related to sun exposure, changing caregivers' behavior related to sun exposure, or changing policies and practices in child care centers. Evidence was insufficient because of (1) limitations in the design and execution of available studies, (2) small numbers of qualifying studies, (3) variability in the interventions evaluated, (4) very short follow-up times, and (5) little substantial or statistically significant improvement in outcomes other than knowledge and attitudes.

Educational and Policy Interventions in Secondary Schools and Colleges: Insufficient Evidence to Determine Effectiveness

Interventions in secondary schools and colleges are potentially important, because adolescents and young adults are more likely to be exposed to UV radiation than younger children and are less likely to adopt sun-protective behaviors; parents and caretakers have less influence in promoting sun protection; and high schools and colleges can provide an infrastructure to support intervention activities. Some data indicate that, although young people know about the potential dangers of unprotected sun exposure, as adolescents they are likely to engage in high-risk behaviors; this presents a unique challenge to health educators.[97-99] Overall, sun-protection programs have reported more success in improving sun-protective practices for infants (provided by parents) and among younger children but less success among adolescents.[98] As primary school children transition to secondary schools, efforts to establish sun-protection education, supportive environments, and policies are difficult to sustain effectively.[100]

Effectiveness

- We found insufficient evidence to determine the effectiveness of interventions in secondary schools or colleges in changing behavior or reducing adverse health effects related to UV exposure.
- Evidence was insufficient because of limitations in the design and execution of available studies, small numbers of qualifying studies, variability in interventions and evaluated outcomes, and short follow-up times.
- Insufficient evidence means that we were not able to determine whether or not the intervention works.

Interventions in secondary schools and colleges involve efforts to promote sun-protective behaviors among adolescents and young adults. These interventions include at least one of the following: providing information to adolescents and young adults through instruction, small media, or both; activities to influence the behavior of adolescents and young adults, such as modeling, demonstration, or role playing; activities intended to change the knowledge, attitudes, or behavior of caregivers (i.e., teachers or parents); and environmental and policy approaches (e.g., providing sunscreen and shade, or scheduling outdoor activities to avoid hours of peak sunlight).

The findings of our systematic review are based on 13 reports[51,101–112] on the effectiveness of educational and policy interventions in secondary schools and colleges. We identified four additional reports,[49,50,113,114] but they did not meet our quality criteria and were excluded from the review. Intervention activities used in these studies included didactic classroom teaching combined with some interactive classroom- and home-based activities; Internet-based activities; small media; and provision of sunscreen samples, extra class credit, or money. One study used a strategy of information dissemination and support of school staff to facilitate policy implementation.

Only four reports (six intervention arms) examined changes in sun-protective behavior or policy, and each report measured different sun-protective behaviors (amount of time spent in the sun, sunscreen use, measure of a composite behavior, and self-reported practices). The inconsistency of the interventions undertaken and outcomes measured did not allow us to determine the effectiveness of the interventions.

We did not conduct formal quantitative analyses of the intermediate outcomes of knowledge, attitudes, or intentions. Nine intervention arms generally showed an increase in knowledge as a result of the intervention. Seven intervention arms measured attitudes and beliefs, with inconsistent results, and seven measured intentions (the majority of which looked only at the intention to use sunscreen); these results were also inconsistent.

Because we could not establish the effectiveness of this intervention, we did not examine situations where it would be applicable, information about economic efficiency, or possible barriers to implementation.

In conclusion, the Task Force found insufficient evidence to determine the effectiveness of interventions in secondary schools or colleges to reduce adverse health effects or to change behavior related to UV exposure. Evidence was insufficient because of (*1*) limitations in the design and execution of available studies, (*2*) small numbers of qualifying studies, (*3*) variability in interventions and evaluated outcomes, and (*4*) short follow-up times.

Programs in Outdoor Occupational Settings: Insufficient Evidence to Determine Effectiveness

Programs in outdoor occupational settings promote sun-protective behaviors among workers. These interventions include at least one of the following: providing information to workers (instruction, education through small media, or both); additional activities intended to change the knowledge, attitudes, beliefs, intentions, or behaviors of workers (i.e., modeling or demonstration); and environmental or policy approaches, including providing sunscreen and shade.

Effectiveness

- We found insufficient evidence to determine the effectiveness of interventions in outdoor occupational settings in reducing UV exposure and promoting sun-protective behaviors.
- Evidence was insufficient because too few reports were available, and those reports provided inconsistent results.
- Insufficient evidence means that we were not able to determine whether or not the intervention works.

The receipt of information about preventing skin cancer is crucial for outdoor workers in the United States. According to the Census Bureau, over 8% of the U.S. national workforce (over 9 million workers) works primarily outdoors, in such occupations as construction, farming, forestry, fishing, land surveying and mapping, gardening, groundskeeping, mail delivery, and amusement park or recreational center attendants.[115] From both scientific and programmatic perspectives, occupational settings are ideal sites for sun-protection programs. High rates of nonmelanoma (basal cell and squamous cell) skin cancer have been found among occupational groups that work outdoors, and these rates are significantly associated with cumulative UV exposure.[116,117] Outdoor workers may receive up to six to eight times the dose of UV radiation that indoor workers receive.[117] A recent Canadian survey[118] found low levels of sun protection among outdoor workers: 44% seek shade, 38% avoid the sun, 58% wear a hat or protective clothing, and 18% to 23% reported using sunscreen while at work. Because outdoor workers receive intense, prolonged exposure to the sun and are at increased risk of developing squamous cell cancer, interventions that educate these workers and modify their work environment are well suited to the workplace and could provide substantial benefit.

The findings of our systematic review are based on eight studies that evaluated the effectiveness of interventions in outdoor occupational settings.[68,72,82,121–125] Three reports provided additional information on studies already included in the review.[79,80,119] Another three reports were identified but did not meet our quality criteria and were excluded from the review.[77,120,126]

The reports in our review involved numerous intervention activities: providing sun-safety training to workers, sun-protection and skin cancer education sessions and skin exams by a physician, promoting covering-up behaviors, role modeling by lifeguards or aquatics instructors, providing sun protection products to outdoor workers (e.g., sunglasses, brimmed hat, and sunscreen), using educational brochures designed for men over the age of 45 and a body chart for self-assessment of pigmented lesions to educate male workers about skin cancer, and use of environmental supports (sunscreen dispensers and shade structures) to promote sun-protective behavior.

The reports also evaluated a variety of outcomes: changes in sun-protective behaviors and UV exposure, incidence of sunburn, knowledge, attitudes or beliefs, and environmental policies at pools. The reports provided insufficient evidence to determine the effectiveness of the intervention in increasing the sun-protective behaviors of covering up or seeking shade, or in decreasing the incidence of sunburn and UV exposure, because of inconsistent results and the limited number of studies that measured outcomes that could form the basis for a recommendation. Three arms from two reports examining sun protection demonstrated desirable effects of the intervention on sun-safety measures and environmental supports (provision of sunscreen dispensers and portable shade structures) at recreational centers and swimming pools. Six arms from five reports demonstrated inconsistent effects on knowledge, and five arms from four reports demonstrated inconsistent effects on attitudes or beliefs.

Because we could not establish the effectiveness of this intervention, we did not examine situations where it would be applicable, information about economic efficiency, or possible barriers to implementation.

Reviewed studies did not include information on other potential effects of these interventions. Other positive effects might include reaching populations who are not otherwise exposed to skin cancer prevention and reducing the risk of overexposure to heat. Potential negative effects of the intervention might include worker requests for reduction in time spent working outdoors.

In conclusion, available reports provide insufficient evidence to determine the effectiveness of interventions in outdoor occupational settings in reducing UV exposure and promoting sun-protective behaviors because of too few reports and inconsistent evidence. Although available reports show that the intervention is effective in improving some sun-protective measures and environmental supports at outdoor recreational centers and swimming pools, this does not necessarily result in decreased UV exposure or better health.

Programs in Healthcare System and Provider Settings:
Insufficient Evidence to Determine Effectiveness

Interventions to reduce UV exposure and promote sun-protective behaviors can take place in healthcare settings (e.g., pharmacies, drugstores, clinics, physicians' offices, and medical schools) or can target healthcare providers (e.g., physicians, nurses, physicians' assistants, medical students, and pharmacists). In our systematic review, we included studies of interventions promoting primary prevention among populations at average risk for skin cancer. Studies usually included at least one of the following: (*1*) activities aimed at providers to increase knowledge or change attitudes and intentions, to increase positive role modeling for patients and clients, or to increase counseling behaviors or information provision to patients and clients or (*2*) activities placed within a healthcare setting to promote increased knowledge and improved attitudes and intentions about sun-protective behaviors among patients and clients, to promote provision of information about skin cancer to patients and clients, and to increase sun-protective behaviors among patients and clients. Our review did not evaluate interventions that focused on early detection of skin cancers or on interventions intended for people who are thought to be at higher than average risk of skin cancer, such as people who have already been diagnosed with one skin cancer.

Effectiveness

- We found insufficient evidence to determine the effectiveness of programs in healthcare system and provider settings in reducing clients' UV exposure or increasing their sun-protective behaviors.
- Evidence was insufficient because of inconsistent results among studies that evaluated these outcomes.
- Insufficient evidence means that we were not able to determine whether or not the intervention works.

People in the United States make an average of 1.7 visits to primary care providers annually,[127] and surveys consistently show that healthcare providers are a trusted and important source of health information. For these reasons, healthcare providers and systems have a special opportunity to affect population knowledge, attitudes, and beliefs about reducing UV exposure and increasing sun-protective behaviors. Through increasing knowledge, changing attitudes and intentions, role-modeling behaviors, and even establishing policies, healthcare providers and healthcare settings can greatly influence the behavior of the people who use their services.

According to the U.S. Preventive Services Task Force (USPSTF),[32] evidence was insufficient to recommend for or against regular counseling by primary care clinicians to decrease sun exposure, avoid sun lamps, use sunscreen or protective clothing, or practice skin self-examination. Our review expands on that of the USPSTF by evaluating a broader range of providers and by including system approaches not limited to providers.

The findings of our systematic review are based on 11 reports[61,128–137] on the effectiveness of interventions oriented to providers and healthcare systems. An additional nine reports[56,129,138–144] were identified but did not meet our quality criteria and were excluded from the review. One report[145] provided additional information on a study already included in the review.

The target audiences of the reviewed interventions were diverse, as was the content of the interventions and the media by which they were delivered. Studies targeting healthcare providers evaluated brief educational sessions for physicians and house staff in a large urban teaching hospital; evaluated a didactic skin cancer prevention module aimed specifically at nurses; provided a skin cancer prevention curriculum for medical students; taught physicians through a triage curriculum (teaching providers when to act on symptoms presented by patients, when to reassure patients, and when to track patients' conditions) how to implement and manage basic skin cancer control practices; used the Internet to train physicians, medical students, and house staff about skin cancer; taught medical students about skin cancer control and then sent them to elementary school classrooms to teach school-children about skin cancer control; and used videotapes and role-modeling training procedures to teach and encourage pharmacists to engage their clients in more skin cancer control behaviors.

Studies oriented to clients in healthcare settings used community drug-stores to promote the message of appropriate sunscreen use and the concept of *sun protective factor* (SPF); used a physician's waiting room to recruit and educate people about the importance of sunscreen; and tested the effects of different message content and sources of messages on client behaviors.

Only two of the studies in our review assessed the outcomes of reducing UV exposure or increasing sun-protective behaviors, and results were inconsistent in direction and statistical significance. Because of the small number of studies and inconsistency in the findings, the evidence was insufficient to determine whether or not programs in healthcare and provider settings are effective in reducing exposure to UV radiation or increasing sun-protective behaviors. Measurements of provider behaviors were diverse in type and inconsistent in direction and statistical significance. None of the studies in the review reported on behaviors or exposures among clients, only on behaviors of providers toward clients. Several but not all reviewed studies showed improvements in intermediate outcomes, such as changes in knowledge, attitudes, beliefs, and intentions of providers. Studies measuring client knowledge, attitudes, beliefs, or intentions tended to show results in the desirable direction, although they did not consistently reach a level of statistical significance.

Because not enough reviewed studies measured changes in the behaviors or health outcomes on which we could base a recommendation, and those that did showed a lack of consistency in results, evidence was insufficient to determine the effectiveness of programs in healthcare system and provider settings in reducing clients' UV exposure or increasing their sun-protective behaviors.

Because we could not establish the effectiveness of this intervention, we did not examine situations where it would be applicable, information about economic efficiency, or possible barriers to implementation.

In conclusion, evidence was insufficient to determine the effectiveness of interventions in healthcare settings or for healthcare providers in reducing UV exposure or increasing sun-protective behaviors because of lack of measurement of key behaviors and health outcomes among clients and lack of consistency in results.

Interventions in Diverse Settings

Mass Media Campaigns Alone: Insufficient Evidence to Determine Effectiveness

Mass media campaigns promote sun-protective behaviors, generally in geographically defined communities. They provide information through mass media (e.g., television, radio, newspapers, magazines, and billboards), small media (e.g., brochures, flyers, newsletters, informational letters, and posters), or both. Mass media have been widely used in public health programs to address behavioral risk factors and are a recognized vehicle for reaching wide audiences, particularly for the purpose of raising awareness and concern about an issue.

Effectiveness

- We found insufficient evidence to determine the effectiveness of mass media campaigns alone in promoting sun-safe behaviors or reducing ultraviolet (UV) exposure.
- Evidence was insufficient because of limitations in the design and execution of available studies, the small number of available studies, and variability in interventions and outcomes evaluated.
- Insufficient evidence means that we were not able to determine whether or not the intervention works.

Several mass media campaigns to prevent and control skin cancer were conducted in the United States over the past decade, including campaigns by the Skin Cancer Foundation (http://www.skincancer.org), the federal government (http://www.chooseyourcover.gov), the American Academy of Dermatology (http://www.aad.org), the American Cancer Society (http://www.cancer.org), and the Weather Channel (http://www.weather.com). These campaigns were launched because of the reported success of Australia's regional programs, which rely heavily on mass media.[146] Ours is the first systematic review of the effectiveness of such campaigns.[147]

The findings of our systematic review are based on three reports[148–150] on the effectiveness of mass media campaigns without other activities in reducing exposure to UV radiation or increasing sun-protective behaviors. An additional seven reports[151–157,157a] were identified but did not meet our quality criteria and were excluded from the review. One report[158] provided additional information on a study already included in the review. We reviewed interventions that included any effort using mass media alone or mass media in combination with small media, with the aim of changing the knowledge, attitudes, beliefs, intentions, or sun-protective behaviors or health outcomes of children or adults. We only reviewed reports that allowed evaluation of the effect of mass media alone on behavior change. Studies that included mass media as part of multicomponent programs are also evaluated in this chapter (see Community-wide Multicomponent Programs, Including Comprehensive Community-wide Interventions).

The reviewed interventions included a three-segment television program emphasizing early detection and the dangers of sun exposure and sunburn; the use of a CD-ROM–based information kiosk housed at sites accessible to the public; media reporting of skin cancer advisories in the form of a UV index; and a rating of sunlight intensity coupled with recommendations for appropriate sun-protective measures. Reported results of these interventions either did not address the outcomes we wanted to measure or did not allow us to separate the specific effects of mass media alone. Thus, these studies provide insufficient evidence to determine the effectiveness of mass media approaches in promoting sun-safe behaviors or reducing UV exposure. All three reports, however, found that mass media campaigns tended to show increases in some aspects of knowledge.

Because we could not establish the effectiveness of this intervention, we did not examine situations where it would be applicable, information about economic efficiency, or possible barriers to implementation.

The studies in this review did not include information on other potential effects of the intervention. Some authors, however, have cited a concern that a primary prevention campaign may result in increased unnecessary excisions of benign skin lesions.[159]

In conclusion, we found insufficient evidence to determine the effectiveness of mass media interventions alone in changing sun exposure behaviors. Evidence was insufficient because of limitations in the design and execution of available studies, the small number of qualifying studies, and variability in the interventions and outcomes evaluated.

Interventions Oriented to Children's Parents and Caregivers:
Insufficient Evidence to Determine Effectiveness

Interventions for parents and caregivers involve activities that primarily promote sun-protective behaviors for children under their care. A caregiver is defined as a nonparental adult (e.g., professional nannies, mother's helpers, babysitters, grandparents, or other family or household members) who assumes responsibility, at least part-time on a regular basis, for the care of at least one child. Occupational or volunteer caregivers such as lifeguards, teachers, coaches, or scout leaders were not included here, but were included in our review of interventions in outdoor occupational settings and in recreational and tourism settings (see Educational and Policy Interventions in Primary Schools, Educational and Policy Interventions in Recreational and Tourism Settings, and Programs in Outdoor Occupational Settings).

Interventions for parents and caregivers include at least one of the following: providing information to parents or caregivers and the children under their care (through instruction, small media education, or both); activities intended to change the knowledge, attitudes, beliefs, intentions, or behavior of parents or caregivers and the children under their care (i.e., modeling, demonstration, or role playing); or environmental or policy approaches, including provision of sunscreen or shade, or scheduling of outdoor activities to avoid hours of peak UV radiation.

Effectiveness

- We found insufficient evidence to determine the effectiveness of interventions for parents or caregivers in reducing UV exposure or increasing sun-protective behaviors.
- Evidence was insufficient because too few reports were available and available reports showed inconsistent evidence.
- Insufficient evidence means that we were not able to determine whether or not the intervention works.

Parents and caregivers play an important role in protecting children from UV radiation. In addition to directly reducing children's UV exposure, parents and caregivers can support sun-protective behaviors by incorporating preventive behaviors into family routines and by serving as role models for the children under their care. Parental beliefs about and involvement in disease prevention are important components of successful skin cancer prevention programs for children, especially young children. Parents control family resources and activities, and the availability of sunscreen and protective clothing.[160]

Children are more likely to use sunscreen if their parents do,[90,161] but this tendency has not been shown with other sun-protective behaviors. Some parents know the risks of skin cancer but do not realize that children are at risk.[86,87] Some parents believe a suntan is a sign of good health; others use sunscreen on their children as their only or preferred skin cancer prevention measure,[91] even when other methods (e.g., shade, appropriate clothing) are available. Sometimes parents apply sunscreen on their children incorrectly and inconsistently[30,162,163] (e.g., only after a child has experienced a painful sunburn). Reports of high sunburn rates among youth[164,165] highlight the need for better education of parents and caregivers about appropriate sun-protective behaviors.

The findings of our systematic review are based on nine reports that evaluated the effectiveness of interventions directed to parents or caregivers in reducing UV exposure.[68,69,71,73,74,166–169] Three additional reports were identified but did not meet our quality criteria and were excluded from the review.[54,77,157] Four reports provided additional information on studies already included in the review.[79,80,170,171]

The reports in our review used numerous activities and evaluated a variety of outcomes in one or both parents and their children. No reports evaluated outcomes among other caregivers. Studies used interactive sun-protective activities (stories, games, puzzles, stamps, arts and crafts) and environmental supports (e.g., providing sunscreen, shade, and signage); educational materials or presentations; a UV exposure-reduction curriculum at poolside; home-based activities for parents and children; giving new mothers sun-protective guidelines, postcard reminders, sunscreen samples, baby sun hats, and sun umbrellas; point-of-purchase prompts and discount coupons for children's hats and sunscreen; and a combination of focused behavioral strategies and community-wide publicity campaigns to change the attitudes and behaviors of parents and their children.

The reports showed insufficient evidence to determine the effectiveness of the intervention in changing parental sun-protective behavior, parental UV exposure, children's sun-protective behavior, children's UV exposure, and the incidence of children's sunburn because too few reports were available (parents' UV exposure and incidence of children's sunburn) or results were inconsistent (parents' sun-protective behavior, children's sun-protective behavior, and children's UV exposure).

Effects of the intervention on parental knowledge, parental attitudes or beliefs, and parental intentions were inconsistent. Effects on children's attitudes or beliefs were desirable and consistent (median increase of 67.6%), as were parent-reported sun-protective measures and environmental supports at outdoor recreational centers or swimming pools (median difference, a 1.3 increase in score using a scale from 0 to 4), but neither of these outcomes, by itself, would have supported a recommendation.

Because we could not establish the effectiveness of this intervention, we did not examine situations in which it would be applicable, information about economic efficiency, or possible barriers to implementation.

We identified other potential effects of interventions for parents or caregivers, but further evaluation is needed to determine if these effects are important. Interventions for parents or caregivers may reduce the risk of overexposure to UV radiation that comes from overreliance on sunscreen. Additionally, a reduction in UV exposure could be associated with reductions in cataract formation. Potential negative effects of the intervention include vitamin D deficiency and reduction in outdoor physical activity.

In conclusion, available reports provide insufficient evidence to determine the effectiveness of interventions for parents or caregivers in reducing UV exposure or increasing sun-protective behaviors. Evidence was insufficient because of too few reports or inconsistent evidence. Additionally, although the following are not outcomes on which we would base a recommendation, the reviewed reports demonstrate that the intervention led to some improvements in children's attitudes or beliefs as well as in sun-safety measures and environmental supports at outdoor recreational centers and swimming pools.

Community-Wide Multicomponent Programs, Including Comprehensive
Community-Wide Interventions: Insufficient Evidence to Determine Effectiveness

Multicomponent sun-protection programs aim to achieve behavioral changes among the people in a defined geographic area (e.g., counties, states, countries). Some are relatively modest efforts, such as combining a setting-specific program with a community-wide mass media or small media effort, whereas others are multilevel and comprehensive, involving entire communities, schools, workplaces, healthcare and recreation settings, mass media, and other organizations. In addition to education, these programs may also include significant efforts to institute sun-protection policies and structural supports.

Programs like these have been in place for two decades in Australia, with the longest-standing and most commonly cited ones being the Slip! Slap! Slop! and SunSmart campaigns in Victoria.[146] Two U.S. programs, the Safe-Sun Project in New Hampshire[55,57] and the Falmouth Safe Skin Project in Massachusetts,[168] have used similar strategies on a smaller scale.

Effectiveness

- We found insufficient evidence to determine the effectiveness of community-wide multicomponent programs that include comprehensive community-wide interventions in reducing UV exposure or increasing sun-protective behaviors.
- Evidence was insufficient because of inconsistent results.
- Insufficient evidence means that we were not able to determine whether or not the intervention works.

We defined *community-wide multicomponent programs* as those that used combinations of individually directed strategies, mass media campaigns, and environmental and policy changes in an integrated effort in a defined geographic area (city, state, province, or country). Such programs are usually delivered with a defined theme, name, logo, and set of messages[146] and sometimes also incorporate setting-specific strategies. We included studies in this review if they occurred in a defined geographic area and had at least two components and two settings. We defined *comprehensive community-wide interventions* to be multilevel (i.e., those that include multiple individually directed, setting-specific, and community-wide components), addressing a substantial proportion of the population in a defined area, and lasting longer than one year.

The findings of our systematic review are based on eight reports[57,168,172-177] that evaluated the effectiveness of multicomponent and comprehensive community-wide interventions in reducing UV exposure or increasing sun-protective behaviors. An additional five studies[178-182] were identified but did not meet our quality criteria and were excluded from the review. Another 22 reports[42,55,56,62,146,147,183-198] provided additional information on studies already included in the review.

Of the seven multicomponent studies that measured covering-up or sun-avoidance behaviors, four showed generally positive outcomes, one showed an increase in risk behaviors, and two others showed essentially no change. Results of comprehensive community-wide programs were generally more positive. All three such studies showed desirable changes in covering-up or sun-avoidance behaviors. These results, all from Australia, are promising but by themselves still provide insufficient evidence to determine the effectiveness of the interventions because of the small number of studies and limitations in study design and execution. Furthermore, available evidence (which comes mostly from sustained programs in Australia, a country with high skin cancer rates) may or may not generalize to the United States, where skin cancer is a less prominent public health concern and the population includes a higher proportion of dark-skinned individuals who are at lower risk of developing skin cancer.

Studies that evaluated self-reported sunscreen use generally reported increased sunscreen use. Many of the comprehensive community-wide studies evaluated changes in school and government policy and changes in the environment. These studies generally showed positive outcomes (e.g., an increase in the number of sun-safe policies in schools or governments, an increase in the number of stores with available low-cost sunscreen, or an increase in the amount of information and the number of posters provided). The effects on the knowledge, attitudes, and beliefs of adults and children were inconsistent.

Because evidence was insufficient to determine effectiveness, we did not fully evaluate situations in which these interventions would be applicable. It should, however, be noted that the most promising results of the available studies are from three long-term, intensive interventions in Australia. The context in which those studies occurred may differ in some important ways from the U.S. context: in some studies the mass media component was heavily subsidized, the incidence and risk of skin cancer are higher in Australia than in the United States, and UV exposure on average is probably higher in Australia than in the United States. Any of these factors might affect the extent to which these results may or may not be applicable in the United States.

Because we could not establish the effectiveness of this intervention, we did not examine information about economic efficiency or possible barriers to implementation.

The studies included in this review did not address potential harms of reducing UV exposure, such as an increase in the incidence of vitamin D deficiency or reduction in physical activity.

In conclusion, available studies provide insufficient evidence to determine the effectiveness of community-wide multicomponent programs in reducing UV exposure or increasing sun-protective behaviors because of inconsistent results. Evidence was also insufficient to determine the effectiveness of comprehensive community-wide programs to reduce UV exposure or increase sun-protective behaviors because of the small number of studies and limitations in their design and execution.

CONCLUSION: SKIN CANCER

This first part of the chapter summarizes Task Force conclusions and recommendations for preventing skin cancer by reducing exposure to ultraviolet (UV) radiation. To reduce exposure to UV radiation, the Task Force recommends educational and policy interventions in primary schools and in recreational and tourism settings. Evidence was insufficient to determine the effectiveness of educational and policy interventions in child care centers, secondary schools, or colleges in reducing exposure to UV radiation. Evidence was also insufficient to determine the effectiveness of programs in outdoor occupational settings, for parents and caregivers, or in healthcare systems and provider settings; of mass media campaigns alone; or of community-wide multicomponent programs (including comprehensive community-wide interventions) in reducing exposure to ultraviolet radiation.

Details of these reviews have been published[33,199,200] and these articles, along with additional information about the reviews, are available at www .thecommunityguide.org/cancer.

PROMOTING INFORMED DECISION MAKING FOR CANCER SCREENING

There was a time when doctors told their patients what tests to have or what procedures to undergo, and patients generally followed their doctors' advice. In twenty-first-century health care, the belief that "the doctor knows what's best" is being supplanted by a belief that patients must be increasingly involved in the decisions made about their care. Two principal approaches to helping clients make decisions about whether to be screened for a disease, have a test, or be treated are informed decision making (IDM) and shared decision making (SDM). Informed decision making interventions should help an individual to understand the nature of the disease or condition being addressed; to understand the clinical service and its likely consequences, including risks, limitations, benefits, alternatives, and uncertainties; to consider his or her preferences as appropriate; to participate in decision making at a personally desirable level; and either to make a decision consistent with his or her preferences and values or to defer a decision to a later time. Shared decision making is one type of IDM, which occurs in the clinical setting. Based on the work of the U.S. Preventive Services Task Force (USPSTF),[201] we have defined SDM as occurring when a patient and his or her healthcare provider(s), in the clinical setting, both express preferences and participate in making treatment decisions. We have defined an IDM intervention as any intervention in a community or healthcare system that promotes IDM, including SDM.

Informed decision making can apply to a range of cancer screening decisions. It sometimes applies to tests that have uncertain effects on health outcomes. Providers and individuals are often compelled to consider such tests because (1) the screening test is highly publicized or widely available; (2) the test addresses a critical public health problem for which no good alternative prevention or treatment exist; or (3) public interest in the test is strong. At times, when publicity fails to fully inform the public about the potential risks and benefits of a given screening test, IDM and SDM interventions can help put potential risks and benefits in context.

Prostate-specific antigen (PSA) testing for prostate cancer is a relevant example. Prostate cancer is the most commonly diagnosed cancer in men other than non-melanoma skin cancer,[1] and the PSA screening test is widely recommended and available.[202] This has led to considerable public interest in the test. However, the effectiveness of PSA screening in reducing cancer morbidity and death is uncertain, and the diagnostic testing and treatment that follow PSA testing may involve important risks.[203,204] Moreover, some of the diagnostic testing may be unnecessary because it results from a false positive screening test or identifies a cancer that would never have become apparent during the individual's lifetime. As a result of these complexities, the balance of the benefits and harms of PSA screening is unclear. Individuals considering PSA screening may find IDM to be an important aid in understanding the benefits, risks, and uncertainties of this screening method, which can help them make an informed choice. In addition, IDM might be applicable to other high-profile cancer screening issues, such as spiral-computed tomography for lung cancer or pelvic ultrasound for ovarian cancer. The importance of IDM for cancer screening tests of uncertain benefit is likely to increase as more and more cancer screening tests become available.

Informed decision making can also apply to tests with proven benefit. Scientific studies have shown that some screening tests produce greater benefit than harm for populations. As a result, these tests are widely recommended. For example, the USPSTF recommends mammography every one to two years for women over 40, because this screening test has been found to reduce breast cancer mortality.[205] However, the benefit among women in their forties is smaller than for older women, and the balance of benefits versus harms increases with age. Women need to be aware of the potential harms, which include false positive test results and unnecessary anxiety, biopsies, and costs from false test results. Nonetheless, the magnitude of the benefit is relatively small; scientific discussion continues about how conclusively the benefit has been proven; the procedure is inconvenient; and the test produces a moderately high rate of false positive results requiring follow-up, for which women should be prepared. For these reasons, balanced information on the benefits and harms should be provided to the public.[205,206]

In addition, for a growing number of healthcare conditions, people must choose among two or more equally valid screening regimens. For example, the recommended interval for cervical cancer screening may be yearly or less frequently (e.g., every two or three years), and older women may safely discontinue use of the test.[13,207] Colon cancer screening can be performed in a variety of ways (fecal occult blood testing, sigmoidoscopy, or colonoscopy)[208] but the relative merits of each method vary, as do the values individuals place on these relative merits.[208,209] An example of an Internet-based tool intended to promote IDM for colorectal cancer screening, including the pros and cons of different screening options, can be found at http://www.med.unc.edu/medicine/edursrc/colon.htm.[210]

We conducted a systematic literature review to assess whether or not IDM interventions in the area of cancer screening have been effective in helping individuals (1) increase their understanding of the cancers and the screening tests, (2) participate in IDM at a comfortable level, or (3) reach decisions consistent with their preferences and values, or if the interventions have been effective in changing healthcare or provider systems or policies to promote greater use of IDM and SDM.

In choosing which health or public health programs to pursue, the goal of making decisions consistent with individuals' values and preferences may conflict with other important social goals (such as improved population health or rational allocation of resources). Goals may include providing treatments that produce the greatest likelihood of good outcomes for the greatest number of individual patients while considering the best available science, rational allocation of societal resources, and organizational financial impact, as well as the need to respect individual autonomy. Decision makers must make trade-offs among such competing goals when choosing which clinical or public health interventions to support. Our review sought to clarify what is known about the likely outcomes of programs to promote IDM about cancer screening so that decision makers can compare the results of these programs with those of other alternatives. For example, some interventions might lead to more rational decisions about prostate cancer screening that may or may not save lives. On the other hand, good conceptual bases and some empirical evidence suggest that informed and involved individuals are more likely to adhere to treatment recommendations[211,212] and less informed patients may have poorer outcomes. Better-informed patients may therefore have more autonomy *and* better health.

OBJECTIVES AND RECOMMENDATIONS FROM OTHER ADVISORY GROUPS

Informed decision making is a broad and growing topic. The *Healthy People 2010*[29] goals shown in Table 4–1 touch on some aspects of IDM.

The USPSTF, which has published a paper clarifying how it envisions the application of SDM in the execution of screening and chemoprevention,[201]

Table 4–1. *Healthy People 2010*[29] Objectives Relevant to Informed Decision Making Interventions

Objective	Population	2010 Objective
Increase the proportion of persons appropriately counseled about management of menopause (females aged 46–56 years) (Objective 1–3h)	Women	Developmental
Increase the proportion of physicians and dentists who counsel their at-risk patients about tobacco use cessation, physical activity, and cancer screening (3–10)	All	Varies by provider type and health area
Increase the proportion of healthcare organizations that provide patient and family education (7–7)	All	Developmental
Increase the proportion of patients who report that they are satisfied with the patient education they receive from their healthcare organization (7–8)	All	Developmental
Increase the proportion of health-related World Wide Web sites that disclose information that can be used to assess the quality of the site (11–4)	All	Developmental
Increase the proportion of persons who report that their healthcare providers have satisfactory communication skills (11–6)	All	Developmental

does not endorse a specific style of decision making but does encourage informed and joint decisions.

In addition to the summary of our systematic review provided in this chapter, we have published an extended discussion of the conceptual aspects of IDM and SDM, along with details of the systematic review[213] (also available at www.thecommunityguide.org/cancer).

METHODS

Methods used for the reviews are summarized in Chapter 10. Specific methods used in the systematic reviews of IDM and cancer screening have been described in detail elsewhere.[213] In our systematic review of IDM interventions for cancer screening, we assessed the extent to which these interventions have been tested and the extent to which potential outcomes have been evaluated empirically. We limited our inquiry to IDM outside of the individual clinical encounter (i.e., excluding SDM) in the areas of prevention and early detection. The USPSTF has published on SDM in the clinical encounter.[201]

Although IDM is relevant to many treatment and prevention topics, we limited this review to cancer screening because different prevention topics may raise unique questions.

The proposed outcomes on which recommendations are based in this review (i.e., knowledge, participation, and consistency with values) differ from those typically identified in *Community Guide* reviews[214] in that they are not health outcomes or established proxies for health outcomes. However, for this novel public health intervention, we considered informed and participatory decisions consistent with preferences and values to be of value by themselves, regardless of whether or not they lead to better health. Since some informed and participatory decisions may not result in better health, we decided that we could not logically require that an intervention result in decisions that are consistent with individuals' preferences and values and also require better health as an outcome.

ECONOMIC EFFICIENCY

A systematic review of economic evaluations is conducted for each recommended intervention in a topic area. Because the Task Force found insufficient evidence to determine if the one intervention reviewed in this area— IDM interventions to promote cancer screening—is effective, no systematic review of economic evaluations was conducted.

RECOMMENDATIONS AND FINDINGS

This section presents a summary of the findings of the systematic review conducted to determine the effectiveness of IDM interventions in promoting skin cancer screening.

Informed Decision Making Interventions to Promote Cancer Screening: Insufficient Evidence to Determine Effectiveness

Informed decision making interventions occur in communities or healthcare systems and help an individual to understand the nature of the disease or condition being addressed; to understand the clinical service and its likely consequences, including risks, limitations, benefits, alternatives, and uncertainties; to consider his or her preferences as appropriate; to participate in decision making at a personally desirable level; and either to make a decision consistent with his or her preferences and values or to defer a decision to a later time.

Effectiveness

- Almost all studies reported increases in knowledge, improved perceptions of risk, or both.
- Evidence, however, was insufficient to determine the effectiveness of IDM interventions in helping individuals participate in IDM at a comfortable level or reach decisions consistent with their preferences or values.

- Evidence was also insufficient to determine the effectiveness of IDM interventions in changing healthcare or provider systems or policies related to IDM or SDM.
- Evidence was insufficient because of the small number of studies measuring relevant outcomes and inconsistent results among studies.
- Insufficient evidence means that we were not able to determine whether or not the intervention works.

The findings of our systematic review are based on 11 reports[210,211,215-223] that provided information on 15 independent intervention arms. Two additional reports[224,225] provided information on studies already included in our review. Of the 15 intervention arms, 10 addressed prostate cancer screening, 3 addressed colorectal cancer screening, and 2 addressed mammography screening. Most studies were directed to clients in clinical settings.

The studies in our review examined several different approaches to providing the information on which informed decisions could be based. Client-oriented interventions used small media alone (including videos, brochures, or written materials; some of the written materials were customized to individual needs and circumstances), one-on-one education (by itself or supported by computer-generated decision aids to help people make choices among options), or small group education. The only provider-oriented intervention we reviewed included aspects of provider education and reminders.

Thirteen of the study arms measured patients' knowledge, beliefs, or perceptions about the risk or natural history of the disease or about the performance of the preventive service. The evidence showed effectiveness in improving these outcomes: almost all of the available studies reported increased knowledge, increased accuracy of beliefs and perceptions, or both. Some but not all of the more intensive interventions produced larger effects.

One study showed self-reported increases in preferences for SDM. Three reports showed increases (of unstated size) in individual or patient participation in decision making. Only a single study reported on whether participation was consistent with expressed preferences for level of participation (i.e., primarily by the patient, primarily by the physician, or shared). That study showed that people in an intensive intervention group were no more likely to adopt a level of participation consistent with pre-intervention preferences than those in a less intensive intervention group. Only a single study measured any outcome related to whether intervention preferences were acted upon; it showed that only 19% of patients who received an intensive intervention actually chose a screening strategy at their next office visit that was consistent with the most highly rated strategy identified during the intervention. The results, therefore, provided insufficient evidence to determine whether IDM interventions resulted in participation in decision making with which the patient was comfortable or decisions consistent with patient values and preferences.

Results of the interventions on screening outcomes were mixed, but effect sizes were generally small. Of the studies of prostate cancer (for which there is no consensus about whether screening provides a net benefit), eight allowed for calculation of percentage point changes in testing and showed a median 8 percentage point decrease (range, 47 percentage point decrease to 14 percentage point increase). Two more prostate cancer studies showed statistically significant decreases in self-reported preferences for screening. Of the five studies of colorectal cancer or breast cancer (where consensus is greater about the benefits of screening), four allowed calculation of the proportion of patients accepting screening after the intervention and showed a median 6 percentage point increase in screening (range, 2 percentage point decrease to 14 percentage point increase). Only the 14 percentage point increase was reported to be statistically significant. The other study showed generally small and nonsignificant increases in intentions to be screened.

Evidence was also insufficient to determine whether IDM interventions increase implementation of policies that promote and facilitate IDM (e.g., increasing time for or reimbursement of providers who participate in SDM or hiring or training non-physician staff to help facilitate SDM); improving providers' knowledge and motivation, attitudes about, and intentions to perform SDM or their participation in SDM; or improvements for clients resulting from changes in provider and healthcare system approaches.

Because we could not establish the effectiveness of IDM interventions, we did not examine situations in which they would be applicable, information about economic efficiency, or possible barriers to implementation.

We considered whether IDM interventions might have negative effects on individuals or community members (e.g., confusion, frustration, positive or negative effects on other preventive care), on healthcare systems or providers (e.g., effects on clinic efficiency), or on whole communities (e.g., adverse effects of competing or contradictory clinical and community approaches). None of the reviewed studies provided information about any of these possible effects.

In conclusion, current evidence was insufficient to determine whether IDM interventions resulted in participation in decision making at a comfortable level or in decisions consistent with patient values and preferences. This insufficiency of evidence applied to individuals in healthcare settings and community members outside of healthcare settings. Evidence was also insufficient to determine whether IDM interventions were effective in changing the knowledge, attitudes, or behaviors of healthcare providers or the policies of healthcare systems. On the other hand, these interventions generally improved knowledge, beliefs, risk perceptions, or a combination of these.

CONCLUSION: INFORMED DECISION MAKING

The finding of this review—that available evidence was insufficient to determine the effectiveness of interventions to promote IDM—does not mean that the interventions do not achieve their objectives. Both IDM and SDM are important emerging trends, and additional studies of these interventions should be conducted. Limitations, costs, uncertainties, and trade-offs should be studied empirically and should be considered when choosing interventions. However, hypothesized costs, barriers, or trade-offs should not limit additional exploration of IDM.

Several criteria may make IDM interventions of higher priority for research and practice, make the provision of more information appropriate, or both. These include:

- High interest in the test(s) in the community or among individuals, especially if combined with uncertainty about effectiveness, uncertainty about the balance of benefits and harms, unavailability of balanced information (e.g., knowing the pros but not the cons of a particular screening test), or high complexity of trade-offs.
- Low demand despite known effectiveness.
- High variability in values or preferences.
- High-stakes issues (e.g., more common or serious conditions; more costly, complex, or dangerous consequences of screening).

This second section in the chapter summarizes Task Force conclusions about IDM interventions. The Task Force found insufficient evidence to determine the effectiveness of IDM interventions in promoting understanding of cancer screening, facilitating participation in decision making about cancer screening at a level comfortable for individuals, or encouraging individuals to make cancer screening decisions consistent with their preferences and values. Details of this review have been published[213] and this article, along with additional information about the reviews, is available at www.thecommunityguide.org/cancer.

Acknowledgments

This chapter was written by the members of the systematic review teams: Peter Briss, MD, MPH, Division of Prevention Research and Analytic Methods (DPRAM), Epidemiology Program Office (EPO), Centers for Disease Control and Prevention (CDC), Atlanta, Georgia; Mona Saraiya, MD, MPH, Division of Cancer Prevention and Control (DCPC), National Center for Chronic Disease Prevention and Health Promotion (NCCDPHP), CDC, Atlanta; Rosalind Breslow, PhD, DCPC/NCCDPHP/CDC, Atlanta; Barbara Rimer, DrPH, National Cancer Institute (NCI), National Institutes of Health (NIH), Bethesda, Maryland; Ralph C. Coates, PhD, DCPC/NCCDPHP/CDC, Atlanta; Nancy C. Lee, MD, DCPC/NCCDPHP/CDC, Atlanta; Jon F. Kerner PhD, NCI/NIH, Bethesda; Patricia D. Mullen, DrPH, University of Texas-Houston School of Public Health and the Task Force on Community Preventive Services; Phyllis Nichols, MPH, DPRAM/EPO/CDC, Atlanta; Cornelia White, PhD, DPRAM/EPO/CDC, Atlanta; Debjani Das, MPH, DCPC/NCCDPHP/ CDC, Atlanta; Bernice Tannor, MPH, DCPC/NCCDPHP/CDC, Atlanta; Nisha Gandhi, MPH, DPRAM/EPO/CDC, Atlanta; Prethibha George, MPH, National Center for Infectious Diseases, CDC, Atlanta; Katherine M. Wilson, PhD, MPH, DCPC/NCCDPHP/CDC, Atlanta; S. Jay Smith, MHPA, DPRAM/EPO/CDC, Atlanta; Angela B. Hutchinson, PhD, MPH, DPRAM/EPO/CDC, Atlanta; Barbara Reilley, RN, PhD, Health Program Development, Houston, Texas; Robert A. Hiatt, MD, PhD, NCI/NIH, Bethesda; Phaedra Corso, PhD, DPRAM/EPO/CDC, Atlanta; Karen Glanz, PhD, MPH, University of Hawaii; Phyllis Rochester, PhD, DCPC/NCCDPHP/CDC, Atlanta; George Isham, MD, HealthPartners, Minneapolis, Minnesota and the Task Force on Community Preventive Services; Steven M. Teutsch, MD, MPH, Merck & Co., Inc., West Point, Pennsylvania and the Task Force on Community Preventive Services; Alan Hinman, MD, MPH, Task Force for Child Survival and Development, Atlanta and the Task Force on Community Preventive Services; Robert Lawrence, MD, MPH, Bloomberg School of Public Health, Johns Hopkins University, Baltimore, Maryland; and Patricia Buffler, PhD, MPH, University of California, Berkeley and the Task Force on Community Preventive Services.

Consultants for skin cancer and IDM reviews: Ross Brownson, PhD, St. Louis University School of Public Health, St. Louis, Missouri; Robert Burack, MD, MPH, Wayne State University, Detroit, Michigan; Linda Burhansstipanov, DrPH, Native American Cancer Research, Pine, Colorado; Allen Dietrich, MD, MPH, Dartmouth Medical School, Hanover, New Hampshire; Russell Harris, MD, MPH, University of North Carolina School of Medicine, Chapel Hill; Thomas D. Koepsell, MD, MPH, University of Washington, Seattle; Howard K. Koh, MD, MPH, Massachusetts Department of Public Health, Boston; Peter Layde, MD, MSc, Medical College of Wisconsin, Milwaukee; Al Marcus, PhD, AMC Cancer Center, Denver, Colorado; Margaret C. Mendez, MPA, Texas Department of Health, Austin; Amilie Ramirez, PhD, Baylor College of Medicine, San Antonio, Texas; Linda Randolph, MD, MPH, National Center for Education on Maternal and Child Health, Arlington, Virginia; Lisa Schwartz, MD, Department of Veterans Affairs Medical Center, White River Junction, Vermont; Jonathan Slater, PhD, Minnesota State Health Department, Minneapolis; Robert A. Smith, PhD, American Cancer Society, Atlanta, Georgia; Stephen Taplin, MD, Group Health Cooperative of Puget Sound, Seattle, Washington; Sally Vernon, PhD, University of Texas School of Public Health, Houston; Fran Wheeler, PhD, School of Public Health, University of South Carolina, Columbia; Daniel B. Wolfson, MHSA, Alliance of Community Health Plans, New Brunswick, New Jersey; Steve Woloshin, MD, Department of Veterans Affairs Medical Center, White River Junction, Vermont; John K. (Kim) Worden, PhD, University of Vermont, Burlington; Jane Zapka, PhD, University of Massachusetts Medical Center, Worcester.

Articles included in the reviews were abstracted by: Carol Wyninger, Nicole Piscatelli, Debjani Das, Nisha Gandhi, Barbara Reilley, and Prethibha George.

References

1. American Cancer Society. Cancer facts and figures—2004. Atlanta, GA: American Cancer Society, 2004.

2. Centers for Disease Control and Prevention. Annual smoking-attributable mortality, years of potential life lost, and economic costs—United States, 1995–1999. MMWR 2002;51(14):300–3.

3. Curry SJ, Byers T, Hewitt ME, National Cancer Policy Board (U.S.). Fulfilling the potential of cancer prevention and early detection. Washington, DC: National Academies Press, 2003.

4. Adami HO, Trichopoulos D. Obesity and mortality from cancer. N Engl J Med 2003; 348(17):1623–4.

5. Calle EE, Rodriguez C, Walker-Thurmond K, Thun MJ. Overweight, obesity, and mortality from cancer in a prospectively studied cohort of U.S. adults. N Engl J Med 2003;348(17):1625–38.

6. International Agency for Research on Cancer. Weight control and physical activity. IARC handbooks of cancer prevention, Vol. 6. Lyon: IARC Press, 2002.

7. Hartman KE, Hall SA, Nanda K, Boggess FJ, Zolnoun D. Screening for cervical cancer: file inventory. Systematic evidence review number 25. Available at: http://www.ahrq.gov/clinic/prev/crvcainv.htm. Accessed April 6, 2004.

8. Humphrey LL, Helfand M, Chan BKS, Woolf SH. Breast cancer screening: summary of the evidence. Ann Intern Med 2002;137:344–6. Also available at: http://www.ahrq.gov/clinic/3rduspstf/breastcancer/bcscrnsum1.htm. Accessed April 6, 2004.

9. Pignone M, Rich M, Teutsch SM, Berg AO, Lohr KN. Screening for colorectal cancer in adults at average risk: summary of the evidence for the U.S. Preventive Services Task Force. Ann Intern Med 2002;137:132–41. Also available at: http://www.ahrq.gov/clinic/3rduspstf/colorectal/colosum1.htm. Accessed April 6, 2004.

10. U.S. Preventive Services Task Force. Screening for breast cancer: recommendations and rationale. Available at: http://www.ahrq.gov/clinic/3rduspstf/breastcancer/brcanrr.htm. Accessed April 6, 2004.

11. U.S. Preventive Services Task Force. Screening for colorectal cancer: recommendations and rationale. Available at: http://www.ahrq.gov/clinic/3rduspstf/colorectal/colorr.htm. Accessed April 6, 2004.

12. U.S. Preventive Services Task Force. Colorectal cancer—screening: Summary of recommendations. Available at: http://www.ahrq.gov/clinic/uspstf/uspscolo.htm. Accessed April 6, 2004.

13. U.S. Preventive Services Task Force. Cervical cancer screening: recommendations and rationale. Available at: http://www.ahrq.gov/clinic/3rduspstf/cervcan/cervcanrr.htm. Accessed April 6, 2004.

14. Greenlee RT, Murray T, Bolden S, Wingo PA. Cancer statistics, 2000. CA Cancer J Clin 2000;50(1):7–33.

15. Armstrong B, Kricker A. How much melanoma is caused by sun exposure? Melanoma Res 1993;3(6):395–401.

16. Whiteman DC, Whiteman CA, Green AC. Childhood sun exposure as a risk factor for melanoma: a systematic review of epidemiologic studies. Cancer Causes Control 2001;12(1):69–82.

17. Westerdahl J, Olsson H, Ingvar C. At what age do sunburn episodes play a crucial role for the development of malignant melanoma? Eur J Cancer 1994;30A(11):1647–54.

18. Elwood JM. Melanoma and sun exposure: contrasts between intermittent and chronic exposure. World J Surg 1992;16(2):157–65.

19. Kricker A, Armstrong BK, English DR, Heenan PJ. Does intermittent sun exposure cause basal cell carcinoma? A case-control study in Western Australia. Int J Cancer 1995; 60(4):489–94.

20. Gallagher R, Hill G, Bajdik CD, et al. Sunlight exposure, pigmentary factors, and risk of nonmelanocytic skin cancer I. Basal cell carcinoma. Arch Dermatol 1995;131: 157–63.

21. Gallagher RP. Sun exposure and non-melanocytic skin cancer. In: Grob JJ, Stern RS, Mackie RM, Weinstock WA, eds. Epidemiology, causes, and prevention of skin diseases. London: Blackwell Science, 1997:72–7.

22. Elwood JM, Jopson J. Melanoma and sun exposure: an overview of published studies. Int J Cancer 1997;73:198–203.

23. Armstrong BK. Melanoma: childhood or lifelong sun exposure. In: Grob JJ, Stern RS, Mackie RM, Weinstock WA, eds. Epidemiology, causes, and prevention of skin diseases. London: Blackwell Science, 1997:63–6.

24. Whiteman D, Green A. Melanoma and sunburn. Cancer Causes Control 1994; 5(6):564–72.

25. Autier P, Dore JF, Cattaruzza MS, et al. Sunscreen use, wearing clothes, and number of nevi in 6- to 7-year-old European children. J Natl Cancer Inst 1998;90(24):1873–80.

26. Autier P, Dore JF, Lejeune F, et al. Recreational exposure to sunlight and lack of information as risk factors for cutaneous malignant melanoma. Results of a European Organization for Research and Treatment of Cancer (EORTC) case-control study in Belgium, France and Germany. Melanoma Res 1994;4:79–85.

27. Diffey BL. Solar ultraviolet radiation effects on biological systems. Phys Med Biol 1991;36(3):299–328.

28. International Agency for Research on Cancer. Solar and ultraviolet radioation. Monographs on the evaluation of carcinogenic risks to humans. Lyon: International Agency for Research on Cancer, 1992:55.

29. U.S. Department of Health and Human Services. Healthy people 2010. 2nd ed. Washington, DC: U.S. Government Printing Office, 2000.

30. IARC Working Group on the Evaluation of Cancer Preventive Agents. IARC handbooks of cancer prevention. Vol. 5: Sunscreens. Vainio H, Bianchini F, eds. Lyon: International Agency for Research on Cancer, 2001.

31. Glanz K, Saraiya M, Wechsler H. Guidelines for school programs to prevent skin cancer. MMWR 2002;51(RR-4):1–18.

32. U.S. Preventive Services Task Force. Counseling to prevent skin cancer: recommendation statement. Available at: http://www.ahrq.gov/clinic/uspstf/uspsskco.htm. Accessed March 1, 2004.

33. Saraiya M, Glanz K, Briss PA, et al. Interventions to prevent skin cancer by reducing exposure to ultraviolet radiation: a systematic review. Am J Prev Med, in press.

34. Bastuji-Garin S, Grob JJ, Grognard C, Grosjean F. Melanoma prevention: evaluation of a health education campaign for primary schools. Arch Dermatol 1999;135:936–40.

35. Buller DB, Buller MK, Beach B, Ertl G. Sunny Days, Healthy Ways: evaluation of a skin cancer prevention curriculum for elementary school-aged children. J Am Acad Dermatol 1996;35(6):911–22.

36. Buller DB, Hall JR, Powers PJ, et al. Evaluation of the "Sunny Days, Healthy Ways" sun safety CD-ROM program for children in grades 4 and 5. Cancer Prev Control 1999;3(3):188–95.

37. Buller MK, Goldberg G, Buller DB. SunSmart Day: A pilot program for photoprotection education. Pediatr Dermatol 1997;14(4):257–63.

38. Buller MK, Loescher LJ, Buller DB. "Sunshine and Skin Health": a curriculum for skin cancer prevention education. J Cancer Educ 1994;9(3):155–62.

39. DeLong M, LaBat K, Gahring S, Nelson N, Leung L. Implications of an educational intervention program designed to increase young adolescents' awareness of hats for sun protection. Clothing Textiles Res J 1999;17(2):73–83.

40. Girgis A, Sanson-Fisher RW, Tripodi DA, Golding T. Evaluation of interventions to improve solar protection in primary schools. Health Educ Q 1993;20(2):275–87.

41. Gooderham MJ, Guenther L. Sun and the skin: evaluation of a sun awareness program for elementary school students. J Cutan Med Surg 1999;3(5):230–5.

42. Grant-Petersson J, Dietrich AJ, Sox CH, Winchell CW, Stevens MM. Promoting sun protection in elementary schools and child care settings: the Sun Safe Project. J Sch Health 1999;69(3):100–6.

43. Hoffmann RG III, Rodrigue JR, Johnson JH. Effectiveness of a school-based program to enhance knowledge of sun exposure: attitudes toward sun exposure and sunscreen use among children. Child Health Care 1999;28(1):69–86.

44. Hornung RL, Lennon PA, Garrett JM, DeVellis RF, Weinberg PD, Strecher VJ. Interactive computer technology for skin cancer prevention targeting children. Am J Prev Med 2000;18(1):69–76.

45. Hughes AS. Sun protection and younger children: lessons from the Living with Sunshine program. J Sch Health 1994;64(5):201–4.

46. Labat KL, DeLong MR, Gahring S. Evaluation of a skin cancer intervention program for youth. J Family Consumer Sci 1996;88:3–10.

47. Milne E, English DR, Johnston R, et al. Improved sun protection behaviour in children after two years of the Kidskin intervention. Aust N Z J Public Health 2000; 24(5):481–7.

48. McWhirter JM, Collins M, Bryant I, Wetton NM, Bishop JN. Evaluating "Safe in the Sun," a curriculum programme for primary schools. Health Educ Res 2000;15(2): 203–17.

49. Reding DJ, Fischer V, Gunderson P, Lappe K. Skin cancer prevention: a peer education model. Wis Med J 1995;94(2):77–81.

50. Reding DJ, Fischer V, Gunderson P, Lappe K, Anderson H, Calvert G. Teens teach skin cancer prevention. J Rural Health 1996;12(4 suppl):265–72.

51. Schofield MJ, Edwards K, Pearce R. Effectiveness of two strategies for dissemination of sun-protection policy in New South Wales primary and secondary schools. Aust N Z J Public Health 1997;21(7):743–50.

52. Thornton C, Piacquadio DJ. Promoting sun awareness: evaluation of an educational children's book. Pediatrics 1996;98(1):52–5.

53. Vitols P, Oates RK. Teaching children about skin cancer prevention: why wait for adolescence? Aust N Z J Public Health 1997;21(6):602–5.

54. Fleming C, Newell J, Turner S, Mackie R. A study of the impact of Sun Awareness Week 1995. Br J Dermatol 1997;136(5):719–24.

55. Dietrich AJ, Olson AL, Sox CH, et al. A community-based randomized trial encouraging sun protection for children. Pediatrics 1998;102(6):E64.

56. Dietrich AJ, Olson AL, Sox CH, Winchell CW, Grant-Petersson J, Collison DW. Sun protection counseling for children: primary care practice patterns and effect of an intervention on clinicians. Arch Fam Med 2000;9(2):155–9.

57. Dietrich AJ, Olson AL, Sox CH, Tosteson TD, Grant-Petersson J. Persistent increase in children's sun protection in a randomized controlled community trial. Prev Med 2000;31(5):569–74.

58. Milne E, Corti B, English DR, Cross D, Costa C, Johnston R. The use of observational methods for monitoring sun-protection activities in schools. Health Educ Res 1999;14(2):167–75.

59. Milne E, English DR, Corti B, et al. Direct measurement of sun protection in primary schools. Prev Med 1999;29(1):45–52.

60. Milne E, English DR, Cross D, Corti B, Costa C, Johnston R. Evaluation of an intervention to reduce sun exposure in children: design and baseline results. Am J Epidemiol 1999;150(2):164–73.

61. Gooderham MJ, Guenther L. Impact of a sun awareness curriculum on medical students' knowledge, attitudes, and behaviour. J Cutan Med Surg 1999;3(4):182–7.

62. Olson AL, Dietrich AJ, Sox CH, Stevens MM, Winchell CW, Ahles TA. Solar protection of children at the beach. Pediatrics 1997;99(6):E1.

63. Speare R, Buettner PG. Hard data needed on head lice transmission. Int J Dermatol 2000;39(11):877–8.

64. Travel Industry Association of America. Domestic travel in the United States. Available at: http://www.tia.org/Travel/tripChar.asp. Accessed March 1, 2004.

65. Armstrong BK, English DR. Cutaneous malignant melanoma. In: Schottenfeld D, Fraumeni JF, eds. Cancer epidemiology and prevention, 2nd ed. New York: Oxford University Press, 1996:1282–312.

66. Detweiler JB, Bedell BT, Salovey P, Pronin E, Rothman AJ. Message framing and sunscreen use: gain-framed messages motivate beach-goers. Health Psychol 1999;18(2):189–96.

67. Dey P, Collins S, Will S, Woodman CB. Randomised controlled trial assessing effectiveness of health education leaflets in reducing incidence of sunburn. BMJ 1995; 311(7012):1062–3.

68. Glanz K, Chang L, Song V, Silverio R, Muneoka L. Skin cancer prevention for children, parents, and caregivers: a field test of Hawaii's SunSmart program. J Am Acad Dermatol 1998;38(3):413–7.

69. Glanz K, Lew RA, Song V, Murakami-Akatsuka L. Skin cancer prevention in outdoor recreation settings: effects of the Hawaii SunSmart Program. Eff Clin Pract 2000; 3(2):53–61.

70. Keesling B, Friedman HS. Interventions to prevent skin cancer: experimental evaluation of informational and fear appeals. Psychol Health 1995;10(6):477–90.

71. Glanz K, Geller AC, Shigaki D, Maddock JE, Isnec MR. A randomized trial of skin cancer prevention in aquatic settings: the Pool Cool Program. Health Psychol 2002; 21(6):579–87.

72. Lombard D, Neubauer TE, Canfield D, Winett RA. Behavioral community intervention to reduce the risk of skin cancer. J Appl Behav Anal 1991;24(4):677–86.

73. Mayer JA, Slymen DJ, Eckhardt L, et al. Reducing ultraviolet radiation exposure in children. Prev Med 1997;26(4):516–22.

74. Mayer JA, Lewis E.C, Eckhardt L, et al. Promoting sun safety among zoo visitors. Prev Med 2001;33(3):162–9.

75. Segan C, Borland R, Hill D. Development and evaluation of a brochure on sun protection and sun exposure for tourists. Health Educ J 1999;58(2):177–91.

76. Weinstock MA, Rossi JS, Redding CA, Maddock JE. Randomized trial of a multicomponent stage-matched intervention to increase sun protection in at-risk beach bathers. Prev Med 2002;35(6):584–92.

77. Parrott R, Duggan A, Cremo J, Eckles A, Jones K, Steiner C. Communicating about youth's sun exposure risk to soccer coaches and parents: a pilot study in Georgia. Health Educ Behav 1999;26(3):385–95.

78. Presant CA, Presant SL, Mack J, Atterbury GB, French RA, Schroeder T. Youth cancer education through a combined American Cancer Society–Boy Scouts of America pilot program. J Cancer Educ 1987;2(4):229–31.

79. Glanz K, Silverio R, Farmer A. Diary reveals sun protective practices. Skin Ca Fdn J 1996;14:27–8.

80. Glanz K, Carbone E, Song V. Formative research for developing targeted skin cancer prevention programs for children in multiethnic Hawaii. Health Educ Res 1999; 14(2):155–66.

81. Glanz K, Lew RA, Song V, Murakami-Akatsuka L. Effects of skin cancer prevention in outdoor recreation settings: the Hawaii SunSmart Program. Eff Clin Pract 2000;3(2):1–5.

82. Glanz K, Maddock JE, Lew RA, Murakami-Akatsuka L. A randomized trial of the Hawaii SunSmart program's impact on outdoor recreation staff. J Am Acad Dermatol 2001;44(6):973–8.

83. Weinstock MA, Rossi JS, Redding CA, Maddock JE, Cottrill S. Sun protection behaviors and stages of change for the primary prevention of skin cancers among beachgoers in southeastern New England. Ann Behav Med 2000;22(4):286–93.

84. Stern RS, Weinstein MC, Baker SG. Risk reduction for nonmelanoma skin cancer with childhood sunscreen use. Arch Dermatol 1986;122(5):537–45.

85. Marks R. Role of childhood in the development of skin cancer. Aust Paediatr J 1988;24(6):337–8.

86. Grob JJ, Guglielmina C, Gouvernet J, Zarour H, Noe C, Bonerandi JJ. Study of sunbathing habits in children and adolescents: application to the prevention of melanoma. Dermatology 1993;186(2):94–88.

87. Maducduc L, Wagner R, Wagner K. Parents' use of sunscreen on beach-going children. Arch Dermatol 1992;128:628–9.

88. Weinstein JM, Yarnold PR, Hornung RL. Parental knowledge and practice of primary skin cancer prevention: gaps and solutions. Pediatr Dermatol 2001;18(6):473–7.

89. Centers for Disease Control and Prevention. Sun-protection behaviors used by adults for their children—United States, 1997. MMWR 1998;47:480–1.

90. Johnson K, Davy L, Boyett T, Weathers L, Roetzheim RG. Sun protection practices for children: knowledge, attitudes, and parent behaviors. Arch Pediatr Adolesc Med 2001;155(8):891–6.

91. Hall HI, Jorgensen CM, McDavid K, Kraft JM, Breslow R. Protection from sun ex-

posure in U.S. white children ages 6 months to 11 years. Public Health Rep 2001;116(4): 353–61.

92. Moise AF, Harrison SL, Gies HP. Solar ultraviolet radiation exposure of infants and small children. Photodermatol Photoimmunol Photomed 1999;15(3–4):109–14.

93. Grin CM, Pennoyer JW, Lehrich DA, Grant-Kels JM. Sun exposure of young children while at day care. Pediatr Dermatol 1994;11(4):304–9.

94. Boldeman C, Jansson B, Holm LE. Primary prevention of malignant melanoma in a Swedish urban preschool sector. J Cancer Educ 1991;6(4):247–53.

95. Boldeman C, Ullen H, Mansson-Brahme E, Holm LE. Primary prevention of malignant melanoma in the Stockholm Cancer Prevention Programme. Eur J Cancer Prev 1993;2:441–6.

96. Loescher LJ, Emerson J, Taylor A, Christensen DH, McKinney M. Educating preschoolers about sun safety. Am J Public Health 1995;85(7):939–43.

97. Marks R, Hill D. Behavioural change in adolescence: a major challenge for skin-cancer control in Australia. Med J Aust 1988;149(10):514–5.

98. Hill D, Dixon H. Promoting sun protection in children: rationale and challenges. Health Educ Behav 1999;26(3):409–17.

99. Arthey S, Clarke VA. Suntanning and sun protection: a review of the psychological literature. Soc Sci Med 1995;40(2):265–74.

100. Dobbinson S, Peipers A, Reading D, Sinclair C. A national approach to skin cancer prevention: the National SunSmart Schools Program. Med J Aust 1998;169(10):513–4.

101. Bernharndt J. Tailoring messages and design in a Web-based skin cancer prevention intervention. Int Electron J Health Educ 2001;4:290–7.

102. Cody R, Lee C. Behaviors, beliefs, and intentions in skin cancer prevention. J Behav Med 1990;13(4):373–89.

103. Jones JL, Leary MR. Effect of appearance-based admonitions against sun exposure on tanning intentions in young adults. Health Psychol 1994;13(1):86–90.

104. Katz RC, Jernigan S. Brief report: an empirically derived educational program for detecting and preventing skin cancer. J Behav Med 1991;14(4):421–8.

105. Lowe JB, Balanda KP, Stanton WR, Gillespie AM. Evaluation of a three-year school-based intervention to increase adolescent sun protection. Health Educ Behav 1999;26(3):396–408.

106. Mahler HI, Fitzpatrick B, Parker P, Lapin A. The relative effects of a health-based versus an appearance-based intervention designed to increase sunscreen use. Am J Health Promot 1997;11(6):426–9.

107. Mermelstein RJ, Riesenberg LA. Changing knowledge and attitudes about skin cancer risk factors in adolescents. Health Psychol 1992;11(6):371–6.

108. Mickler TJ, Rodrigue JR, Lescano CM. A comparison of three methods of teaching skin self-examinations. J Clin Psychol Med Settings 1999;6(3):273–86.

109. Kamin CS, O'Neill PN, Ahearn MJ. Developing and evaluating a cancer prevention teaching module for secondary education: Project SAFETY (Sun Awareness for Educating Today's Youth). J Cancer Educ 1993;8(4):313–8.

110. Prentice-Dunn S, Jones JL, Floyd DL. Persuasive appeals and the reduction of skin cancer risk: the roles of appearance concern, perceived benefits of a tan, and efficacy information. J Appl Soc Psychol 1997;27(12):1041–7.

111. Rothman AJ, Salovey P, Antone C, Keough K. The influence of message framing on intentions to perform health behaviors. J Exp Soc Psychol 1993;29(5):408–33.

112. Stephenson MT, Witte K. Fear, threat, and perceptions of efficacy from frightening skin cancer messages. Public Health Rev 1998;26(2):147–74.

113. Castle CM, Skinner TC, Hampson SE. Young women and suntanning: an evaluation of a health education leaflet. Psychol Health 1999;14(3):527.

114. Hughes BR, Altman DG, Newton JA. Melanoma and skin cancer: evaluation of a health education programme for secondary schools. Br J Dermatol 1993;128(4):412–7.

115. U.S. Census Bureau. Statistical abstract of the United States: 2000. Available at: http://www.census.gov/prod/2001pubs/statab/sec13.pdf. Accessed March 1, 2004.

116. Scotto J, Fears TR, Fraumeni JF Jr. Incidence of nonmelanoma skin cancer in the United States. Bethesda, MD: National Cancer Institute, National Institutes of Health, 1983. No. 83–2433.

117. Holman CD, Gibson IM, Stephenson M, Armstrong BK. Ultraviolet irradiation of human body sites in relation to occupation and outdoor activity: field studies using personal UVR dosimeters. Clin Exp Dermatol 1983;8(3):269–77.

118. Shoveller JA, Lovato CY, Peters L, Rivers JK. Canadian National Survey on Sun Exposure and Protective Behaviours: outdoor workers. Can J Public Health 2000;91(1): 34–5.

119. Azizi E, Modan M, Fuchs Z, Kushelevsky AP. Skin cancer risk of Israeli workers exposed to sunlight. Harefuah 1990;118:508–11.

120. Borland RM, Hocking B, Godking GA, Gibbs AF, Hill DJ. The impact of a skin cancer educational package for outdoor workers. Med J Aust 1991;154:686–8.

121. Dobbinson S, Borland R, Anderson M. Sponsorship and sun protection practices in lifesavers. Health Promot Int 1999;14(2):167–76.

122. Geller AC, Glanz K, Shigaki D, Isnec MR, Sun T, Maddock J. Impact of skin cancer prevention on outdoor aquatics staff: the Pool Cool program in Hawaii and Massachusetts. Prev Med 2001;33(3):155–61.

123. Girgis A, Sanson-Fisher RW, Watson A. A workplace intervention for increasing outdoor workers' use of solar protection. Am J Public Health 1994;84(1):77–81.

124. Hanrahan PF, Hersey P, Watson AB, Callaghan TM. The effect of an educational brochure on knowledge and early detection of melanoma. Aust J Public Health 1995; 19(3):270–4.

125. Azizi E, Flint P, Sadetzki S, et al. A graded work site intervention program to improve sun protection and skin cancer awareness in outdoor workers in Israel. Cancer Causes Control 2000;11(6):513–21.

126. Novick M. To burn or not to burn: use of computer-enhanced stimuli to encourage application of sunscreens. Cutis 1997;60(2):105–8.

127. Nelson C, Woodwell D. National Ambulatory Medical Care Survey: 1993 summary. Vital Health Stat 1998;13:136.

128. Dolan NC, Ng JS, Martin GJ, Robinson JK, Rademaker AW. Effectiveness of a skin cancer control educational intervention for internal medicine housestaff and attending physicians. J Gen Intern Med 1997;12(9):531–6.

129. Gerbert B, Wolff M, Tschann JM, et al. Activating patients to practice skin cancer prevention: response to mailed materials from physicians versus HMOs. Am J Prev Med 1997;13(3):214–20.

130. Harris JM, Salasche SJ, Harris RB. Can Internet-based continuing medical education improve physicians' skin cancer knowledge and skills? J Gen Intern Med 2001; 16(1):50–6.

131. Harris JM Jr, Salasche SJ, Harris RB. Using the Internet to teach melanoma management guidelines to primary care physicians. J Eval Clin Pract 1999;5(2):199–211.

132. Johnson EY, Lookingbill DP. Sunscreen use and sun exposure. Trends in a white population. Arch Dermatol 1984;120(6):727–31.

133. Liu KE, Barankin B, Howard J, Guenther LC. One-year followup on the impact of a sun awareness curriculum on medical students' knowledge, attitudes, and behavior. J Cutan Med Surg 2001;5(3):193–200.

134. Mayer JA, Slymen DJ, Eckhardt L, et al. Skin cancer prevention counseling by pharmacists: specific outcomes of an intervention trial. Cancer Detect Prev 1998;22(4): 367–75.

135. McCormick LK, Masse L, Cummings SS, Burke C. Evaluation of skin cancer prevention module for nurses: change in knowledge, self-efficacy, and attitudes. Am J Health Promot 1999;13(5):282–9.

136. Mikkilineni R, Weinstock MA, Goldstein MG, Dube CE, Rossi JS. The impact of the basic skin cancer triage curriculum on provider's skin cancer control practices. J Gen Intern Med 2001;16(5):302–7.

137. Palmer RC, Mayer JA, Eckhardt L, Sallis JF. Promoting sunscreen in a community drugstore. Am J Public Health 1998;88(4):681.

138. Azurdia RM, Pagliaro JA, Rhodes LE. Sunscreen application technique in photosensitive patients: a quantitative assessment of the effect of education. Photodermatol Photoimmunol Photomed 2000;16(2):53–6.

139. Brandberg Y, Bergenmar M, Michelson H, Mansson-Brahme E, Sjoden P. Six-month follow-up of effects of an information programme for patients with malignant melanoma. Patient Educ Couns 1996;28(2):201–8.

140. Brodkin RH, Altman EM. Controlling malignant melanoma: a focus on pediatricians. Am J Dis Child 1993;147(8):875–81.

141. Leinweber CE, Campbell HS, Trottier DL. Is a health promotion campaign successful in retail pharmacies? Can J Public Health 1995;86(6):380–3.

142. Robinson JK. Behavior modification obtained by sun protection education coupled with removal of a skin cancer. Arch Dermatol 1990;126(4):477–81.

143. Robinson JK. Compensation strategies in sun protection behaviors by a population with nonmelanoma skin cancer. Prev Med 1992;21(6):754–65.

144. Robinson JK, Rademaker AW. Skin cancer risk and sun protection learning by helpers of patients with nonmelanoma skin cancer. Prev Med 1995;24(4):333–41.

145. Mayer JA, Eckhardt L, Stepanski BM, et al. Promoting skin cancer prevention counseling by pharmacists. Am J Public Health 1998;88(7):1096–9.

146. Montague M, Borland R, Sinclair C. Slip! Slop! Slap! and SunSmart, 1980–2000: skin cancer control and 20 years of population-based campaigning. Health Educ Behav 2001;28(3):290–305.

147. Smith BJ, Ferguson C, McKenzie J, Bauman A, Vita P. Impacts from repeated mass media campaigns to promote sun protection in Australia. Health Promot Int 2002; 17(1):51–60.

148. Geller AC, Hufford D, Miller DR, et al. Evaluation of the Ultraviolet Index: media reactions and public response. J Am Acad Dermatol 1997;37(6):935–41.

149. Kiekbusch S, Hannich HJ, Isacsson A, et al. Impact of a cancer education multimedia device on public knowledge, attitudes, and behaviors: a controlled intervention study in Southern Sweden. J Cancer Educ 2000;15(4):232–6.

150. Theobald T, Marks R, Hill D, Dorevitch A. "Goodbye Sunshine": effects of a television program about melanoma on beliefs, behavior, and melanoma thickness. J Am Acad Dermatol 1991;25(4):717–23.

151. Boutwell WB. Under Cover: a community-based skin cancer prevention initiative. Cancer Bull 1993;45:279–81.

152. Boutwell WB. The Under Cover Skin Cancer Prevention Project. A community-based program in four Texas cities. Cancer 1995;75(2 suppl):657–60.

153. Cameron IH, McGuire C. "Are you dying to get a suntan?" The pre- and post-campaign survey results. Health Educ J 1990;49(4):166–70.

154. King PH, Murfin GD, Yanagisako KL, et al. Skin cancer/melanoma knowledge and behavior in Hawaii: changes during a community-based cancer control program. Prog Clin Biol Res 1982;130:135–44.

155. Putnam GL, Yanagisako KL. Skin cancer comic book: evaluation of a public educational vehicle. J Audiov Media Med 1985;8(1):22–5.

156. McGee R, Williams S. Adolescence and sun protection. N Z Med J 1992;105(943): 401–3.

157. Pfahlberg A, Gefeller O, Kolmel KF. Public awareness of malignant melanoma risk factors in Germany. J Epidemiol Commun Health 1997;51(6):698–700.

157a. Gelb BD, Boutwell WB, Cummings S. Using mass media communication for health promotion: results from a cancer center effort. Hosp Health Serv Adm 1994;39(3): 283–93.

158. Anonymous. Media dissemination of and public response to the Ultraviolet Index—United States, 1994–1995. MMWR 1997;46(17):370–3.

159. Del Mar CB, Green AC, Battistutta D. Do public media campaigns designed to increase skin cancer awareness result in increased skin excision rates? Aust N Z J Public Health 1997;21(7):751–4.

160. Buller DB, Callister MA, Reichert T. Skin cancer prevention by parents of young children: health information sources, skin cancer knowledge, and sun-protection practices. Oncol Nurs Forum 1995;22(10):1559–66.

161. Foltz AT. Parental knowledge and practices of skin cancer prevention: a pilot study. J Pediatr Health Care 1993;7(5):220–5.

162. Vail-Smith K, Watson CL, Felts WM, Parrillo AV, Knight SM, Hughes JL. Childhood sun exposure: parental knowledge, attitudes, and behaviors. J Health Educ 1997; 28(3):149–55.

163. Robinson JK, Rigel DS, Amonette RA. Summertime sun protection used by adults for their children. J Am Acad Dermatol 2000;42(5 pt 1):746–53.

164. Davis KJ, Cokkinides VE, Weinstock MA, O'Connell MC, Wingo PA. Summer sunburn and sun exposure among U.S. youths ages 11 to 18: national prevalence and associated factors. Pediatrics 2002;110(1 pt 1):27–35.

165. Hall HI, McDavid K, Jorgensen CM, Kraft JM. Factors associated with sunburn in white children aged 6 months to 11 years. Am J Prev Med 2001;20(1):9–14.

166. Bolognia JL, Berwick M, Fine JA, Simpson P, Jasmin M. Sun protection in newborns. A comparison of educational methods. Am J Dis Child 1991;145(10):1125–9.

167. Buller DB, Burgoon M, Hall JR, et al. Using language intensity to increase the success of a family intervention to protect children from ultraviolet radiation: predictions from language expectancy theory. Prev Med 2000;30(2):103–13.

168. Miller DR, Geller AC, Wood MC, Lew RA, Koh HK. The Falmouth Safe Skin Pro-

ject: evaluation of a community program to promote sun protection in youth. Health Educ Behav 1999;26(3):369–84.

169. Rodrigue JR. Promoting healthier behaviors, attitudes, and beliefs toward sun exposure in parents of young children. J Consult Clin Psychol 1996;64(6):1431–6.

170. Buller DB, Borland R, Burgoon M. Impact of behavioral intention on effectiveness of message features: evidence from the family sun safety project. Hum Commun Res 1998;24:433–53.

171. Buller DB, Burgoon M, Hall JR, et al. Long-term effects of language intensity in preventive messages on planned family solar protection. Health Commun 2000;12(3):2000–275.

172. Anti-Cancer Council of Victoria. Sunsmart evaluation studies, 2000–2003. Carlton: Anti-Cancer Council of Victoria, 2003.

173. Biger C, Epstein LM, Hagoel L, Tamir A, Robinson E. An evaluation of an education programme, for prevention and early diagnosis of malignancy in Israel. Eur J Cancer Prev 1994;3(4):305–12.

174. Carmel S, Shani E, Rosenberg L. The role of age and an expanded Health Belief Model in predicting skin cancer protective behavior. Health Educ Res 1994;9(4):433–47.

175. NSW Cancer Council. Report on the Seymour Snowman Sun Protection Campaign (1997–1998). (unpublished). New South Wales, Australia: 1998.

176. Rassaby J, Larcombe I, Hill D, Wake R. Slip Slop Slap: health education about skin cancer. Cancer Forum 1983;7(63):69.

177. Sanson-Fisher R. Me No Fry 1994/1995 summer campaign evaluation report. New South Wales, Australia: NSW Department of Health, 1995.

178. Fielder H, Lo SV, Shorney S, Roberts DL. Skin, sun and sense: an evaluation of a skin cancer prevention campaign. Health Educ J 1996;55(4):431–8.

179. Holtrop JS. Sticking to it: a multifactor cancer risk-reduction program for low-income clients. J Health Educ 2000;31(3):122–7.

180. Kelly PP. Skin cancer and melanoma awareness campaign. Oncol Nurs Forum 1991;18(5):927–31.

181. Ramsdell WM, Kelly P, Coody D, Dany M. The Texas Skin Cancer/Melanoma Project. Tex Med 1991;87(10):70–3.

182. Richard MA, Martin S, Gouvernet J, Folchetti G, Bonerandi JJ, Grob JJ. Humour and alarmism in melanoma prevention: a randomized controlled study of 3 types of information leaflet. Br J Dermatol 1999;140(5):909–14.

183. Anti-Cancer Council of Victoria. Sunsmart evaluation studies 1. Carlton: Anti-Cancer Council of Victoria, 1994.

184. Anti-Cancer Council of Victoria. Sunsmart evaluation studies 2. Carlton: Anti-Cancer Council of Victoria, 1995.

185. Anti-Cancer Council of Victoria. Sunsmart evaluation studies 3. Carlton: Anti-Cancer Council of Victoria, 1996.

186. Anti-Cancer Council of Victoria. Sunsmart evaluation studies 4. Carlton: Anti-Cancer Council of Victoria, 1997.

187. Anti-Cancer Council of Victoria. SunSmart evaluation studies 5. Carlton: Anti-Cancer Council of Victoria, 1998.

188. Anti-Cancer Council of Victoria. SunSmart evaluation studies 6. Carlton: Anti-Cancer Council of Victoria, 1999.

189. Borland R, Hill D, Noy S. Being SunSmart: changes in community awareness

and reported behaviour following a primary prevention program for skin cancer control. Behav Change 1990;7:126–35.

190. Carmel S, Shani E, Rosenberg L. Skin cancer protective behaviors among the elderly: explaining their response to a health education program using the Health Belief Model. Educ Gerontol 1996;22(7):651–8.

191. Chapman S, Marks R, King M. Trends and tans and skin protection in Australian fashion magazines, 1982 through 1991. Am J Public Health 1992;82(12):1677–82.

192. Geller AC, Sayers L, Koh HK, Miller DR, Steinberg BL, Crosier-Wood M. The New Moms Project: educating mothers about sun protection in newborn nurseries. Pediatr Dermatol 1999;16(3):198–200.

193. Hill D, White V, Marks R, Theobald T, Borland R, Roy C. Melanoma prevention: behavioral and nonbehavioral factors in sunburn among an Australian urban population. Prev Med 1992;21(5):654–69.

194. Hill D, White V, Marks R, Borland R. Changes in sun-related attitudes and behaviours, and reduced sunburn prevalence in a population at high risk of melanoma. Eur J Cancer Prev 1993;2(6):447–56.

195. Marks R. Melanoma prevention: is it possible to change a population's behavior in the sun? Pigment Cell Res 1994;7(2):104–6.

196. Sanson-Fisher R. Me No Fry 1992/93 summer campaign evaluation report. New South Wales, Australia: NSW Department of Health, 1993.

197. Sanson-Fisher R. Me No Fry 1993/1994 summer campaign evaluation report. New South Wales, Australia: NSW Department of Health, 1994.

198. Staples M, Marks R, Giles G. Trends in the incidence of non-melanocytic skin cancer (NMSC) treated in Australia 1985–1995: are primary prevention programs starting to have an effect? Int J Cancer 1998;78:144–8.

199. Centers for Disease Control and Prevention. Preventing skin cancer. Findings of the Task Force on Community Preventive Services on reducing exposure to ultraviolet light. MMWR 2003;52(RR-15):1–12.

200. Task Force on Community Preventive Services. Recommendations to prevent skin cancer by reducing exposure to ultraviolet radiation. Am J Prev Med, in press.

201. Sheridan SL, Harris RP, Woolf SH. Shared decision making about screening and chemoprevention: a suggested approach from the U.S. Preventive Services Task Force. Am J Prev Med 2004;26(1):56–66.

202. Ross LE, Coates RJ, Breen N, Uhler RJ, Potosky AL, Blackman D. Prostate-specific antigen (PSA) test use reported in the 2000 National Health Interview Survey. Prev Med 2004; 38(6): 732–44..

203. Harris R, Lohr KN. Screening for prostate cancer: an update of the evidence for the U.S. Preventive Services Task Force. Ann Intern Med 2002;137(11):917–29.

204. U.S. Preventive Services Task Force. Recommendations and rationale: screening for prostate cancer. Available at: http://www.ahcpr.gov/clinic/3rduspstf/prostatescr/prostaterr.htm. Accessed April 6, 2004.

205. U.S. Preventive Services Task Force. Recommendations and rationale: screening for breast cancer. Available at: http://www.ahcpr.gov/clinic/3rduspstf/breastcancer/brcanrr.htm. Accessed April 21, 2003.

206. Smith RA, Saslow D, Sawyer KA, et al. American Cancer Society guidelines for breast cancer screening: update 2003. CA Cancer J Clin 2003;53(3):141–69.

207. Saslow D, Runowicz CD, Solomon D, et al. American Cancer Society guideline

for the early detection of cervical neoplasia and cancer. CA: Cancer J Clin 2002;52(6): 342–62.

208. U.S. Preventive Services Task Force. Recommendations and rationale: screening for colorectal cancer. Available at: http://www.ahcpr.gov/clinic/3rduspstf/colorectal/colorr.htm. Accessed April 21, 2003.

209. Woolf SH. The best screening test for colorectal cancer-a personal choice. N Engl J Med 2000;343(22):1641–3.

210. Pignone M, Harris R, Kinsinger L. Videotape-based decision aid for colon cancer screening. A randomized, controlled trial. Ann Intern Med 2000;133(10):761–9.

211. Rimer BK, Halabi S, Sugg SC, et al. Effects of a mammography decision-making intervention at 12 and 24 months. Am J Prev Med 2002;22(4):247–57.

212. Greenfield S, Kaplan SH, Ware JE Jr, Yano EM, Frank HJ. Patients' participation in medical care: effects on blood sugar control and quality of life in diabetes. J Gen Intern Med 1988;3(5):448–57.

213. Briss PA, Rimer BK, Reilley B, et al. Promoting informed decisions about cancer screening in communities and healthcare systems. Am J Prev Med 2004;26(1):67–80.

214. Briss PA, Zaza S, Pappaioanou M, et al. Developing an evidence-based Guide to Community Preventive Services—methods. Am J Prev Med 2000;18(1S):35–43.

215. Davison BJ, Kirk P, Degner LF, Hassard TH. Information and patient participation in screening for prostate cancer. Patient Educ Couns 1999;37(3):255–63.

216. Dolan JG, Frisina S. Randomized controlled trial of a patient decision aid for colorectal cancer screening. Med Decis Making 2002;22(2):125–39.

217. Flood A, Wennberg J, Nease R, Fowler F, Ding J, Hynes L. The importance of patient preference in the decision to screen for prostate cancer. J Gen Intern Med 1996; 11:342–9.

218. Frosch DL, Kaplan RM, Felitti V. The evaluation of two methods to facilitate shared decision making for men considering the prostate-specific antigen test. J Gen Intern Med 2001;16(6):391–8.

219. Schapira MM, VanRuiswyk J. The effect of an illustrated pamphlet decision-aid on the use of prostate cancer screening tests. J Fam Pract 2000;49(5):418–24.

220. Volk R, Cass A, Spann S. A randomized controlled trial of shared decision making for prostate cancer screening. Arch Fam Med 1999;8:333–40.

221. Wilt TJ, Paul J, Murdoch M, Nelson D, Nugent S, Rubins HB. Educating men about prostate cancer screening. A randomized trial of a mailed pamphlet. Eff Clin Pract 2001;4(3):112–20.

222. Wolf AM, Nasser JF, Wolf AM, Schorling JB. The impact of informed consent on patient interest in prostate-specific antigen screening. Arch Intern Med 1996;156(12): 1333–6.

223. Wolf AM, Schorling JB. Does informed consent alter elderly patients' preferences for colorectal cancer screening? Results of a randomized trial. J Gen Intern Med 2000; 15(1):24–30.

224. Rimer BK, Halabi S, Sugg SC, et al. The short-term impact of tailored mammography decision-making interventions. Patient Educ Couns 2001;43(3):269–85.

225. Wolf AM, Schorling JB. Preferences of elderly men for prostate-specific antigen screening and the impact of informed consent. J Gerontol A Biol Sci Med Sci 1998;53(3): M195–M200.

Chapter 5

Diabetes

Diabetes mellitus (diabetes) is a prevalent, costly condition that causes significant illness, disability, and premature death. An estimated 15.7 million people (5.9% of the total U.S. population) have diabetes,[1] of whom 5.4 million are undiagnosed. In 1997 alone, 789,000 new cases were diagnosed.[1] Moreover, according to 1996 death certificates, diabetes is the seventh leading cause of death in the United States.[1] The costs of diabetes to the American healthcare system are enormous, with total (direct and indirect) costs estimated at $98 billion in 1997.[2]

Our systematic reviews focused on population-based strategies to improve the care of people with either type 1 or type 2 diabetes. (Type 1 diabetes results from destruction of the β-cells of the pancreas, and type 2 is charac-

---

*Insufficient evidence means that we were not able to determine whether or not the intervention works.

The Task Force approved the recommendations in this chapter in 2000–2001. The research on which the findings are based was conducted between 1966 and December 2000. This information has been previously published in the American Journal of Preventive Medicine (2002; 22[4S]:10–14, 15–38, and 39–66) and the MMWR Recommendations and Reports (2001; 50[No. RR-16]:1–15).

terized by insulin resistance and relative insulin deficiency.[3]) The interventions reviewed were conducted both in healthcare systems and in community settings.

OBJECTIVES AND RECOMMENDATIONS FROM OTHER ADVISORY GROUPS

Reducing illness, disability, and premature death and improving the quality of life for people with diabetes is a major public health objective. *Healthy People 2010*[4] objectives have been set to prevent diabetes, increase early diagnosis, improve rates of screening for its complications, and decrease morbidity and mortality. Objectives that address issues specifically covered in this chapter are shown in Table 5–1.

Recommendations for clinical care of persons with diabetes can be obtained from the American Diabetes Association (ADA),[5] and screening recommendations are available from the U.S. Preventive Services Task Force's *Guide to Clinical Preventive Services.*[6]

METHODS

Methods used for the reviews are summarized in Chapter 10. Specific methods used in the systematic reviews of diabetes have been described elsewhere[7] and are available at www.thecommunityguide.org/diabetes. The analytic frameworks depicting the conceptual approach used in the reviews are presented in Figures 5–1 and 5–2.

ECONOMIC EFFICIENCY

A systematic review of available economic evaluations was conducted for all recommended interventions, and a summary of each review is presented with the related intervention. The methods used to conduct these economics reviews are summarized in Chapter 11.

RECOMMENDATIONS AND FINDINGS

This section presents a summary of the findings of the systematic reviews conducted to determine the effectiveness of the selected interventions in this topic area. We reviewed two interventions appropriate for use in healthcare systems (disease management and case management) and five situations in which diabetes self-management education (DSME) may be appropriate (in community gathering places, in the home, in summer camps, at the worksite, and in the education of school personnel).

Table 5–1. *Healthy People 2010*[4] Objectives for Improving Diabetes Outcomes

Objective	Population	Baseline	2010 Objective
Increase the proportion of persons with diabetes who receive formal diabetes education (Objective 5–1)	All diabetics	45% (1998[a])	60%
Reduce the frequency of foot ulcers in persons with diabetes (5–9)	All diabetics	Developmental	
Reduce the rate of lower extremity amputations per 1000 persons with diabetes (5–10)	All diabetics	4.1% (1997[a])	1.8
Increase the proportion of persons with diabetes who obtain an annual urinary microalbumin measurement (5–11)	All diabetics	Developmental	
Increase the proportion of adults ≥18 years with diabetes who have a glyco-sylated hemoglobin measurement at least once a year (5–12)	Adult diabetics	24% (1998[a,b])	50%
Increase the proportion of adults ≥18 years with diabetes who have an annual dilated eye examination (5–13)	Adult diabetics	47% (1998[a])	75%
Increase the proportion of adults ≥18 years with diabetes who have at least an annual foot examination (5–14)	Adult diabetics	55% (1998[a,b])	75%
Increase the proportion of adults ≥40 years with diabetes who take aspirin at least 15 times per month (5–16)	Adult diabetics	20% (1988–94[a])	30%
Increase the proportion of adults ≥18 years with diabetes who perform blood-glucose self-monitoring at least once daily (5–17)	Adult diabetics	42% (1998[a,b])	60%

[a]Age adjusted to the year 2000 standard population.

[b]Mean of data from 39 states.

Healthcare System Interventions

Traditional methods of healthcare delivery do not adequately address the needs of individual people or populations with diabetes. For example, in a survey of the care received by patients of primary care providers, people with diabetes were receiving only 64% to 74% of the services recommended by the ADA Provider Recognition Program.[8] A chart audit covering one year in a health maintenance organization (HMO) setting showed that, despite the ADA recommendation of two to four glycated hemoglobin (GHb) measure-

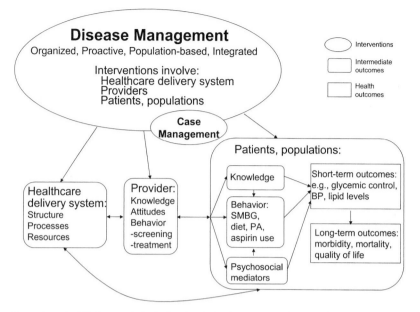

Figure 5–1. Analytic framework illustrating the relationships between disease and case management and short- and long-term health care, system, provider, and client outcomes. (BP = blood pressure, PA = physical activity, SMBG = self-monitoring blood glucose.) (Reprinted from Am J Prev Med, Vol. 22, No. 4S, Norris SL et al., The effectiveness of disease and case management for people with diabetes: a systematic review, p. 17, Copyright 2002, with permission from American Journal of Preventive Medicine.)

ments per year, values were documented for only 44% of people with diabetes and annual urine protein measurements were performed on only 48% of patients.[9]

Improving care for people with diabetes reduces healthcare costs. In a review of economic analyses of interventions for diabetes, eye care and preconception care were found to be cost-saving, and preventing neuropathy in type 1 diabetes and improving glycemic control for either type 1 or type 2 diabetes were found to be clearly cost-effective.[10] Using modeling techniques at an HMO, it was found that every percentage point increase in A1c (a test that measures a person's average blood glucose level over the past two to three months) above normal was associated with a significant increase in costs over the next three years.[11] Decreases in A1c result in cost savings: one study noted that improved glycemic control was associated with short-term decreases in the use of healthcare services, increased productivity, and enhanced quality of life,[12] and another found that achieving and sustaining glycemic control for one to two years was associated with cost savings among adults with diabetes.[13]

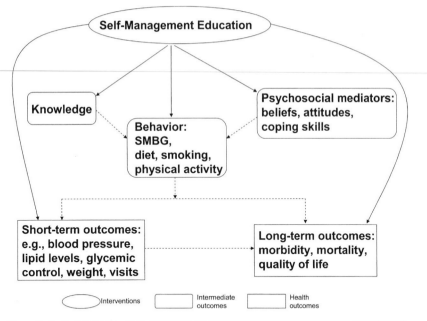

Figure 5–2. Analytic framework illustrating the relationships between self-management education and short- and long-term client outcomes. (SMBG = self-monitoring blood glucose.) (Reprinted from Am J Prev Med, Vol. 22, No. 4S, Norris SL et al., Increasing diabetes self-management education in community settings: a systematic review, p. 40, Copyright 2002, with permission from American Journal of Preventive Medicine.)

In the 1990s, innovative interventions for healthcare delivery emerged, which show promise for improving care, improving health outcomes, and reducing costs for individuals and populations with diabetes. Disease and case management are two such new interventions.

Our conceptual approach to the reviews of disease and case management interventions, as well as the relationships between the interventions and provider and patient outcomes, are shown in Figure 5–1. Disease management involves many factors in the health-care delivery system and among providers and patients, as illustrated in Figure 5–1. Case management can be implemented along with disease management, by itself, or with other interventions.

Disease and case management can affect patient knowledge[14] and such psychosocial factors as motivation,[15] social support,[16] and health beliefs,[16,17] which in turn predict how well a patient will care for him- or herself. Patient self-care behaviors (e.g., self-monitoring of blood glucose) and lifestyle directly affect blood pressure, lipid concentrations, glycemic control, renal function, lesions of the feet, and diabetic retinopathy,[18–26] which, in turn, affect long-term health, quality of life, and mortality.[18,27–31]

Disease Management: Recommended (Strong Evidence of Effectiveness)

These interventions use organized, proactive, multicomponent approaches to healthcare delivery for people with diabetes. Care is focused on, and integrated across, the spectrum of the disease and its complications, the prevention of comorbid conditions, and the relevant aspects of the delivery system, with the goal of improving both short- and long-term health or economic outcomes.

Effectiveness

- Disease management is effective in reducing GHb by approximately 0.5 percentage points.
- Disease management is also effective in improving provider monitoring of GHb by approximately 16 percentage points and lipid levels by approximately 24 percentage points.
- Disease management is also effective in improving provider screening for retinopathy by approximately 9 percentage points, foot lesions and peripheral neuropathy by approximately 27 percentage points each, and urine protein (proteinuria) by approximately 10 percentage points.

Applicability

- These findings should be applicable to adults with diabetes in managed care organizations and community clinics in the United States and Europe.

Disease management has played a prominent role in innovative systems of clinical care over the past two decades. The earliest application of a disease-focused intervention involved prescription drugs,[32] and the first use of the term *disease management* appears to have been in the late 1980s at the Mayo Clinic.[33] In the mid-1990s the term emerged in the general medical literature, and by 1999 approximately 200 companies offered disease management services.[34] The initial focus of disease management was cost control, but more recently, quality and economic efficiency have driven disease management interventions. These interventions are used in several clinical care areas, primarily for costly chronic diseases or conditions such as heart failure,[35,36] arthritis,[37] and depression.[38,39]

We define disease management[40] as an organized, proactive, multicomponent approach to healthcare delivery that involves all members of a population with a specific disease such as diabetes. The essential components of disease management are (*1*) identification and management of people with diabetes or a subset with certain risk factors for poor outcomes (e.g., cardiovascular disease risk factors), (*2*) guidelines or performance standards for care, (*3*) information systems for tracking and monitoring, and (*4*) measurement and management of outcomes. Disease management can be combined with interventions that focus on the patient or population (e.g., DSME), the provider (e.g., reminders or continuing education), or the healthcare system or practice (e.g., practice redesign). For example, a small group of providers might initiate the following as a disease management program: People with diabetes are identified from billing records or provider and support staff recollection. Patients' names are placed in an electronic file (e.g., a spreadsheet, a relational database, or software specifically designed for this purpose). This database records A1c, the last visit, and the last retinal and foot exams. Once a month, a nurse or support staff member reviews the database and calls or mails reminders to patients who are in need of visits and screening. A team of providers, including a nurse whose role is to coordinate and monitor the care of people with diabetes, then delivers care that follows evidence-based diabetes care guidelines.

Our definition of disease management excludes many programs that may refer to themselves as *disease management.* This review and its recommendations apply only to programs that encompass the four components of disease management in our definition. We did not examine the effectiveness of individual components or the effectiveness of various other combinations of interventions.

The findings of our systematic review are based on 27 studies (in 28 reports) that evaluated the effectiveness of disease management in improving patient health and provider practices.[41–68] An additional eight studies were identified but did not meet our quality criteria and were excluded from the review.[69–76] The 27 studies provided evidence of effectiveness for several patient and provider outcomes. Glycated hemoglobin improved in 18 of 19 studies, with a median absolute decrease of 0.5 percentage points (interquartile range, 0.1 to 1.35). We found strong evidence of improvement in the percentage of providers who performed annual monitoring of GHb and retinopathy screening, and sufficient evidence of improvement in screening for foot lesions or peripheral neuropathy, lipid concentrations, and proteinuria. A small number of studies examined the effectiveness of disease management on other important patient outcomes, including weight and body mass index, blood pressure, and lipid concentrations. These studies reported inconsistent results, and therefore provided insufficient evidence to determine the effectiveness of the intervention on these outcomes.

The improvements in glycemic control as measured by GHb, as well as an increase in the percentage of providers who perform annual monitoring of GHb and retinopathy and other screening, show that disease management is effective in improving patient health and provider practices.

These findings should be applicable to adults with diabetes in managed care organizations and community clinics. No studies examined children with diabetes. Studies were conducted predominantly in urban centers in the United States and Europe.

Although type 1 diabetes patients were not examined exclusively in any study, these results should apply to adults with type 1 diabetes. Despite important differences between people with type 1 and type 2 diabetes, the goals of treatment and general management guidelines are identical. Thus, effective methods of population management are likely to be similar for adults with type 1 and type 2 diabetes. Disease management has been studied in minority and racially mixed populations, but it remains unclear how cultural characteristics might affect outcomes. One possible difference could be varying levels of access to health care. Gestational diabetes (which develops in 2% to 3% of all pregnant women and disappears with delivery[1]) was not specifically studied, but disease management interventions should also apply to affected individuals.

Studies generally involved the entire population of providers in a facility, although in some studies the researchers selected specific providers to participate or the providers volunteered. Researcher- or self-selected providers may have more of a commitment to change or have greater skills in systems change, the use of practice guidelines, or team approaches to care, thus limiting the applicability of these studies to other providers.

Studies were conducted in a variety of managed care organizations (including network or primary care–based models and staff or group model HMOs as well as community clinics). Other settings (academic centers, a hospital clinic, and the Indian Health Service)[67] were examined, but the data were insufficient to determine the effectiveness of disease management in those settings. Where community clinics and managed care delivery systems differ from other delivery systems, applicability to those other types of delivery systems could be limited. However, findings in HMOs may be applicable to other organized systems, such as the Indian Health Service.

The findings of our systematic review of economic evaluations are based on two studies. The first study, a cost analysis conducted in Scotland, reported the average cost for adult patients of an integrated care disease management intervention versus traditional hospital clinic care.[49] Integrated care patients were seen in a general practice every three or four months and in the hospital clinic annually. General practitioners and patients received consultation reminders, patient records were consistently updated, and practices received care guidelines. Traditional care patients were seen at the clinic every four months and received appointment reminders. Costs included those associated with general practice and clinic visits (staff, administrative, overhead, and supply costs). The annual average adjusted costs were $143–$185 for integrated care and $101 for traditional care. After two years, no significant difference was seen between the two groups for GHb, body mass index, creatinine, or blood pressure. The integrated care patients, however, had higher annual rates compared with the traditional care group for routine diabetes care visits (5.3 versus 4.8) and frequency of screening and monitoring of GHb (4.5 versus 1.3), blood pressure (4.2 versus 1.2), and visual acuity (2.6 versus 0.7). The applicability of these findings is limited to general practice and hospital clinic settings.

The second study was a cost–benefit analysis of preconception plus prenatal care versus prenatal care only for women with established diabetes.[1] Preconception care involves close interaction between the patient and an interdisciplinary healthcare team (primary care and specialist physicians, nurse educator, dietitian, and social worker), intensive evaluation, follow-up, testing, and monitoring to optimize glycemic control and reduce adverse maternal and infant outcomes. The analysis modeled the program's costs and benefits, or savings, from reduced adverse maternal and neonatal outcomes. Program costs included personnel, laboratory and other tests, supplies, outreach, delivery, and time of the patient and a significant other. Costs for maternal and neonatal adverse outcomes were for hospital, physician, and subsequent neonatal care. Costs attributable to future lost productivity of the mother and child were not included. The preconception care intervention's adjusted cost saving (net benefit) of $2702 per enrollee was the difference between estimated prenatal care only and the preconception and prenatal care intervention costs (program costs plus maternal and neonatal adverse outcome costs). The savings resulted largely from preventing the most expensive adverse events—congenital anomalies. The incremental benefit–cost ratio of 1.86 was the adverse outcome cost savings of the preconception plus prenatal care intervention versus the prenatal only program divided by the difference in program costs. This ratio represents the savings for each additional dollar invested in the preconception and prenatal care program versus the prenatal care only program.

Although not evaluated in the literature, we also identified potential barriers to implementing disease management interventions among organizations, providers or support staff, and patients. Organizations may lack the leadership to support these interventions and the financial resources needed for implementation and maintenance, or they may lack practice guidelines and the necessary skills and resources to develop guidelines. (Several practice guidelines are publicly available, such as the guidelines published annually by the ADA.[5]) Providers practicing in the traditional mode of reactive care may find that the switch to proactive, organized management requires the redesign of much of their practice and approach to patient care, including appointment and follow-up scheduling; allocation of clinic time to review registries and practice guidelines; delineation of the roles of support staff and providers; the delegation of care traditionally performed by physicians to other professionals, such as nurses; team organization; and the use of planned visits and patient reminders.[77-79] Providers may find disease management time-consuming, particularly initially, and they may be inexperienced or uncomfortable with information systems. Barriers to using practice guidelines, described elsewhere,[80] include lack of awareness of or familiarity with them, disagreement with the guidelines, lack of confidence that patient outcomes can be improved, inability to overcome the inertia of previous routines, and external barriers such as inconvenience and insufficient time. In addition, there may be little or no reimbursement for delivering patient reminders and other proactive care strategies. Identifying patients to participate in these interventions, also often difficult, can be accomplished through provider and staff memory, hospital discharge summaries, claims data,[81,82] visit encounter forms, laboratory test results, patient-initiated visits, or pharmacy activity. Patient barriers include difficulties in maintaining a healthy lifestyle and the complexity of diabetes self-management.[83]

In conclusion, the Task Force recommends disease management on the basis of strong evidence of effectiveness in reducing GHb and of increasing the percentage of patients screened annually for diabetic retinopathy. Sufficient evidence was also found for improving provider screening for foot lesions or peripheral neuropathy, lipid concentrations, and proteinuria. These findings should be applicable to adults with diabetes in managed care organizations and community clinics in the United States and Europe.

Case Management: Recommended (Strong Evidence of Effectiveness)

Case management identifies people at risk for excessive use of healthcare resources, poor coordination of healthcare services, or poor health outcomes and addresses their needs through improved planning, coordination, and provision of care. Authority is assigned to one professional (the case manager) who is not the direct healthcare provider, but who oversees and is responsible for coordinating all of the patient's care. Case management can stand alone as a single-component intervention, can be combined with other clinical care interventions (e.g., practice guidelines or patient reminders), or can be part of a disease management intervention.

Effectiveness

- Case management is effective both when delivered in conjunction with disease management and when delivered with one or more educational, reminder, or support interventions.

- Glycated hemoglobin improved when case management was part of a disease management intervention (approximate decrease 0.5 percentage points) or alone (approximate decrease 0.4 percentage points).
- Case management is effective in improving provider monitoring of GHb by approximately 33 percentage points as part of a disease management intervention.

Applicability

- These findings should be applicable primarily to adults in managed care settings in community clinics in the United States.

Case management is an important intervention for people at high risk for adverse outcomes and excessive use of healthcare services.[84] It usually involves the assignment of authority to a professional (the case manager) who is not the provider of direct health care, but who oversees and is responsible for coordinating and implementing care. In interventions involving diabetes, the case manager is generally a non-physician, most commonly a nurse.

Case management was first used in nursing and social work as early as the 1850s,[85] and the terminology has evolved. The term *care management* is often used instead (the American Geriatrics Society prefers this term to others[86]). The effectiveness of case management has been examined in a number of diseases, conditions, and situations other than diabetes, including psychiatric disorders,[87] chronic heart failure,[88] geriatric care,[89] and care initiated at the time of hospital discharge.[90,91]

Case management in diabetes has five essential features:

- Identification of eligible people—those at high risk for excessive resource use, poor outcomes, or poor coordination of services. All people with diabetes might be targeted, but more commonly a subset with specific disease risk factors (e.g., coexisting cardiovascular disease or poor glycemic control) or high healthcare usage (e.g., as determined by visits or costs) is targeted.
- Comprehensive assessment of each individual's needs.
- Development of an individual care plan.
- Implementation of the care plan.
- Monitoring of outcomes. Monitoring of the individual patient or population may involve several outcomes, including process (e.g., client satisfaction, service usage), health, quality of life, or economic (e.g., cost, hospital admissions) outcomes.

Case management interventions are often incorporated into multicomponent interventions, making it difficult to assess the effectiveness of case management alone. Interventions that can be combined with case management include self-management education (DSME, reviewed in this chapter), home visits, telephone call outreach, telemedicine, and client reminders.

The findings of our systematic review are based on 15 studies (in 18 reports) that examined the effectiveness of diabetes case management.[42,45,46,50,51,55,58,60–62,64,70,92–97] Nine additional studies were identified but did not meet our quality criteria or did not report on relevant outcomes and were excluded from the review.[72,98–105] The 15 reviewed studies provided data on numerous provider and client outcomes. Improvement in GHb was similar when case management was delivered with disease management and when it was not. When delivered with disease management, the evidence of its effect on provider monitoring of GHb was sufficient to show its effectiveness. When delivered either alone or in combination with disease management, the evidence was insufficient to determine the effect of case management on lipid concentrations, weight or body mass index, and blood pressure, as studies were few, with inconsistent results. The quality of life improved in two studies.

These results show that case management, whether combined with disease management or with another educational, reminder, or support intervention, is effective in improving both monitoring of GHb levels and GHb levels themselves.

These findings should be applicable to adults in U.S. managed care settings. All but one study was performed in the United States. Settings were primarily managed care organizations, although an academic center, community clinics, a military clinic, and a veterans' hospital were also studied. In most studies, the entire eligible population of providers at a clinic or in a healthcare organization was recruited to participate, except for three studies that used a subset of providers.

Study populations, mainly adults with type 2 diabetes, were predominantly mixed by sex and race. One study was of children with type 1 diabetes (mean age, 9.8 years). Demographic information, including age and type of diabetes, was not reported in many studies.

Case management was implemented along with disease management in many of the studies. Other studies included such additional interventions as DSME, telemedicine support, insulin-adjustment algorithms, group support, client reminders, and hospital discharge assessment and follow-up. It was therefore not possible to determine the isolated effect of case management in these studies.

We did not find any economic evaluations of case management.

Possible barriers to implementation are discussed above under Disease Management.

In conclusion, the Task Force recommends case management on the basis of strong evidence of effectiveness in improving glycemic control. When combined with disease management, case management is also effective in improving provider monitoring of GHb. These findings are applicable primarily to adults in managed care settings in the United States.

Diabetes Self-Management Education

Diabetes self-management education (DSME), the process of teaching people to manage their diabetes,[106] has been considered an important part of the clinical management of diabetes since the 1930s.[107] The American Diabetes Association (ADA) recommends assessing self-management skills and knowledge of diabetes at least annually and providing or encouraging continuing education.[108] Diabetes self-management education is considered "the cornerstone of treatment for all people with diabetes" by the Task Force to Revise the National Standards for Diabetes Self-Management Education Programs,[106] a group representing national public health and diabetes-related organizations. This need is also recognized in objective 5–1 of *Healthy People 2010*:[4] to increase to 60% (from the 1998 baseline of 40%) the proportion of people with diabetes who receive formal diabetes education.

The goals of DSME are to achieve optimal metabolic control and quality of life and to prevent acute and chronic complications while keeping costs acceptable.[109] Unfortunately, 50% to 80% of people with diabetes have significant knowledge and skill deficits,[110] and mean glycated hemoglobin (GHb) levels are unacceptably high both in people with type 1[111] and those with type 2[112] diabetes. Furthermore, less than half of the people with type 2 diabetes achieve ideal glycemic control[113] (A1c $< 7.0\%$).[108]

The abundant literature on diabetes education and its effectiveness includes several important reviews demonstrating the positive effects of DSME on a variety of outcomes, particularly at short-term follow-up.[83,110,114–118] These reviews, however, and most of the existing literature focus primarily on clinical settings.

Our conceptual approach to the reviews of diabetes self-management interventions is shown in Figure 5–2. We reviewed the effectiveness of DSME delivered outside of traditional clinical settings, in community centers, faith institutions, and other community gathering places; the home; the worksite; recreational camps; and schools. We did not examine evidence on the effectiveness of clinical care interventions for the individual patient; recommendations on clinical care may be obtained from the ADA,[5] and screening recommendations are available from the U.S. Preventive Services Task Force.[6] Our review focused on people who have diabetes and did not address primary prevention of diabetes. For prevention of type 2 diabetes, the best strategies are weight control and adequate physical activity among high-risk people, including those with impaired glucose tolerance.[119]

Diabetes Self-Management Education in Community Gathering Places:
Recommended for Adults with Type 2 Diabetes (Sufficient Evidence of Effectiveness)

Diabetes self-management education for people 18 years of age or older can be provided in such community gathering places as community centers, libraries, private facilities (e.g., cardiovascular risk reduction centers), and faith institutions. Although recommended for improving glycemic control, the interventions reviewed were rarely coordinated with the individual's clinical care provider, and the nature and extent of care in the clinical setting was unclear. These interventions should be coordinated with the individual's primary care provider and are not meant to replace education delivered in the clinical setting.

Effectiveness

- Diabetes self-management education in community gathering places is effective in decreasing GHb by approximately 2 percentage points.

Applicability

- These findings should be applicable to adults with type 2 diabetes, with a range of racial and ethnic backgrounds, in a variety of settings.
- Applicability may be limited, however, because study populations were self-selected, had high attrition rates, and had high baseline GHb levels.

We reviewed DSME interventions in which people aged 18 or older were educated in settings outside the home, clinic, school, or worksite because clinic settings may not be ideal for DSME, the home setting is conducive only to individual and family teaching, and the worksite is available only to people who work outside the home. Thus, DSME in community gathering places may reach people who would not normally receive this education. Church-based health education and screening programs are effective in helping African Americans,[120] particularly women 65 years of age and older, to adopt new behaviors.[121] Community interventions often offer the benefit of cultural relevance, possibly because the diverse learning styles of different cultures are better addressed in the community setting. The increased cultural relevance may increase acceptance of diabetes education.[122] Interventions in community gathering places also may be more convenient, especially for those in rural areas, and may thus promote attendance.

The findings of our systematic review are based on eight studies (in 12 reports) that evaluated the effectiveness of DSME in community gathering places.[123-134] Three additional studies were identified but did not meet our quality criteria or did not report on relevant outcomes and were excluded from the review.[135-137] The reviewed studies evaluated changes in GHb levels (four studies); knowledge (one study); fasting blood glucose (four studies); physical activity (one study); dietary intake (one study); or changes in weight (six studies), blood pressure (two studies), and lipid concentrations (three studies). The improvements in glycemic control (pooled estimate [weighted average], a decrease of 1.9%, 95% CI: 1.4, 2.4; four studies) provided sufficient evidence of effectiveness to recommend DSME in community gathering places. Evidence, however, was insufficient to determine the effectiveness of this intervention in improving dietary intake, physical activity, weight, blood pressure, or lipid levels because of the small number of studies and inconsistent effects.

These results should be applicable to adults with type 2 diabetes, with a range of racial and ethnic backgrounds, in a variety of settings. Applicability may be limited, however, by the fact that those studied chose to be in the studies and had high attrition rates as well as high baseline GHb levels. The mean age of the study populations ranged from 43 to 71 years in the seven studies that reported age. Seven studies examined both male and female populations, and five studies reported racial and ethnic backgrounds: Native American (two studies) and Mexican American (three studies). The six studies that reported the type of diabetes all involved people with type 2 diabetes. Baseline mean GHb levels were high, with a mean of 12.3% (range, 11.7% to 15.8%). The population in six studies consisted of self-selected volunteers, with randomly selected populations in the other two. All eight studies were performed in the United States, three in rural areas.

The interventions were conducted in a variety of settings: faith-based institutions (two studies), community centers (five studies), and a Pritikin residential treatment center (one study). Interventions focused on a variety of issues: general diabetes education and self-care, diet, physical activity, and diet combined with physical activity. The interventions in three studies were coordinated with primary care providers, but the nature and extent of clinical care was unclear. Attrition rates varied from 0% to 79%; in four studies these rates exceeded 20%, and no study compared dropouts to completers.

A lack of quality control and accountability could negatively affect the quality of programs in community settings, although no studies in our review examined this issue.

We did not find any economic evaluations of DSME in community gathering places.

We identified several potential barriers to implementing these interventions. In community settings, it may be difficult to find people who should receive DSME training. Participants are generally self-selected, and more general recruitment may be difficult. Another issue may be coordinating these interventions with the patient's primary care team.

In conclusion, the Task Force recommends DSME in community gathering places for adults with type 2 diabetes, on the basis of sufficient evidence that DSME is effective in improving glycemic control among people of varying ages and ethnic or racial backgrounds. Several precautions should, however, be noted. (*1*) Applicability may be limited because study populations were self-selected and had high attrition rates and high baseline GHb levels. (*2*) The studies rarely reported coordination with the clients' clinical care provider, and the nature and extent of care in the clinical setting was unclear. DSME for adults delivered in community gathering places should be coordinated with the individual's primary care provider, and should not be considered a replacement for education in the clinical setting until adequate coordination is established.

Diabetes Self-Management Education in the Home: Recommended for Children and Adolescents with Type 1 Diabetes (Sufficient Evidence of Effectiveness) Insufficient Evidence to Determine Effectiveness for People with Type 2 Diabetes

The home can be a good setting for DSME training, allowing the educator to address issues that may be more difficult to deal with in clinical settings, such as cultural, family, and environmental factors affecting lifestyle, self-monitoring of blood glucose, and barriers to optimal self-care.

Effectiveness

- Diabetes self-management education in the home is effective in improving glycemic control among children and adolescents with type 1 diabetes, whether conducted through home visits or computer-assisted instruction.
- Evidence was insufficient to determine the effectiveness of DSME in the home for people of any age with type 2 diabetes.
- Insufficient evidence means that we were not able to determine whether or not the intervention works.

Applicability

- The recommendation should be applicable to children and adolescents with type 1 diabetes.

In most of these home-based interventions, educators come to the home of the person with diabetes to assess and address issues that may not be apparent or may be more difficult to manage in the clinical setting. These issues include cultural, family, and environmental factors affecting lifestyle (particularly diet and physical activity), problem solving, self-monitoring of blood glucose, glycemic control, and the prevention and management of complications. Information and support can also be provided through computer-assisted instruction and electronic communication with healthcare professionals.

The findings of our systematic review are based on 10 randomized controlled trials that evaluated the effectiveness of DSME interventions in the home.[97,138-146] An additional eight studies were identified but either did not meet our quality criteria or did not report on relevant outcomes and were excluded from the review.[103,147-153] The reviewed studies examined knowledge, self-care skills, self-concept, use of healthcare services, birthweight and gestational age, quality of life, weight, foot appearance, blood glucose, and GHb levels.

Six studies examined GHb levels and were stratified by type of diabetes. Evidence of the effectiveness of DSME in the home on glycemic control was sufficient to recommend use of this approach for adolescents with type 1 diabetes (pooled estimate [weighted average], a decrease of 1.1%, 95% CI, 0.6, 1.6; four studies) but not for adults with type 2 diabetes (pooled estimate, a decrease of 0.5%, 95% CI, -0.1, 1.1; two studies). Evidence of the effectiveness of DSME in the home was insufficient to determine its effectiveness on other psychosocial, behavioral, or health outcomes for people with both type 1 and type 2 diabetes because of the small number of studies that examined these outcomes.

The recommendation should be applicable to children or adolescents with type 1 diabetes. Studies of young people with a mean age of 9 to 14 years were performed in the United States, Canada, and Australia; race or ethnicity was not reported in any of them. The recommendation, however, does not extend to people with type 2 diabetes because only two studies examined this population and their findings were inconsistent.

We identified other potential positive effects of DSME in the home. It could increase the involvement and support of the family and thereby improve lifestyle, knowledge level, and social support for people with diabetes. It could also lead to positive changes in diet and physical activity for family members, which could both help the person with diabetes maintain these new behaviors and prevent development of diabetes in relatives. People who have difficulty visiting a clinic may especially benefit from DSME in the home. We did not find any harms of this intervention.

The findings of our systematic review of economic evaluations of DSME in the home are based on one study.[154] This cost analysis study at the Montreal Children's Hospital in Canada reported the average cost of intensive home care, including insulin adjustment and DSME, for a group of children aged 2 to 17 years. Following diagnosis and hospitalization to stabilize their metabolic condition, home-care patients were discharged, whereas traditional-care patients remained hospitalized for insulin adjustment and DSME. Education content was similar in the two settings. The home-care intervention consisted of visits by a specially trained nurse who was also available by telephone and an extra post-discharge clinic visit. Costs measured included those for health system resources (hospital supplies, services, and non-physician staff time, and physician and counseling services) and parent out-of-pocket and time costs for 24 months. Costs not included were an identical family monthly government allowance for insulin and medical supplies, diabetes-related health services not provided by the hospital, and overhead and residents' and interns' services at the hospital. The average program costs for the home intervention (adjusted to the *Community Guide* reference case) were $50 per child more than for traditional-care patients (a nonsignificant difference between groups). Mean GHb levels were 10% lower for the home-care patients at 24 and 36 months. The two groups differed little in the use of hospital and physician services during the 24 months. The findings in this study are applicable to hospital settings with post-discharge home-care support.

Several potential barriers to implementing this intervention should be noted. Identifying people who would benefit from DSME in the home may be difficult because they may rarely be seen in a clinic and thus would not be well known to the healthcare team. Similarly, in the clinic it may be difficult to identify those patients whose families and living situations present barriers to self-management.

In conclusion, the Task Force recommends DSME in the home on the basis of sufficient evidence of effectiveness in improving glycemic control among children and adolescents with type 1 diabetes. This recommendation should be applicable to all children or adolescents with type 1 diabetes. Evidence was insufficient, however, to determine the effectiveness of this intervention on glycemic control or other outcomes for people with type 2 diabetes because of the small number of studies that examined these outcomes.

Diabetes Self-Management Education in Summer Camps:
Insufficient Evidence to Determine Effectiveness

Diabetes self-management education in summer camps for young people with diabetes exposes children and adolescents with diabetes to intensive self-management education. Summer camp sessions usually last one or two weeks. At camp, DSME can be readily integrated into daily routines, optimal compliance with educational and medical treatment can be achieved, food intake is controlled, medical expertise is usually readily available, and children can safely pursue physical activity.

Effectiveness

- Although 10 qualifying studies were identified, evidence was insufficient to determine the effectiveness of DSME in summer camps in improving health outcomes such as glycemic control because of the limited number of studies that measured this outcome.
- The studies also had limitations in study design and execution, as well as inconsistent results.
- Insufficient evidence means that we were not able to determine whether or not the intervention works.

Children with diabetes need to follow the same regimen of care year-round, and summer is often a challenging time for these children and their parents. With diverse outdoor activities and inconsistent routines, children may find it difficult to follow their schedule of daily monitoring, injections, and specific meal plans, or they may simply lose interest in doing so. To accommodate children and adolescents, the first residential summer camp for children with diabetes was established in 1925.[155] The camp's mission was to give these children a camping experience in a safe environment while enabling them to share their experiences and learn to be more personally responsible for the care of their disease.[156] Recreational camps are now frequently used for DSME of children and adolescents; in the United States over 90 camps serve more than 10,000 people.[155]

In the camp setting, the recreational, educational, social, and healthcare needs of children can be met in a safe, enjoyable, and productive environment. Diabetes self-management education can be readily integrated into daily routines, optimal compliance with educational and medical treatment can be achieved, food intake is controlled, medical expertise is usually readily available, and children can safely pursue physical activity.

The findings of our systematic review are based on 10 studies that evaluated the effectiveness of DSME interventions in recreational summer camps.[157-166] An additional five studies were identified but did not meet our quality criteria or did not report on relevant outcomes and were excluded from the review.[167-171]

Study participants, identified as having type 1 diabetes, ranged in age from 8 to 15 years and were both male and female. Three studies were conducted among an all-white population, and one study reported a racially mixed population. All interventions were performed in the United States.

Although seven studies did provide sufficient evidence of a positive effect on knowledge (part of the mission of these summer camps), with significant improvement in four studies, this evidence was insufficient to determine the effectiveness of recreational camps in improving glycemic control because of the limited number of studies that measured this outcome. Glycated hemoglobin levels improved in one of two studies where this outcome was measured, glycated albumin improved in a third study, and psychosocial mediators improved in three studies.

Because we could not establish the effectiveness of this intervention, we did not examine situations in which it would be applicable, information about economic efficiency, or possible barriers to implementation.

Other potential benefits of DSME in summer camps include the ability to combine DSME with recreational activities (e.g., give instruction about insulin adjustment just before physical activity), nutritious meals and snacks to help campers develop healthy eating habits, and peer support to help improve self-esteem and motivation. Through the relaxed, fun, non-clinical atmosphere of the camp setting, young people can come to associate DSME with a positive experience. We did not identify any harms of this intervention.

In conclusion, although sufficient evidence demonstrated a positive effect on knowledge for children and adolescents with type 1 diabetes, this improvement alone will not necessarily improve health. Because too few studies examined health outcomes such as glycemic control, the Task Force found insufficient evidence to determine the effectiveness of DSME in recreational camps.

Diabetes Self-Management Education at the Worksite: Insufficient Evidence to Determine Effectiveness

Because workers with diabetes spend a significant portion of their time at work, DSME at the worksite can improve their access to health promotion efforts. In addition, education of supervisors, managers, and coworkers about diabetes can create a supportive environment and prepare them to respond appropriately to diabetes-related emergencies. It can also minimize discrimination against those with special needs created by diabetes.

Effectiveness

- The evidence was insufficient to determine the effectiveness of DSME at worksites in improving the health of workers with diabetes because it consisted of only one study, which had design limitations.
- Insufficient evidence means that we were not able to determine whether or not the intervention works.

Although the 1992 Americans with Disabilities Act prohibits employer discrimination against qualified people with disabilities and requires employers to provide reasonable accommodations, worksites still present many challenges to people with diabetes. These people are more likely to experience difficulty getting a job and staying employed than are people without diabetes,[172,173] and they experience more employer discrimination than do non-disabled workers.[174,175] Workers with diabetes often find it difficult to reconcile their daily diabetes-related routines with their job requirements, making the worksite a potentially important place for DSME. Bringing DSME to the worksite may make it easier for people with diabetes to attend and may provide valuable information for supervisors, managers, and coworkers. Supervisors and managers need to support healthy lifestyles; make allowances for meal and snack-time requirements, self-monitoring of blood glucose, and medical appointments; and promote understanding, tolerance, and support among coworkers.

The findings of our systematic review are based on one study that examined the effectiveness of DSME at the worksite.[176] Two other studies were identified but did not meet our quality criteria and were excluded from the review.[177,178] Although improvement was shown in GHb levels (a decrease of 1.4 percentage points), this single study did not provide strong enough evidence of effectiveness for the Task Force to determine whether or not DSME at the worksite is effective in improving the health of people with diabetes.

Because we could not establish the effectiveness of this intervention, we did not examine situations in which it would be applicable, information about economic efficiency, or possible barriers to implementation.

We identified other potential effects, although these have not been evaluated in the literature. Education of coworkers could increase tolerance for and understanding of diabetes and other chronic diseases and minimize disability-related discrimination. Both the employee with diabetes and the employer could benefit from the increased employee productivity resulting from improvements in the work environment. Potential negative effects include labeling of workers with diabetes and issues related to the confidentiality of health information. Coworkers who learn about diabetes may be uncomfortable or fearful about how to respond to diabetes-related emergencies.

In conclusion, the Task Force found insufficient evidence to determine the effectiveness of DSME at the worksite in improving the health of workers with diabetes, as only a single study, with limitations in its design, was identified. Evidence of the effectiveness of educating coworkers about diabetes is also insufficient, as no studies were identified.

Educating School Personnel about Diabetes: Insufficient Evidence to Determine Effectiveness

Educating teachers and other school professionals about diabetes can create a supportive environment for a student's self-management of diabetes, can minimize the disruptions in educational routines attributable to diabetes, and can teach school personnel appropriate ways of responding to diabetes-related emergencies.

Effectiveness

- The evidence was insufficient to determine the effectiveness of educating school personnel about diabetes in improving the health of students with diabetes.
- Only one study, with design limitations, showed variable effects on knowledge and did not report on outcomes other than knowledge.
- Insufficient evidence means that we were not able to determine whether or not the intervention works.

To improve the health and well-being of students with diabetes, professionals in schools can be educated about the disease and the needs of their students. Most of the 125,000 children in the United States who have diabetes[179] attend school, and they need special accommodation at school to ensure their immediate safety, long-term physical and psychological well-being, and opportunities for optimal scholastic achievement. School personnel are required by law to provide health-related services to children who demonstrate an identified need.[180] Unfortunately, the level of teacher knowledge about diabetes, especially of life-threatening emergencies such as hypoglycemia, is inadequate and poses a serious threat to the safety and well-being of children who require assistance.[181] School personnel, particularly teachers, receive inadequate or no training to prepare them for dealing with children who have chronic health conditions.[182-184] When school personnel fail to respond to diabetes-related emergencies promptly and appropriately, the child with diabetes may suffer serious health consequences.[185]

The findings of our systematic review are based on one study, which evaluated the effectiveness of educating teachers and other school personnel about diabetes.[181] A second study was identified but did not meet our quality criteria and was excluded from the review.[186] The one qualifying study, with limitations in design and execution, showed varied effects on knowledge and did not report on any other outcomes. Therefore, the evidence was insufficient to determine whether or not educating school personnel about diabetes is effective in improving the health of students with diabetes.

Because we could not establish the effectiveness of this intervention, we did not examine situations in which it would be applicable, information about economic efficiency, or possible barriers to implementation.

We identified, but did not evaluate, other potential effects of this intervention. Education about diabetes could make teachers and students more tolerant not only of the needs of students with diabetes but also of the needs of students with other chronic conditions. Possible negative effects could include labeling or ostracism of the child with diabetes, issues of confidentiality, the opportunity cost of teacher education (using money for diabetes education that could be spent on preventing and treating more common health problems), and teacher anxiety associated with feeling personally responsible and potentially liable for a child's health and well-being.

In conclusion, the Task Force found insufficient evidence to determine the effectiveness of educating school personnel about diabetes in improving the health and well-being of students with diabetes. Only one study was included in the review: it had design limitations and only reported on changes in knowledge, where the effect was inconsistent.

REDUCING THE BURDEN OF DIABETES THROUGH USE OF THESE RECOMMENDATIONS

Diabetes affects children, adolescents, and adults of every racial and ethnic group everywhere in the United States. In addition to those who have the disease, the people with whom they live, learn, and work are also affected. Management of diabetes requires knowledge and a willingness to make lifestyle changes and special accommodations. The interventions recommended in this chapter can help people with diabetes manage their disease, which can result in fewer diabetes-related emergencies, overall better health, and, hopefully, greater enjoyment of life.

Healthcare systems can do a lot to help people with diabetes. Offering a combination of disease management and case management can both improve the health of people with diabetes and potentially reduce the costs of caring for diabetes and its related complications (e.g., cardiovascular disease, kidney disease, frequent use of health services in emergencies). A good starting point is to assess the current burden of diabetes, the level of care and education provided for clients with diabetes, and complication rates. This information can then be compared with the care guidelines and goals of treatment presented by organizations such as the American Diabetes Association (ADA) (www.diabetes.org).

In selecting and implementing interventions, communities and healthcare systems should strive to develop a comprehensive strategy for people with diabetes, which includes improving blood pressure, lipid concentrations, and glycemic control; decreasing complications and mortality; and improving the quality of life. Choosing effective interventions that are well matched to local culture, needs, and capabilities, and implementing those interventions well, are vital steps for improving outcomes among people with diabetes. In setting priorities for interventions to meet local objectives, recommendations and other evidence provided in the *Community Guide* should be considered along with such local information as resource availability; administrative structures; and the cultural, economic, social, and regulatory environments of organizations and practitioners. Information on applicability is provided to help decision makers determine if recommended interventions are appropriate in their particular settings. Although the Task Force generally does not use economic information to modify recommendations, this information can help in the decision-making process by identifying (*1*) resource requirements for interventions and (*2*) interventions that meet public health goals more efficiently than other available options.

If local goals and resources permit, the use of recommended interventions should be initiated or increased. Even though the Task Force found insufficient evidence to determine the effectiveness of DSME in summer camps, schools, and worksites, and in the home for adults with type 2 diabetes, the ADA (www.diabetes.org) provides useful information about many aspects of living with the disease. Until sufficient evidence becomes available to determine the effectiveness of these approaches, readers are encouraged to become better informed about aspects of diabetes relevant to their situations. "Insufficient evidence to determine effectiveness" only means that too little evidence was available to determine whether or not the intervention is effective; it doesn't mean that the intervention doesn't work.

CONCLUSION

This chapter summarizes Task Force conclusions and recommendations on interventions to reduce the burden of diabetes. For interventions in the healthcare system, the Task Force recommends both disease management and case management. To improve DSME, the Task Force recommends delivering DSME in community gathering places for adults with type 2 diabetes and in the home for adolescents with type 1 diabetes. Evidence was insufficient to determine the effectiveness of DSME interventions in the home for people with type 2 diabetes, in camps, or at the worksite. Evidence was also insufficient to determine the effectiveness of interventions to educate school personnel about diabetes. Details of these reviews have been published[7,187–189] and these articles, along with additional information about the reviews, are available at www.thecommunityguide.org/diabetes.

Acknowledgments

This chapter was written by members of the systematic review development team: Susan L. Norris, MD, MPH, Division of Diabetes Translation (DDT), National Center for Chronic Disease Prevention and Health Promotion (NCCDPHP), Centers for Disease Control and Prevention (CDC), Atlanta, Georgia; Phyllis J. Nichols, MPH, DDT/NCCDPHP/CDC, Atlanta; Carl J. Caspersen, PhD, MPH, DDT/NCCDPHP/CDC, Atlanta; Russell E. Glasgow, PhD, AMC Cancer Research Center, Denver, Colorado; Vilma G. Carande-Kulis, PhD, MS, Division of Prevention Research and Analytic Methods (DPRAM), Epidemiology Program Office (EPO), CDC, Atlanta; Susan Snyder, PhD, DPRAM/EPO/CDC, Atlanta; Michael M. Engelgau, MD, MSc, DDT/NCCDPHP/CDC, Atlanta; Leonard Jack, Jr., PhD, MSc, DDT/NCCDPHP/CDC, Atlanta; George Isham, MD, HealthPartners, Minneapolis, Minnesota and the Task Force on Community Preventive Services; Sanford Garfield, MD, Diabetes Program Branch, National Institute of Diabetes and Digestive and Kidney Diseases, National Institutes of Health, Bethesda, Maryland; and David McCulloch, MD, Group Health Cooperative of Puget Sound, Seattle, Washington.

Consultants for the reviews were: Tanya Agurs-Collins, PhD, Howard University Cancer Center, Washington, DC; Ann Albright, PhD, RD, California Department of Health Services, Sacramento; Pam Allweiss, MD, University of Kentucky, Lexington, Kentucky; Elizabeth Barrett-Connor, MD, University of California, San Diego; Peter A. Briss, MD, MPH, DPRAM/EPO/CDC, Atlanta; Richard Eastman, MD, Cygnus, San Francisco, California; Luis Escobedo, MD, New Mexico Department of Health, Las Cruces; Wilfred Fujimoto, MD, University of Washington, Seattle; Richard Kahn, PhD, American Diabetes Association, Alexandria, Virginia; Robert Kaplan, PhD, University of California, San Diego; Shiriki Kumanyika, PhD, University of Pennsylvania, Philadelphia; David Marrerro, PhD, Indiana University, Indianapolis; Marjorie Mau, MD, University of Hawai'i, Honolulu; Nicolaas P. Pronk, PhD, HealthPartners, Minneapolis, Minnesota; Laverne Reid, PhD, MPH, North Carolina Central University, Durham; Yvette Roubideaux, MD, MPH, University of Arizona, Tucson.

Articles included in the reviews were abstracted by: Semra Aytur, MPH; Inkyung Baik, PhD; Holly Murphy MD, MPH; Cora Roelofs, ScD; and Kelly Welch, BSc.

References

1. Centers for Disease Control and Prevention. National diabetes fact sheet: general information and national estimates on diabetes in the United States, 2003. Available at: http://www.cdc.gov/diabetes/pubs/factsheet.htm. Accessed January 23, 2004.

2. American Diabetes Association. Economic consequences of diabetes mellitus in the U.S. in 1997. Diabetes Care 1998;21:296–309.

3. Expert Committee on the Diagnosis and Classification of Diabetes Mellitus. Report of the Expert Committee on the Diagnosis and Classification of Diabetes Mellitus. Diabetes Care 2003;26(suppl 1):S5–S20.

4. U.S. Department of Health and Human Services. Healthy people 2010. 2nd ed. Washington, DC: U.S. Government Printing Office, 2000.

5. American Diabetes Association. Clinical practice recommendations 2003. Diabetes Care 2003;26(suppl 1):S1–S156.

6. Harris R, Donahue K, Salf SR, Frame P, Woolf SH, Lohr KN. Screening adults for

type 2 diabetes: a review of the evidence for the U.S. Preventive Services Task Force. Ann Intern Med 2003;138(3):215–29.

7. Norris SL, Nichols PJ, Caspersen CJ, et al. The effectiveness of disease and case management for people with diabetes: a systematic review. Am J Prev Med 2002;22(4S): 15–38.

8. Glasgow RE, Strycker LA. Preventive care practices for diabetes management in two primary care samples. Am J Prev Med 2000;19(1):9–14.

9. Peters AL, Legorreta AP, Ossorio RC, Davidson MB. Quality of outpatient care provided to diabetic patients. A health maintenance organization experience. Diabetes Care 1996;19(6):601–6.

10. Klonoff DC, Schwartz DM. An economic analysis of interventions for diabetes. Diabetes Care 2000;23(3):390–404.

11. Gilmer TP, O'Connor PJ, Manning WG, Rush WA. The cost to health plans of poor glycemic control. Diabetes Care 1997;20(12):1847–53.

12. Testa MA, Simonson DC. Health economic benefits and quality of life during improved glycemic control in patients with type 2 diabetes mellitus. JAMA 1998;280:1490–6.

13. Wagner EH, Sandhu N, Newton KM, McCulloch DK, Ramsey SD, Grothaus LC. Effect of improved glycemic control on health care costs and utilization. JAMA 2001; 285:182–9.

14. Lockington TJ, Farrant S, Meadown KA, Dowlatshahi D, Wise PH. Knowledge profile and control in diabetic patients. Diabet Med 1988;5:381–6.

15. Grembowski D, Patrick D, Diehr P, et al. Self-efficacy and health behavior among older adults. J Health Soc Behav 1993;34:89–104.

16. Wilson W, Ary DV, Biglan A, Glasgow RE, Toobert DJ, Campbell DR. Psychosocial predictors of self-care behaviors (compliance) and glycemic control in non-insulin-dependent diabetes mellitus. Diabetes Care 1986;9(6):614–22.

17. Peyrot M. Behavior change in diabetes education. Diabetes Educ 1999;25 (suppl 6):62–73.

18. The Diabetes Control and Complications Trial Research Group. The effect of intensive treatment of diabetes on the development and progression of long-term complications in insulin-dependent diabetes mellitus. N Engl J Med 1993;329:977–86.

19. Ohkubo Y, Kishikawa H, Araki E, et al. Intensive insulin therapy prevents the progression of diabetic microvascular complications in Japanese patients with non-insulin-dependent diabetes mellitus: a randomized prospective 6-year study. Diabetes Res Clin Pract 1995;28:103–17.

20. Wake N, Hisashige A, Katayama T, et al. Cost-effectiveness of intensive insulin therapy for type 2 diabetes: a 10-year follow-up of the Kumamoto study. Diabetes Res Clin Pract 2000;48:201–10.

21. Reaven GM. Beneficial effect of moderate weight loss in older patients with non-insulin-dependent diabetes mellitus poorly controlled with insulin. J Am Geriatr Soc 1985;33:93–5.

22. Wing RR, Koeske R, Epstein LH, Nowalk MP, Gooding W, Becker D. Long-term effects of modest weight loss in type II diabetic patients. Arch Intern Med 1987;147: 1749–53.

23. Watts NB, Spanheimer RG, DiGirolamo M, et al. Prediction of glucose response to weight loss in patients with non-insulin-dependent diabetes mellitus. Arch Intern Med 1990;150:803–6.

24. American Diabetes Association. Nutrition recommendations and principles for people with diabetes mellitus. Diabetes Care 2001;24(suppl 1):S44–S47.

25. American Diabetes Association. Diabetes mellitus and exercise. Diabetes Care 2001;24(suppl 1):S51–S55.

26. Early Treatment Diabetic Retinopathy Study Research Group. Early photocoagulation for diabetic retinopathy. ETDRS Report Number 9. Ophthalmology 1991;98:766–85.

27. UK Prospective Diabetes Study (UKPDS) Group. Intensive blood-glucose control with sulphonylureas or insulin compared with conventional treatment and risk of complications in patients with type 2 diabetes (UKPDS 33). Lancet 1998;352:837–53.

28. UK Prospective Diabetes Study Group. Tight blood pressure control and risk of macrovascular and microvascular complications in type 2 diabetes (UKPDS 38). BMJ 1998;317:703–13.

29. Bakris GL, Williams M, Dworkin L, et al. Preserving renal function in adults with hypertension and diabetes: a consensus approach. National Kidney Foundation Hypertension and Diabetes Executive Committees Working Group. Am J Kidney Dis 2000; 36(3):646–61.

30. Fontbonne A, Eschwege E, Cambien F, et al. Hypertriglyceridaemia as a risk factor of coronary heart disease mortality in subjects with impaired glucose tolerance or diabetes. Results from the 11-year follow-up of the Paris Prospective Study. Diabetologia 1989;32:300–4.

31. American Diabetes Association. Management of dyslipidemia in adults with diabetes. Diabetes Care 2001;24(suppl 1):S58–S61.

32. Kesteloot K. Disease management. A new technology in need of critical assessment. Int J Technol Assess Health Care 1999;15(3):506–19.

33. Zitter M. A new paradigm in health care delivery: disease management. Todd WE, Nash D, eds. Chicago: American Hospital Publishing, 1996.

34. Bodenheimer T. Disease management in the American market. BMJ 2000;320: 563–6.

35. Roglieri JL, Futterman R, McDonough KL, et al. Disease management interventions to improve outcomes in congestive heart failure. Am J Manag Care 1997;3:1831–9.

36. Rich MW, Beckham V, Wittenberg C, Leven CL, Freedland KE, Carney RM. A multidisciplinary intervention to prevent the readmission of elderly patients with congestive heart failure. N Engl J Med 1995;333(18):1190–5.

37. Lorig KR, Sobel DS, Stewart AL, et al. Evidence suggesting that a chronic disease self-management program can improve health status while reducing hospitalization: a randomized trial. Med Care 1999;37:5–14.

38. Lin EH, VonKorff M, Russo J, et al. Can depression treatment in primary care reduce disability? A stepped care approach. Arch Fam Med 2000;9:1052–8.

39. Wells KB, Sherbourne C, Schoenbaum M, et al. Impact of disseminating quality improvement programs for depression in managed primary care: a randomized controlled trial. JAMA 2000;283(2):212–20.

40. Norris SL, Glasgow RE, Engelgau MM, O'Connor PJ, McCulloch D. Chronic disease management: a definition and systematic approach to component interventions. Disease Manag Health Outcomes 2003;11(8):477–88.

41. Acton K, Valway S, Helgerson S, et al. Improving diabetes care for American Indians. Diabetes Care 1993;16(suppl 1):372–5.

42. Aubert RE, Herman WH, Waters J, et al. Nurse case management to improve glycemic control in diabetic patients in a health maintenance organization. A randomized, controlled trial. Ann Intern Med 1998;129(8):605–12.

43. Carlson A, Rosenqvist U. Diabetes care organization, process, and patient outcomes: effects of a diabetes control program. Diabetes Educ 1991;17(1):42–8.

44. Casey DE Jr, Egede LE. Effect of a disease management tool on residents' compliance with American Diabetes Association standard of care for type 2 diabetes mellitus. American Diabetes Association. Md Med J 1999;48:119–21.

45. Chicoye L, Roethel CR, Hatch MH, Wesolowski W. Diabetes care management: a managed care approach. WMJ 1998;97(3):32–4.

46. Cook CB, Ziemer DC, El-Kebbi IM, et al. Diabetes in urban African-Americans. XVI. Overcoming clinical inertia improves glycemic control in patients with type 2 diabetes. Diabetes Care 1999;22:1494–500.

47. de Sonnaville JJ, Bouma M, Colly LP, Deville W, Wijkel D, Heine RJ. Sustained good glycaemic control in NIDDM patients by implementation of structured care in general practice: 2-year follow-up study. Diabetologia 1997;40:1334–40.

48. Deichmann R, Castello E, Horswell R, Friday KE. Improvements in diabetic care as measured by HbA1c after a physician education project. Diabetes Care 1999;22(10):1612–6.

49. Diabetes Integrated Care Evaluation Team. Integrated care for diabetes: clinical, psychosocial, and economic evaluation. BMJ 1994;308:1208–12.

50. Domurat ES. Diabetes managed care and clinical outcomes: the Harbor City, California Kaiser Permanente diabetes care system. Am J Manag Care 1999;5(10):1299–307.

51. Foulkes A, Kinmonth AL, Frost S, MacDonald D. Organized personal care—an effective choice for managing diabetes in general practice. J R Coll Gen Pract 1989;39:444–7.

52. Friedman NM, Gleeson JM, Kent MJ, Foris M, Rodriguez DJ, Cypress M. Management of diabetes mellitus in the Lovelace Health Systems' Episodes of Care program. Eff Clin Pract 1998;1(1):5–11.

53. Goldfracht M, Porath A. Nationwide program for improving the care of diabetic patients in Israeli primary care centers. Diabetes Care 2000;23(4):495–9.

54. Johnston C, Ponsonby E. Northwest Herts diabetic management system. Comput Methods Programs Biomed 2000;62(3):177–89.

55. Legorreta A, Peters A, Ossorio RC, Lopez R, Jatulis D, Davidson M. Effect of a comprehensive nurse-managed diabetes program: an HMO prospective study. Am J Manag Care 1996;2:1024–30.

56. McCulloch DK, Price MJ, Hindmarsh M, Wagner EH. A population-based approach to diabetes management in a primary care setting: early results and lessons learned. Eff Clin Pract 1998;1(1):12–22.

57. North Tyneside Diabetes Team. The diabetes annual review as an educational tool: assessment and learning integrated with care, screening, and audit. Diabet Med 1992;9:389–94.

58. O'Connor PJ, Rush WA, Peterson J, et al. Continuous quality improvement can improve glycemic control for HMO patients with diabetes. Arch Fam Med 1996;5:502–6.

59. Payne TH, Galvin M, Taplin SH, Austin B, Savarino J, Wagner EH. Practicing population-based care in an HMO: evaluation after 18 months. HMO Pract 1995;9(3):101–6.

60. Peters AL, Davidson MB. Application of a diabetes managed care program. The feasibility of using nurses and a computer system to provide effective care. Diabetes Care 1998;21(7):1037–43.

61. Rubin RJ, Dietrich KA, Hawk AD. Clinical and economic impact of implementing a comprehensive diabetes management program in managed care. J Clin Endocrinol Metab 1998;83(8):2635–42.

62. Sadur CN, Moline N, Costa M, et al. Diabetes management in a health maintenance organization. Efficacy of care management using cluster visits. Diabetes Care 1999;22(12):2011–7.

63. Sidorov J, Gabbay R, Harris R, et al. Disease management for diabetes mellitus: impact on hemoglobin A1c. Am J Manag Care 2000;6:1217–26.

64. Sikka R, Waters J, Moore W, Sutton DR, Herman WH, Aubert RE. Renal assessment practices and the effect of nurse case management of health maintenance organization patients with diabetes. Diabetes Care 1999;22(1):1–6.

65. Sperl-Hillen J, O'Connor PJ, Carlson RR, et al. Improving diabetes care in a large health care system: an enhanced primary care approach. Jt Commun J Qual Improv 2000; 26:615–22.

66. Taplin S, Galvin MS, Payne T, Coole D, Wagner E. Putting population-based care into practice: real option or rhetoric? J Am Board Fam Pract 1998;11:116–26.

67. Tom-Orme L. Chronic disease and the social matrix: a Native American diabetes intervention. Recent Adv Nurs 1988;22:89–109.

68. Varroud-Vial M, Mechaly P, Joannidis S, et al. Cooperation between general practitioners and diabetologists and clinical audit improve the management of type 2 diabetic patients. Diabetes Metab 1999;25:55–63.

69. Anonymous. Disease management program improves diabetes outcomes, curbs hospital costs, utilization. Health Care Cost Reengineering Rep 1998;3(3):42–5.

70. Davidson MB. Incorporating diabetes care into a health maintenance organization setting: a practical guide. Disease Manage Health Outcomes 1998;3:71–80.

71. Day JL, Humphreys H, Alban-Davies H. Problems of comprehensive shared diabetes care. BMJ 1987;294:1590–2.

72. Joshi MS, Bernard DB. Clinical performance improvement series. Classic CQI integrated with comprehensive disease management as a model for performance improvement. Jt Commun J Qual Improv 1999;25:383–95.

73. Kelling DG, Wentworth JA, Wright JB. Diabetes mellitus. Using a database to implement a systematic management program. N C Med J 1997;58:368–71.

74. Rosenthal MM, Carlson A, Rosenqvist U. Beyond CME: diabetes education fieldinteractive strategies from Sweden. Diabetes Educ 1988;14:212–7.

75. Wells S, Benett I, Holloway G, Harlow V. Area-wide diabetes care: the Manchester experience with primary health care teams 1991–1997. Diabet Med 1998;15(suppl 3):S49–S53.

76. Williams DR, Munroe C, Hospedales CJ, Greenwood RH. A three-year evaluation of the quality of diabetes care in the Norwich community care scheme. Diabet Med 1990;7(1):74–9.

77. Wagner EH, Austin BT, Von Korff M. Improving outcomes in chronic illness. Manag Care Q 1996;4(2):12–25.

78. Wagner EH. Care of older people with chronic illness. In: Calkins E, Boult C, Wagner EH, Pacala JT, eds. New ways to care for older people. New York: Springer, 1998:39–64.

79. Wagner EH, Davis C, Schaefer J, Von Korff M, Austin B. A survey of leading chronic disease management programs: are they consistent with the literature? Manag Care Q 1999;7:56–66.

80. Cabana MD, Rand CS, Power NR, et al. Why don't physicians follow clinical practice guidelines? A framework for improvement. JAMA 1999;282:1458–65.

81. Roos LL, Sharp SM, Cohen MM. Comparing clinical information with claims data: some similarities and differences. J Clin Epidemiol 1991;44:881–8.

82. O'Connor PJ, Rush WA, Pronk NP, Cherney LM. Identifying diabetes mellitus or heart disease among health maintenance organization members: sensitivity, specificity, predictive value, and cost of survey and database methods. Am J Manag Care 1998;4:335–42.

83. Norris SL, Engelgau MM, Venkat Narayan KM. Effectiveness of self-management training in type 2 diabetes: systematic review of randomized controlled trials. Diabetes Care 2001;24:561–87.

84. Institute for Clinical Systems Integration. Technology assessment: care management for chronic illness, the frail elderly, and acute myocardial infarction. Bloomington, MN: Institute for Clinical Systems Integration (ICSI), 1998. Report No. 44.

85. Ward MD, Rieve JA. The role of case management in disease management. In: Todd WE, Nash E, eds. Disease management: a systems approach to improving patient outcomes. Chicago: American Hospital Publishing, 1997:235–59.

86. American Geriatric Society Public Policy Committee. Care management. J Am Geriatr Soc 1991;39:429–30.

87. Holloway F, Oliver N, Collins E, Carson J. Case management: a critical review of the outcome literature. Eur Psychiatry 1995;10:113–28.

88. Brass-Mynderse NJ. Disease management for chronic congestive heart failure. J Cardiovasc Nurs 1996;11:54–62.

89. Bernabei R, Landi F, Gambassi G, et al. Randomised trial of impact of model of integrated care and case management for older people living in the community. BMJ 1998;316:1348–51.

90. Naylor MD, Brooten D, Campbell R, et al. Comprehensive discharge planning and home follow-up of hospitalized elders; a randomized clinical trial. JAMA 1999;281: 613–20.

91. Fitzgerald JF, Smith DM, Martin DK, Freedman JA, Katz BP. A case manager intervention to reduce readmissions. Arch Intern Med 1994;154:1721–9.

92. Caravalho JY, Saylor CR. Continuum of care. An evaluation of a nurse case-managed program for children with diabetes. Pediatr Nurs 2000;26(3):296–300,328.

93. Humphry J, Jameson LM, Beckham S. Overcoming social and cultural barriers to care for patients with diabetes. West J Med 1997;167(3):138–44.

94. Peters AL, Davidson MB, Ossorio RC. Management of patients with diabetes by nurses with support of subspecialists. HMO Pract 1995;9(1):8–13.

95. Weinberger M, Kirkman MS, Samsa GP, et al. A nurse-coordinated intervention for primary care patients with non-insulin-dependent diabetes mellitus: impact on glycemic control and health-related quality of life. J Gen Intern Med 1995;10:59–66.

96. Weinberger M, Oddone EZ, Henderson WG. Does increased access to primary care reduce hospital readmissions? Veterans Affairs Cooperative Study Group on Primary Care and Hospital Readmission. N Engl J Med 1996;334:1441–7.

97. Whitlock WL, Brown A, Moore K, et al. Telemedicine improved diabetic management. Mil Med 2000;165:579–84.

98. Beyerman K. Casefinder program IDs 1,500 at risk for diabetes. Hosp Case Manag 1999;7:204–6.

99. Day JL, Johnson P, Rayman G, Walker R. The feasibility of a potentially 'ideal' system of integrated diabetes care and education based on a day centre. Diabet Med 1988;5:70–5.

100. Day JL, Metcalfe J, Johnson P. Benefits provided by an integrated education and clinical diabetes centre: a follow-up study. Diabet Med 1992;9:855–9.

101. Edelstein EL, Cesta TG. Nursing case management: an innovative model of care for hospitalized patients with diabetes. Diabetes Educ 1993;19(6):517–21.

102. Ginn M, Frate DA, Keys L. A community-based case management model for hypertension and diabetes. J Miss State Med Assoc 1999;40:226–8.

103. Giordano B, Rosenbloom AL, Heller D, Weber FT, Gonzalez R, Grgic A. Regional services for children and youth with diabetes. Pediatrics 1977;60(4):493–8.

104. Lorber D. What works? The Diabetes Care and Information Center. Diabet Med 1998;15(suppl 4):S24–S27.

105. Lowes L. Evaluation of a paediatric diabetes specialist nurse post. Br J Nurs 1997;6(11):625–6, 628–33.

106. Task Force to Revise the National Standards, the American Diabetes Association. National standards for diabetes self-management education programs. Diabetes Educ 1995;21(3):189–93.

107. Bartlett EE. Historical glimpses of patient education in the United States. Patient Educ Couns 1986;8:135–49.

108. American Diabetes Association. Standards of medical care for patients with diabetes mellitus. Diabetes Care 2001;24(suppl 1):S33–S55.

109. de Weerdt I, Visser AP, van der Veen EA. Attitude behaviour theories and diabetes education programmes. Patient Educ Couns 1989;14:3–19.

110. Clement S. Diabetes self-management education. Diabetes Care 1995;18(8):1204–14.

111. Rosilio M, Cotton JB, Wieliczko MC, et al. Factors associated with glycemic control. A cross-sectional nationwide study in 2,579 French children with type 1 diabetes. Diabetes Care 1998;21(7):1146–53.

112. Harris MI. Health care and health status and outcomes for patients with type 2 diabetes. Diabetes Care 2000;23(6):754–8.

113. Harris MI, Eastman RC, Cowie CC, Flegal KM, Eberhardt MS. Racial and ethnic differences in glycemic control of adults with type 2 diabetes. Diabetes Care 1999;22:403–8.

114. Brown SA. Effects of educational interventions in diabetes care: a meta-analysis of findings. Nurs Res 1988;37(4):223–30.

115. Brown SA. Studies of educational interventions and outcomes in diabetic adults: a meta-analysis revisited. Patient Educ Couns 1990;16:189–215.

116. Padgett D, Mumford E, Hynes M, Carter R. Meta-analysis of the effects of educational and psychosocial interventions on management of diabetes mellitus. J Clin Epidemiol 1988;41:1007–30.

117. Norris SL, Lau J, Smith SJ, Schmid CH, Engelgau MM. Self-management education for adults with type 2 diabetes. Diabetes Care 2002;25(7):1159–71.

118. Hampson SE, Skinner TC, Hart J, et al. Behavioral interventions for adolescents with type 1 diabetes: how effective are they? Diabetes Care 2000;23:1416–22.

119. Helmrich JP, Ragland DR, Leung RW, Paffenbarger RS. Physicial activity and reduced occurrence of non-insulin-dependent diabetes mellitus. N Engl J Med 1991;325: 147–52.

120. Irwin C, Braithwaite R. Church-based diabetes education program for older, African-American women. Am J Health Studies 1997;13(1):1–7.

121. Kumanyika SK, Charleston JB. Lose weight and win: a church-based weight loss program for blood pressure control among black women. Patient Educ Couns 1992;19: 19–32.

122. Carter JS, Gilliland SS, Perez GE, et al. Native American Diabetes Project: designing culturally relevant education materials. Diabetes Educ 1997;23:133–4,139.

123. Barnard RJ, Lattimore L, Holly RG, Cherny S, Pritikin N. Response of non-insulin-dependent diabetic patients to an intensive program of diet and exercise. Diabetes Care 1982;5:370–4.

124. Barnard RJ, Jung T, Inkeles SB. Diet and exercise in the treatment of NIDDM: the need for early emphasis. Diabetes Care 1994;17(12):1469–72.

125. Brown SA, Hanis CL. A community-based, culturally sensitive education and group-support intervention for Mexican Americans with NIDDM: pilot study of efficacy. Diabetes Educ 1995;21(3):203–10.

126. Brown SA, Upchurch SL, Garcia AA, Barton SA, Hanis CL. Symptom-related self-care of Mexican Americans with type 2 diabetes: preliminary findings of the Starr County Diabetes Education Study. Diabetes Educ 1998;24:331–9.

127. Brown SA, Hanis CL. Culturally competent diabetes education for Mexican Americans: the Starr County Study. Diabetes Educ 1999;25(2):226–36.

128. Elshaw EB, Young EA, Saunders MJ, McGurn WC, Lopez LC. Utilizing a 24-hour dietary recall and culturally specific diabetes education in Mexican Americans with diabetes. Diabetes Educ 1994;20:228–35.

129. Hahn JM, Gordon DH. "Learn, taste, and share": a diabetes nutrition education program developed, marketed, and presented by the community. Diabetes Educ 1998; 24:153–4,161.

130. Heath GW, Wilson RH, Smith J, Leonard BE. Community-based exercise and weight control: diabetes risk reduction and glycemic control in Zuni Indians. Am J Clin Nutr 1987;53(suppl 6):1642S–6S.

131. Pratt C, Wilson W, Leklem J, Kingsley L. Peer support and nutrition education for older adults with diabetes. J Nutr Elder 1987;6:31–43.

132. Wang CY, Abbott LJ. Development of a community-based diabetes and hypertension preventive program. Public Health Nurs 1998;15(6):406–14.

133. Wilson W, Pratt C. The impact of diabetes education and peer support upon weight and glycemic control of elderly persons with noninsulin dependent diabetes mellitus (NIDDM). Am J Public Health 1987;77:634–5.

134. Wilson R, Hoy W. Short-term effects of participation in a community-based exercise program: a study in the pueblo of Zuni. IHS Prim Care Provid 1993;18(7):126–31.

135. Drainville SG, Sevier RE. One community's approach to diabetes education. N C Med J 1984;45(3):169–71.

136. Irvine AA, Mitchell CM. Impact of community-based diabetes education on program attenders and nonattenders. Diabetes Educ 1992;18(1):29–33.

137. Sullivan ED, Joseph DH. Practice point. University/community partnership to improve the lives of people with diabetes. Practical Diabetes Int 2000;17(1):26–30.

138. Basch CE, Walker EA, Howard CJ, Shamoon H, Zybert P. The effect of health education on the rate of ophthalmic examinations among African Americans with diabetes mellitus. Am J Public Health 1999;89(12):1878–82.

139. Brown SJ, Lieberman DA, Germeny BA, Fan YC, Wilson DM, Pasta DJ. Educational video game for juvenile diabetes: results of a controlled trial. Med Inform 1997; 22:77–89.

140. Mazzuca KB, Farris NA, Mendenhall J, Stoupa RA. Demonstrating the added value of community health nursing for clients with insulin-dependent diabetes. J Commun Health Nurs 1997;14:211–24.

141. Rettig BA, Shrauger DG, Recker RR, Gallagher TE, Wiltse H. A randomized study of the effects of a home diabetes education program. Diabetes Care 1986;9:173–8.

142. York R, Brown LP, Samuels P, et al. A randomized trial of early discharge and nurse specialist transitional follow-up care of high-risk childbearing women. Nurs Res 1997;46(5):254–61.

143. Couper JJ, Taylor J, Fotheringham MJ, Sawyer M. Failure to maintain the benefits of home-based intervention in adolescents with poorly controlled type 1 diabetes. Diabetes Care 1999;22(12):1933–7.

144. Turnin MC, Beddok RH, Clottes JP, et al. Telematic expert system Diabeto. New tool for diet self-monitoring for diabetic patients. Diabetes Care 1992;15:204–12.

145. Manning RM, Jung RT, Leese GP, Newton RW. The comparison of four weight reduction strategies aimed at overweight diabetic patients. Diabet Med 1995;12:409–15.

146. Dougherty G, Schiffrin A, White D, Soderstrom L, Sufrategui M. Home-based management can achieve intensification cost-effectively in type I diabetes. Pediatrics 1999;103(1):122–8.

147. Anderson RM, Fitzgerald JT, Funnell MM, et al. Evaluation of an activated patient diabetes education newsletter. Diabetes Educ 1994;20(1):29–34.

148. Dammacco F, Torelli C, Frezza E, Misuraca A, Perrotta P. Computer based instruction of diabetic children and adolescents. Techniques and results. J Endocrinol Invest 1989;12(8(suppl 3)):141–2.

149. Hanstine S, Fanning V. Teaching patients to manage diabetes safely in the home. Home Health Care Manag Pract 2000;12(4):40–8.

150. Horan PP, Yarborough MC, Besigel G, Carlson DR. Computer-assisted self-control of diabetes by adolescents. Diabetes Educ 1990;16:205–11.

151. Johnston B, Wheeler L, Deuser J, Sousa KH. Outcomes of the Kaiser Permanente Tele-Home Health Research Project. Arch Fam Med 2000;40–5.

152. Ledda MA, Walker EA, Basch CE. Development and formative evaluation of a foot self-care program for African Americans with diabetes. Diabetes Educ 1997;23:48–50.

153. Strock E, Jacobson J, Reader D, Hollander P. Managing diabetes in the home: a model approach. Caring 1988;7(2):50–6.

154. Dougherty GE, Soderstrom L, Schiffrin A. An economic evaluation of home care for children with newly diagnosed diabetes: results from a randomized controlled trial. Med Care 1998;36:586–98.

155. Mimura G. Summer camp. Diabetes Res Clin Pract 1994;24(suppl):S287–S290.

156. American Diabetes Association. Management of diabetes at diabetes camps. Diabetes Care 1999;22(1):167–9.

157. Harkavy J, Johnson SB, Silverstein J, Spillar R, McCallum M, Rosenbloom A. Who learns what at diabetes summer camp. J Pediatr Psychol 1983;8:143–53.

158. Kaplan RM, Chadwick MW, Schimmel LE. Social learning intervention to promote metabolic control in type I diabetes mellitus: pilot experiment results. Diabetes Care 1985;8:152–5.

159. Kemp SF, Canfield ME, Kearns FS, Elders MJ. The effect of short-term intervention on long-term diabetes management. J Ark Med Soc 1986;83:241–4.

160. Massouh SR, Steele TM, Alseth ER, Diekmann JM. The effect of social learning intervention on metabolic control of insulin-dependent diabetes mellitus in adolescents. Diabetes Educ 1989;15:518–21.

161. Misuraca A, Di Gennaro M, Lioniello M, Duval M, Aloi G. Summer camps for diabetic children: an experience in Campania,Italy. Diabetes Res Clin Pract 1996; 32(1–2):91–6.

162. Pichert JW, Murkin SA, Snyder GM, Boswell EJ, Kinzer CK. Problem-based diabetes education using a video anchor. Diabetes Spectrum 1993;6:160–4.

163. Pichert JW, Smeltzer C, Snyder GM, Gregory RP, Smeltzer R, Kinzer CK. Traditional vs anchored instruction for diabetes-related nutritional knowledge, skills, and behavior. Diabetes Educ 1994;20:45–8.

164. Pichert J, Snyder G, Kinzer C, Boswell E. Problem solving anchored instruction about sick days for adolescents with diabetes. Patient Educ Couns 1994;23:115–24.

165. Smith KE, Schreiner BJ, Brouhard BH, Travis LB. Impact of a camp experience on the choice of coping strategies by adolescents with insulin-dependent diabetes mellitus. Diabetes Educ 1991;17:49–53.

166. Zimmerman E, Carter MC, Sears JH, Lawson JS, Howard CP, Hassanein RE. Diabetic camping: effect on knowledge, attitude, and self-concept. Issues Compr Pediatr Nurs 1987;10:99–111.

167. Lebovitz FL, Ellis GJ, Skyler JS. Performance of technical skills of diabetes management: increased independence after a camp experience. Diabetes Care 1978;1:23–6.

168. Maryniuk MD, Kauwell GP, Thomas RG. A test of instructional approaches designed to influence food selection. Diabetes Educ 1986;12:34–6.

169. McFarlane J, Hames CC. Children with diabetes. Learning self-care in camp. Am J Nurs 1973;73(8):1362–5.

170. Pichert JW, Meek JM, Schlundt DG, et al. Impact of anchored instruction on problem-solving strategies of adolescents with diabetes. J Am Diet Assoc 1994;94: 1036–8.

171. Warzak WJ, Ayllon T, Delcher HK. Peer instruction of home glucose monitoring. Diabetes Care 1982;5:44–6.

172. Robinson N, Bush L, Protopapa LE, Yateman NA. Employers' attitudes to diabetes. Diabet Med 1989;6:692–7.

173. Songer TJ, LaPorte RE, Corman JS, Orchard TJ, Becker DJ, Drash AL. Employment spectrum of IDDM. Diabetes Care 1989;12(9):615–21.

174. Heins JM, Arfken CL, Nord WR, Houston CA, McGill JB. The Americans with Disabilites Act and diabetes. Diabetes Care 1994;17(5):453.

175. Fisher JN. Diabetics need not apply. Diabetes Care 1989;12(9):659–60.

176. Burton WN, Connerty CM. Evaluation of a worksite-based patient education intervention targeted at employees with diabetes mellitus. J Occup Environ Med 1998;40: 702–6.

177. Simmons D, Fleming C, Cameron M, Leakehe L. A pilot diabetes awareness and exercise programme in a multiethnic workforce. N Z Med J 1996;109:373–6.

178. Reynolds WB. Health education for the diabetic. Occup Health Nurs 1978; 26:7–14.

179. LaPorte RE, Tajima N, Dorman JS, et al. Differences between blacks and whites in the epidemiology of insulin-dependent diabetes mellitus in Allegheny County, Pennsylvania. Am J Epidemiol 1986;123:592–603.

180. Gray D, Ingersoll G, Lawlor R, Golden M. Status of IDDM care in schools. Diabetes 1985;34(suppl):41a.

181. Jarrett L, Hillam K, Bartsch C, Lindsay R. The effectiveness of parents teaching elementary school teachers about diabetes mellitus. Diabetes Educ 1993;19(3):193–7.

182. Krier JJ. Involvement of educational staff in the healthcare of medically fragile children. Pediatr Nurs 1993;19(3):251–4.

183. Bradbury AJ, Smith CS. An assessment of the diabetic knowledge of school teachers. Arch Dis Child 1983;58:692–6.

184. Challen AH, Davies AG, Williams RJW, Baum JD. Support for families with diabetic children: parents' views. Practical Diabetes 1990;7:26–31.

185. Rewers M, LaPorte RE, King H, Tuomilehto J. Trends in the prevalence and incidence of diabetes: insulin-dependent diabetes mellitus in childhood. World Health Stat Q 1988;41:179–89.

186. Gesteland HM, Sims S, Lindsay RN. Evaluation of two approaches to educating elementary school teachers about insulin-dependent diabetes mellitus. Diabetes Educ 1989;15:510–3.

187. Centers for Disease Control and Prevention. Strategies for reducing morbidity and mortality from diabetes through health-care system interventions and self-management training and education in community settings. A report on recommendations of the Task Force on Community Preventive Services. MMWR 2001;50 (RR-16):1–15.

188. Norris SL, Nichols PJ, Caspersen CJ, et al. Increasing diabetes self-management education in community settings: a systematic review. Am J Prev Med 2002;22(4S):39–66.

189. Task Force on Community Preventive Services. Recommendations for healthcare system and self-management education interventions to reduce morbidity and mortality from diabetes. Am J Prev Med 2002;22(4S):10–4.

Chapter 6

Vaccine-Preventable Diseases

In this chapter, we report on the effectiveness of interventions to increase the use of both *universally recommended* and *targeted* vaccines. As the name implies, universally recommended vaccines are those that should be administered to all people in a given age group, whereas targeted vaccines are those given to specific groups because of factors that make those groups particularly susceptible to a disease. Note that it is not actually the vaccines themselves that change, but rather their indicated use. For example, the influenza vaccine is *universally recommended* for all people over 50 years of age and is also *targeted* to people under 50 who have specific health problems. Interventions and policies to promote targeted vaccines are likely to be much more complex than similar interventions to promote universally recommended vaccines. For example, programs to improve coverage with universally recommended vaccines might need no more information about the target population than age, whereas programs to promote targeted vaccines might require information on age, risk factors, and vaccination history. Therefore, although the distinction between universally recommended and targeted vaccines is not clear, we have discussed these issues separately in Sections I and II, respectively. (The term *vaccination coverage* refers to the proportion of people who have received a particular vaccination.)

SECTION I: UNIVERSALLY RECOMMENDED VACCINATIONS

Increasing Community Demand for Vaccinations

RECOMMENDED INTERVENTIONS

The Task Force approved the recommendations in this chapter for universally recommended vaccines in 1997–1998. The research on which the findings are based was conducted from 1980 to 1997. The recommendations in Section I of this chapter have been previously published in the American Journal of Preventive Medicine [2000;18(1S):92–96 and 97–140] and the MMWR Recommendations and Reports series [1999; 48(No. RR-8):1–15].

In 2001, based on seven additional studies published between 1995 and 2000, the Task Force updated the finding for vaccination programs in schools from "Insufficient evidence to determine effectiveness" to "Recommended with sufficient evidence of effectiveness."

Some of the background information included in the chapter has been updated since the original publications.

SECTION II: TARGETED VACCINES: IMPROVING TARGETED INFLUENZA, PNEUMOCOCCAL POLYSACCHARIDE, AND HEPATITIS B VACCINATION COVERAGE AMONG HIGH-RISK ADULTS

*Insufficient evidence means that we were not able to determine whether or not the intervention works.

†This intervention is recommended to increase coverage with universally recommended vaccines. See Section I of this chapter for complete information.

The Task Force approved the recommendations in this chapter for targeted vaccines in 2002. The research on which the findings are based was conducted from 1980 to 2001. This information is being prepared for publication, and more information will be available at www.thecommunityguide.org as it becomes available.

In the first section of this chapter we review approaches to increasing coverage of universally recommended vaccines (those that should be administered to all people in a given age group). In the second section, we look at targeted vaccinations, those given to specific groups with factors that make them particularly susceptible to a disease (*at-risk* or *high-risk* populations). We present these separately because interventions and policies to improve targeted vaccination coverage may be more complex than similar interventions and policies for universally recommended vaccines for a number of reasons. For example, it may be more difficult to identify the people who should receive targeted vaccines and to determine whether they have been previously vaccinated.

Vaccine-preventable diseases are still major causes of illness and death for people of all ages in the United States.[1] Despite great successes in the use of vaccines to prevent childhood disease—over the past 50 years the occurrence of the vaccine-preventable diseases of childhood has decreased by more than 95%—more than 400,000 children and adults in the United States become ill (Centers for Disease Control and Prevention, unpublished data) and approximately 50,000 still die each year from preventable diseases.[2] Influenza and pneumonia in the elderly account for most of the mortality.

Vaccines are available to prevent many diseases in people of all ages. The primary vaccine-preventable diseases of childhood are diphtheria, invasive diseases caused by the *Haemophilus influenzae* type b (Hib) bacterium, measles, poliomyelitis (polio), rubella ("German" measles), tetanus, mumps, varicella (chickenpox), and pertussis (whooping cough). The primary vaccine-preventable diseases of adulthood are influenza, diseases caused by the *Streptococcus pneumoniae* bacterium, and hepatitis B. The distinctions between diseases of childhood and those of adulthood, however, have become less clear in recent years. Several diseases formerly considered childhood diseases (e.g., measles and pertussis) are now being found among adults, and hepatitis B vaccinations are now routinely recommended for infants and adolescents.

These preventable diseases are still much too common in the United States. Each year, more than 50,000 children contract varicella, the most common vaccine-preventable disease of childhood.[3] Influenza, pneumococcal infections, and hepatitis B affect hundreds of thousands of adults annually.[4] Each year approximately 500 people die of childhood vaccine-preventable diseases and more than 40,000 adults die of influenza, pneumococcal infections, and hepatitis B.[1,5] Influenza is the leading killer among these diseases,[5] with most deaths occurring among people age 65 or older.

Vaccination not only protects individuals but also limits the spread of disease in the general population. Therefore, the more people who receive a vaccination, the better the protection for everyone, including those who have not been vaccinated.

OBJECTIVES AND RECOMMENDATIONS FROM OTHER ADVISORY GROUPS

The interventions recommended in this chapter can be used to reach objectives set out in *Healthy People 2010*[6] (Table 6–1). In addition, the recommendations complement information from other advisory groups, including the following:

Recommendations for Childhood Vaccinations

These recommendations are issued regularly by the Advisory Committee on Immunization Practices (ACIP) of the U.S. Department of Health and Human Services (DHHS)/Centers for Disease Control and Prevention (CDC),[7] the American Academy of Pediatrics (AAP),[8] and the American Academy of Family Physicians (AAFP).[9] The AAP, AAFP, and ACIP work together to develop a common childhood vaccination schedule.

Table 6–1. *Healthy People 2010*[6] Objectives for Improving Vaccination
Coverage and Reducing the Incidence of Vaccine-Preventable Diseases

Objective	*Population*	*Baseline*	*2010 Objective*
Improving Vaccination Coverage			
Achieve and maintain effective vaccination coverage levels for universally recommended vaccines among young children (Objective 14–22)	Young children	Varies by vaccine regimen	90%
Maintain vaccination coverage levels for children in licensed day care facilities and children in kindergarten through first grade (14–23)	Children	Varies by vaccine	95%
Increase the proportion of young children and adolescents who receive all vaccines that have been recommended for universal administration for at least five years (four DTaP, three polio, one MMR, three Hib, three hepatitis B):			
• Among children aged 19–35 months (14–24a)	Young children	73% (1998)	80%
• Among adolescents aged 13–15 years (14–24b)	Adolescents	Developmental	
Increase the proportion of providers who have measured the vaccination coverage levels among children in their practice population within the past two years:			
• Public health providers (14–25a)	Children	66% (1997)	90%
• Private providers (14–25b)		6% (1997)	90%
Increase the proportion of children who participate in fully operational population-based immunization registries (14–26)	Children under 6 years	32% (1999)	95%
Increase routine vaccination coverage levels for adolescents aged 13–15 years (14–27)	Adolescents	Varies by vaccine	90%
Increase hepatitis B vaccine coverage among high-risk groups:			
• Dialysis patients (14–28a)	High-risk groups	35% (1995)	90%
• Men having sex with men (14–28b)		9% (1995)	60%
• Occupationally exposed workers (14–28c)		71% (1995)	98%

continued next page

Table 6–1. *Continued*

Objective	Population	Baseline	2010 Objective
Improving Vaccination Coverage (continued)			
Increase the proportion of adults who are vaccinated annually against influenza and ever vaccinated against pneumococcal disease (14–29)	Adults	Varies by vaccine and population	Varies by vaccine and population
Reducing the Incidence of Vaccine-Preventable Diseases			
Reduce or eliminate indigenous cases of vaccine-preventable diseases (14–1)	All	Varies by disease	Varies by disease
Reduce chronic hepatitis B virus infections in infants and young children (perinatal infections) (14–2)	Infants/ young children	1682 (1995)	400
Reduce hepatitis B cases per 100,000 population (14–3)	All	Varies by population	Varies by population
Reduce bacterial meningitis cases per 100,000 young children (14–4)	Young children (1–23 months)	13.0 (1998)	8.6
Reduce invasive pneumococcal infections (14–5)	All	Varies by age of population	Varies by population

Recommendations for Adolescent and Adult Vaccinations

These recommendations are published by ACIP,[10,11] the American College of Physicians,[12] Infectious Disease Society of America,[12,13] AAFP,[9] and the American College of Obstetricians and Gynecologists.[14] Vaccination recommendations for adolescents are now coordinated among ACIP, AAP, AAFP, and the American Medical Association.

Recommendations for Interventions to Improve Vaccination Coverage

These recommendations have been developed by the Canadian Community Health Practice Guidelines Working Group,[15,16] ACIP,[17,18] and the National Vaccine Advisory Committee.[19]

METHODS

Methods used for the reviews are summarized in Chapter 10. Specific methods used in the systematic reviews for universally recommended vaccinations have been described elsewhere[20] and are available at www.thecommunityguide

.org/vaccine. The logic framework depicting the conceptual approach used in reviews of both universally recommended and targeted vaccines is presented in Figure 6–1.

For purposes of our reviews, we did not consider certain activities that might improve vaccination coverage to be interventions. Activities that provide useful information for public health action (e.g., immunization registries) may incorporate or lead to such interventions as client reminders and recalls, provider reminders and recalls, and assessment plus feedback for vaccination providers. Consequently, we considered registries to represent part of the public health infrastructure rather than being interventions themselves. Similarly, improving vaccines (e.g., developing vaccines that are less likely to cause adverse reactions or increasing the number of antigens contained in a vaccine, thus reducing the number of injections required) can lead to improvements in vaccination coverage. However, improvements are made primarily for other reasons (e.g., reducing potential harm or allowing administration of more antigens than would otherwise be feasible) and therefore, for purposes of our systematic reviews, we did not consider them to be interventions.

ECONOMIC EFFICIENCY

A systematic review of available economic evaluations was conducted for all recommended interventions, and a summary of each review is presented with the related intervention. The methods used to conduct these economics reviews are summarized in Chapter 11.

RECOMMENDATIONS AND FINDINGS

This section presents a summary of the findings of the systematic reviews conducted to determine the effectiveness of interventions to increase coverage with universally recommended vaccines. Interventions are grouped into three categories: increasing community demand for vaccinations, enhancing access to vaccination services, and provider- or system-based interventions.

Universally Recommended Vaccines: Increasing Community Demand for Vaccinations

Interventions to increase community demand for vaccinations are designed to work in several ways: they can educate communities about the importance of vaccinations and about which vaccinations are appropriate and at what ages; remind families directly when vaccinations are due; make vaccinations

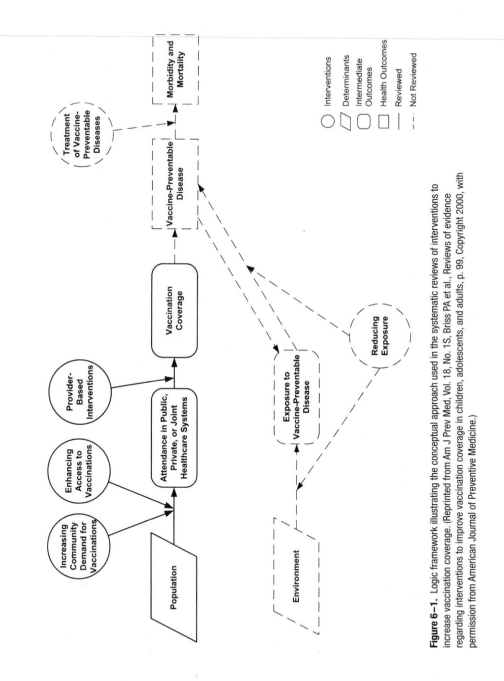

Figure 6–1. Logic framework illustrating the conceptual approach used in the systematic reviews of interventions to increase vaccination coverage. (Reprinted from Am J Prev Med, Vol. 18, No. 1S, Briss PA et al., Reviews of evidence regarding interventions to improve vaccination coverage in children, adolescents, and adults, p. 99, Copyright 2000, with permission from American Journal of Preventive Medicine.)

a requirement for child care, school, and college attendance; and provide families with take-home vaccination records and schedules. We reviewed client reminder and recall systems; vaccination requirements for child care, school, and college attendance; community-wide education and clinic-based education as single-component interventions; multicomponent interventions that include education; client or family incentives; and client-held medical records.

Client Reminder and Recall Systems to Increase Coverage with Universally Recommended Vaccines: Recommended (Strong Evidence of Effectiveness)

(See also Client Reminder Systems When Used Alone to Increase Targeted Vaccines Coverage: Insufficient Evidence to Determine Effectiveness, in Section II of this chapter.)

Community organizations, providers, and healthcare systems can help clients remember to come in for vaccinations through reminders (if it's time for the vaccination) and recalls (if the vaccination is overdue). These messages— delivered by telephone, letter, post card, or e-mail—can be either specific (i.e., telling the client to come in by a certain date to receive a specific vaccination) or general (i.e., telling the client to get in touch with the provider or healthcare system to make an appointment for needed vaccinations). Providers and systems that must reach a large number of clients may choose to use an autodialing system to help deliver phone messages.

(Client reminder and recall systems are also used in conjunction with home visits. See the review of Home Visits in this section for more information about this use.)

Effectiveness

- Client reminder and recall systems alone are effective in increasing coverage for universally recommended vaccines by approximately 8 percentage points.
- Client reminder and recall systems combined with other activities are effective in increasing coverage for universally recommended vaccines by approximately 16 percentage points.

Applicability

- These findings should be applicable to most adults and children in the United States for whom universally recommended vaccines are appropriate where improvements in coverage are needed.

The findings of our systematic review of client reminder and recall systems are based on 42 studies that evaluated the effectiveness of these systems.[21-62] An additional 18 studies were identified but did not meet our quality criteria and were excluded from the review.[63-80] Nine additional reports provided information on studies already included in the review.[81-89] We examined the use of reminders and recalls alone, as well as reminder and recall systems combined with one or more of the following activities: expanding access in healthcare settings; provider reminders; provider education; assessment plus feedback for vaccination providers; clinic-based education; community-wide education; client incentives; client-held medical records; reducing out-of-pocket costs; women, infants, and children (WIC) programs; home visits; or standing orders.

Most studies evaluated the effectiveness of reminders; some evaluated either recalls only or a combination of reminders and recalls. Telephone, post card, and letter reminders were evaluated; e-mail reminders would have been included, but we identified no studies of the use of these reminders. Two studies compared mailed and telephone reminders and found no difference between them. More intensive or more specific reminders were found to generate greater increases in vaccination coverage (e.g., more vs. fewer reminders, specific vs. general, personalized vs. generic, and letters signed by a physician) in five of six studies.

Client reminder and recall systems used alone showed an overall median difference of 8 percentage points (range, −7 to +31; 31 intervention arms). When used in conjunction with other activities, the median difference was 16 percentage points (range, −8 to +47; 23 intervention arms). Therefore, whether used alone or in combination with other interventions, and across a range of intervention content and delivery, client reminder and recall systems are effective in increasing vaccination coverage.

These findings should be applicable to most adults and children in the United States for whom universally recommended vaccines are appropriate where improvements in coverage are needed. Studies were conducted among white, African-American, and Hispanic people, poor and non-poor, in cities, suburbs, or rural areas. The findings are also applicable in a variety of settings: private practice, managed care, pharmacies, academic clinics, and community-wide. We also found effectiveness in increasing delivery of a broad range of vaccinations: measles, mumps, and rubella (MMR); diphtheria, tetanus, pertussis (DTP); oral poliovirus (OPV); *Haemophilus influenzae* type B Hib; influenza; pneumococcal polysaccharide; and the adult formulation of diphtheria and tetanus toxoids (Td).

No studies in this review of universally recommended vaccines examined the use of reminders and recalls to increase delivery of vaccinations to adolescents or specific delivery of hepatitis B vaccinations.

We did not look for or find any other positive or negative effects of client reminders and recalls.

The findings of our systematic review of economic evaluations are based on 11 studies of client reminder and recall interventions.[28,33,38,44,46,65,88,90-93] Median adjusted cost per additional vaccination for single-component interventions was $9 (range, $3 to $46). Adjusted cost per additional vaccination for multicomponent interventions was $4 for a combination of client and provider reminders; $51 for a combination of reminders and a lottery-type incentive; and $43 for a combination of mailed reminders and free vaccinations. Adjusted average costs varied from $0.65 to $5.75 per child.

The burden placed on providers or healthcare systems, or the lack of an information infrastructure (e.g., computerized records), can present a barrier to implementation of client reminders and recalls.

In conclusion, the Task Force recommends client reminders and recalls on the basis of strong evidence of effectiveness in increasing vaccination coverage, whether used alone or combined with other activities. The findings of this review should be applicable to most children and adults in the United States for whom universally recommended vaccines are appropriate where improvements in coverage are needed.

Multicomponent Interventions That Include Education to Increase Coverage with Universally Recommended Vaccines: Recommended (Strong Evidence of Effectiveness)

(Multicomponent interventions implemented in combination, which are related to but not identical to this intervention, are recommended to increase coverage with targeted vaccines. See Section II of this chapter.)

Education of clients or providers, when combined with other activities, can be very effective in increasing vaccination coverage. This education can be combined with one or more of the following: client reminders; provider reminders; longer hours of operation or improved access to clinics; reducing out-of-pocket costs; client-held vaccination records; providing information, incentives, or vaccinations to clients receiving WIC benefits; medical and psychosocial assessments; nutrition services; or home visits.

Effectiveness

- These interventions are effective in increasing coverage with universally recommended vaccines by approximately 16 percentage points in clinical settings.
- The interventions are also effective in increasing vaccination coverage with universally recommended vaccines by approximately 12 percentage points in community settings.
- It was not possible to separate the independent effects of specific intervention components.

Applicability

- These findings should be applicable to most adults and children in the United States for whom universally recommended vaccines are appropriate where improvements in coverage are needed.

Other Effects

- Multicomponent interventions that include education may also improve delivery of other preventive or clinical care.

The findings of our systematic review of multicomponent interventions that include education are based on 17 studies.[27,36,39,48–50,52,53,61,70,94–100] An additional 17 studies were identified but did not meet our quality criteria and were excluded from the review.[64–66,101–114] Three additional reports provided information on studies already included in the review.[81–83] All studies evaluated community or client education, along with other activities: client reminders; provider reminders; provider education; longer hours of operation or improved access to clinics; reducing out-of-pocket costs; client-held vaccination records; providing information, incentives, or vaccinations to clients receiving WIC benefits; medical and psychosocial assessments; nutrition services; or home visits.

These interventions make community members and clients in clinics aware of available vaccination services and the usefulness and relevance of these services, and provide information about how to access and use them. In the reviewed studies, information was provided in many ways, including mailed reminders, community outreach activities, media reports, posters in waiting rooms, other print materials in waiting rooms (e.g., flyers, brochures), educational sessions led by nursing staff, home visits, and client questionnaires that were reviewed by providers. Fifteen studies with follow-up periods of up to five years found a median difference in vaccination coverage of 16 percentage points (range, −4 to +29). The median difference in clinics was 16 percentage points (range, −4 to +25) and in community settings it was 12 percentage points (range, 5 to 29). In both clinic and community settings, these multicomponent approaches were effective in increasing vaccination coverage.

Although we could not attribute incremental improvements to the specific components, it appears that combined activities improve vaccination coverage. Why is there more solid evidence of the effectiveness of multicomponent approaches than of education alone? It could be because:

- the combined activities reinforce one another (e.g., education alone might not be enough to increase acceptance of vaccinations, but it could make clients more receptive to other components);

- multicomponent interventions are delivered more intensively than single-component interventions;
- more studies have been done of multicomponent interventions than of single-component interventions; or
- multicomponent interventions might increase the likelihood of a client's exposure to at least one component.

These results should be applicable to adults and children of any socioeconomic status for whom universally recommended vaccines are appropriate where improvements in coverage are needed. The reviewed studies were conducted among white, African-American, and Hispanic populations. The findings are also applicable in a variety of settings: academic clinics, private practice, public health clinics, and managed care. These interventions increased delivery of a broad range of vaccinations: influenza; pneumococcal polysaccharide; the adult formulation of diphtheria and tetanus toxoids (Td); diphtheria, tetanus, pertussis (DTP); oral poliovirus (OPV); measles, mumps, and rubella (MMR); and *Haemophilus influenzae* type B (Hib).

No studies in this review of universally recommended vaccines examined the use of multicomponent interventions that include education to increase delivery of vaccinations to adolescents or specific delivery of hepatitis B vaccinations.

An additional benefit of these multicomponent interventions may be improved delivery of other preventive or clinical care through reduction of client-, access-, provider-, or system-related barriers to such care.

The findings of our systematic review of economic evaluations of these multicomponent interventions are based on two studies,[109,115] both cost analyses. One study evaluated the costs of an intervention that included assembling a community task force, undertaking a media campaign, and implementing a school-based program that assessed students' immunization status and delivered vaccinations. The adjusted program costs for that study were $23 per child vaccinated. Another study estimated the costs of an intervention that included expanding access to vaccination services, multiple education and health promotion activities, and evaluation of the functioning of the clinics established as part of the intervention. The adjusted estimate of program costs for that study was $7.65 per vaccination delivered. Children in the first study could have received more than one vaccination, so the estimates might be more similar than they appear.

The difficulties of coordinating activities among several programs or administrative systems could present a barrier to the implementation of these multicomponent interventions.

In conclusion, the Task Force recommends multicomponent interventions that include education on the basis of strong evidence of effectiveness in increasing vaccination coverage in both clinical and community settings. The findings of this review should be applicable to most children and adults in the United States for whom universally recommended vaccines are appropriate where improvements in coverage are needed. These interventions may also improve delivery of other preventive or clinical care.

Vaccination Requirements for Child Care, School, and College Attendance to Increase Coverage with Universally Recommended Vaccines: Recommended (Sufficient Evidence of Effectiveness)

(See also Vaccination Requirements When Used Alone to Increase Targeted Vaccines Coverage: Insufficient Evidence to Determine Effectiveness in Section II of this chapter.)

Preschools and day care centers, elementary and high schools, and colleges and universities often require proof that incoming attendees or students have had certain vaccinations. In the 1970s–1980s, most primary and secondary schools began requiring vaccination of students. This led to consistent vaccination of more than 95% of students. For preschoolers and college-age students, laws and enforcement are more recent and vary greatly from state to state.

Effectiveness

- Vaccination requirements for child care, school, and college attendance are effective in increasing coverage with universally recommended vaccines by approximately 15 percentage points.

Applicability

- These findings should be applicable to most children and young adults in the United States for whom universally recommended vaccines are appropriate where improvements in coverage are needed.

The findings of our systematic review are based on 9 studies.[116–124] One additional study was identified but did not meet our quality criteria and was excluded from the review.[125] Another report provided information on a study already included in the review.[126] Six studies examined how effective these requirements were in reducing disease. Of these, three national studies found that the incidence of measles and mumps was lower in states that required school-age children to be vaccinated against these diseases; one of these also showed that officials in low-incidence areas are more likely to enforce the laws by excluding unvaccinated students from school attendance. Three additional studies measured diverse characteristics of laws and enforcement and generally found lower rates of disease. In jurisdictions where the incidence of measles was lower, laws banning unvaccinated children from entering school were more likely to be enforced. During an outbreak of mumps in New Jersey, children in schools that required vaccination were much less likely to have the disease than were other children. In New York State, the decline in Hib was greater for children in day care centers that required Hib vaccinations (even without any provision for enforcement) than for the state overall. We did not attempt a quantitative combination of these disparate outcomes and effect measures, but consider the pattern of results to be consistent with a conclusion that these requirements are effective in increasing coverage with universally recommended vaccines and decreasing rates of disease.

Three studies (one of which also measured disease rates) looked for changes in vaccination coverage and found a median difference of 15 percentage points (range, 5 to 35).

These findings should be applicable to most children and young adults in the United States who attend child care, school, or college, for whom universally recommended vaccines are appropriate and where improvements in coverage are needed. Studies were conducted in all 50 states, mostly in primary and high schools, but also in two- and four-year colleges as well as statewide in New York and California. Although no studies provided specific race and ethnicity data, studies in these large, diverse state populations should include, and apply to, diverse populations including racial and ethnic minorities.

Studies assessed the effectiveness of these laws in improving delivery of vaccinations against measles, mumps, and rubella (MMR), in reducing the occurrence of measles and mumps and the incidence of *Haemophilus influenzae* type B (Hib) and in increasing coverage of diphtheria, tetanus (DT), diphtheria, tetanus, pertussis (DTP), and oral poliovirus (OPV) vaccinations. No studies in this review of universally recommended vaccines examined the effectiveness of these laws in improving delivery of hepatitis B vaccinations.

We did not look for or find any other positive or negative effects of vaccination requirements for day care, school, and college attendance. We also did not find any economic evaluations of the effects of these laws. The difficulties of passing laws, and then of administering them and coordinating among various programs, can present barriers to implementation.

In conclusion, the Task Force recommends vaccination requirements for day care, school, and college attendance on the basis of sufficient evidence of effectiveness in increasing vaccination coverage. These results should be applicable to most children and young adults in the United States for whom universally recommended vaccines are appropriate where improvements in coverage are needed.

Community-Wide Education When Used Alone to Increase Coverage with Universally Recommended Vaccines: Insufficient Evidence to Determine Effectiveness

(See also Community-wide Education When Used Alone to Increase Coverage with Targeted Vaccines: Insufficient Evidence to Determine Effectiveness in Section II of this chapter.)

The goal of community-wide education about vaccinations is to help people within a specified geographic area learn more about vaccinations in the hope that they (and their children) will get the vaccinations they need. Healthcare providers can often be additional targets of these education programs. Community-wide education efforts can use one or more approaches, including mail, radio, television, newspaper, and posters.

Community-wide education can be one component in a multicomponent intervention. A number of the interventions reviewed in this section include community-wide education (see Client Reminder and Recall Systems; Multicomponent Interventions That Include Education; Vaccination Programs in Women, Infants, and Children (WIC) Settings; and Provider Reminder and Recall Systems).

Effectiveness

- We found insufficient evidence to determine the effectiveness of community-wide education, when used alone, to increase vaccination coverage.
- Evidence was insufficient because the only qualifying study had limitations in its design and execution and showed inconsistent results in different subpopulations.
- Insufficient evidence means that we were not able to determine whether or not the intervention works.

We found only one study that qualified for the systematic review of this intervention.[52] An additional five studies were identified but did not meet our quality criteria and were excluded from the review.[71,78,127–129] The reviewed study showed inconsistent results, with improvements in measles vaccination coverage among 6-year-olds but not among 14- to 18-month-olds. The evidence is therefore insufficient to determine the effectiveness of community-wide education alone to increase vaccination coverage. We did not look for other harms or benefits of education-only programs.

Because we could not establish the effectiveness of these programs, we did not examine situations in which the programs would be applicable, information about economic efficiency, or possible barriers to implementation.

In conclusion, although educational components can be part of effective multicomponent interventions, the Task Force found insufficient evidence to determine the effectiveness of community-wide education, when used alone, to increase vaccination coverage. Only a single qualifying study was identified, which had limitations in its design and execution and showed inconsistent results in different subpopulations.

Clinic-Based Education When Used Alone to Increase Coverage with Universally Recommended Vaccines: Insufficient Evidence to Determine Effectiveness

(See also Clinic-based Client Education When Used Alone to Increase Coverage with Targeted Vaccines: Insufficient Evidence to Determine Effectiveness in Section II of this chapter.)

Clinic-based education about vaccinations is directed to clients coming to medical or public health clinics to let them know about services and recommended vaccinations available at the clinic. Educational materials often take the form of standardized "Vaccine Information Statements," which are available to all vaccination providers for distribution to clients (and can be found at www.cdc.gov/nip/publications/VIS/default.htm). These statements include both information and consent forms for vaccinations.

Clinic-based education can be one component in a multicomponent intervention. A number of the multicomponent interventions reviewed in this section include clinic-based education (see Client Reminder and Recall Systems; Multicomponent Interventions That Include Education; and Provider Reminder and Recall Sytems).

Effectiveness

- We found insufficient evidence to determine the effectiveness of clinic-based education, when used alone, to increase vaccination coverage.
- Evidence was insufficient because the small number of studies showed no consistent effect on vaccine coverage or knowledge and attitudes.
- Insufficient evidence means that we were not able to determine whether or not the intervention works.

The findings of our systematic review are based on three studies.[98,130,131] An additional two studies were identified but did not meet our quality criteria and were excluded from the review.[132,133] In a randomized trial, provider education plus clinic-based education produced no significant increases in receipt of influenza and pneumococcal vaccines compared with provider education alone. Two before-and-after studies looked at the effects of Vaccine Information Statements on parents' knowledge about and attitudes toward vaccinations: one found a significant increase in both parental knowledge and willingness to have children vaccinated, but the other found no significant difference in either knowledge or attitude. We did not look for other harms or benefits of clinic-based education programs. The small number of studies and the inconsistent results in those studies provide insufficient evidence to determine the effectiveness of clinic-based education, by itself, in increasing vaccination coverage.

Because we could not establish the effectiveness of these programs, we did not examine situations in which they would be applicable, information about economic efficiency, or possible barriers to implementation.

In conclusion, the Task Force found insufficient evidence to determine the effectiveness of clinic-based education, when used alone, to increase vaccination coverage because of the small numbers of studies and lack of consistent demonstration of an effect.

Client or Family Incentives to Increase Coverage with Universally Recommended Vaccines: Insufficient Evidence to Determine Effectiveness

(See also Client or Family Incentives When Used Alone to Increase Targeted Vaccines Coverage: Insufficient evidence to Determine Effectiveness in Section II of this chapter.)

One approach to getting clients to agree to be vaccinated or to have their children vaccinated is to offer either positive or negative incentives (e.g., money, baby toys, discount coupons for retailers, or exclusion from a particular program).

Some programs that focus on other approaches to increasing coverage of universally recommended vaccines also include incentives. For the results of these reviews see Vaccination Requirements for Child Care, School, and College Attendance and Vaccination Programs in Women, Infants, and Children (WIC) Settings.

Effectiveness

- We found insufficient evidence to determine the effectiveness of client or family incentives in increasing vaccination coverage.
- Evidence was insufficient because the small number of studies showed no consistent effect.
- Insufficient evidence means that we were not able to determine whether or not the intervention works.

The findings of our systematic review of client or family incentives are based on three studies.[27,44,62] One additional report provided information on a study already included in the review.[84] All the studies in our review included the use of both positive incentives (e.g., gift certificates or lotteries for cash prizes) and other activities (e.g., client and provider reminders, home visits, or transportation assistance). In one study, one intervention arm evaluated incentives alone. No studies of negative incentives were evaluated.

These studies all showed an increase in vaccine coverage in response to offers of gift certificates or cash prizes, but some changes were small and many were not statistically significant. The small number of studies, with inconsistent effects, provided insufficient evidence to determine the effectiveness of incentives in increasing coverage. (We also found insufficient evidence to determine whether or not client or family incentives are effective in increasing hepatitis B vaccine coverage. See Section II of this chapter.)

Because we could not establish the effectiveness of these programs, we did not examine situations in which they would be applicable or information about economic efficiency.

A possible barrier to implementation of such programs would be ethical concerns about whether incentives constitute coercion.

We did not look for other harms or benefits of client or family incentives.

In conclusion, the Task Force found insufficient evidence to determine the effectiveness of incentives in increasing receipt of vaccinations because the small number of studies showed no consistent effect.

Client-Held Medical Records to Increase Coverage with Universally Recommended Vaccines: Insufficient Evidence to Determine Effectiveness

The idea behind encouraging clients to keep a record of their vaccinations is that they will be more aware of when their vaccinations are due or overdue and may request the vaccinations themselves. And when a client can bring a copy of his or her vaccination record to a healthcare provider, the provider may be prompted to deliver a vaccination that might otherwise be missed. Some state and local health departments and private provider offices have distributed medical records to clients.

Effectiveness

- We found insufficient evidence to determine the effectiveness of client-held medical records in increasing vaccination coverage.
- Evidence was insufficient because of the small number of studies, the variability in the programs evaluated, and the lack of statistical significance in the results of some studies.
- Insufficient evidence means that we were not able to determine whether or not the intervention works.

The findings of our systematic review are based on four studies.[48,94,134,135] An additional four studies were identified but did not meet our quality criteria and were excluded from the review.[108,136-138] One study compared a combination of client-held medical records and provider reminders with provider reminders alone. Other studies evaluated client-held medical records combined with clinic-based education, client reminders, or multiple approaches. Although three studies reported median increases in coverage of 5 to 15 percentage points, not all of these were statistically significant improvements. Therefore, the small number of studies, the variety of evaluated programs, the small effect sizes, and the lack of statistical significance in some of the findings provide insufficient evidence to determine the effectiveness of client-held medical records in increasing vaccination coverage.

Because we could not establish effectiveness of these programs, we did not examine situations in which such programs would be applicable or information about economic efficiency.

A possible barrier to implementation could be the burden placed on providers. In one survey, 80% of providers had positive reactions to client-held medical records, but 17% felt that such records had a negative effect on clinic efficiency.

In conclusion, although four studies were reviewed, the differences among the evaluated programs and the fact that several of the results were neither substantial nor significantly different from zero provide insufficient evidence to determine the effectiveness of client-held medical records in increasing vaccination coverage.

Universally Recommended Vaccines: Enhancing Access to Vaccination Services

Even if community demand for vaccinations can be increased through the interventions reviewed above, other barriers to vaccination may still remain. Costs that are too high for clients to pay, or inconvenient locations or hours for vaccination, are typical barriers. The strategy reviewed here, enhancing access to vaccination services, focuses on reducing such barriers by making it as easy as possible for individuals and families to get the vaccinations they need. Interventions that enhance access to vaccination services work by reducing the cost of vaccinations or by making vaccinations very easy to obtain. We reviewed interventions that reduce the price consumers pay for vaccinations; expand availability of vaccinations in healthcare settings; and provide vaccinations in nonmedical settings, including women, infants, and children (WIC) programs, home visits, schools, and child care centers.

Reducing Out-of-Pocket Costs to Increase Coverage with Universally Recommended Vaccines: Recommended (Strong Evidence of Effectiveness)

(See also Reducing Client Out-of-Pocket Costs to Increase Coverage with Targeted Vaccines: Recommended as Part of a Combination Approach, as well as Reducing Client Out-of-Pocket Costs When Used Alone, to Increase Coverage with Targeted Vaccines: Insufficient Evidence to Determine Effectiveness in Section II of this chapter.)

The cost of vaccinations often stops clients and their family members from being vaccinated. Covering the cost of the vaccines or their administration either directly or through insurance coverage, or reducing clients' co-payments for vaccinations, can increase the number of clients who get appropriate vaccinations. Programs to reduce costs and increase vaccine coverage have been used by the federal government (e.g., the Vaccines for Children Program), state governments (e.g., providing free vaccinations), and managed care organizations (e.g., reducing co-payments).

Effectiveness

- Reducing out-of-pocket costs alone is effective in increasing coverage with universally recommended vaccines by approximately 10 percentage points.
- Reducing out-of-pocket costs combined with other activities is effective in increasing coverage with universally recommended vaccines by approximately 16 percentage points.

Applicability

- These findings should be applicable in a broad range of settings, among populations for whom universally recommended vaccines are appropriate, where improvements in coverage are needed.

The findings of our systematic review are based on 19 studies.[42,46,48,50,54,70,97,139-150] An additional seven studies were identified but did not meet our quality criteria and were excluded from the review.[71,101,103,107,110,151,152] Two additional reports provided information on a study already included in the review.[153,154] The reviewed studies evaluated improvement in vaccination outcomes, reduction in the likelihood that providers would refer clients elsewhere to get needed vaccines, or both.

Five surveys of providers' likelihood to refer clients elsewhere for needed vaccinations (including two nationally representative surveys of pediatricians and family physicians) consistently found that limited insurance coverage (public or private) for children was a key factor in providers' decisions to refer children to other sites for vaccinations.

Efforts to improve vaccination outcomes (earlier or increased vaccination) were either single-component or multicomponent. Findings of the five single component studies that could be expressed with a percentage point improvement showed a median improvement in vaccination outcomes of 10 percentage points (range, −1 to +29). The eight multicomponent studies looked at reducing out-of-pocket costs along with client reminders and recalls, community-wide education, expanding access in healthcare settings, provider education, clinic-based education, client-held medical records, WIC interventions, or provider reminders and recalls. The median improvement in these studies was 16 percentage points (range, −8 to +47).

The evidence therefore shows that reducing clients' out-of-pocket costs is effective in increasing vaccination coverage.

These results should be applicable to adults and children of low or mixed socioeconomic status for whom universally recommended vaccines are appropriate and improvements in coverage are needed, in rural and urban settings, in hospitals, clinics, private offices, WIC settings, and emergency departments.

The findings of our systematic review of economic evaluations of interventions to reduce out-of-pocket cost for vaccinations are based on one study.[46] That study evaluated the cost effectiveness of a multicomponent intervention to encourage influenza vaccination, which consisted of mailed reminders and free vaccinations. The adjusted cost per additional vaccination in this intervention was $43.

We questioned whether reducing out-of-pocket costs would have any negative effects on vaccine research and development but did not find any studies that examined this issue. We did not look for any other positive or negative effects of reducing out-of-pocket costs.

A possible barrier to reducing out-of-pocket costs could be the complexities and fragmentation of mechanisms for payment of vaccinations.

In conclusion, the Task Force recommends reducing out-of-pocket costs on the basis of strong evidence of effectiveness in increasing vaccination coverage. The components of the interventions reviewed varied considerably, yet these findings should be applicable in a variety of settings to a variety of populations for whom universally recommended vaccines are appropriate and improvements in coverage are needed.

Expanding Access in Healthcare Settings, to Increase Coverage with Universally Recommended Vaccines: Recommended as Part of a Multicomponent Intervention (Strong Evidence of Effectiveness) Insufficient Evidence to Determine Effectiveness When Used Alone

(See also Expanding Access in Healthcare Settings to Increase Coverage with Targeted Vaccines: Recommended as Part of a Combination Approach, as well as Expanding Access in Healthcare Settings When Used Alone to Increase Coverage with Targeted Vaccines: Insufficient Evidence to Determine Effectiveness, in Section II of this chapter.)

Barriers to clients seeking and obtaining vaccinations for themselves or their children are common, and include limited hours during which vaccination services are available (e.g., while most people must be at work or in school), distances to travel to vaccination locations, and difficulties in arranging for vaccinations. Financially disadvantaged families are particularly burdened by the challenges of child care and transportation. These barriers can be reduced by administering vaccines in additional locations (e.g., emergency departments, inpatient units in hospitals, or subspecialty clinics), especially if these are closer to where clients live and work; expanding the hours of facilities that offer vaccinations; or easing the process of getting a vaccination (e.g., in a "drop-in" clinic or an "express lane" vaccination service).

Effectiveness

- Expanding access in healthcare settings is effective in increasing coverage with universally recommended vaccines by approximately 13 percentage points when used as part of a multicomponent intervention.
- We found insufficient evidence to determine the effectiveness of this intervention when used alone because the small number of studies did not show statistically significant improvement.
- Insufficient evidence means that we were not able to determine whether or not the intervention works when used alone.

Applicability

- Review findings should be applicable to adults and children for whom universally recommended vaccines are appropriate in diverse clinical and community settings where improvements in coverage are needed.

The findings of our systematic review are based on 16 studies that examined expanding access alone and expanding access combined with other activities.[27,35,36,39,40,42,47,53,61,62,77,96,99,147,155,156] An additional nine studies were identified but did not meet our quality criteria and were excluded from the review.[65,101,103,105,107,110,113,136,157] Four additional reports provided information on studies already included in the review.[81,83,84,86]

Approaches to expanding access were drop-in clinics; increased night and weekend hours; making vaccinations available in emergency departments; special vaccination clinics; special vaccination appointments; inpatient vaccination stations; and transportation assistance. The activities combined with expanded access were client reminder and recall, provider education, clinic-based education, standing orders, community-wide education, client incentives, vaccination programs in WIC settings, home visits, or assessment plus feedback for vaccination providers. Overall, 12 of the studies of expanded access combined with another intervention showed a median improvement of 13 percentage points (range, −8 to +35) in vaccination coverage, indicating the effectiveness of the multicomponent interventions in increasing vaccination coverage.

No statistically significant improvement was found in two studies that examined expanding access by itself, although these efforts could help to make other approaches (e.g., standing orders or client reminders) more effective. The small number of studies showing no statistically significant improvement provided insufficient evidence to determine the effectiveness of expanded access alone in increasing vaccination coverage.

Multicomponent approaches may be generally more effective because they are more intense or because the combined effects of the various components increase the overall effectiveness of each one.

These findings should be applicable to most adults and children for whom universally recommended vaccines are appropriate where improvements in coverage are needed. Studies were conducted in managed care settings, public health clinics, community clinics, private practices, Veterans Administration hospitals and clinics, academic settings, and as part of community-wide programs.

We did not look for any other positive or negative effects of expanding access in healthcare settings.

The findings of our systematic review of economic evaluations of this multicomponent intervention are based on one study.[115] The study, a cost analysis, estimated the costs of an intervention that included expanding access to vaccination services, multiple education and health promotion activities, and evaluation of the functioning of the clinics established as part of the intervention. The adjusted program costs were $7.65 per vaccination delivered.

Efforts to expand access to vaccination services can encounter several barriers, presented either by clients or by the settings in which they might seek vaccinations. These barriers include the problems of coordinating between settings and of having appropriate records available, the lack of a relationship between vaccination programs and the primary purpose of the setting in which they are offered, clients' inability to remember which vaccinations they or their children have received, and contraindications to receiving vaccinations in some situations (e.g., feverish children being brought to emergency departments).

In conclusion, the Task Force recommends multicomponent interventions to expand access in healthcare settings on the basis of strong evidence of effectiveness in increasing vaccination coverage. When used alone, however, evidence was insufficient to determine the effectiveness of the intervention because of a small number of studies that showed no statistically significant improvement in coverage. The findings of this review should be applicable to adults and children for whom universally recommended vaccines are appropriate in most clinical and community settings where improvements in coverage are needed.

Access to vaccination services can be expanded in nonmedical settings, too. Assessing immunization status and referring or vaccinating children or adults in places where they go on a regular basis may be effective ways to increase vaccination coverage. These nonmedical settings can also offer education about, and incentives to accept, vaccinations.

The Task Force recommends expanding access to include WIC settings, home visiting, and school-based programs (based on sufficient evidence of effectiveness). Evidence was insufficient, however, to determine if expanding access in child care centers is effective. The findings of our reviews of these four settings follow.

Vaccination Programs in Women, Infants, and Children (WIC) Settings to Increase Coverage with Universally Recommended Vaccines: Recommended (Sufficient Evidence of Effectiveness)

The Special Supplemental Nutrition Program for Women, Infants, and Children (WIC) provides supplemental foods, health care referral, and nutrition education for low-income women, infants, and children who are at nutritional risk. Administered by the U.S. Department of Agriculture, this single largest point of access to health-related services for low-income preschool children reaches 45% of all U.S. infants; in some cities, up to 80% of all infants participate in WIC. Participants in the WIC programs visit program sites every 2 to 3 months for nutrition services and food vouchers, and receive comprehensive health status evaluations every 6 to 12 months. The programs are required to serve as a gateway to, and coordinator for, other health services, including vaccinations.

Programs that promote vaccinations in WIC settings require assessment of each child's immunization status. They may refer underimmunized children to a healthcare provider or provide vaccinations onsite. These programs can also include education or incentives to accept vaccinations. One such incentive is the voucher restriction or *monthly voucher pick up,* which require clients at high risk of not receiving the vaccines they need to come to the WIC site more frequently, usually monthly.

Effectiveness

- Vaccination programs in WIC settings used alone increased vaccination coverage by approximately 9 percentage points.
- Vaccination programs in WIC settings combined with other activities increased vaccination coverage by approximately 12 percentage points.

Applicability

- These findings should be applicable to WIC participants of any race for whom universally recommended vaccines are appropriate, in urban and rural settings, where improvements in coverage are needed.

Other Effects

- We found no evidence to support the possible harm that vaccination requirements or monthly voucher pick up increase WIC dropout rates.

The findings of our systematic review are based on four studies that examined the effectiveness of vaccination programs in WIC settings in increasing vaccination coverage.[61,141,158,159] An additional six studies were identified but did not meet our quality criteria and were excluded from the review.[160-165] One additional report provided information on a study already included in the review.[166] Three of the reviewed studies were conducted entirely among WIC clients. These studies (1) compared a combination of education, assessment, and referral with the same combination plus monthly voucher pick up or an escort to a vaccination clinic, resulting in small but significant increases in vaccination coverage, or (2) compared WIC programs with no program. Various combinations of education, assessment, referral, free vaccinations, monthly voucher pick up, and regular care produced a median increase of 9 percentage points (range, 4 to 34) in vaccination coverage over regular care alone. Education, assessment, monthly voucher pick up, free vaccinations, and various combinations of vaccination referrals or onsite vaccinations resulted in a median increase of 34 percentage points in vaccination coverage; the specific strategies used for vaccination or referral produced no differences in effectiveness. The fourth study looked at programs in WIC settings as part of a comprehensive multicomponent program and found that the components combined produced a median increase of 12 percentage points in vaccination coverage. The four reviewed studies provide sufficient evidence that a variety of vaccination programs, delivered in WIC settings, are effective in increasing vaccination coverage.

Although studies in this review looked at minority children in urban areas, the results should be applicable to all WIC clients, of any race, for whom universally recommended vaccines are appropriate in either rural or urban settings where improvements in coverage are needed.

Despite concerns on the part of many WIC providers that vaccination requirements or monthly voucher pick up could negatively affect WIC participation, two studies suggested that these effects may not be large. The first found that the dropout rates remained constant among those receiving the vaccine program but increased in the group receiving no such program. The second found small dropout rates (~ 1 percentage point) when comparing children who received assessment and escort, assessment and referral, or assessment and monthly voucher pick up. These findings do not suggest substantial effects of these programs on dropout rates.

The findings of our systematic review of economic evaluations of WIC interventions are based on two studies.[141,166] One of these reported cost per fully vaccinated child of three variations of a WIC intervention that differed primarily in the way referrals were handled and how vaccines were provided. Adjusted cost per fully vaccinated child ranged from $34 to $84. Adjusted cost of assessing immunization status, based on a second study, were $2.65 per assessment for interventions using an onsite vaccination nurse and $1.28 per assessment for interventions using other strategies to promote vaccination.

Difficulties in coordinating WIC programs with vaccination programs can present barriers to implementation of the latter, as can objections among WIC providers and managers to the concept of monthly voucher pick up requirements.

In conclusion, the Task Force recommends vaccination programs in WIC settings on the basis of sufficient evidence of effectiveness in increasing vaccination coverage. These findings should be applicable to WIC clients of any race for whom universally recommended vaccines are appropriate, in rural and urban settings, where improvements in coverage are needed. No evidence was found to support the possible harm that vaccination requirements or monthly voucher pick up increase WIC dropout rates.

Vaccination Programs in Schools to Increase Coverage with Universally Recommended Vaccines: Recommended (Sufficient Evidence of Effectiveness)

The goal of school-based vaccination programs is to improve vaccination delivery to students aged 5–18 years. At this time, the only vaccination programs that would be appropriate in schools are those for newly recommended vaccines, such as hepatitis B vaccine. School-based vaccination programs offer a unique opportunity for providing vaccinations and other preventive services to young people. In the United States, for example, approximately 99% of children aged 11 and 12 years attend school. The vaccination programs we reviewed were almost always multicomponent, and included efforts to increase demand (through educating students, parents, teachers, and other school staff about vaccines and providing reminders or recalls when students were due or past due for vaccinations) and access (by providing free vaccines, incentives, and special vaccination hours and locations). Written consent from parents or guardians was usually required. The programs often involved collaboration among schools, local health departments, community clinics, and private health providers. (Vaccination requirements for school attendance are reviewed elsewhere in this section; see Vaccination Requirements for Child Care, School, and College Attendance.)

Effectiveness

- Vaccination programs in schools are effective in increasing immunization coverage by approximately 58 percentage points.

Applicability

- These findings should be applicable to adolescents for whom universally recommended vaccines are appropriate, of any socioeconomic status and race, in most schools where improvements in coverage are needed.
- These findings should also be applicable to newly recommended vaccines (e.g., hepatitis B vaccine).

The findings of our systematic review are based on nine studies (in multiple reports).[167-183] All of the studies except one[183] were conducted to assess the acceptance of hepatitis B vaccine at a time when the vast majority of students were unvaccinated. Only one of these studies had a concurrent comparison group in which vaccination was available but not promoted in a special program.[172] We therefore included before-and-after studies in our review as long as an assessment of the baseline vaccination coverage of the entire target student population (usually the entire school) was included. An additional 11 studies were identified (in two reports) but did not meet our quality criteria and were excluded from the review.[176,184]

The nine studies of school-based programs reported a median increase in vaccination coverage of 58 percentage points (range, 11 to 92). This improvement shows that vaccination programs in schools are effective in increasing coverage. Although exact dates of these programs were not always provided, follow-up was generally one school year.

These results should be applicable to adolescents of any socioeconomic status and race for whom universally recommended vaccines are appropriate and where improvements in coverage are needed. They are also applicable in a variety of types of schools. Because the studies only evaluated newly introduced or recommended (but not required) vaccines, and because coverage with vaccines already recommended for children in the United States is greater than 90% by the time children enter school, school-based programs can only be recommended for the introduction of new vaccines (e.g., hepatitis B vaccine).

One positive effect of vaccinating adolescents in schools is that they do not then need to make special visits to their providers to receive vaccinations. However, not visiting providers for vaccinations could have the unintended negative effect of reducing the provision of other recommended adolescent health services that might be offered when vaccines are delivered in a clinical setting. We did not find empirical studies of this suggested harm.

The findings of our systematic review of economic evaluations of school-based vaccination programs are based on one study.[185] That study included a cost analysis and a cost-effectiveness analysis of a school-based universal hepatitis B vaccination program for sixth graders in British Columbia. The adjusted program cost per fully vaccinated child (three vaccinations) was US$47.11. Considering direct costs only, the adjusted cost per life-year saved was US$2316 compared with the policy in place prior to the program (screening mothers and vaccinating children born to carrier mothers, in addition to vaccinating high-risk individuals).

Need for special staff, difficulties coordinating school-based health programs in each school, potential disruption of school routines, and concerns about confidentiality are potential barriers to the implementation of these programs.

In conclusion, the Task Force recommends vaccination programs in schools on the basis of sufficient evidence of effectiveness in increasing vaccination coverage. These findings should be applicable to most schools and students for whom newly recommended vaccines are indicated (e.g., hepatitis B vaccine) where improvements in coverage are needed.

Vaccination Programs in Child Care Centers to Increase Coverage with Universally Recommended Vaccines: Insufficient Evidence to Determine Effectiveness

In 1997, approximately 32% of preschool children were cared for in child care centers.[186] These children, mostly under the age of five, are at increased risk of contracting communicable diseases.[187] Programs to encourage vaccination of children who are in child care assess a child's immunization status either when the child enrolls in the center or one or more times while the child is attending the center. The efforts can be combined with education or notification of parents, referrals to healthcare providers, and even providing needed vaccinations at the center. Some centers require proof that children have received certain vaccinations before they can be enrolled (see Vaccination Requirements for Child Care, School, and College Attendance).

Effectiveness

- We found insufficient evidence to determine the effectiveness of vaccination programs in child care centers in increasing vaccination coverage.
- Evidence was insufficient because no studies met the quality standards required for review.
- Insufficient evidence means that we were not able to determine whether or not the intervention works.

We found no studies that qualified for our systematic review of vaccination programs in child care centers. One study was identified but did not meet our quality criteria and was not included in the review.[188] We therefore had insufficient evidence to determine whether or not these programs are effective in increasing vaccination coverage. We did not look for other harms or benefits of these programs.

Because we could not establish the effectiveness of these programs, we did not examine situations in which such programs would be applicable, information about economic efficiency, or possible barriers to implementation.

In conclusion, the Task Force found insufficient evidence to determine the effectiveness of vaccination programs in child care centers in increasing vaccination coverage because no qualifying studies were identified.

Home Visits to Increase Coverage with Universally Recommended Vaccines: Recommended (Sufficient Evidence of Effectiveness)

Home visits to promote receipt of vaccinations consist of face-to-face services delivered to clients in their homes, including education, assessment of need for vaccinations, referral to a vaccination provider, or providing vaccinations in the clients' homes. Telephone or mail reminders can also be used. Home visits are usually directed to subpopulations that are difficult to reach, such as people living in public housing communities or rural areas. (Home visits are also used to address other public health issues such as violence [see Chapter 9]).

Effectiveness

- Home visits combined with other activities are effective in increasing vaccination coverage by approximately 13 percentage points.

Applicability

- These findings should be applicable to adults and children for whom universally recommended vaccines are appropriate, including those of low socioeconomic status, in urban and rural settings where improvements in coverage are needed.

Economic Efficiency

- Although effective in increasing vaccination coverage, home visits solely for this purpose can have very high resource costs for the benefits achieved.

The findings of our systematic review are based on seven studies that examined the effectiveness of home visits alone or combined with other activities to promote vaccinations.[27,77,189-193] An additional eight studies were identified but did not meet our quality criteria and were excluded from the review.[194-201] One additional report provided information on a study already included in the review.[84] Five of the reviewed studies looked at home visiting with or without client reminders and case management, and two studies looked at home visits along with other activities, including community outreach, education, transportation assistance, or provider education with feedback (see Assessment plus Feedback for Vaccination Providers). These seven studies showed a median increase of 10 percentage points in vaccination coverage (range, −1 to +49). The generally positive changes in the reviewed studies provide sufficient evidence of the effectiveness of home visits in increasing vaccination coverage.

These findings should be applicable to most adults and children, including those of low socioeconomic status, living in urban or rural areas, for whom universally recommended vaccines are appropriate and where improvements in coverage are needed.

The findings of our systematic review of economic evaluations of home visits are based on four studies.[191,193,197,202] Adjusted cost per child vaccinated was $22[197] and $130.[202] Adjusted cost per additional vaccination was $513[191] and $13,020.[193]

The need to train those who will conduct home visits, and concerns about their safety, present potential barriers to use of this approach.

In conclusion, the Task Force recommends home visits on the basis of sufficient evidence of effectiveness in increasing coverage with universally recommended vaccines. These findings should be applicable to most adults and children, including those of low socioeconomic status, in both urban and rural settings where improvements in coverage are needed. Although home visits are an effective way to increase vaccination coverage, when made solely for this purpose they can have very high resource costs for the benefits achieved.

Universally Recommended Vaccines: Provider- or System-Based Interventions

Healthcare providers and systems can also help to ensure that their clients receive recommended vaccinations. Unfortunately, they often miss such opportunities. Provider- or system-based interventions, which are implemented primarily through healthcare systems, are designed to encourage healthcare providers to actively ensure that clients get needed vaccinations. These interventions educate providers about vaccinations, remind providers when individual clients are due for vaccinations, and give feedback to providers on how well they are doing in terms of providing specific vaccinations. An additional intervention—*standing orders*—removes a potential barrier to vaccination (heavy physician workload) by increasing the number of personnel in healthcare settings qualified to give vaccinations.

Provider Reminder and Recall Systems to Increase Coverage with Universally Recommended Vaccines: Recommended (Strong Evidence of Effectiveness)

(See also Provider Reminder Systems to Increase Coverage with Targeted Vaccines: Recommended as Part of a Combination Approach, as well as Provider Reminder Systems When Used Alone to Increase Coverage with Targeted Vaccines: Recommended in Section II of this chapter.)

Through provider reminder and recall systems, providers are reminded that clients are due (reminder) or overdue (recall) for specific vaccinations. Reminders can take many forms, including notes in clients' charts, mailings, checklists, flowcharts, or computer notification. The content of the reminders varies, ranging from a simple notation that a vaccination is due or late to such a reminder combined with additional information. Providers most often receive the information during a scheduled appointment with a client, but can also receive it before or after the appointment.

Provider reminder and recall can be used alone or combined with other activities including clinic-based education, assessment plus feedback for vaccination providers, provider education, community-wide education, or expanded access to vaccination services.

(Provider reminders can also be combined with standing orders. See Standing Orders for more information about this use.)

Effectiveness

- Provider reminder and recall systems, when used alone, are effective in increasing vaccination coverage by approximately 17 percentage points.
- Various combinations of interventions that include provider reminder and recall systems are effective in increasing vaccination coverage by approximately 14 percentage points.

Applicability

- These findings should be applicable to clients of any age for whom universally recommended vaccines are appropriate, for a range of providers and healthcare settings, where improvements in coverage are needed.

Other Effects

- The use of provider reminder and recall systems may lead to improvements in outcomes other than vaccine coverage, such as improved delivery of other preventive services or clinical care.

The findings of our systematic review are based on 30 studies.[24,25,33,36,39,41, 51,52,95,100,156,191,203–220] An additional 30 studies were identified but did not meet our quality criteria and were excluded from the review.[56,68,75,104,106,110–112,114,]

[136,137,151,152,195,221-236] Eight additional reports provided information on studies already included in the review.[81,85,87,88,237-240] Reviewed studies evaluated reminder and recall alone, in combination with other activities, or both. Provider reminder and recall systems used alone showed an overall median increase of 17 percentage points (range, 1 to 67; 17 intervention arms). When combined with other activities, the median increase was 14 percentage points (range, 1 to 36; 12 intervention arms). Whether used alone or in combination with other activities, provider reminder and recall systems were effective in increasing vaccination coverage.

These results should be applicable, where improvements in coverage are needed, to clients for whom universally recommended vaccines are appropriate and to diverse providers in a wide range of settings. The findings are applicable to several kinds of providers—residents, physicians who have completed their training, and non-physician providers of vaccinations—in academic clinics, managed care facilities, private practice, community health centers, community hospitals, and community-wide settings. Physicians who practice internal medicine, family medicine, and pediatrics were studied. Clients were either outpatients or inpatients of any age. Reminder and recall systems were effective in increasing delivery of vaccines for measles, mumps, and rubella (MMR); diphtheria, tetanus, pertussis (DTP); oral poliovirus (OPV); *Haemophilus influenzae* type B (Hib); influenza; pneumococcal disease; and the adult formulation of diphtheria and tetanus toxoids (Td). Studies of universally recommended vaccines did not examine provider reminder and recall system effectiveness in increasing delivery of hepatitis B vaccinations.

Some studies found additional benefits of provider reminder and recall systems in the form of improved delivery of other preventive services or clinical care, perhaps owing to improved performance of providers and systems in delivering preventive care. We did not look for other positive or negative effects of provider reminder and recall systems.

The findings of our systematic review of economic evaluations are based on three studies.[33,88,221] The first study showed that the adjusted cost per additional vaccination for provider reminders only[88] was $0.70. This cost is probably an underestimate because it does not include the cost of producing reminders. The second study estimated the cost of an intervention that included both client and provider reminders.[33] The adjusted cost per additional child vaccinated in that study was $4. The third study[221] estimated the cost of a program that assessed the immunization status of hospitalized children by contacting the children's usual physicians and by reminding hospital physicians to vaccinate the children before they were discharged. The adjusted cost per fully vaccinated child was $300.

We found two potential barriers to implementing provider reminder and recall systems: the burden placed on administrative systems (e.g., difficulty in placing reminders in clients' charts or providers' difficulty in using the reminders) and lack of an information infrastructure (e.g., computerized records) to generate reminders and recalls.

In conclusion, the Task Force recommends provider reminder and recall systems alone or in combination with other activities on the basis of strong evidence of effectiveness in increasing vaccination coverage. These findings should apply to clients of any age, for whom universally recommended vaccines are appropriate and where improvements in coverage are needed, and should also apply to diverse providers in most settings where vaccinations are provided.

Assessment Plus Feedback for Vaccination Providers to Increase Coverage with Universally Recommended Vaccines: Recommended (Strong Evidence of Effectiveness)

(See also Assessment Plus Feedback for Vaccination Providers to Increase Coverage with Targeted Vaccines: Recommended as Part of a Combination Approach, as well as Assessment Plus Feedback for Vaccination Providers, When Used Alone, to Increase Coverage with Targeted Vaccines: Insufficient Evidence to Determine Effectiveness, in Section II of this chapter.)

Assessment and feedback programs for vaccination providers involve assessing the provider's performance in delivering one or more vaccinations to clients and giving information about that assessment to the provider. Goals of these programs can include changing the provider's knowledge, attitudes, and behavior and stimulating other changes in the way vaccinations are delivered (e.g., use of provider reminders [see Provider Reminder and Recall Systems] or standing orders [see Standing Orders]). Program activities can also include use of financial or other incentives (positive or negative) or benchmarking (comparing a provider's performance to a goal or standard of performance).

Assessments can be conducted for providers in private practices, group practices, managed care organizations, teaching hospitals, or other settings and may be conducted by the provider's staff, the staff of the organization that manages the setting, insurance companies, or others with an interest in improving provider and system success in delivering vaccinations. One good example of provider assessment and feedback can be found at www.cdc.gov/nip/afix/default.htm.

Effectiveness

- Provider assessment plus feedback, when used alone, is effective in increasing vaccination coverage by approximately 16 percentage points.

- Various combinations of provider assessment plus feedback with other activities are effective in increasing vaccination coverage by approximately 17 percentage points.

Applicability

- These findings should be applicable to clients of any age, for universally recommended vaccinations delivered by most providers, in most settings where vaccinations are provided and where improvements in coverage are needed.

Other Effects

- Provider assessment plus feedback can lead to improvements other than vaccine coverage, such as improved delivery of other preventive services or clinical care.

The findings of our systematic review are based on 14 studies that evaluated the effectiveness of provider assessment plus feedback, either alone or in combination with other activities[24,29,36,72,191,209,210,214,219,224,241–244] (most often provider reminder and recall systems, as well as provider education, client reminders, clinic-based education, or incentives). An additional 13 studies were identified but did not meet our quality criteria and were excluded from the review.[75,79,136,223,228,229,234,235,245–249] Four additional reports provided information on studies already included in the review.[81,89,101,250] Provider feedback plus assessment was effective in increasing vaccination coverage, whether used alone (median increase of 16 percentage points; range, 9 to 41) or in combination with other activities (median increase of 17 percentage points; range, 1 to 43). Several studies showed that these improvements could be maintained or increased over several subsequent years.

These results should be applicable to clients of any age for whom universally recommended vaccines are appropriate, seen by many kinds of providers (residents; physicians in internal medicine, family medicine, and general practice; and non-physician providers) in settings where vaccinations are commonly delivered (private practice, managed care organizations, public health clinics, community health centers, and university or other teaching hospitals) and where improvements in coverage are needed. Provider assessment plus feedback was effective in increasing delivery of several vaccines: measles, mumps, and rubella (MMR); diphtheria, tetanus, pertussis (DTP); oral poliovirus (OPV); *Haemophilus influenzae* type B (Hib); influenza; pneumococcal; and the adult formulation of diphtheria and tetanus toxoids (Td). Studies of universally recommended vaccines did not examine the effectiveness of provider assessment plus feedback in increasing delivery of hepatitis B vaccinations.

Some studies looked at additional benefits of provider assessment plus feedback (e.g., improved delivery of other preventive services or clinical care) and found some improvements in these areas. We did not look for other positive or negative effects of provider assessment plus feedback.

We did not find any economic evaluations of these programs.

The lack of an adequate information infrastructure (e.g., computerized records) and the administrative burden placed on providers and systems are potential barriers to implementing provider assessment plus feedback programs.

In conclusion, the Task Force recommends assessment plus feedback for vaccination providers either alone or in combination with other activities, on the basis of strong evidence of effectiveness in increasing vaccination coverage. These findings should be applicable to clients of any age, for whom universally recommended vaccines are appropriate, for many kinds of providers, in settings where vaccines are usually delivered and where improvements in coverage are needed.

Provider Education Only to Increase Coverage with Universally Recommended Vaccines: Insufficient Evidence to Determine Effectiveness

(See also Provider Education When Used Alone to Increase Targeted Vaccines Coverage: Insufficient Evidence to Determine Effectiveness in Section II of this chapter.)

Provider education seeks to increase providers' knowledge and change their attitudes about vaccinations, to get them to deliver more of the appropriate vaccinations to their clients, to stimulate them to use additional approaches to increasing vaccine coverage (e.g., client or provider reminder and recall systems or standing orders), or to improve their interactions with clients so that clients are more willing to accept vaccinations. Educational information for providers can be made available through written materials, computer software, videos, lectures, or continuing medical education programs.

(For more information on provider education programs that include other activities to increase universally recommended vaccine coverage, see Provider Reminder and Recall Systems and Assessment Plus Feedback for Vaccination Providers.)

Effectiveness

- We found insufficient evidence to determine the effectiveness of provider education alone in increasing vaccination coverage or improving providers' knowledge and attitudes about vaccinations.
- Evidence was insufficient because of the small number of studies, small effect sizes, variable statistical significance, and few studies measuring outcomes other than knowledge and attitudes.

- Insufficient evidence means that we were not able to determine whether or not the intervention works.
- Provider education combined with provider reminders or provider assessment and feedback, however, can be effective in increasing coverage with universally recommended vaccines.

The findings of our systematic review are based on four studies.[206,251–253] An additional two studies were identified but did not meet our quality criteria and were excluded from the review.[232,254] One additional report provided information on a study already included in the review.[240] Two studies evaluated improvements in vaccination coverage among adults. One found a small and nonsignificant improvement, and the other found that provider education alone produced less improvement in vaccination coverage than did standing orders or provider reminders. The two other studies found small improvements in provider knowledge and attitudes. The programs evaluated in three of the studies were not very intensive. Overall, the evidence was insufficient to determine whether or not provider education, by itself, is effective in increasing vaccination coverage.

Because we could not establish the effectiveness of these programs, we did not examine situations in which they would be applicable, information about economic efficiency, or possible barriers to implementation.

In conclusion, the small number of studies, small effect sizes, variable statistical significance, and few studies measuring outcomes other than knowledge and attitudes provided insufficient evidence for the Task Force to determine the effectiveness of provider education alone in increasing vaccination coverage or improving providers' knowledge and attitudes about vaccinations. It should be noted, though, that provider education can be effective in increasing vaccine coverage when used in combination with provider reminders or provider assessment and feedback (see Provider Reminder and Recall Systems and Assessment Plus Feedback for Vaccination Providers).

Standing Orders to Increase Coverage with Universally Recommended Vaccines:
Recommended for Adults (Strong Evidence of Effectiveness)
Insufficient Evidence to Determine Effectiveness for Children

(See also Standing Orders to Increase Coverage with Targeted Vaccines: Recommended as Part of a Combination Approach, as well as Standing Orders When Used Alone to Increase Coverage with Targeted Vaccines: Insufficient Evidence to Determine Effectiveness in Section II of this chapter.)

Standing orders allow professionals who are not physicians (e.g., nurses or pharmacists) to give vaccinations without direct physician involvement at the time of the vaccination. The goal of standing orders is to increase vaccination coverage by reducing missed opportunities and overcoming existing barriers, such as requirements for a physical examination before vaccinating a client or unavailability of physicians due to other demands on their time.

We reviewed the use of standing orders in clinics, hospitals, and nursing homes. Although dedicated vaccination clinics often operate using standing orders, we did not consider this use to be a provider or system intervention and therefore did not include this setting in our review.

Effectiveness

- Standing orders, when used alone, were effective in increasing vaccine coverage of adults by approximately 51 percentage points.
- Various combinations of interventions that include standing orders are effective in increasing vaccination of adults by approximately 16 percentage points.
- We found insufficient evidence to determine the effectiveness of standing orders in increasing vaccination coverage among children: the only study included in our review found no overall improvement in vaccination coverage.
- Insufficient evidence means that we were not able to determine whether or not the intervention works to increase vaccination of children through standing orders.

Applicability

- The recommended intervention should be applicable to adults for whom universally recommended vaccines are appropriate in both inpatient and outpatient settings where improvements in coverage are needed.

The findings of our systematic review are based on 11 studies (in 12 reports) that examined standing orders either alone or combined with other activities.[36,40,47,81,98,155,206,255–259] An additional five studies were identified but did not meet our quality criteria and were excluded from the review.[110,152,233,260,261] Two additional reports provided information on a study already included in the review.[86,262] Used alone, standing orders increased adult vaccination coverage by a median of 51 percentage points (range, 30 to 81). Used in combination—with expanding access in healthcare settings, client reminder and recall systems, clinic-based education, provider education, provider reminder and recall systems, or provider assessment plus feedback—standing orders increased adult vaccination coverage by a median of 16 percentage points (range, 6 to 26). Most studies were less than a year long, but one found that improvement continued over a five-year period. Alone or combined with other interventions, standing orders are effective in increasing adult vaccination coverage.

We found only one study that evaluated standing orders for vaccinations for children, which showed no overall improvement in vaccination coverage.

Because vaccination protocols in children are more complex than such protocols in adults, and because the single available study showed no improvement in coverage, the evidence was insufficient to determine the effectiveness of standing orders in increasing vaccination coverage among children.

These findings should be applicable to delivery of influenza and pneumococcal polysaccharide vaccines to adults in hospitals, nursing homes, and outpatient settings including private practices, managed care organizations, Veterans' Administration clinics, and university-related clinics where improvements in coverage are needed. No studies looked at using standing orders to increase delivery of vaccines to adolescents or to increase delivery of hepatitis B vaccinations or the adult formulation of diphtheria and tetanus toxoids (Td).

We did not look for any other positive or negative effects of standing orders and did not find any economic evaluations of these programs.

The burden placed on providers and healthcare systems, difficulties in fostering inter-professional communication and sharing of responsibilities, and challenges of reconciling these programs with local legal and regulatory structures can present barriers to implementing standing orders programs.

In conclusion, the Task Force recommends standing orders to increase vaccination coverage among adults on the basis of strong evidence of effectiveness. This finding should be applicable to adults in both inpatient and outpatient settings where improvements in coverage are needed.

The Task Force, however, found insufficient evidence to determine the effectiveness of standing orders in increasing vaccination coverage among children.

CONCLUSION: UNIVERSALLY RECOMMENDED VACCINES

This first section of the chapter summarizes Task Force conclusions and recommendations on interventions to increase delivery of universally recommended vaccines for children, adolescents, and adults. To increase community demand for these vaccinations the Task Force recommends client reminder and recall systems; multicomponent interventions that include education; and vaccination requirements for child care, school, and college attendance; insufficient evidence exists at this time to determine the effectiveness of community-wide education; clinic-based education; client or family incentives; or client-held medical records. To enhance access to vaccination services, the Task Force recommends reducing client out-of-pocket costs, expanding access as part of a multicomponent intervention, vaccination programs in WIC settings, vaccination programs in schools, and home visits; insufficient evidence is available to determine the effectiveness of expanding access as a single-component intervention or of vaccination programs in child care centers. To improve the performance of providers and systems in delivering vaccines, the Task Force recommends provider reminder and recall systems, assessment plus feedback for vaccination providers, and standing orders for adults; insufficient evidence was found to determine the effectiveness of either standing orders for children or provider education by itself. Details of these reviews have been published[20,263,264] and these articles, along with additional information about the reviews, are available at www.thecommunity guide.org/vaccine. Updates and expansions of this chapter are in progress and will also be available at that site. Additional information about using these recommendations is available at the end of this chapter.

SECTION II: TARGETED VACCINES: IMPROVING TARGETED INFLUENZA, PNEUMOCOCCAL POLYSACCHARIDE, AND HEPATITIS B VACCINATION COVERAGE AMONG HIGH-RISK ADULTS

(See summary list of interventions at the beginning of this chapter.)

Section I of this chapter considered effective approaches to increasing coverage of universally recommended vaccines (those that should be administered to all people in a given age group). Now we turn to targeted vaccines, those given to specific groups with factors that make them particularly susceptible to a disease (at-risk or high-risk populations). Note that it is not actually the vaccines themselves that change, but rather their indicated use. For example, the influenza vaccine is *universally recommended* for all people over age 50 and is also *targeted* to people under age 50 who have specific health problems. Interventions and policies to promote targeted vaccines are likely to be more complex than similar interventions to promote universally recommended vaccines. For example, interventions to improve coverage with universally recommended vaccines might need no more information about the target population than age; programs to promote targeted vaccines might require information on age, risk factors, and vaccination history.

Three vaccine-preventable diseases—influenza, pneumococcal infections, and hepatitis B—cause significant illness and premature death each year in the United States. The people most likely to develop these diseases can be identified by specific risk factors, and prevention of the diseases can be enhanced by increasing vaccine coverage in the at-risk groups.[265]

Annually, influenza may cause as many as 36,000 deaths in the United States[5] and hospitalize as many as 114,000 people.[266] The most vulnerable groups are adults age 65 and older, and younger people with medical conditions such as diabetes, heart disease, or lung disease.[267-269]

More than 7000 people in the United States die every year as a result of invasive pneumococcal disease.[270] Pneumococcal infections account for more than 100,000 hospitalizations for pneumonia and more than 60,000 cases of bacteremia and other forms of invasive pneumococcal diseases annually.[271-273] Risk factors for complications of pneumococcal infections are similar to those for influenza, and include age and chronic illnesses such as diabetes, heart disease, and lung disease.[267,268,274]

As many as 1.25 million people in the United States are chronically infected with hepatitis B virus (HBV),[275] and 5000 die of HBV-related cirrhosis or liver cancer annually.[276,277] An estimated 73,000 new HBV infections occurred in 2000.[278] The most commonly reported risk factors for hepatitis B include heterosexual activity (39.8%), sexual activity between men (14.6%), and injection drug use (13.8%).[279] Infection with HBV is also an occupational risk for health, rescue, and law enforcement personnel who deliver either routine or emergency care.

Annual vaccination to prevent influenza is recommended[280] for people over 50 years of age and for younger people with certain chronic conditions, especially during the active flu season between October and March. Influenza coverage rates among adults under 65 years of age with high-risk conditions remain well below the *Healthy People 2010*[6] goal of 60%.[281] In 2000, vaccination coverage for adults aged 18–49 years with high-risk conditions was 24.7%, and among adults aged 50–64 with high-risk conditions, coverage rates were only 43.9%.[266]

Similarly, in 2000, only 12.3% of people aged 18–49 years with high-risk conditions had ever been vaccinated with the pneumococcal polysaccharide vaccine, and only 26% of those aged 50–64 with high-risk conditions had been vaccinated; in contrast, coverage among people over the age of 65 was 52.9%.[282] It is worth noting, however, that vaccination coverage rates among people over the age of 65 largely reflect vaccination coverage of non-Hispanic whites, 56.8% of whom have been vaccinated, whereas only 30.4% of Hispanics and 30.7% of non-Hispanic blacks have received the vaccine.

The impact of a policy to deliver hepatitis B vaccine routinely to healthcare workers can be seen in the dramatic decline of HBV infections among these workers after such vaccination became routine: from 17,000 in 1983 to only 400 in 1995.[283] Despite the availability of this effective vaccine, vaccination coverage rates for HBV still remain low in most targeted populations. Two small local studies showed vaccination coverage rates of only 9% of men who have sex with men in 1998[284] and only 6% among injection drug users in 1998–2001.[285]

Over the past decade, improvements in vaccination coverage for adults have also been unevenly distributed. Although coverage rates for influenza and pneumococcal polysaccharide vaccines have steadily improved among adults over 65 years of age, improvements in vaccination coverage among younger adults with risk conditions have been less dramatic and coverage rates remain low.[281] Similarly, significant increases in vaccination coverage for HBV among healthcare workers have not been matched in harder-to-reach populations engaging in high-risk behaviors.

OBJECTIVES AND RECOMMENDATIONS FROM OTHER ADVISORY GROUPS

The interventions recommended in this chapter can be used to reach objectives set out in *Healthy People 2010*[6] (Table 6-1). These targeted vaccines objectives are also priorities for the National Immunization Program (NIP) of the Centers for Disease Control and Prevention (CDC). In addition, the recommendations complement information from other advisory groups, including the following:

Recommendations for Adolescent and Adult Vaccinations

These recommendations are published by the Advisory Committee on Immunization Practices (ACIP) of the U.S. Department of Health and Human Services (DHHS)/CDC,[10,11] the American College of Physicians,[12] Infectious Disease Society of America,[12,13] the American Academy of Family Physicians (AAFP),[9] and the American College of Obstetricians and Gynecologists.[14] Vaccination recommendations for adolescents are now coordinated among ACIP, AAFP, and the American Medical Association.

Recommendations for Interventions to Improve Vaccination Coverage

These recommendations have been developed by the Canadian Community Health Practice Guidelines Working Group,[15,16] ACIP,[17,18] and the National Vaccine Advisory Committee.[19]

METHODS

Methods used for the reviews are summarized in Chapter 10. Specific methods used in the systematic reviews are described elsewhere[286] and are available at www.thecommunityguide.org/vaccine. For this review of interventions to increase targeted vaccines coverage among high-risk adults, we adopted the conceptual approach used in the reviews of evidence on effectiveness of interventions to improve universally recommended vaccines coverage, the topic of the first section of this chapter (see also Briss et al., 2000[20]). The logic framework (Figure 6–1) shows the strategy and intervention options available for efforts to increase targeted vaccination coverage in populations at high risk, which is the same as that for universally recommended vaccines.

In interpreting the results of our systematic reviews of interventions to increase targeted vaccine coverage, we found that only 1 of 11 interventions, when implemented alone, provided evidence of effectiveness strong enough for the Task Force to recommend use of the intervention (Provider Reminders, described below). Among the other 10 interventions, too few studies with sufficient quality of design and execution were available to formulate a recommendation (all described below). Many of the studies in the review evaluated the use of more than one intervention (multicomponent interventions). In these published reports of multicomponent interventions, we found that the effects of the individual interventions could not be calculated separately from the overall effect. Yet, as we worked with the data on the effectiveness of the multicomponent interventions, we saw that they frequently combined interventions from at least two of our three categories: increasing client demand for vaccinations, enhancing access to vaccination services, and provider- or system-based interventions. We analyzed the various combinations used, and discovered that the effective combinations usually combined one or more interventions to enhance access with one or more provider- or system-based interventions and/or one or more interventions to increase client demand (a more complete discussion of this process can be found elsewhere[286]). This qualitative approach to data analysis allowed us to formulate a recommendation that encompasses the three categories and provides a "menu" of options from which users can choose (see Increasing Targeted Vaccines Coverage Through Multiple Interventions Implemented in Combination below).

ECONOMIC EFFICIENCY

We found no economic evaluations of interventions recommended for increasing targeted vaccine coverage and therefore present no economic data in this section of the chapter.

RECOMMENDATIONS AND FINDINGS

This section presents a summary of the findings of the systematic reviews conducted to determine the effectiveness of interventions to increase coverage with vaccinations targeted to high-risk populations. These interventions are grouped into four categories: increasing community demand for vaccinations; enhancing access to vaccination services; provider- or system-based interventions; and increasing targeted vaccines coverage through multiple interventions implemented in combination.

Targeted Vaccines: Increasing Community Demand for Vaccinations

Interventions to increase demand for vaccination services provide information and advice to individual clients or to people within a community who are at risk. Within this category, we reviewed interventions that use clinic-based or community-wide client education, client reminder systems, client incentives, and vaccination requirements.

Clinic-Based Client Education When Used Alone to Increase Coverage with Targeted Vaccines: Insufficient Evidence to Determine Effectiveness

(See also Clinic-Based Education When Used Alone to Increase Coverage with Universally Recommended Vaccines: Insufficient Evidence to Determine Effectiveness in Section I of this chapter.)

Clinic-based education interventions provide information on vaccinations to clients while they are being served in a medical or public health clinic setting. These interventions help clients to identify their risk status and determine whether they should get specific vaccines. The interventions also educate clients about the potential benefits of vaccination. Such education can reduce or remove barriers to vaccination by changing negative attitudes and beliefs. These interventions may use a variety of formats such as letters, newsletters, brochures, and posters.

Effectiveness

- We found insufficient evidence to determine the effectiveness of clinic-based client education alone in increasing targeted vaccines coverage.
- Evidence was insufficient because of the small number of available studies.
- Insufficient evidence means that we were not able to determine whether or not the intervention works.

The findings of our systematic review are based on two studies that examined the effectiveness of clinic-based client education when used alone.[287,288] In both studies, brochures were used to provide education to clients. One study also evaluated two versions of health information brochures given to healthcare providers for use with their clients. The two brochure versions were associated with increases of 2 and 10 percentage points, respectively, in the proportion of clients screened or vaccinated for hepatitis B. The second study evaluated the effect on subsequent receipt of pneumococcal vaccination of an educational brochure given to clients. In this study, vaccination rates among clients with at-risk medical conditions improved by 16.1 percentage points compared with rates among clients who were not given the brochure. The small number of studies, however, does not provide enough evidence to determine the effectiveness of the intervention.

Because we could not establish the effectiveness of these programs, we did not examine situations in which they would be applicable, information about economic efficiency, or possible barriers to implementation.

In conclusion, the Task Force found insufficient evidence to determine the effectiveness of clinic-based client education when used alone to increase vaccination coverage among adult populations at high risk. The evidence was considered insufficient because of the small number of available studies. (Clinic-based client education when combined with additional interventions is reviewed below. See Increasing Targeted Vaccines Coverage through Multiple Interventions Implemented in Combination.)

Client Reminder Systems When Used Alone to Increase Coverage with Targeted Vaccines: Insufficient Evidence to Determine Effectiveness

(Client reminder and recall systems are recommended for increasing coverage with universally recommended vaccines. See Section I of this chapter.)

Client reminder systems for targeted vaccines provide information or advice directly to individual clients at high risk to encourage them to obtain appropriate vaccinations. Examples of client reminders include letters or postcards sent from a provider's office, healthcare system, or insurance carrier. In this review, we categorized as client reminders those interventions that identified and notified individual clients at high risk and included a vaccination recommendation developed for the client by his or her healthcare provider or system.

Effectiveness

- We found insufficient evidence to determine the effectiveness of client reminder systems alone in increasing targeted vaccination coverage.
- Evidence was insufficient because of the small number of available studies.
- Insufficient evidence means that we were not able to determine whether or not the intervention works.

The findings of our systematic review are based on one study evaluating the effectiveness of client reminder systems when used alone.[37] In this study, clients identified as being at high risk for influenza received a postcard with a personal message signed by their physician. At follow-up, self-reported vaccination for influenza improved by 3.7 percentage points compared with clients who did not receive a postcard reminder. This single study, however, provided insufficient evidence to determine whether or not client reminders, by themselves, are effective in increasing vaccination coverage.

Because we could not establish the effectiveness of these interventions, we did not examine situations in which they would be applicable, information about economic efficiency, or possible barriers to implementation.

In conclusion, the Task Force found insufficient evidence to determine the effectiveness of client reminder systems when used alone to increase vaccination coverage among high-risk adults because of the small number of available studies. (Client reminder systems when combined with additional interventions are reviewed below. See Increasing Targeted Vaccines Coverage through Multiple Interventions Implemented in Combination.)

Community-Wide Education When Used Alone to Increase Coverage with Targeted Vaccines: Insufficient Evidence to Determine Effectiveness

(See also Community-wide Education When Used Alone to Increase Coverage with Universally Recommended Vaccines: Insufficient Evidence to Determine Effectiveness in Section I of this chapter.)

Community-wide education interventions provide information to most or all of a target group of people in a geographic area, which can include vaccination providers in addition to clients. Educational messages can be delivered by various methods (e.g., mail, radio, newspapers, television, and posters). The goal of community-wide education is to increase or improve the availability of information about vaccinations and increase people's knowledge, thereby increasing their acceptance of and demand for vaccinations and, ultimately, increasing vaccination coverage.

Effectiveness

- We found insufficient evidence to determine the effectiveness of community-wide education interventions alone in increasing targeted vaccines coverage.
- Evidence was insufficient because no studies were available.
- Insufficient evidence means that we were not able to determine whether or not the intervention works.

We did not find any studies that evaluated community-wide education when used alone, and therefore had insufficient evidence to determine whether or not this intervention is effective in increasing vaccination coverage.

Because we could not establish the effectiveness of these interventions, we did not examine situations in which they would be applicable, information about economic efficiency, or possible barriers to implementation.

In conclusion, the Task Force found insufficient evidence to determine the effectiveness of community-wide education when used alone to increase targeted vaccines coverage among high-risk adults because no studies were available.

Client or Family Incentives When Used Alone to Increase Coverage with Targeted Vaccines: Insufficient Evidence to Determine Effectiveness

(See also Client or Family Incentives to Increase Coverage with Universally Recommended Vaccines: Insufficient Evidence to Determine Effectiveness in Section I of this chapter.)

These interventions use financial or other incentives to motivate people at risk to accept vaccinations. Incentives may be positive (rewards) or negative (penalties). This approach is based on the idea that clients will be motivated to seek vaccinations if they receive rewards (e.g., money or discount coupons for retail establishments) or face penalties (e.g., being excluded from participation in a program).[289]

Effectiveness

- We found insufficient evidence to determine the effectiveness of client or family incentives alone in increasing targeted vaccines coverage.
- Evidence was insufficient because of the small number of available studies.
- Insufficient evidence means that we were not able to determine whether or not the intervention works.

The findings of our systematic review are based on one study evaluating the effectiveness of client incentives when used alone.[289] This study evaluated the implementation of a $10 incentive to increase hepatitis B vaccination coverage among recruited injection drug users; the incentive increased vaccinations by 35 percentage points. Although this is a relatively large increase, this single study alone did not provide enough evidence for the Task Force to determine whether or not client incentives by themselves are effective in increasing vaccination coverage.

Because we could not establish the effectiveness of these interventions, we did not examine situations in which they would be applicable, information about economic efficiency, or possible barriers to implementation.

In conclusion, the Task Force found insufficient evidence to determine the effectiveness of client incentives when used alone to increase targeted vaccines coverage among adults at high risk because of the small number of available studies.

Vaccination Requirements When Used Alone to Increase Coverage with Targeted Vaccines: Insufficient Evidence to Determine Effectiveness

(Vaccination requirements for child care, school, and college attendance are recommended to increase coverage with universally recommended vaccines. See Section I of this chapter.)

These laws or policies require vaccinations or other documentation of immunity (or documentation of refusing a vaccination) as a condition of attendance, participation, or employment. Although some hospitals have policies requiring staff to be vaccinated against influenza, no state or federal laws in the United States require high-risk adults to receive influenza, pneumococcal polysaccharide, or hepatitis B vaccines. Current standards of the Occupational Safety and Health Administration[290] mandate that employers offer the hepatitis B vaccination series, at no cost, to any employee whose work is likely to include exposure to blood or other potentially infectious materials,[291] although employees can decline the vaccination. The impact of this policy can be seen in the dramatic decline of HBV infections among healthcare workers, from 17,000 in 1983 to only 400 in 1995.[283]

Effectiveness

- We found insufficient evidence to determine the effectiveness of vaccination requirements, when used alone, in increasing targeted vaccines coverage.
- Evidence was insufficient because there were no qualifying studies.
- Insufficient evidence means that we were not able to determine whether or not the intervention works.

We found no studies that qualified for our systematic review, and therefore had insufficient evidence to determine whether or not vaccination requirements, by themselves, are effective in increasing vaccination coverage.

Because we could not establish the effectiveness of these policies, we did not examine circumstances in which they would be applicable, information about economic efficiency, or possible barriers to implementation.

In conclusion, the Task Force found insufficient evidence to determine the effectiveness of vaccination requirements alone in increasing vaccination coverage among high-risk adults because no qualifying studies were identified.

Targeted Vaccines: Enhancing Access to Targeted Vaccination Services

Interventions that enhance access to vaccination services are designed to reduce the cost or to increase the convenience of being vaccinated. We reviewed interventions that reduce out-of-pocket costs to the client and those that expand access to vaccination services in healthcare settings.

Reducing Client Out-of-Pocket Costs When Used Alone to Increase Targeted Vaccines Coverage: Insufficient Evidence to Determine Effectiveness

(Reducing out-of-pocket costs is recommended to increase coverage with universally recommended vaccines. See Section I of this chapter.)

Methods to reduce out-of-pocket vaccination costs to clients include paying for vaccinations or administration, providing insurance coverage, or reducing co-payments for vaccinations at the point of service. Reducing client out-of-pocket costs can increase vaccination coverage by improving availability of vaccinations, by increasing the demand for them, or both.

Effectiveness

- We found insufficient evidence to determine the effectiveness of reducing out-of-pocket vaccination costs alone in increasing targeted vaccines coverage.
- Evidence was insufficient because no studies were identified.
- Insufficient evidence means that we were not able to determine whether or not the intervention works.

We did not find any studies that evaluated reducing client out-of-pocket costs and therefore had insufficient evidence to determine whether or not these programs are effective in increasing vaccination coverage.

Because we could not establish the effectiveness of these programs, we did not examine situations in which they would be applicable, information about economic efficiency, or possible barriers to implementation.

In conclusion, the Task Force found insufficient evidence to determine the effectiveness of reducing client out-of-pocket costs, when used alone, in increasing targeted vaccines coverage among high-risk adults, because no studies were identified. (Reducing client out-of-pocket costs when combined with additional interventions is reviewed below. See Increasing Targeted Vaccines Coverage through Multiple Interventions Implemented in Combination.)

Expanding Access in Healthcare Settings When Used Alone to Increase Coverage with Targeted Vaccines: Insufficient Evidence to Determine Effectiveness

(Expanding access in healthcare settings to increase coverage with universally recommended vaccines is recommended as part of a multicomponent intervention; when used alone, we found insufficient evidence to determine effectiveness in increasing coverage with universally recommended vaccines. See Section I of this chapter.)

Interventions that expand access focus on increasing the availability of vaccinations in medical or public health clinic settings. These interventions are designed to remove important barriers to obtaining vaccinations, including inconvenient clinic hours or locations and burdensome administrative requirements. These barriers are particularly significant among clients who do not visit clinics on a regular basis or who have transportation problems or other difficulties getting to appointments. Interventions to expand access in healthcare settings do so by (1) reducing the distance from the healthcare setting to the population, (2) increasing or changing hours for vaccination services, (3) delivering vaccinations in clinical settings that did not previously provide them (e.g., emergency departments, inpatient units, or subspecialty clinics), or (4) reducing administrative barriers to obtaining vaccination services within clinics (e.g., by developing a drop-in clinic or an express lane vaccination service).

Effectiveness

- We found insufficient evidence to determine the effectiveness of expanding access in healthcare settings, when used alone, in increasing targeted vaccines coverage among high-risk clients.
- Evidence was insufficient because no studies were identified for review.
- Insufficient evidence means that we were not able to determine whether or not the intervention works.

We did not find any studies that evaluated expanding access in healthcare settings, when used alone, and therefore had insufficient evidence to determine whether or not these programs, by themselves, are effective in increasing vaccination coverage.

Because we could not establish the effectiveness of these interventions, we did not examine situations in which they would be applicable, information about economic efficiency, or possible barriers to implementation.

In conclusion, the Task Force found insufficient evidence to determine the effectiveness of expanding access in healthcare settings, when used alone, in increasing vaccination coverage of high-risk adults because no studies were identified for review. (Expanded access in healthcare settings when combined with additional interventions is reviewed below. See Increasing Targeted Vaccines Coverage through Multiple Interventions Implemented in Combination.)

Targeted Vaccines: Provider- or System-Based Interventions

Healthcare providers can play a vital role in ensuring that high-risk adults receive appropriate vaccinations. Unfortunately, for a variety of reasons, providers often miss opportunities to vaccinate clients. Provider-based interventions, implemented primarily through healthcare systems, are designed to encourage healthcare providers to actively ensure that clients who are at risk get needed vaccinations. We reviewed four provider- or system-based interventions used alone: provider reminder systems, provider education, assessment plus feedback for vaccination providers, and standing orders.

Provider Reminder Systems When Used Alone to Increase Coverage with Targeted Vaccines: Recommended (Strong Evidence of Effectiveness)

(Provider reminder and recall systems are also recommended to increase coverage with universally recommended vaccines. See Section I of this chapter.)

Provider reminders to administer vaccines to high-risk clients let providers or other appropriate staff know when individual clients are due for vaccinations. Reminder techniques can include notations in clients' charts, stickers or other prompts attached to clients' charts, standardized checklists generated by clinical staff, or computer databases and registries. Reminders can be directed at the primary healthcare provider or clinic staff. All of the reminder systems we reviewed provided information to the provider at the time of the scheduled appointment.

Effectiveness

- When used alone, provider reminder systems are effective in increasing targeted vaccines coverage among high-risk adults by approximately 22 percentage points.

Applicability

- These findings should be applicable to providers and staff in most healthcare settings where improvements in coverage are needed.

Other Effects

- Provider reminder systems can also improve delivery of other preventive services or clinical care through use of additional reminders.

The findings of our systematic review are based on seven studies that examined the effectiveness of provider reminder systems alone in increasing targeted vaccines coverage.[25,203,207,211,213,237,238] Several types of provider reminder systems were examined in the qualifying studies, including attachments to clients' charts generated by computer programs or clinic staff and a reminder questionnaire designed as a letter from a colleague.

Two studies measured changes in influenza vaccine coverage, and one study measured differences or changes in pneumococcal vaccine coverage. Four studies provided measurements of differences or changes in coverage for both influenza and pneumococcal vaccinations. Overall, the nine study arms in the seven qualifying studies reported a median improvement in targeted vaccines coverage of 22 percentage points (range, 8 to 72), indicating that provider reminder systems, by themselves, are effective in increasing vaccination coverage.

These findings should be applicable to providers and staff in most healthcare settings where improvements in coverage are needed. All studies were implemented and evaluated in academic healthcare settings, including hospitals and clinics, and all evaluated the effectiveness of provider reminder systems on resident and faculty physicians and nurses. The client populations in the qualifying studies were patients with chronic illnesses. It should be noted, however, that none of the studies identified in this review evaluated outcomes of hepatitis B vaccination coverage in high-risk populations.

Provider reminder systems may provide an additional benefit in that they allow for prompts to deliver additional preventive services or clinical care. In three of the reviewed studies, provider reminder systems also included prompts for fecal occult blood tests (FOBT), Pap tests, mammography, dental exams, tetanus boosters, cancer screening, and measurements of serum cholesterol. Our review did not find any harms associated with provider reminder systems.

We did not find any economic evaluations of this intervention.

Potential barriers to the implementation of provider reminder systems include the concerns of some providers about the efficacy[211,257] and safety[207] of pneumococcal vaccination. Clients may also refuse to receive vaccinations.[203,207] The costs associated with implementation of reminder systems can also be a barrier.

In conclusion, the Task Force recommends provider reminder systems, when used alone, on the basis of strong evidence of effectiveness in increasing targeted vaccines coverage among high-risk adults. These findings should be applicable to providers and staff in most healthcare settings where improvements in coverage are needed. (Provider reminder systems when combined with additional interventions are also recommended. See Increasing Targeted Vaccines Coverage through Multiple Interventions Implemented in Combination.)

Provider Education When Used Alone to Increase Coverage with Targeted Vaccines: Insufficient Evidence to Determine Effectiveness

(See also Provider Education When Used Alone to Increase Coverage with Universally Recommended Vaccines: Insufficient Evidence to Determine Effectiveness in Section I of this chapter.)

Provider education seeks to increase providers' knowledge and change their attitudes about vaccinations, to get them to deliver more of the appropriate vaccinations to their clients or improve their interactions with clients so that clients are more willing to accept vaccinations. Giving information to providers can result in fewer missed vaccination opportunities and a greater proportion of eligible clients receiving appropriate vaccinations. Information can be delivered through written materials, videos, lectures, continuing medical education programs, and computerized software.

Effectiveness

- We found insufficient evidence to determine the effectiveness of provider education alone in increasing targeted vaccines coverage.
- Evidence was insufficient because no studies were identified for review.
- Insufficient evidence means that we were not able to determine whether or not the intervention works.

We did not find any studies that evaluated provider education interventions when used alone, and therefore had insufficient evidence to determine whether or not these programs are effective in increasing vaccination coverage.

Because we could not establish the effectiveness of these interventions, we did not examine situations in which they would be applicable, information about economic efficiency, or possible barriers to implementation.

In conclusion, the Task Force found insufficient evidence to determine the effectiveness of provider education, when used alone, in increasing targeted vaccines coverage among high-risk adults because no studies were identified for review.

Standing Orders When Used Alone to Increase Coverage with Targeted Vaccines: Insufficient Evidence to Determine Effectiveness

(Standing orders to increase coverage with universally recommended vaccines are recommended for adults; for children, we found insufficient evidence to determine effectiveness. See Section I of this chapter.)

Standing orders allow professionals who are not physicians (e.g., nurses or pharmacists) to give vaccinations without direct physician involvement at the time of the vaccination. Standing orders can increase vaccination coverage by reducing missed opportunities and overcoming existing barriers, such as a requirement for a physical exam before receiving a vaccination or limited availability of physicians due to other demands.

Effectiveness

- We found insufficient evidence to determine the effectiveness of standing orders alone in increasing targeted vaccines coverage.
- Evidence was insufficient because no studies were identified for review.
- Insufficient evidence means that we were not able to determine whether or not the intervention works.

We did not find any studies that evaluated standing orders when used alone, and therefore had insufficient evidence to determine whether or not these programs are effective in increasing vaccination coverage.

Because we could not establish the effectiveness of these interventions, we did not examine situations in which they would be applicable, information about economic efficiency, or possible barriers to implementation.

In conclusion, the Task Force found insufficient evidence to determine the effectiveness of standing orders, when used alone, in increasing targeted vaccines coverage among high-risk adults, because no studies were identified in this review. (The effectiveness of standing orders when combined with additional interventions is reviewed below. See Increasing Targeted Vaccines Coverage through Multiple Interventions Implemented in Combination.)

Assessment Plus Feedback for Vaccination Providers When Used Alone, to Increase Coverage with Targeted Vaccines: Insufficient Evidence to Determine Effectiveness

(Assessment plus feedback for vaccination providers is recommended to increase coverage with universally recommended vaccines. See Section I of this chapter.)

Assessment plus feedback programs for vaccination providers assess the provider's performance in delivering one or more vaccinations to clients and provide assessment results to the provider. Assessment plus feedback can result in improvements in vaccination coverage by changing provider knowledge, attitudes, and behaviors and by stimulating additional improvements in the vaccination delivery system (e.g., through reminders or standing orders).

Effectiveness

- We found insufficient evidence to determine the effectiveness of provider assessment plus feedback programs alone in increasing targeted vaccines coverage.
- Evidence was insufficient because only one study was identified for review, and it had limitations in the quality of execution.
- Insufficient evidence means that we were not able to determine whether or not the intervention works.

The findings of our systematic review are based on one study evaluating the effectiveness of assessment plus feedback for vaccination providers when used alone.[242] This study evaluated the effect on influenza and pneumococcal polysaccharide vaccine coverage of annual chart reviews and feedback to resident physicians. Vaccination coverage improved among at-risk patients by 32 percentage points for influenza vaccine and 18 percentage points for pneumococcal polysaccharide vaccine. Although the findings from this study are encouraging, they do not, in themselves, provide adequate evidence for the Task Force to determine whether or not assessment plus feedback for providers is effective in increasing vaccination coverage when used alone, because the study had limitations in the quality of its execution.

Because we could not establish the effectiveness of these interventions, we did not examine situations in which they would be applicable, information about economic efficiency, or possible barriers to implementation.

In conclusion, the Task Force found insufficient evidence to determine the effectiveness of assessment plus feedback for vaccination providers, when used alone, in increasing targeted vaccines coverage among high-risk patients, because only one study with limitations in the quality of study execution was identified for review. (The effectiveness of assessment plus feedback for vaccination providers when combined with additional interventions is reviewed below. See Increasing Targeted Vaccines Coverage through Multiple Interventions Implemented in Combination.)

Increasing Targeted Vaccines Coverage through Multiple Interventions Implemented in Combination

Interventions to Increase Vaccine Coverage When Implemented in Combination: Recommended (Strong Evidence of Effectiveness)

Most of the available evidence on effectiveness identified in this review comes from studies evaluating interventions implemented in combination rather than alone. The limited evidence on the effectiveness of interventions when used alone, and the variety of intervention combinations evaluated, led us to develop a "menu option" approach (discussed above under "Methods" and in greater detail in Ndiaye et al.[286]). The complete Task Force recommendation is written as follows, and the options themselves are shown in Table 6–2:

> The Task Force recommends one or more interventions to enhance access to targeted vaccination services combined or coordinated with one or more provider- or system-based interventions and/or one or more interventions to increase community demand for targeted vaccination services, on the basis of strong evidence of effectiveness in increasing targeted vaccination coverage.

Effectiveness

- The combinations of interventions described in Table 6–2 were consistently effective in increasing targeted vaccines coverage.

Table 6–2. Menu Format of Intervention Combinations Recommended by the Task Force on Community Preventive Services to Increase Targeted Vaccinations

One or both of these interventions to enhance access to vaccination services	Expanded access in healthcare settings Reducing client out-of-pocket costs
Plus	
One or more of these provider- or system-based interventions	Standing orders Provider reminder systems Provider assessment and feedback
And/Or	
One or both of these interventions to increase client demand for vaccination services	Client reminder systems Client education

- Only one of these interventions (provider reminder systems), when used alone, had sufficient evidence to determine effectiveness (see Provider Reminder Systems When Used Alone to Increase Coverage with Targeted Vaccines).

Applicability

- These results should be applicable in most client and provider populations and most settings where improvements in coverage are needed.

The findings of our systematic review are based on 23 studies evaluating interventions to increased targeted vaccines coverage when implemented in combination (multicomponent interventions).[24–26,31,37,44,47,57,135,257,262,290,292–302] Twenty-four other studies were identified but did not meet our quality criteria and were excluded from the review.[112,114,137,206,224,225,232,236,256,303–317] Two additional papers provided information on studies already included in the review.[86,152]

Overall, the 23 qualifying studies provided 26 study arms evaluating 22 different combinations of interventions. A total of seven study arms in seven studies evaluated one of three specific intervention combinations: two studies evaluated a combination of client reminders and provider reminders; two used a combination of client education, client reminders, and expanded access in a healthcare setting; and three used a combination of client education, client reminders, expanded access, and reduced client out-of-pocket costs. In the remaining 19 study arms, the intervention combinations evaluated were unique.

As mentioned above, we conducted additional analyses to examine the combinations of interventions described in the qualifying studies. The effectiveness of interventions combined across two or three conceptual categories of vaccination demand and delivery was evaluated in 21 of the 23 qualifying studies (24 of 26 study arms). A total of 19 study arms from 16 qualifying studies evaluated the effectiveness of combinations that included one or more interventions to enhance access to vaccination services with one or more interventions from one or both of the other two categories. Within this subset of combined interventions, the median improvement in vaccination coverage was 16.5 percentage points (range, −5.9 to +67.0). This combined approach is recommended by the Task Force on the basis of strong evidence of effectiveness.

The reviewed studies provided insufficient evidence to determine the effectiveness of the following combinations because of the small number of qualifying studies or inconsistent effects on vaccination coverage among populations at high risk. Only two qualifying studies evaluated interventions combined *within* conceptual categories: the combination of client education and client reminders showed an improvement of 13.6 percentage points, and the combination of provider education and provider assessment plus feedback showed an improvement of 11 percentage points. In five studies, an intervention to increase client demand was combined with one or two provider- or system-based interventions. The median increase in vaccination coverage reported in these studies was 3.7 percentage points (range, −2.0 to +28.9).

In addition, the available studies provided insufficient evidence to determine the effectiveness of client incentives or community-wide education as options for interventions to increase demand for vaccination because of the small number of qualifying studies.

Finally, the available studies provided insufficient evidence to assess the effectiveness of provider education as an option for provider- or system-based interventions because the small number of qualifying studies reported results that were inconsistent and small in magnitude when compared with other intervention combinations.

Although we could not attribute incremental improvements in vaccine coverage to the specific components, we did find that combined activities improved vaccination coverage. This could reflect any of the following:

- The combined activities reinforce one another (e.g., education alone might not be enough to increase acceptance of vaccinations but could make clients more receptive to other components);
- Multicomponent interventions are delivered more intensively than single-component interventions;
- More studies have been done of multicomponent than of single-component interventions; or
- Multicomponent interventions might increase the likelihood of a client's exposure to at least one component.

These results should be applicable in most client and provider populations and most settings where improvements in coverage are needed. Interventions were evaluated among outpatients, inpatients, healthcare workers, nurses, and faculty physicians. Evaluated healthcare settings included academic programs, outpatient clinics, hospitals, and long-term care facilities.

No additional positive or negative effects specific to the combination of interventions were identified in this review. (Positive or negative effects of single-component interventions, which may remain relevant, are examined above for each intervention.)

We found economic evaluations of the effects of these combined interventions, but none of them met our quality criteria. We did not, therefore, report results of these economic evaluations.

Barriers to the implementation of single-component interventions (described above) are likely to be relevant to combinations of interventions. Additional barriers, such as lack of infrastructure, may also be encountered in efforts to combine and coordinate two or more interventions.

In conclusion, the Task Force recommends one or more interventions to enhance access to targeted vaccination services combined or coordinated with one or more provider- or system-based interventions, and/or one or more interventions to increase community demand for targeted vaccination services, on the basis of strong evidence of effectiveness in increasing targeted vaccines coverage among adult populations at high risk. These findings should be applicable to most client populations for which targeted vaccines are indicated and where improvements in coverage are needed, and to diverse provider populations and healthcare settings.

CONCLUSION: TARGETED VACCINES

The second section of this chapter summarizes Task Force conclusions and recommendations on interventions to increase delivery of targeted vaccines for adolescents and adults. The most effective interventions were provider reminders and those that combined one or more interventions to enhance access to vaccination services (expanded access in healthcare settings, reducing client out-of-pocket costs) with at least one provider- or system-based intervention (standing orders, provider reminder systems, provider assessment plus feedback) and/or at least one intervention to increase client demand for vaccination services (client reminder systems, client education). The Task Force found insufficient evidence to determine the effectiveness of all but one intervention when used alone to increase targeted vaccines coverage: among provider- or system-based interventions, the Task Force found strong evidence of the effectiveness of provider reminders. Evidence was insufficient to determine the effectiveness of any of the following interventions when used alone: increasing community demand for targeted vaccines through client reminders, clinic-based education, community-wide education, client or family incentives, or vaccination requirements; enhancing access to targeted vaccination services by expanding access in healthcare settings or reducing client out-of-pocket costs; or improving provider- or system-based delivery of targeted vaccines through assessment plus feedback for vaccination providers, provider education, or standing orders. Details of these reviews are being published[265,286,318] and these articles, along with additional information about the reviews, are available at www.thecommunityguide.org/vaccine. Updates and expansions of this chapter are in progress and will also be available at that site.

INCREASING VACCINATION COVERAGE THROUGH USE OF THESE RECOMMENDATIONS

Putting the recommendations in this chapter into practice offers many opportunities for increasing vaccination coverage among children, adolescents, and adults. Many decision makers, policy makers, planners, and implementers in communities and healthcare systems can carry out recommended interventions. A detailed list of interventions and potential implementers is shown in Table 6–3. Following the four steps shown below can help ensure that recommended interventions will achieve their goals.

Assess Activities, Coverage, and Vaccine-Preventable Disease in the Community

As a first step, states, communities, and healthcare systems can assess the current vaccination-related activities, levels of vaccination coverage, and rates of vaccine-preventable disease, both within their organizations or groups and throughout the community as well. To help determine where local changes and improvements are needed, these rates can be compared with relevant goals, such as those in *Healthy People 2010* (Table 6–1). Next, the recommendations in this chapter can be compared with current interventions and activities to answer two questions: Are the interventions already in place adequately implemented and funded? and What other recommended interventions, if any, should we try?

Another key question to ask is whether special efforts should be made to reach and vaccinate groups at high risk of not receiving the vaccinations they need, of being exposed to a disease, or both. For example, most vaccine-preventable diseases are primarily spread by person-to-person contact among unvaccinated people. Crowding and low vaccination coverage levels can be

Table 6–3. Examples of Implementers and
Specific Interventions That Might Benefit Them

Healthcare Systems

Client reminder and recall systems (managed care and provider offices)

Multicomponent interventions that include education

Reducing out-of-pocket costs

Expanding access plus multicomponent intervention

Home visits

Provider reminder and recall systems (managed care and provider offices)

Assessment plus feedback for providers (managed care and provider offices)

Standing orders for adult vaccinations (managed care, provider offices, and hospitals)

Insurers

Client reminder and recall systems

Reducing out-of-pocket costs

Assessment plus feedback for providers

Employers

Client reminder and recall systems

Reducing out-of-pocket costs

Public Health Departments

Multicomponent interventions that include education

Vaccination requirements for child care, school, and college attendance

Expanding access plus multicomponent intervention

Vaccination programs in schools

Home visits

Community Organizations

Multicomponent interventions that include education

Home visits

Legislatures

Vaccination requirements for child care, school, and college attendance

Reducing out-of-pocket costs

Schools

Vaccination requirements for child care, school, and college attendance

Vaccination programs in schools

Government Agencies

Reducing out-of-pocket costs

Vaccination programs in women, infants, and children (WIC) settings
(U.S. Department of Agriculture/Food and Nutrition Service)

particularly common among urban and low socioeconomic populations. Therefore, improving coverage of the urban poor should be a top priority. In general, the lower the vaccination coverage rate and the higher the burden of vaccine-preventable diseases in a population, the greater the need to increase coverage.

Assess Applicable Barriers to Vaccination

It is also important to identify the barriers that may keep people from getting the vaccinations they need. Success in delivering vaccinations requires participation from both those who need vaccines and the people and systems that provide them. Individuals may lack knowledge about vaccinations or have negative attitudes or fear of vaccination; they may also have little or no contact with the healthcare system. And, although most people in the United States accept the need for vaccinations and are seen periodically in healthcare settings, providers and systems often miss opportunities to vaccinate. In addition, people must have financial and physical access to the healthcare system.

Select Approaches that Address Applicable Barriers

Assessing and diagnosing your local barriers—in as simple or complex a way as your resources will allow—can help you select the most effective choices to reduce those barriers. If a key barrier is individuals' lack of knowledge or negative attitudes, coverage might be improved by implementing interventions that increase community demand, such as client reminder and recall systems; vaccination requirements for child care, school, and college attendance; or multicomponent interventions including education. If lack of access to the healthcare system is a key barrier, improvements might come from reducing out-of-pocket costs; implementing programs in non-healthcare settings such as WIC settings, schools, or homes; or enhancing access to the healthcare system using multicomponent programs that include expanding access. Finally, if providers or healthcare systems are missing opportunities to vaccinate, provider reminder and recall systems, provider assessment plus feedback, or standing orders might be useful. You may also find barriers in more than one area, in which case implementing a combination of interventions may be appropriate.

Conversely, using additional interventions when vaccine coverage is already high, or using additional interventions that are poorly matched to local problems (e.g., provider-oriented interventions when the undervaccinated population lacks access to services), are unlikely to result in important benefits.

Monitor Program Progress and Effects

After selecting and implementing one or more interventions, keep track of whether each is being implemented as planned and evaluate its progress to see if it is achieving its objectives—in as simple or complex a way as your resources will allow. Remember that efforts to increase coverage are likely to be most effective and cost effective when baseline coverage rates are low because of the large number of people needing vaccines; when baseline rates are high, there is literally less room for improvement. Single approaches alone often will not reach goals if baseline coverage is very low. For example, most of the effective interventions we reviewed showed improvements of 10– 20 percentage points. If your baseline coverage is low, such improvements may not be sufficient. Therefore, you may need to use more than one approach, change your approach, or make corrections to programs in progress.

Additional Issues in Increasing the Use of Targeted Vaccines

Use of recommendations to increase targeted vaccines coverage has much in common with use of recommendations for increasing universally recommended vaccines coverage. The following specific considerations related to increasing targeted vaccines coverage may also be helpful.

Although coverage rates for influenza and pneumococcal polysaccharide vaccines have steadily improved among adults over 65 years of age in the past decade, improvements in vaccination coverage among younger adults with risk conditions have been less dramatic, and coverage rates remain low.[281] Similarly, significant increases in vaccination coverage for HBV among healthcare workers have not been matched in harder-to-reach populations engaging in high-risk behaviors. To close these gaps, communities, healthcare systems, and providers may consider implementing or adding one or more interventions to improve vaccination coverage among adults at high risk.

These reviews looked at three different vaccines, a number of at-risk populations, and a variety of community and healthcare settings. Despite some limitations in the available evidence, the Task Force recommendations, except as noted below, should be broadly applicable. For example, although few studies of population-based interventions to increase hepatitis B vaccine coverage among healthcare workers were identified, the Task Force recommendation reflects confidence that effective efforts to increase influenza coverage among healthcare workers are potentially applicable.

Significant gaps exist, however, in the evidence on effectiveness of community-based efforts to increase vaccination coverage of people with high-risk behaviors for hepatitis B. The Task Force notes that efforts to address significant differences in the vaccination requirements (a series of three injections), the target populations (people with such high-risk behaviors as injection drug use), and the settings for intervention (limited access to health care and healthcare settings), which have not been evaluated in depth in the published literature, are unlikely to be successful through the application of effective healthcare system strategies developed for use with other populations and settings. (Areas in which additional research is needed are described elsewhere.[265])

In 2000, the Advisory Committee on Immunization Practices (ACIP) extended the universal recommendation for annual influenza vaccination to include adults between the ages of 50 and 64 (in addition to adults 65 years of age and older).[280] Efforts to increase coverage with influenza vaccine in this "new" population can benefit from recommendations for both universally recommended and targeted vaccines. For initial efforts, the recommendations in the universal review may provide a number of effective and flexible intervention options. Those wishing to enhance initial program efforts may find the information on interventions implemented in combination in the review of targeted vaccines helpful.

Finally, some studies included in these reviews evaluated interventions or combinations of interventions to increase vaccine coverage among *all* adult clients within a healthcare system (those with both universal and high-risk indications). To match effective interventions to local needs, existing disparities, if any, in vaccine coverage among adult patients with universal and targeted indications should be considered.

Acknowledgments

This chapter was written by the members of the systematic review development teams: Peter A. Briss, MD, MPH, Division of Prevention Research and Analytic Methods (DPRAM), Epidemiology Program Office (EPO), Centers for Disease Control and Prevention (CDC), Atlanta, Georgia; Serigne M. Ndiaye, PhD, National Immunization Program (NIP)/CDC, Atlanta; Lance E. Rodewald, MD, NIP/CDC, Atlanta; Alan R. Hinman, MD, MPH, Task Force for Child Survival and Development, Atlanta and the Task Force on Community Preventive Services; Abigail M. Shefer, MD, NIP/CDC, Atlanta; David P. Hopkins, MD, MPH, DPRAM/EPO/CDC, Atlanta; Raymond A. Strikas, MD, NIP/CDC, Atlanta; Roger R. Bernier, PhD, NIP/CDC, Atlanta; Vilma G. Carande-Kulis, MS, PhD, DPRAM/EPO/CDC, Atlanta; Angela B. Hutchinson, PhD, MPH, DPRAM/EPO/CDC, Atlanta ; Hussain R. Yusuf, MBBS, MPH, NIP/CDC, Atlanta; Sheree M. Williams, PhD, National Center for Chronic Disease Prevention and Health Promotion, CDC, Atlanta; Margaret S. Coleman, PhD, NIP/CDC, Atlanta; Daniel B. Fishbein, MD, NIP/CDC, Atlanta; and Bayo Willis, MPH, NIP/CDC, Atlanta.

Consultants for the reviews of universally recommended vaccines were: David Atkins, MD, MPH, Agency for Health Care Policy and Research, Rockville, Maryland; Joseph Chin, MD, MS, Health Care Financing Administration, Baltimore, Maryland; Caswell A. Evans, DDS, MPH, National Institutes of Health, Bethesda, Maryland; Theresa W. Gyorkos, PhD, Montreal General Hospital and McGill University, Montreal, Quebec, Canada; George J. Isham, MD, HealthPartners, Minneapolis, Minnesota and the Task Force on Community Preventive Services; Susan M. Lett, MD, MPH, Massachusetts Department of Public Health, Boston; Rose Marie Matulionis, MSPH, Association of State and Territorial Directors of Health Promotion and Public Health Education, Washington, DC; Lloyd F. Novick, MD, MPH, Onondaga County Health Department, Syracuse, New York; Thomas N. Saari, MD, University of Wisconsin, Madison; William Schaffner II, MD, Vanderbilt University, Nashville, Tennessee; and Susan C. Scrimshaw, PhD, University of Illinois, Chicago and the Task Force on Community Preventive Services.

Consultants for the reviews of targeted vaccines were: Bob Gunn, MD, National Center for HIV, STD and TB Prevention, CDC, Atlanta; Joseph Chin, MD, MS, Center for Medicare Services, Baltimore; Lloyd Novick, MD, Onondaga County Health Department, Syracuse, New York; Rose Marie Matulionis, MSPH, Association of State and Territorial Directors of Health Promotion and Public Health Education, Washington, DC; Susan Lett, MD, MPH, Massachusetts Department of Health, Boston; Tracy Lieu, MD, Harvard University, Cambridge, Massachusetts; Theresa W. Gyorkos, PhD, Montreal General Hospital and McGill University, Montreal; Tom Saari, MD, University of Wisconsin, Madison; William Schaffner II, MD, Vanderbilt University, Nashville; Peter Szilagyi, MD, University of Rochester, New York.

Articles included in the reviews of universally recommended vaccines were abstracted by: Sania Amr, MD, MS; Judith E. Gendler, MS; Richard J. Gugelman, MD, MPH; Alan R. Hinman, MD, MPH; Thomas N. Saari, MD; Sarah E. Teagle, DrPH; Peter A. Briss, MD; Nino Khetsuriani, MD, PhD; C. Dexter (Bo) Kimsey, PhD, MSEH; Serigne M. Ndiaye, PhD; Abigail M. Shefer, MD; Raymond A. Strikas, MD; Benedict I. Truman, MD, MPH; Seymour G. Williams; Sheree M. Williams, PhD; and Hussain R. Yusuf, MBBS, MPH.

Articles included in the reviews of targeted vaccines were abstracted by: Bayo Willis, MPH and Iddrisu Sulemana, MPH.

References

1. Fedson DS. Adult immunization: summary of the national vaccine advisory committee. JAMA 1994;272:1133–7.

2. Mokdad AH, Marks JS, Stroup DF, Gerberding JL. Actual causes of death in the United States, 2000. JAMA 2004;291(10):1238–45.

3. Centers for Disease Control and Prevention. Prevention of varicella: Recommendations of the Advisory Committee on Immunization Practices (ACIP). Centers for Disease Control and Prevention. MMWR 1996;45(RR-11):1–36.

4. Centers for Disease Control and Prevention. Prevention and control of influenza: recommendations of the Advisory Committee on Immunization Practices (ACIP). MMWR 1998;47(RR-6):1–26.

5. Thompson WW, Shay DK, Weintraub E, et al. Mortality associated with infleunza and respiratory syncytial virus in the United States. JAMA 2003;289(2):179–86.

6. U.S. Department of Health and Human Services. Healthy people 2010. 2nd ed. Washington, DC: U.S. Government Printing Office; 2000.

7. Centers for Disease Control and Prevention. Recommended childhood immunization schedule—United States, 1998. MMWR 1998;47(1):8–12.

8. American Academy of Pediatrics. Report of the Committee on Infectious Diseases.

Peter G, Halsey NA, Marcuse EK, Pickering LK, eds. Elk Grove Village, IL.: American Academy of Pediatrics, 1997.

9. American Academy of Family Physicians. Summary of policy recommendations for periodic health examination. Kansas City, MO: American Academy of Family Physicians, 1996.

10. Centers for Disease Control and Prevention. Update on adult immunization. Recommendations of the Immunization Practices Advisory Committee (ACIP). MMWR 1991; 40(RR-12):1–94.

11. Centers for Disease Control and Prevention. Immunization of adolescents. Recommendations of the Advisory Committee on Immunization Practices, the American Academy of Pediatrics, the American Academy of Family Physicians, and the American Medical Association. MMWR 1996;45(RR-13):1–16.

12. American College of Physicians, Task Force on Adult Immunization, Infectious Disease Society of America. Guide for adult immunizations, 3rd ed. Philadelphia: American College of Physicians, 1994.

13. Gershon AA, Gardner P, Peter G, Nichols K, Orenstein W. Quality standards for immunization.Guidelines from the Infectious Diseases Society of America. Clin Infect Dis 1997;25(4):782–6.

14. American College of Obstetricians and Gynecologists. The obstetrician-gynecologist and primary-preventive care. Washington, DC: American College of Obstetricians and Gynecologists, 1993.

15. Gyorkos TW, Tannenbaum TN, Abrahamowicz M, et al. Evaluation of the effectiveness of immunization delivery methods. Can J Public Health 1994;85(suppl 1): S14–S30.

16. Tannenbaum TN, Gyorkos TW, Abrahamowicz M, et al. Immunization delivery methods: practice recommendations. Can J Public Health 1994;85(suppl 1):S37-S40.

17. Centers for Disease Control and Prevention. Recommendations of the Advisory Committee on Immunization Practices: programmatic strategies to increase vaccination rates—assessment and feedback of provider-based vaccination coverage information. MMWR 1996;45(10):219–20.

18. Centers for Disease Control and Prevention. Recommendations of the Advisory Committee on Immunization Practices: programmatic strategies to increase vaccination coverage by age 2 years—linkage of vaccination and WIC services. MMWR 1996;45(10): 217–8.

19. Centers for Disease Control and Prevention/National Immunization Program. Standards for pediatric immunization practices. Atlanta, GA: U.S. Department of Health and Human Services, 1996.

20. Briss PA, Rodewald LE, Hinman AR, et al. Reviews of evidence regarding interventions to improve vaccination coverage in children, adolescents, and adults. Am J Prev Med 2000;18(1S):97–140.

21. Alemi F, Alemagno SA, Goldhagen J, et al. Computer reminders improve on-time immunization rates. Med Care 1996;34(10 suppl):OS45-OS51.

22. Alto WA, Fury D, Condo A, Doran M, Aduddell M. Improving the immunization coverage of children less than 7 years old in a family practice residency. J Am Board Fam Pract 1994;7(6):472–7.

23. Barnas GP, McKinney WP. Postcard reminders and influenza vaccination. J Am Geriatr Soc 1989;37(2):195.

24. Barton MB, Schoenbaum SC. Improving influenza vaccination performance in an HMO setting: the use of computer-generated reminders and peer comparison feedback. Am J Public Health 1990;80(5):534–66.

25. Becker DM, Gomez EB, Kaiser DL, Yoshihasi A, Hodge RH. Improving preventive care at a medical clinic: how can the patient help? Am J Prev Med 1989;5(6):353–9.

26. Brimberry R. Vaccination of high-risk patients for influenza: a comparison of telephone and mail reminders. J Fam Pract 1988;26(4):397–400.

27. Browngoehl K, Kennedy K, Krotki K, Mainzer H. Increasing immunization: a Medicaid managed care model. Pediatrics 1997;99(1):E4.

28. Buchner DM, Larson EB, White RF. Influenza vaccination in community elderly. A controlled trial of postcard reminders. J Am Geriatr Soc 1987;35(8):755–60.

29. Buffington J, Bell KM, LaForce FM. A target-based model for increasing influenza immunizations in private practice. Genesee Hospital Medical Staff. J Gen Intern Med 1991;6(3):204–9.

30. Campbell JR, Szilagyi PG, Rodewald LE, Doane C, Roughmann KJ. Patient-specific reminder letters and pediatric well-child-care show rates. Clin Pediatr 1994;1994:268–72.

31. Carter WB, Beach LR, Inui TS. The flu shot study: using multiattribute utility theory to design a vaccination intervention. Organ Behav Hum Decis Process 1986;38(3):378–91.

32. Centers for Disease Control and Prevention. Increasing influenza vaccination rates for Medicare beneficiaries—Montana and Wyoming, 1994. MMWR 1995;44(40):744–6.

33. Frame P, Zimmer J, Werth P, Hall J, Eberly S. Computer-based vs. manual health maintenance tracking. Arch Fam Med 1994;3:581–8.

34. Grabenstein JD, Hartzema AG, Guess HA, Johnston WP. Community pharmacists as immunisation advocates: A pharmacoepidemiologic experiment. Int J Pharm Pract 1993;2:5–10.

35. Hutchison BG, Shannon HS. Effect of repeated annual reminder letters on influenza immunization among elderly patients. J Fam Pract 1991;33(2):187–9.

36. Karuza J, Calkins E, Feather J, Hershey CO, Katz L, Majeroni B. Enhancing physician adoption of practice guidelines. Dissemination of influenza vaccination guideline using a small- group consensus process. Arch Intern Med 1995;155(6):625–32.

37. Larson EB, Bergman J, Heidrich F, Alvin BL, Schneeweiss R. Do postcard reminders improve influenza compliance? A prospective trial of different postcard "cues." Med Care 1982;20(6):639–48.

38. Lieu TA, Black SB, Ray P, et al. Computer-generated recall letters for under-immunized children: how cost-effective? Pediatr Infect Dis J 1997;16(1):28–33.

39. Lukasik MH, Pratt G. The telephone: an overlooked technology for prevention in family medicine. Can Fam Physician 1987;33:1997–2001.

40. Margolis KL, Nichol KL, Wuorenma J, Von Sternberg TL. Exporting a successful influenza vaccination program from a teaching hospital to a community outpatient setting. J Am Geriatr Soc 1992;40(10):1021–3.

41. McDowell I, Newell C, Rosser W. Comparison of three methods of recalling patients for influenza vaccination. Can Med Assoc J 1986;135(9):991–7.

42. Moran WP, Nelson K, Wofford JL, Velez R. Computer-generated mailed reminders for influenza immunization: a clinical trial. J Gen Intern Med 1992;7(5):535–7.

43. Moran WP, Wofford JL, Velez R. Assessment of influenza immunization of com-

munity elderly: illustrating the need for community-level health information. Carolina Health Serv Rev 1995;3:21–9.

44. Moran WP, Nelson K, Wofford JL, Velez R, Case LD. Increasing influenza immunization among high-risk patients: education or financial incentive? Am J Med 1996; 101(6):612–20.

45. Mullooly JP. Increasing influenza vaccination among high-risk elderly: a randomized controlled trial of a mail cue in an HMO setting. Am J Public Health 1987; 77(5):626–7.

46. Nexoe J, Kragstrup J, Ronne T. Impact of postal invitations and user fee on influenza vaccination rates among the elderly. A randomized controlled trial in general practice. Scand J Prim Health Care 1997;15(2):109–12.

47. Nichol KL, Korn JE, Margolis KL, Poland GA, Petzel RA, Lofgren RP. Achieving the national health objective for influenza immunization: success of an institution-wide vaccination program. Am J Med 1990;89(2):156–60.

48. O'Sullivan AL, Jacobsen BS. A randomized trial of a health care program for first-time adolescent mothers and their infants. Nurs Res 1994;41(4):210–5.

49. Oeffinger KC, Roaten SP, Hitchcock MA, Oeffinger PK. The effect of patient education on pediatric immunization rates. J Fam Pract 1992;35(3):288–93.

50. Ohmit SE, Furumoto-Dawson A, Monto AS, Fasano N. Influenza vaccine use among an elderly population in a community intervention. Am J Prev Med 1995;11(4):271–6.

51. Ornstein SM, Garr DR, Jenkins RG, Rust PF, Arnon A. Computer-generated physician and patient reminders. Tools to improve population adherence to selected preventive services. J Fam Pract 1991;32(1):82–90.

52. Paunio M, Virtanen M, Peltola H, et al. Increase of vaccination coverage by mass media and individual approach: intensified measles, mumps, and rubella prevention program in Finland. Am J Epidemiol 1991;133(11):1152–60.

53. Pierce C, Goldstein M, Suozzi K, Gallaher M, Dietz V, Stevenson J. The impact of the standards for pediatric immunization practices on vaccination coverage levels. JAMA 1996;276(8):626–30.

54. Satterthwaite P. A randomised intervention study to examine the effect on immunisation coverage of making influenza vaccine available at no cost. Impact of postal invitations and user fee on influenza vaccination rates among the elderly. A randomized controlled trial in general practice. N Z Med J 1997;110(1038):58–60.

55. Siebers MJ, Hunt VB. Increasing the pneumococcal vaccination rate of elderly patients in a general internal medicine clinic. J Am Geriatr Soc 1985;33:175–8.

56. Soljak MA, Handford S. Early results from the Northland immunisation register. N Z Med J 1987;100(822):244–6.

57. Spaulding SA, Kugler JP. Influenza immunization: the impact of notifying patients of high-risk status. J Fam Pract 1991;33(5):495–8.

58. Stehr-Green PA, Dini EF, Lindegren ML, Patriarca PA. Evaluation of telephoned computer-generated reminders to improve immunization coverage at inner-city clinics. Public Health Rep 1993;108(4):426–30.

59. Tollestrup K, Hubbard BB. Evaluation of a follow-up system in a county health department's immunization clinic. Am J Prev Med 1991;7(1):24–8.

60. Tucker JB, DeSimone JP. Patient response to mail cues recommending influenza vaccine. Fam Med 1987;19:209–12.

61. Waterman SH, Hill LL, Robyn B, et al. A model immunization demonstration for

preschoolers in an inner-city barrio, San Diego, California, 1992–1994. Am J Prev Med 1996;12(4S):8–13.

62. Yokley JM, Glenwick DS. Increasing the immunization of preschool children; an evaluation of applied community interventions. J Appl Behav Anal 1984;17(3):313–25.

63. Bell JC, Whitehead P, Chey T, Smith W, Capon AG, Jalaludin B. The epidemiology of incomplete childhood immunization: an analysis of reported immunization status in outer western Sydney. J Paediatr Child Health 1993;29(5):384–8.

64. Carter H. Measles and rubella immunisation in Fife. Midwife Health Visit Commun Nurse 1988;24(3):72–4.

65. Chiu TT, Barata SL, Unsicker DM, Brennan L. Community mobilization for preschool immunizations: the "Shots by Two" Project. Am J Public Health 1997;87(3):462–3.

66. Cooling N, Sturge G, Meumann F. Flu vaccination recall database. Med J Aust 1993;159(6):427.

67. Ferson MJ, Fitzsimmons G, Christie D, Woollett H. School health nurse interventions to increase immunisation uptake in school entrants. Public Health 1995;109(1):25–9.

68. Garr DR, Ornstein SM, Jenkins RG, Zemp LD. The effect of routine use of computer-generated preventive reminders in a clinical practice. Am J Prev Med 1993;9(1): 55–61.

69. Gerace TM, Sangster JF. Influenza vaccination: a comparison of two outreach strategies. Fam Med 1988;20(1):43–5.

70. Holtmann AG. The economics of U.S. immunization policy. In: Pauly MV, Robinson CA, Sepe SJ, Sing M, Willian MK, eds. Supplying vaccine: an economic analysis of critical issues. Washington, DC: IOS Press, 1996:153–74.

71. Honkanen PO, Keistinen T, Kivela SL. The impact of vaccination strategy and methods of information on influenza and pneumococcal vaccination coverage in the elderly population. Vaccine 1997;15(3):317–20.

72. Kouides RW, Lewis B, Bennett NM, et al. A performance-based incentive program for influenza immunization in the elderly. Am J Prev Med 1993;9(4):250–5.

73. Leirer VO, Morrow DG, Pariante G, Doksum T. Increasing influenza vaccination adherence through voice mail. J Am Geriatr Soc 1989;37(12):1147–50.

74. Mansoor OD. Ask and you shall be given: practice based immunisation coverage information. N Z Med J 1993;106(968):504–5.

75. Murphy AW, Harrington M, Bury G, et al. Impact of a collaborative immunisation programme in an inner city practice. Ir Med J 1996;89(6):220–1.

76. Newman CP. Immunization in childhood and computer scheme participation. Public Health 1983;97(4):208–13.

77. Nicholson KG, Wiselka MJ, May A. Influenza vaccination of the elderly: perceptions and policies of general practitioners and outcome of the 1985–86 immunization programme in Trent, UK. Vaccine 1987;5(4):302–6.

78. Peterson L. Prevention and community compliance in immunization schedules. Prev Health: Dir Pol Pract 1987;5:79–95.

79. Thompson RS. What have HMOs learned about clinical prevention services? An examination of the experience at Group Health Cooperative of Puget Sound. Milbank Q 1996;74(4):469–509.

80. Young SA, Halpin TJ, Johnson DA, Irvin JJ, Marks JS. Effectiveness of a mailed reminder on the immunization levels of infants at high risk of failure to complete immunizations. Am J Public Health 1980;70(4):422–4.

81. Calkins E, Katz LA, Karuza J, Wagner A. The small group consensus process for changing physician practices: influenza vaccination. HMO Pract 1995;9(3):107-10.

82. Carter H, Jones IG. Measles immunisation: results of a local programme to increase vaccine uptake. Br Med J (Clin Res Ed) 1985;290(6483):1717-9.

83. Frank JW, Henderson M, McMurray L. Influenza vaccination in the elderly: 1. Determinants of acceptance. Can Med Assoc J 1985;132(4):371-5.

84. Kennedy KM, Browngoehl K. A "high tech" "soft-touch" immunization program for members of a Medicaid managed care organization. HMO Pract 1994;8(3):115-21.

85. McDowell I, Newell C, Rosser W. A follow-up study of patients advised to obtain influenza immunizations. Fam Med 1990;22(4):303-6.

86. Nichol KL. Long-term success with the national health objective for influenza vaccination: an institution-wide model. J Gen Intern Med 1992;7(6):595-600.

87. Rosser WW, McDowell I, Newell C. Use of reminders for preventive procedures in family medicine. Can Med Assoc J 1991;145(7):807-14.

88. Rosser WW, Hutchison BG, McDowell I, Newell C. Use of reminders to increase compliance with tetanus booster vaccination. Can Med Assoc J 1992;146(6):911-7.

89. Thompson RS, Taplin TH, McAfee TA, Mandelson MT, Smith AE. Primary and secondary prevention services in clinical practice. Twenty years experience in development, implementation, and evaluation. JAMA 1995;273(14):1130-5.

90. Frank JW, McMurray L, Henderson M. Influenza vaccination in the elderly: 2. The economics of sending reminder letters. Can Med Assoc J 1992;132(5):516-8.

91. Grabenstein JD, Hartzema AG, Guess HA, Johnston WP, Rittenhouse BE. Community pharmacists as immunization advocates. Cost-effectiveness of a cue to influenza vaccination. Med Care 1992;30(6):503-13.

92. Lieu TA, Capra AM, Makol J, Black SB, Shinefield HR. Effectiveness and cost-effectiveness of letters, automated telephone messages, or both for underimmunized children in a health maintenance organization. Pediatrics 1998;101(4):E3.

93. McLeod D, Bowie RD, Kljakovic M. The cost of childhood immunisation in general practice. N Z Med J 1998;111(1061):73-6.

94. Dickey LL, Petitti D. A patient-held minirecord to promote adult preventive care. J Fam Pract 1992;34(4):457-63.

95. Elangovan S, Kallail KJ, Vargo G. Improving pneumococcal vaccination rates in an elderly population by patient education in an outpatient clinic. J Am Board Fam Pract 1996;9(6):411-3.

96. Elster AB, Lamb ME, Tavare J, Ralston CW. The medical and psychosocial impact of comprehensive care on adolescent pregnancy and parenthood. JAMA 1987;258:1187-92.

97. Etkind P, Simon M, Shannon S, et al. The impact of the Medicare Influenza Demonstration Project on influenza vaccination in a county in Massachusetts, 1988-1992. J Commun Health 1996;21(3):199-209.

98. Herman CJ, Speroff T, Cebul RD. Improving compliance with immunization in the older adult: results of a randomized cohort study. J Am Geriatr Soc 1994;42:1154-9.

99. Macdonald H, Roder D. The planning, implementation and evaluation of an immunization promotion campaign in South Australia. Hygie 1985;4(2):13-7.

100. Turner B, Day S, Borenstein B. A controlled trial to improve delivery of preventive care: physician or patient reminders. J Gen Intern Med 1989;4:403-9.

101. Bennett NM, Lewis B, Doniger AS, et al. A coordinated, communitywide pro-

gram in Monroe County, New York, to increase influenza immunization rates in the elderly. Arch Intern Med 1994;154(15):1741–5.

102. Bloom HG, Bloom JS, Krasnoff L, Frank AD. Increased utilization of influenza and pneumococcal vaccines in an elderly hospitalized population. J Am Geriatr Soc 1988;36(10):897–901.

103. Broussard LA, Blankenship FB. Shots for tots: Louisiana's infant immunization initiative. J Soc Pediatr Nurs 1996;1(3):113–6.

104. Brownlee HJ, Brown DL, D'Angelo RJ. Utilization of pneumococcal vaccine in a family practice residency. J Fam Pract 1982;15(6):1111–4.

105. Campbell JF, Donohoe MA, Nevin-Woods C, et al. The Hawaii Pneumococcal Disease Initiative. Am J Public Health 1993;83:1175–6.

106. Cates CJ. A handout about tetanus immunisation: influence on immunisation rate in general practice. BMJ 1990;300(6727):789–90.

107. Centers for Disease Control and Prevention. Pneumococcal immunization program—California, 1986–1988. MMWR 1989;38(30):517–9.

108. Centers for Disease Control and Prevention. National Coalition for Adult Immunization: activities to increase influenza vaccination levels, 1989–1991. MMWR 1992; 41(41):772–5.

109. Hand JS, Anderson D, Feffer D, Day C. A successful school immunization program—or not? J School Health 1980;50(1):50.

110. Knoell KR, Leeds AL. Influenza vaccination program for elderly outpatients. Am J Hosp Pharm 1991;48(2):256–9.

111. Madlon-Kay DJ. Improving the periodic health examination: use of a screening flow chart for patients and physicians. J Fam Pract 1987;25(5):470–3.

112. Ratner ER, Fedson DS. Influenza and pneumococcal immunization in medical clinics, 1978–1980. Arch Intern Med 1983;143(11):2066–9.

113. Rodriguez RM, Baraff LJ. Emergency department immunization of the elderly with pneumococcal and influenza vaccines. Ann Emerg Med 1993;22(11):1729–32.

114. Williams DM, Daugherty LM, Aycock DG, Lindley CM, Harris MJ. Effectiveness of improved targeting efforts for influenza immunization in an ambulatory care setting. Hosp Pharm 1987;22(5):462–4.

115. Westman S, Halbert RJ, Walton LG, Henneman CE. A "clinic without walls": the Los Angeles Immunization Demonstration Project. Am J Public Health 1997;87(2): 293–4.

116. Baughman AL, Williams WW, Atkinson WL, Cook LG, Collins M. The impact of college prematriculation immunization requirements on risk for measles outbreaks. JAMA 1994;272(14):1127–32.

117. Carlson JA, Lewis CA. Effect of the immunization program in Ontario schools. Can Med Assoc J 1985;133(3):215–6.

118. Centers for Disease Control and Prevention. School immunization requirements for measles—United States, 1981. MMWR 1981;30(13):158–60.

119. Chaiken BP, Williams NM, Preblud SR, Parkin W, Altman R. The effect of a school entry law on mumps activity in a school district. JAMA 1987;257(18):2455–8.

120. Nelson DB, Layde MM, Chatton TB. Rubella susceptibility in inner-city adolescents: the effect of a school immunization law. Am J Public Health 1982;72(7):710–3.

121. Robbins KB, Brandling-Bennett D, Hinman AR. Low measles incidence: associ-

ation with enforcement of school immunization laws. Am J Public Health 1981;71(3): 270–4.

122. Scheiber M, Halfon N. Immunizing California's children. Effects of current policies on immunization levels. West J Med 1990;153(4):400–5.

123. Schulte EE, Birkhead GS, Kondracki SF, Morse DL. Patterns of Haemophilus influenzae type b invasive disease in New York State, 1987 to 1991: the role of vaccination requirements for day-care attendance. Pediatrics 1994;94(6 pt 2):1014–6.

124. van Loon FP, Holmes SJ, Sirotkin BI, et al. Mumps surveillance—United States, 1988–1993. Centers for Disease Control and Prevention Surveillance Summaries. MMWR 1995;44(no. SS-3):1–14.

125. Anonymous. Comparison of measles experience in Ottawa, Ontario and Hull, Quebec. Can Dis Wkly Rep 1990;16(24):111–3.

126. Schum TR, Nelson DB, Duma MA, Sedmak GV. Increasing rubella seronegativity despite a compulsory school law. Am J Public Health 1990;80(1):66–9.

127. Anonymous. Expanded programme on immunization. Sentinel school surveillance programme for immunization status and vaccine-preventable diseases. Wkly Epidemiol Rec 1992;67(36):268–70.

128. Mukherji PS, Ryan MP, Howie JG, Stevenson JS. Consultation behaviour and the influence of the media. J R Coll Gen Pract 1982;32(237):242–4.

129. Centers for Disease Control and Prevention. Increasing pneumococcal vaccinationa rates among patients of a national health-care alliance—United States, 1993. JAMA 1995;274:1333–4.

130. Clayton EW, Hickson GB, Miller CS. Parents' responses to vaccine information pamphlets. Pediatrics 1994;93(3):369–72.

131. Lieu TA, Glauber JH, Fuentes-Afflick E, Lo B. Effects of vaccine information pamphlets on parents' attitudes. Arch Pediatr Adolesc Med 1994;148(9):921–5.

132. Esernio-Jenssen D, Turow V. Parents' understanding of the Centers for Disease Control and Prevention's vaccine information material. Am J Public Health 1996;86(11): 1648–9.

133. Henry RL, Adler JA. Missed immunization—are doctors to blame? Med J Aust 1988;148(4):212.

134. Dietrich AJ, Duhamel M. Improving geriatric preventive care through a patient-held checklist. A patient-held minirecord to promote adult preventive care. Fam Med 1989;21(3):195–8.

135. Turner RC, Waivers LE, O'Brien K. The effect of patient-carried reminder cards on the performance of health maintenance measures. Arch Intern Med 1990;150(3): 645–7.

136. Belcher DW. Implementing preventive services. Success and failure in an outpatient trial. Arch Intern Med 1990;150(12):2533–41.

137. Klachko DM, Wright DL, Gardner DW. Effect of a microcomputer-based registry on adult immunizations. J Fam Pract 1989;29(2):169–72.

138. McCormick MC, Shapiro S, Starfield BH. The association of patient-held records and completion of immunizations: A patient-held minirecord to promote adult preventive care. Clin Pediatr 1981;20(4):270–4.

139. Arnold PJ, Schlenker TL. The impact of health care financing on childhood immunization practices. Am J Dis Child 1992;146(6):728–32.

140. Combs SP, Walter EB, Drucker RP, Clements DA. Removing a major barrier to universal hepatitis B immunization in infants. Arch Pediatr Adolesc Med 1996;150(1): 112–4.

141. Hutchins SS, Rosenthal J, Eason P, et al. Effectiveness and cost-effectiveness of linking the special supplemental program for women, infants and children (WIC) and immunization activities. Unpublished 1997.

142. Ives DG, Lave JR, Traven ND, Kuller LH. Impact of Medicare reimbursement on influenza vaccination rates in the elderly. Prev Med 1994;23(2):134–41.

143. Lurie N, Manning WG, Peterson C, Goldberg GA, Phelps CA, Lillard L. Preventive care: do we practice what we preach? Am J Public Health 1987;77(7):801–4.

144. Mainous AG 3rd, Hueston WJ. Medicaid free distribution programs and availability of childhood immunizations in rural practices. Fam Med 1995;27(3):166–9.

145. Rodewald LE, Szilagyi PG, Holl J, Shone LR, Zwanziger J, Raubertas RF. Health insurance for low-income, working families: impact on the delivery of immunizations to preschool children. Arch Pediatr Adolesc Med 1997;151:798–803.

146. Ruch-Ross HS, O'Connor KG. Immunization referral practices of pediatricians in the United States. Pediatrics 1994;94(4 pt 1):508–13.

147. Szilagyi PG, Rodewald LE, Humiston SG, et al. Effect of two urban emergency department immunization programs on childhood immunization rates. Arch Pediatr Adolesc Med 1997;151(10):999– 1006.

148. Taylor JA, Darden PM, Slora E, Hasemeier CM, Asmussen L, Wasserman R. The influence of provider behavior, parental characteristics, and a public policy initiative on the immunization status of children followed by private pediatricians: a study from pediatric research in office settings. Pediatrics 1997;99:209–15.

149. Zimmerman RK, Janosky JE. Immunization barriers in Minnesota private practices: the influence of economics and training on vaccine timing. Fam Pract Res J 1993; 13(3):213–24.

150. Zimmerman RK, Medsger AR, Ricci EM, Raymund M, Mieczkowski TA, Grufferman S. Impact of free vaccine and insurance status on physician referral of children to public vaccine clinics. JAMA 1997;278(12):996–1000.

151. Merkel PA, Caputo GC. Evaluation of a simple office-based strategy for increasing influenza vaccine administration and the effect of differing reimbursement plans on the patient acceptance rate. J Gen Intern Med 1994;9(12):679–83.

152. Scarbrough ML, Landis SE. A pilot study for the development of a hospital-based immunization program. Clin Nurse Spec 1997;11(2):70–5.

153. Hueston WJ, Mainous AG 3rd, Farrell JB. Childhood immunization availability in primary care practices. Effects of programs providing free vaccines to physicians. Arch Fam Med 1994;3(7):605–9.

154. Lave JR, Ives DG, Traven ND, Kuller LH. Evaluation of a health promotion demonstration program for the rural elderly. Health Serv Res 1996;31:261–82.

155. Nichol KL. Improving influenza vaccination rates for high-risk inpatients. Am J Med 1991;91(6):584–8.

156. Rodewald LE, Szilagyi PG, Humiston SG, et al. Effect of emergency department immunizations on immunization rates and subsequent primary care visits. Arch Pediatr Adolesc Med 1996;150(12):1271–6.

157. Polis MA, Davey VJ, Collins ED, Smith JP, Rosenthal RE, Kaslow RA. The emer-

gency department as part of a successful strategy for increasing adult immunization. Ann Emerg Med 1988;17(10):1016–8.

158. Birkhead GS, LeBaron CW, Parsons P, et al. The immunization of children enrolled in the Special Supplemental Food Program for Women, Infants, and Children (WIC). The impact of different strategies. JAMA 1995;274(4):312–6.

159. Golden RE. Evaluation of three immunization interventions among families participating in the Special Supplemental Nutrition Program for Women, Infants, and Children in South Central and South East Los Angeles (dissertation). Los Angeles: UCLA, 1997.

160. Guerra FA, Gonzalez HF, Woehler KS, Pruski C, Pfeil D. San Antonio Age-Appropriate Immunization Demonstration Project. Proceedings of the 27th National WIC/Immunization Conference. Washington, DC: U.S. Department of Health and Human Services, 1993:61–5.

161. Lazorik D, Larzelere M. Improvement in immunization levels following enhanced immunization activities at WIC sites in Massachusetts, 1995–96. Presented at the 31st National Immunization Conference, Atlanta, Georgia, May 19–22, 1997. [Abstract]. 1997.

162. Needham D. Effect of WIC/Immunization coordination on immunization coverage levels. Presented at the 31st National Immunization Conference, Atlanta, Georgia, May 19–22, 1997. [Abstract]. 1997.

163. Stevenson J, Dietz V, Dini G, et al. Working with the women, infants, and children program (WIC) to raise vacination coverage levels in Georgia's public health clinics. Presented at the 30th National Immunization Conference, Washington, DC, April 9–12, 1996. [Abstract]. 1996.

164. Watson JC, Flatt K, Rosenthal J, Anderson K. Improving vaccination coverage among children in the WIC supplemental food program, Dallas, 1992–94. Abstracts of the 123rd annual meeting and exposition of the American Public Health Association; 1995 October; Dallas, Texas. Washington, DC: American Public Health Association, 1995.

165. Hoekstra E, Megaloeconomou Y, Guerrero H, Johnson-Partlow T, Mize J, Devier JR. Citywide implementation of WIC/immunization linkage in Chicago. Presented at the 31st National Immunization Conference, Atlanta, Georgia, May 19–22, 1997. [Abstract]. 1997.

166. Flatt K, Watson JC, Anderson K, Logan L, Nguyen V. A cost comparison of methods used to increase immunization levels at a WIC setting. Abstracts of the 124th annual meeting and exposition of the American Public Health Association; 1996 November 17–21, New York, Session 3299. Washington, DC: American Public Health Association, 1996.

167. Au L, Tso A, Chin K. Asian-American adolescent immigrants: the New York City schools experience. J Sch Health 1997;67(7):277–9.

168. Cassidy WM, Moran-Bell D, Williams K. From university to community: the Baton Rouge experience. J Sch Health 1997;67(7):280–2.

169. Cassidy WM, Mahoney FJ. A hepatitis B vaccination program targeting adolescents. J Adolesc Health 1995;17(4):244–7.

170. Cassidy WM. School-based adolescent hepatitis B vaccination. J La State Med Soc 1999;151(12):622–6.

171. Dobson S, Scheifele D, Bell A. Assessment of a universal, school-based hepatitis B vaccination program. JAMA 1995;274(15):1209–13.

172. Lancman H, Pastore D, Steed N, Maresca A. Adolescent hepatitis B vaccination:

comparison among two high school–based health centers and an adolescent clinic. Arch Pediatr Adolesc Med 2000;154(11):1085–8.

173. Molliconi SA, Zink T. Managed care organizations and public health: exploring collaboration on adolescent immunizations. J Sch Health 1997;67(7):286-9.

174. Unti LM, Coyle KK, Woodruff BA, Boyer-Chuanroong L. Incentives and motivators in school-based hepatitis B vaccination programs. J Sch Health 1997;67(7):265–8.

175. Woodruff BA, Unti L, Coyle K, Boyer-Chuanroong L. Parents' attitudes toward school-based hepatitis B vaccination of their children. Pediatrics 1996;98(3 pt 1):410–3.

176. Unti L, Coyle K, Woodruff BA. A review of adolescent school-based hepatitis B vaccination projects. Washington, DC: U.S. Department of Health and Human Services, Public Health Service, 1996.

177. Cassidy WM. School-based adolescent immunization programs in the United States: stategies and successes. Pediatr Infect Dis J 1998;17(7 suppl):S43–S46.

178. Cassidy W. Factors associated with accepting school-based hepatitis B vaccination. Abstract 300, National Immunization Conference, May 19–22, 1997, Detroit, Michigan. 1999.

179. Goldstein ST, Cassidy WM, Hodgson W, Mahoney FJ. Factors associated with student participation in a school-based hepatitis B immunization program. J Sch Health 2001;71(5):184–7.

180. Peavey L, Roy J, Baron-Cyr M, Dumas W, Etkind P. Vaccinating high school students against hepatitis B: a school/STD clinic collaboration. Am J Public Health 1999; 89(3):412–3.

181. Wilson T, Harman S. Analysis of a bi-state, multi-district, school-based hepatitis B immunization program. J Sch Health 2000;70(10):408–12.

182. Wilson T. Economic evaluation of a metropolitan-wide, school-based hepatitis B vaccination program. Public Health Nurs 2000;17(3):222–7.

183. Andrews G, Marinan LM, Alsop-Shields L, Dugdale AE. Update of rubella immunisation in a school-based campaign. Med J Aust 1990;153(11–12):741–2.

184. Skinner SR, Imberger A, Nolan T, Lester R, Glover S., Bowes G. Randomised controlled trial of an educational strategy to increase school-based adolescent hepatitis B vaccination. Aust N Z J Public Health 2000;24(3):298–304.

185. Krahn M, Guasparini R, Sherman M, Detsky AS. Costs and cost-effectiveness of a universal, school-based hepatitis vaccination program. Am J Public Health 1998;88(11): 1638–44.

186. Capizzano J, Adams G, Sonenstein F. Child care arrangements for children under five: variation across states. Available at: http://www.urban.org/url.cfm?ID=309438. Accessed March 22, 2004.

187. Lopez J, DiLiberto J, McGuckin M. Infection control in day-care centers: present and future needs. Am J Infect Control 1988;16(1):26–9.

188. O'Mara LM, Isaacs S. Evaluation of registered nurses follow-up on the reported immunization status of children attending child care centres. Can J Public Health 1993;84(2):124–7.

189. Black ME, Ploeg J, Walter SD, Hutchinson BG, Scott EA, Chambers LW. The impact of a public health nurse intervention on influenza vaccine acceptance. Am J Public Health 1993;83(12):1751–3.

190. Bond L, Nolan T, Lester R. Home vaccination for children behind in their immunisation schedule: a randomized controlled trial. Med J Aust 1998;168:487–90.

191. Rodewald LE, Szilagyi PG, Humiston SG, Barth R, Kraus R, Raubertas RF. A randomized study of tracking with outreach and provider prompting to improve immunization coverage and primary care. Pediatrics 1999;103(1):31–8.

192. Rosenberg Z, Findley S, McPhillips S, Penachio M, Silver P. Community-based strategies for immunizing the "hard-to-reach" child: the New York State immunization and primary health care initiative. Am J Prev Med 1995;11(S3):14–20.

193. Wood D, Halfon N, Donald-Sherbourne C, et al. Increasing immunization rates among inner-city, African American children. JAMA 1998;279(1):29–34.

194. Begg NT, White JM. A survey of pre-school vaccination programmes in England and Wales. Commun Med 1988;10(4):344–50.

195. Clark J, Day J, Howe E, Williams P, Biley A. Developing an immunisation protocol for the primary health care team. Health Visit 1995;68(5):196–8.

196. Crittenden P, Rao M. The immunisation coordinator: improving uptake of childhood immunisation. Commun Dis Rep CDR Rev 1994;4(7):R79–81.

197. Jefferson N, Sleight G, Macfarlane A. Immunisation of children by a nurse without a doctor present. Br Med J (Clin Res Ed) 1987;294(6569):423–4.

198. McKeith D. Parents attitudes to measles immunization. J R Coll Gen Pract 1987; 37(297):182.

199. Moore BJ, Morris DW, Burton B, Kilcrease DT. Measuring effectiveness of service aides in infant immunization surveillance program in North Central Texas. Am J Public Health 1981;71(6):634–6.

200. Salmond CE, Soljak MA, Bandaranayake DR, Stehr-Green P. Impact of a promotion program for hepatitis B immunisation. Aust J Public Health 1994;18(3):253–7.

201. While AE. Health visitor contribution to pre-school child prophylaxis. Public Health 1987;101(4):229–32.

202. Jones AE. Domiciliary immunisation for preschool child defaulters. Br Med J (Clin Res Ed) 1984;289(6456):1429–31.

203. Chambers CV, Balaban DJ, Carlson BL, Grasberger DM. The effect of microcomputer-generated reminders on influenza vaccination rates in a university-based family practice center. J Am Board Fam Pract 1991;4(1):19–26.

204. Cheney C, Ramsdell JW. Effect of medical records' checklists on implementation of periodic health measures. Am J Med 1987;83(1):129–36.

205. Cohen DI, Littenberg B, Wetzel C, Neuhauser D. Improving physician compliance with preventive medicine guidelines. Med Care 1982;20(10):1040–5.

206. Crouse BJ, Nichol K, Peterson DC, Grimm MB. Hospital-based strategies for improving influenza vaccination rates. J Fam Pract 1994;38(3):258–61.

207. Gelfman DM, Witherspoon JM, Buchsbaum DG, Centor RM. Short-term results of an immunization compliance program. Va Med 1986;113(9):532–4.

208. Hahn DL, Berger MG. Implementation of a systematic health maintenance protocol in a private practice. J Fam Pract 1990;31(5):492–502.

209. Harper PG, Murray DM. An organizational strategy to improve adolescent measles-mumps- rubella vaccination in a low socioeconomic population. A method to reduce missed opportunities. Arch Fam Med 1994;3(3):257–62.

210. Harper PG, Madlon-Kay DJ, Luxenberg MG, Tempest R. A clinic system to improve preschool vaccinations in a low socioeconomic status population. Arch Pediatr Adolesc Med 1997;151:1220–3.

211. Harris RP, O'Malley MS, Fletcher SW, Knight BP. Prompting physicians for pre-

ventive procedures: a five-year study of manual and computer reminders. Am J Prev Med 1990;6(3):145–52.

212. Hutchison BG. Effect of computer-generated nurse/physician reminders on influenza immunization among seniors. Fam Med 1989;21(6):433–7.

213. Klein RS, Adachi N. Pneumococcal vaccine in the hospital. Improved use and implications for high-risk patients. Arch Intern Med 1983;143(10):1878–81.

214. Korn JE, Schlossberg LA, Rich EC. Improved preventive care following an intervention during an ambulatory care rotation: carryover to a second setting. J Gen Intern Med 1988;3(2):156–60.

215. McDonald CJ, Hui SL, Smith DM, et al. Reminders to physicians from an introspective computer medical record. A two-year randomized trial. Ann Intern Med 1984; 100(1):130–8.

216. Shreiner DT, Petrusa ER, Rettie CS, Kluge RM. Improving compliance with preventive medicine procedures in a house staff training program. South Med J 1988;81: 1553–7.

217. Szilagyi PG, Rodewald LE, Humiston SG, et al. Reducing missed opportunities for immunizations. Easier said than done. Arch Pediatr Adolesc Med 1996;150(11): 1193–200.

218. Tape TG, Givner N, Wigton RS. Process in ambulatory care: a controlled clinical trial of computerized records. Symp Comput Applications Med Care 1988;749–52.

219. Tierney WM, Hui SL, McDonald CJ. Delayed feedback of physician performance versus immediate reminders to perform preventive care. Effects on physician compliance. Med Care 1986;24(8):659–66.

220. Weingarten MA, Bazel D, Shannon HS. Computerized protocol for preventive medicine: a controlled self- audit in family practice. Fam Pract 1989;6:120–4.

221. Bell LM, Pritchard M, Anderko R, Levenson R. A program to immunize hospitalized preschool-aged children: evaluation and impact. Pediatrics 1997;100(2):192–6.

222. Brink SG. Provider reminders. Changing information format to increase infant immunizations. Med Care 1989;27(6):648–53.

223. Carlin E, Carlson R, Nordin J. Using continuous quality improvement tools to improve pediatric immunization rates. Jt Comm J Qual Improv 1996;22(4):277–88.

224. Chodroff CH. Cancer screening and immunization quality assurance using a personal computer. QRB Qual Rev Bull 1990;16(8):279–87.

225. Clancy CM, Gelfman D, Poses RM. A strategy to improve the utilization of pneumococcal vaccine. J Gen Intern Med 1992;7(1):14–8.

226. Gill JM, Fisher JA. Improving childhood immunizations in a family practice office. Del Med J 1997;69(1):13–9.

227. Loeser H, Zvagulis I, Hercz L, Pless IB. The organization and evaluation of a computer-assisted, centralized immunization registry. Am J Public Health 1983;73(11): 1298–301.

228. Mandel I, Franks P, Dickinson J. Improving physician compliance with preventive medicine guidelines. J Fam Pract 1985;21(3):223–4.

229. Payne TH, Galvin M, Taplin SH, Austin B, Savarino J, Wagner EH. Practicing population-based care in an HMO: evaluation after 18 months. HMO Pract 1995;9:101–10.

230. Ravet J. Opportunistic recall—a plateau. Med J Aust 1988;148(4):211.

231. Reading R, Colver A, Openshaw S, Jarvis S. Do interventions that improve immunisation uptake also reduce social inequalities in uptake? BMJ 1994;308(6937):1142–4.

232. Rodney WM, Chopivsky P, Quan M. Adult immunization: the medical record design as a facilitator for physician compliance. J Med Educ 1983;58(7):576–80.

233. Setia U, Serventi I, Lorenz P. Factors affecting the use of influenza vaccine in the institutionalized elderly. J Am Geriatr Soc 1985;33:856–8.

234. Shank JC, Powell T, Llewelyn J. A five-year demonstration project associated with improvement in physician health maintenance behavior. Fam Med 1989;21(4):273–8.

235. Stets K, Harper P, Christensen R. Immunization audits and protocols. Valuable tools to improve rates. Minn Med 1996;79(8):43–5.

236. Tobacman JK. Increased use of pneumococcal vaccination in a medicine clinic following initiation of a quality assessment monitor. Infect Control Hosp Epidemiol 1992;13(3):144–6.

237. Davidson RA, Fletcher SW, Retchin S, Duh S. A nurse-initiated reminder system for the periodic health examination. Implementation and evaluation. Arch Intern Med 1984;144(11):2167–70.

238. McDonald CJ, Hui SL, Tierney WM. Effects of computer reminders for influenza vaccination on morbidity during influenza epidemics. MD Comput 1992;9(5):304–12.

239. Ravet J. Tetanus immunization. Med J Aust 1987;146(3):170.

240. Rodney WM, Johnson R, Beaber RJ, Jonokuchi C, Kujubu D. Residency chart review: preventive medicine practice as noted in the medical record. Fam Pract Res J 1982; 1:140–51.

241. Carey TS, Levis D, Pickard CG, Bernstein J. Development of a model quality-of-care assessment program for adult preventive care in rural medical practices. QRB Qual Rev Bull 1991;17(2):54–9.

242. Kern DE, Harris WL, Boekeloo BO, Barker LR, Hogeland P. Use of an outpatient medical record audit to achieve educational objectives: changes in residents' performances over six years. J Gen Intern Med 1990;5(3):218–24.

243. LeBaron CW, Chaney M, Baughman AL, et al. Impact of measurement and feedback on vaccination coverage in public clinics, 1988–1994. JAMA 1997;277(8):631–5.

244. Lynch ML. The uptake of childhood immunization and financial incentives to general practitioners. Health Econ 1994;3(2):117–25.

245. Colver AF. Health surveillance of preschool children: four years experience. Br Med J 1990;300:1246–8.

246. Fleming DM, Lawrence MS. Impact of audit on preventive measures. Br Med J (Clin Res Ed) 1994;1983(6408):1852–4.

247. Kelly SD. The impact of a microcomputer on a general practice immunisation clinic. Practitioner 1988;232(1443):197–201.

248. Morrow RW, Gooding AD, Clark C. Improving physicians' preventive health care behavior through peer review and financial incentives. Arch Fam Med 1995;4(2):165–9.

249. Ritchie LD, Bisset AF, Russell D, Thomson I. Primary and preschool immunisation in Grampian: progress and the 1990 contract. Br Med J 1992;304:816–9.

250. Dini EF, Chaney M, Moolenaar RL, LeBaron CW. Information as intervention: how Georgia used vaccination coverage data to double public sector vaccination coverage in seven years. J Public Health Manag Pract 1996;2(1):45–9.

251. Cowan JA, Heckerling PS, Parker JB. Effect of a fact sheet reminder on performance of the periodic health examination: a randomized controlled trial. Am J Prev Med 1992;8(2):104–9.

252. Freed GL, Bordley WC, Clark SJ, Konrad TR. Universal hepatitis B immunization

of infants: reactions of pediatricians and family physicians over time. Pediatrics 1994; 93(5):747–51.

253. Zimmerman RK, Barker WH, Strikas RA, et al. Developing curricula to promote preventive medicine skills: the teaching immunization for medical education (TIME) project. JAMA 1997;278(9):705–11.

254. Bannerman B, Schram K. Influenza immunization program in long term care facilities. Can J Infect Control 1992;7(1):13–5.

255. Christy C, McConnochie KM, Zernik N, Brzoza S. Impact of an algorithm-guided nurse intervention on the use of immunization opportunities. Arch Pediatr Adolesc Med 1997;151(4):384–91.

256. Hoey JR, McCallum HP, LePage EM. Expanding the nurse's role to improve preventive service in an outpatient clinic. CMAJ 1982;127:27–8.

257. Klein RS, Adachi N. An effective hospital-based pneumococcal immunization program. Arch Intern Med 1986;146(2):327–9.

258. Margolis KL, Lofgren RP, Korn JE. Organizational strategies to improve influenza vaccine delivery. A standing order in a general medicine clinic. Arch Intern Med 1988; 148(10):2205–7.

259. Morton MR, Spruill WJ, Cooper JW. Pharmacist impact on pneumococcal vaccination rates in long-term- care facilities. Am J Hosp Pharm 1988;45(1):73.

260. Fedson DS, Kessler HA. A hospital-based influenza immunization program, 1977–78. Am J Public Health 1983;73(4):442–5.

261. Nichol KL, Grimm MB, Peterson DC. Immunizations in long-term care facilities: policies and practice. J Am Geriatr Soc 1996;44(4):349–55.

262. Landis S, Scarbrough ML. Using a vaccine manager to enhance in-hospital vaccine administration. J Fam Pract 1995;41(4):364–9.

263. Centers for Disease Control and Prevention. Vaccine-preventable diseases: improving vaccination coverage in children, adolescents, and adults. A report on recommendations of the Task Force on Community Preventive Services. MMWR 1999;48 (no. RR-8):1–15.

264. Task Force on Community Preventive Services. Recommendations regarding interventions to improve vaccination coverage in children, adolescents, and adults. Am J Prev Med 2000;18(1S):92–6.

265. Ndiaye SM, Hopkins DP, Shefer AM, et al. Reviews of evidence regarding interventions to improve influenza, pneumococcal polysaccharide, and hepatitis B coverage in high risk adults. Am J Prev Med; in press.

266. Bridges CB, Fukuda K, Uyeki T, Cox N, Singleton J. Prevention and control of influenza. Recommendations of the Advisory Committee on Immunization Practices (ACIP). MMWR 2002;51(RR03):1–31.

267. Barker W, Mullooly J. Impact of epidemic type A influenza in a defined adult population. Am J Epidemiol 1980;112:798–811.

268. Barker W. Excess pneumonia and influenza associated hospitalization during influenza epidemics in the United States, 1970–78. Am J Public Health 1986;76:761–5.

269. Glezen WP, Couch R. Interpandemic influenza in the Houston area, 1974–76. N Engl J Med 1978;298(11):587–92.

270. Centers for Disease Control and Prevention. Pneumococcal disease. In: Atkinson W, ed. Epidemiology and prevention of vaccine-preventable diseases, 6th ed. Atlanta,

GA: Department of Health and Human Services, Public Health Service, Centers for Disease Control and Prevention, 2000:249–63.

271. Centers for Disease Control and Prevention. Active Bacterial Core Surveillance (ABCs) report, Emerging Infections Program Network (EIP). Available at: http://www.cdc.gov/ncidod/dbmd/abcs/survreports/spneu00prelim.pdf. Accessed December 8, 2003.

272. Feikin DR, Schuchat A, Kolczak M, et al. Mortality from invasive pneumococcal pneumonia in the era of antibiotic resistance, 1995–1997. Am J Public Health 2000; 90:223–9.

273. Robinson KA, Baughman W, Rothrock G, et al. Epidemiology of invasive Streptococcus pneumoniae infections in the United States, 1995–1998. JAMA 2001;285(13): 1729–35.

274. Glezen WP. Serious morbidity and mortality associated with influenza epidemics. Epidemiol Rev 1982;4:25–44.

275. Jiles R, Daniels D, Yusuf H, McCauley M, Chu S. Undervaccination with hepatitis B vaccine: missed opportunities or choice? Am J Prev Med 2001;20(4S):75–83.

276. Bloom BS, Hillman AL, Fendrick AM, Schwartz JS. A reappraisal of hepatitis B virus vaccination strategies using cost-effectiveness analysis. Ann Intern Med 1993; 118(4):298–306.

277. Margolis H, Coleman PJ, Brown RE, Mast EE, Sheingold SH, Arevalo JA. Prevention of hepatitis B virus transmission by immunization. An economic analysis of current recommendations. JAMA 1995;274(15):1201–8.

278. National Center for HIV, STD and TB Prevention. Viral hepatitis and injection drug users. Atlanta, GA: Centers for Disease Control and Prevention, 2002.

279. Goldstein ST, Alter MJ, Williams IT, et al. Incidence and risk factors for acute hepatitis B in the United States, 1982–1998: implications for vaccination programs. J Infect Dis 2002;185(6):713–9.

280. Centers for Disease Control and Prevention. Prevention and control of influenza: recommendations of the Advisory Committee on Immunization Practices (ACIP). MMWR 2000;49(RR-03):1–38.

281. Institute of Medicine. Calling the shots: immunization finance policies and practices. Washington, DC: National Academy Press, 2002.

282. National Center for Health Statistics. Early release of selected estimates based on data from the 2002 national Health Interview Survey. Available at: http://www.cdc.gov/nchs/about/major/nhis/released200306.htm. Accessed September 12, 2003.

283. Mahoney FJ, Stewart K, Hu H, Coleman P, Alter MJ. Progress towards elimination of hepatitis B virus transmission among health care workers in the United States. Arch Intern Med 1997;157(22):2601–1605.

284. MacKellar DA, Valleroy LA, Secura GM, et al. Two decades after vaccine license: hepatitis B immunization and infection among young men who have sex with men. Am J Public Health 2001;91(6):965–71.

285. Centers for Disease Control and Prevention. Achievements in public health: hepatitis B vaccination—United States, 1982—2002. MMWR 2002;51(25):549–52,563.

286. Ndiaye SM, Hopkins DP, Smith SJ, et al. Methods for conducting systematic reviews of targeted vaccination strategies for the Guide to Community Preventive Services. Am J Prev Med; in press.

287. Clancy CM, Cebul RD, Williams SV. Guiding individual decisions: a randomized, controlled trial of decision analysis. Am J Med 1988;84(2):283–8.

288. Jacobson TA, Thomas DM, Morton FJ, Offutt G, Shevlin J, Ray S. Use of a low-literacy patient education tool to enhance pneumococcal vaccination rates. A randomized controlled trial. JAMA 1999;282(7):646–50.

289. Trubatch B, Paschane D, Fisher D, Cagle H, Fenaughty K, Schlicting E. Economic incentives: vaccination compliance among drug users. Poster session 3089. 126th Annual Meeting and Exposition of the APHA, November 15–18, Washington, DC, 1997.

290. Yassi A, Khokhar JB, Marceniuk M, McGill ML. Hepatitis B vaccination for health care workers: evaluation of acceptance rate and program strategy at a large tertiary care hospital. Can J Infect Control 1993;8(4):94–7.

291. Department of Labor, Occupational Safety and Health Administration. Occupational exposure to bloodborne pathogens; final rule. Fed Reg 1991;56(29 CFR part 1910. 1030):64004–182.

292. Baker AM, McCarthy B, Gurley VF, Yood MU. Influenza immunization in a managed care organization. J Gen Intern Med 1998;13(7):469–75.

293. Coyne DW, Taylor LF, Yelton S, Long C, Preston SD. Network 12 hepatitis B vaccination quality improvement program: an educational program directed at physicians, staff, and patients. Adv Ren Replace Ther 2000;7(4 suppl 1):S71–S75.

294. Fedson DS. Influenza vaccination of medical residents at the University of Virginia: 1986 to 1994. Infect Control Hosp Epidemiol 1996;17(7):431–3.

295. Harbarth S, Siegrist C, Schira J, Wunderli W, Pittet D. Influenza immunization: improving compliance of healthcare workers. Infect Control Hosp Epidemiol 1998;19(5): 337–42.

296. Hogg WE, Bass M, Calonge N, Crouch H, Satenstein G. Randomized controlled study of customized preventive medicine reminder letters in a community practice. Can Fam Physician 1998;44:81–8.

297. Jans MP, Schellevis FG, Van Hensbergen W, Van Eijk JT. Improving general practice care of patients with asthma or chronic obstructive pulmonary disease: evaluation of a quality system. Eff Clin Pract 2000;3(1):16–24.

298. Nichol KL. Ten-year durability and success of an organized program to increase influenza and pneumococcal vaccination rates among high-risk adults. Am J Med 1998; 105(5):385–92.

299. Overhage JM, Tierney WM, McDonald CJ. Computer reminders to implement preventive care guidelines for hospitalized patients. Arch Intern Med 1996;156:1551–6.

300. Sellors J, Pickard L, Mahony JB, et al. Understanding and enhancing compliance with the second dose of hepatitis B vaccine: a cohort analysis and a randomized controlled trial. Can Med Assoc J 1997;157(2):143–8.

301. Thomas DR, Winsted B, Koontz C. Improving neglected influenza vaccination among healthcare workers in long-term care. J Am Geriatr Soc 1993;41(9):928–30.

302. van Essen GA, Kuyvenhoven MM, de Melker RA. Implementing the Dutch College of General Practitioners' guidelines for influenza vaccination: an intervention study. Br J Gen Pract 1997;47:25–9.

303. Berry BB, Murthy VS. Exceeding the Healthy People 2000 goal for influenza vaccination through a collaborative effort at eight primary care clinics. Wis Med J 1996; 95(10):705–10.

304. Davidson M, Chamblee C, Campbell HG, et al. Pneumococcal vaccination in a remote population of high-risk Alaska Natives. Public Health Rep 1993;108(4):439–46.

305. Girasek DC. Increasing hospital staff compliance with influenza immunization recommendations. Am J Public Health 1990;80(10):1272–3.

306. Grob PJ, Ridao M, Wagner S, Pelzer JO. An account of a pilot hepatitis B vaccination programme for high-risk individuals in Zurich. J Infect 1983;7(suppl 1):85–92.

307. Hak E, Hermens RP, Hoes AW, Verheij TJ, Kuyvenhoven MM, van Essen GA. Effectiveness of a coordinated nationwide programme to improve influenza immunisation rates in The Netherlands. Scand J Prim Health Care 2000;18(4):237–41.

308. Haley N, Roy E, Bélanger L, Crago A. A hepatitis B vaccination outreach project for street youth in Montreal. Can J Hum Sex 1998;7(4):331–8.

309. Helcl J, Cástková J, Benes C, Novotna L, Sepkowitz KA, DeHovitz JA. Control of occupational hepatitis B among healthcare workers in the Czech Republic, 1982 to 1995. Infect Control Hosp Epidemiol 2000;21(5):343–6.

310. Kleschen MZ, Holbrook J, Rothbaum AK, Stringer RA, McInerney MJ, Helgerson SD. Improving the pneumococcal immunization rate for patients with diabetes in a managed care population: a simple intervention with a rapid effect. Jt Comm J Qual Improv 2000;26(9):538–46.

311. Manian FA. Improving hepatitis B vaccination rates among surgeons. Infect Control Hosp Epidemiol 1994;15(9):581.

312. Margolis HS, Handsfield HH, Jacobs RJ, Gangi JE. Evaluation of office-based intervention to improve prevention counseling for patients at risk for sexually acquired hepatitis B virus infection. Am J Obstet Gynecol 2000;182(1 pt 1):1–6.

313. Ohrt CK, McKinney P. Achieving compliance with influenza immunization of medical house staff and students. JAMA 1992;267(10):1377–80.

314. Shannon CS. Community hospitals can increase staff influenza vaccination rates. Am J Public Health 1993;83(8):1174.

315. Slobodkin D, Zielske PG, Kitlas JL, McDermott MF, Miller S, Rydman R. Demonstration of the feasibility of emergency department immunization against influenza and pneumococcus. Ann Intern Med 1998;32(5):537–43.

316. Spruill WJ, Cooper JW, Taylor WJ. Pharmacist-coordinated pneumonia and influenza vaccination program. Am J Hosp Pharm 1982;39(11):1904–6.

317. Wuorenma J, Nichol K, Vonsternberg T. Implementing a mass influenza vaccination program. Nurs Manage 1994;25(5):81–2–84–5.

318. Task Force on Community Preventive Services. Recommendations regarding interventions to improve targeted vaccination coverage in high risk adults. Am J Prev Med; in press.

Chapter 7

Oral Health

In the twentieth century, most people in the United States experienced substantial improvements in their oral health, yet more than an estimated $70 billion is still spent annually on dental services.[1] Each year, people make about 500 million visits to dental offices,[2] and estimated hospital charges for inpatient treatment of diseases of the mouth and disorders of the teeth and jaw were $451 million in 1996.[2] In addition, young people (5–24 years old) make about 600,000 visits to hospital emergency departments for sports-related craniofacial injuries each year.[3] In most cases, dental caries (tooth decay), oral (mouth) and pharyngeal (throat) cancers, and sports-related craniofacial injuries can be prevented. These conditions impose significant financial and human costs and sometimes result in facial disfigurement, disability, or death. For these reasons, we wanted to find effective means to prevent the illness and death associated with these oral and craniofacial conditions.

---

*Insufficient evidence means that we were not able to determine whether or not the intervention works.

The Task Force approved the recommendations in this chapter in 2000. The research on which the findings are based was conducted between 1966 and December 2000. This information has been previously published in the American Journal of Preventive Medicine (2002; 23(1S):16–20, and 21–54) and the MMWR Recommendations and Reports (2001; 50(RR-21):1–13).

OBJECTIVES AND RECOMMENDATIONS FROM OTHER ADVISORY GROUPS

Many of the proposed *Healthy People 2010*[4] objectives in chapters 3, 15, and 21 (Cancer, Injury and Violence Prevention, and Oral Health, respectively) relate directly to preventing and controlling oral and craniofacial diseases, conditions, and injuries and improving access to related services (Table 7–1).

The Surgeon General's Report on Oral Health,[5] published in June 2000, described the principal components of a National Oral Health Plan (National Call To Action To Promote Oral Health, www.surgeongeneral.gov/topics/oralhealth/nationalcalltoaction.htm) to promote and improve oral health: increasing awareness (among the public, policymakers, and health providers) that the health of the mouth and of other parts of the body are related, accelerating the growth of research and application of scientific evidence on intervention effectiveness, building an integrated infrastructure, removing barriers between services and people in need, and using public–private partnerships to reduce disparities. This model of oral health promotion aims to achieve universal oral health literacy through education; prevention and control of common or life-threatening craniofacial diseases, disorders, and injuries; and improvement in general health through better oral health.

A comparison of *Community Guide* oral health recommendations and recommendations recently developed by others has been made by Gooch et al.[6] and is available at www.thecommunityguide.org/oral.

METHODS

Methods used for the reviews are summarized in Chapter 10. Specific methods used in the systematic reviews of oral health interventions have been described (see Appendix A in Truman et al., 2002,[7] also available at www.thecommunityguide.org/oral). The logic framework depicting the conceptual approach used in the oral health reviews is presented in Figure 7–1.

ECONOMIC EFFICIENCY

A systematic review of economic evaluations was conducted for the two recommended interventions (i.e., those shown to be effective), and a summary of each economic review is presented with the related intervention. The methods used to conduct these economics reviews are summarized in Chapter 11.

RECOMMENDATIONS AND FINDINGS

This section presents a summary of the findings of the systematic reviews conducted to determine the effectiveness of the selected interventions in this

Table 7–1. Selected *Healthy People 2010*[4] Oral Health Objectives

Objective	Population	Baseline[a]	2010 Objective
Dental Caries			
Dental caries experience (i.e., life-time number of decayed, missing, or filled teeth measured at a single point in time) in primary or permanent teeth	2–4-year-olds 6–8-year-olds 15-year-olds	18% (1988–94) 52% (1988–94) 61% (1988–94)	11% 42% 51%
Untreated dental decay	2–4-year-olds	16% (1988–94)	9%
	6–8-year-olds	29% (1988–94)	21%
	15-year-olds	20% (1988–94)	15%
	35–44-year-olds	27% (1988–94)	15%
Never had a permanent tooth extracted because of dental caries or periodontal disease	35–44-year-olds	31% (1988–94)	42%
Have had all their natural teeth extracted	65–74-year-olds	26%[b] (1997)	20%
Proportion of children who have received dental sealants on their molar teeth	8-year-olds 14-year-olds	23% (1988–94) 15% (1988–94)	50% 50%
Proportion of the U.S. population served by community water systems with optimally fluoridated water	All	62% (1992)	75%
Oral and Pharyngeal Cancers			
Proportion of oral and pharyngeal cancers detected at the earliest stage (stage 1, localized)	All	35% (1990–95)	50%
Proportion of adults who, in the past 12 months, report having had an examination to detect oral and pharyngeal cancers	Adults >40 years	13%[b] (1998)	20%
Annual oropharyngeal cancer deaths per 100,000 population	All	3.0 (1998)	2.7%
Sports-Related Craniofacial Injuries			
Increase the proportion of public and private schools that require use of appropriate head, face, eye, and mouth protection for students participating in school-sponsored physical activities	Students	Developmental	

[a]Years indicate when the data were analyzed to establish baseline estimates. Some estimates are age-adjusted to the year 2000 standard population.

[b]Based on self-report in National Health Interview Survey, 1997 or 1998.

Reprinted from Am J Prev Med, Vol. 23, No. 1S, Truman BI et al., Reviews of evidence on interventions to prevent dental caries, oral and pharyngeal cancers, and sports-related craniofacial injuries, p. 23, Copyright 2002, with permission from American Journal of Preventive Medicine.

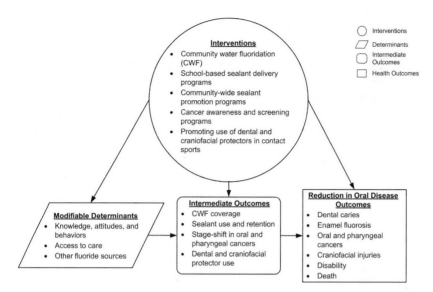

Figure 7–1. Logic framework illustrating the conceptual approach used in the systematic reviews of interventions to improve oral health. (Reprinted from Am J Prev Med, Vol. 23, No. 1S, Truman BI et al., Reviews of evidence on interventions to prevent dental caries, oral and pharyngeal cancers, and sports-related craniofacial injuries, p. 24, Copyright 2002, with permission from American Journal of Preventive Medicine.)

topic area. Interventions are grouped into three categories: preventing or controlling dental caries, preventing or controlling oral and pharyngeal cancers, and preventing or controlling sports-related craniofacial injuries.

Preventing or Controlling Dental Caries

Dental caries—commonly known as *tooth decay*—affect people of all ages, causing tooth loss if not treated. The number of people with decayed, missing, or filled permanent teeth increases with age. Among children 5–11 years of age, 1 in 4 has one or more decayed, missing, or filled permanent teeth; by the time they are adolescents (12–17 years old), 2 out of 3 are affected, and among adults the prevalence rises to over 9 out of 10 people.[8,9]

The prevalence of dental caries is not evenly distributed throughout the population. In the United States, 80% of decayed, missing, or filled permanent teeth are found in 25% of children 5–17 years of age who have at least one permanent tooth.[4,8,10] Lower income, Mexican-American, and African-American children have more untreated decayed teeth than their higher-income or non-Hispanic white counterparts. Among low-income or poor children, more than one third have untreated caries in their primary teeth, which may be linked to eating difficulties and being underweight.[11]

Comprehensive population-based strategies to prevent or control dental caries aim to:[5]

- increase public and professional awareness of caries and ways to address the problem;
- promote practices that support oral health (such as reducing consumption of refined sugar and brushing with toothpaste that contains fluoride);
- ensure optimal exposure to fluoride from all sources (including community water fluoridation); and
- ensure access to and efficient use of regular preventive and restorative dental care, including optimal use of sealants delivered in school-based or school-linked settings.

This section reports on three community interventions to prevent and control dental caries: community water fluoridation, school-based or school-linked pit and fissure sealant delivery programs, and statewide or community-wide sealant promotion programs.

Community Water Fluoridation: Recommended (Strong Evidence of Effectiveness)

Community water fluoridation (CWF), the basis for primary prevention of dental caries (tooth decay) for over 50 years, is the controlled addition of a fluoride compound to a public water supply to achieve an optimal fluoride concentration (since 1962, the U.S. Public Health Service has recommended that community drinking waters contain 0.7–1.2 ppm [parts per million] of fluoride[12]). Community water fluoridation has been recognized as 1 of 10 great achievements in public health of the twentieth century because it has been linked to large reductions in tooth decay in many industrialized countries during the latter half of the century.[12,13]

In 2000 approximately 162 million people in the United States (65.8% of the population served by public water systems) were being supplied with water containing the optimal level of fluoride to protect teeth from caries.[14] The national objective is for at least 75% of the population to be served by community water systems providing optimal levels of fluoride by the year 2010.[4]

Effectiveness

- Starting or continuing CWF is effective in reducing dental caries by 30%–50% in communities.
- Stopping CWF results in increases in dental caries in some communities.

Applicability

- These findings should be applicable to most people in the United States and other industrialized countries who use public water systems, regardless of race, ethnicity, or socioeconomic status.

The findings of our systematic review are based on 21 studies.[15-35] An additional nine studies were identified but did not meet our quality criteria and were excluded from the review.[36-44]

Overall, we found that CWF reduces dental caries approximately 30% to 50% over expected estimates for communities with nonfluoridated water. Further, stopping CWF in situations where other sources of fluoride are inadequate can be expected to result in increases in dental caries (median estimate from our review, 17.9%).[7] All of the study populations were children 4–17 years old, and dental decay was measured in both primary and permanent teeth.

These findings should be applicable to all people in the United States and most industrialized countries. Studies were conducted in many settings; among different cultures; from the 1950s to 2000; on five continents—Europe, North America, Asia, Australia, and Africa; on the effects of starting, continuing, and stopping CWF; and using differing levels of CWF (fluoride concentrations varied from 0.6 to 1.8 ppm in fluoridated water supplies and from 0 to 0.8 ppm in comparison [nonfluoridated] water supplies).

Potential benefits of CWF include reducing the disparity in caries risk and prevalence across socioeconomic, racial, ethnic, and other groups[45] and a *halo effect,* which can spread the effects of CWF to residents of nonfluoridated communities who consume processed food and beverages made with fluoridated water.[46]

A recent review of potential adverse effects of CWF showed no clear association between water fluoridation and incidence of mortality from bone cancers, thyroid cancer, or all cancers.[45]

The findings of our systematic review of economic evaluations of CWF are based on nine studies—four in the United States, one in Canada, two in the United Kingdom, and two in Australia.[47-55] Seven studies reported the annual fluoridation cost per person for 75 water systems of various sizes,[47,49-51,53-55] and five studies calculated net cost (program cost less cost of averted decay) or net cost per tooth surface saved from decay.[48,49,52-54] In general, reporting was based on CWF systems that served three population categories: less than 5000, between 5000 and 20,000, and over 20,000.

The results pointed to economies of scale as the main source of variation in the cost per person per year. The median cost per person was $2.70 for 19 systems serving populations less than 5000; $1.41 for 21 systems serving populations between 5000 and 20,000; and $0.40 for 35 systems serving populations greater than 20,000. From a societal perspective, CWF was cost saving in all studies for populations above 20,000.[48,49,52-54]

Major barriers to the adoption or maintenance of CWF include limited knowledge among the general population and some health professionals of oral health promotion, some organized opposition to CWF (based on fear of adverse effects and appeals for personal autonomy in controlling exposure to fluoride), and some continuing debate about the net balance of benefits and risk of harm from excess fluoride ingested from all sources (of which CWF is one).

In conclusion, the Task Force recommends CWF on the basis of strong evidence of effectiveness in reducing dental decay. This finding should be applicable to most people in the United States who use public water systems, regardless of age, race, ethnicity, or socioeconomic status.

School-Based or School-Linked Pit and Fissure Sealant Delivery Programs: Recommended (Strong Evidence of Effectiveness)

These programs provide pit and fissure sealants directly to children who might not otherwise receive them. *School-based* programs usually are conducted entirely in school settings. *School-linked* programs are conducted partially in the schools (e.g., patient selection and parental permission) but generally provide sealants at private dental practices or other clinics outside of schools. Many programs target *high-risk* children (those unlikely to receive dental care, often those eligible for free or reduced-cost lunch programs) or high-risk teeth (all teeth with deep pits and fissures, especially the first and second permanent molars, which erupt around ages 6 and 12, respectively). A school-based or school-linked component often is an integral part of a community-wide sealant application program.

The appropriate application of pit and fissure sealants to at-risk teeth is one of many complementary strategies for preventing dental caries (tooth decay). Although sealants are necessary to further reduce pit and fissure caries, fluoride is necessary to prevent caries on all types of tooth surfaces.

Effectiveness

- These programs are effective in reducing dental caries by approximately 60% among children aged 6–17 years, of varying socioeconomic levels and baseline caries levels.

Applicability

- Our findings should be applicable to school-age children in a variety of school settings.

Sealants are clear or opaque plastic materials applied to the pits and fissures of teeth to prevent dental caries (tooth decay). When applied properly, sealants prevent food, bacteria, and debris from collecting within the pits and fissures of vulnerable teeth (mainly molars). Because sealants are effective in preventing caries only as long as the sealant material remains in place, ongoing monitoring of retention and periodic re-application of sealant may be necessary to ensure long-term effectiveness.

Since 1998, federal agencies—including the Centers for Disease Control and Prevention (CDC), the National Institute of Dental and Craniofacial Research (NIDCR), the National Institutes of Health (NIH), the Health Resources and Services Administration (HRSA), and the Indian Health Service (IHS)—have supported state-level partnerships (including departments of health and education and private sector businesses and organizations) to develop, expand, and evaluate school-based and school-linked models integrating oral health into their existing coordinated school health programs.

The findings of our systematic review are based on 10 studies that measured the effectiveness of school-based or school-linked sealant delivery programs in reducing tooth decay among children.[56–65] An additional 27 studies were identified but did not meet our quality criteria and were excluded from the review.[66–92]

The studies in our review compared pit and fissure dental caries of children who received sealants in a school-based or school-linked program with children who did not receive sealants. Seven of the 10 studies reported on the effects of using bisphenol A glycidyl methacrylate (bis-GMA) sealant resin as the only caries preventive intervention, and 3 reported on the effects of using bis-GMA sealant combined with other caries preventive interventions (e.g., fluoride gel or rinse, fluoridated water, or health education). In the 10 studies, receiving sealants in a school-based or school-linked program was associated with a median decrease in dental caries of 60% (range, 5% to 93%). School-based programs showed a higher median decrease (65%; range, 23% to 93%) than school-linked programs (37%; range, 5% to 93%). Programs in which sealants were re-applied at some point between initial application and follow-up showed a higher median decrease (65%; range, 23% to 93%) than programs in which sealants were not re-applied (30%; range, 5% to 93%). Overall, these results show that school-based and school-linked pit and fissure sealant programs are effective in reducing dental caries.

The findings should be applicable to school-age children in a range of settings. Studies varied by time, place, population characteristics, number of times sealant was applied to the same tooth surface, and duration of follow-up between sealant application and evaluation of caries status. Studies were conducted in the United States, Guam, the United Kingdom, Australia, Spain, Thailand, and Colombia. All of the study populations involved children aged 6–17 years, and the prevalence of caries was measured in both primary and permanent teeth.

Other potential positive effects of school-based or school-linked sealant delivery programs include increased support for coordinated school-based programs to address related dental and non-dental needs of children from low-income families (e.g., immunization and better nutrition) and increased willingness of third-party payers to pay for sealants applied in other settings. Potential negative effects include competition for time and resources between sealant programs and other school-related activities. In addition, some dentists in private practice are concerned that children who receive dental services in school-based programs may be less likely to keep appointments for regularly scheduled checkups.

The findings of our systematic review of economic evaluations of school-based and school-linked pit and fissure sealant delivery programs are based on six studies—four in the United States, one in Australia, and one in Canada— from the early 1970s to the mid-1990s.[50,53,60,93–95] Two of the U.S. studies limited their analyses to the costs of school-based and school-linked sealant programs.[93] In addition to sealant program costs,[50] the remaining four studies also provided sufficient data on rates of tooth decay and treatment costs to calculate the net cost per tooth surface saved from decay.[53,60,94,95]

Although the number of teeth sealed and resealed varied among school-based and school-linked sealant programs, sealant program costs per child ranged from $18.54[93] to $59.83,[60] with a median cost of $39.10. The net cost per surface saved from decay ranged from less than $0 (cost saving) to $487.

Major barriers to the adoption or maintenance of school-based or school-linked sealant delivery programs include limited knowledge of the availability and value of dental sealants among the general population and some health professionals; limited resources and limited political and administrative support in some school districts; state dental practice laws and regulations that limit the authority to apply sealants to selected categories of dental care professionals; and resistance of some dentists in private practice.

In conclusion, the Task Force recommends school-based and school-linked pit and fissure sealant programs on the basis of strong evidence of effectiveness in reducing decay in pits and fissures of children's teeth. These findings should be applicable to most children of school age.

Statewide or Community-Wide Sealant Promotion Programs:
Insufficient Evidence to Determine Effectiveness

These programs encourage sealant use among private practitioners and through community-based programs (often including school-based programs). Program activities can include continuing education courses for dental health professionals; educational campaigns for consumers, community leaders, and third-party payers; and efforts to promote school-based or school-linked sealant delivery programs.

Effectiveness

- We found insufficient evidence to determine the effectiveness of statewide or community-wide sealant promotion programs in increasing sealant use or reducing tooth decay.
- Evidence was insufficient because the only available data did not show the effects of these programs on the stated outcomes.
- Insufficient evidence means that we were not able to determine whether or not the intervention works.

Statewide or community-wide sealant promotion programs aim to increase public and professional awareness of the health benefits of sealants, appropriate use of sealants by dental practitioners, and access to sealants (e.g., through school-based programs) for disadvantaged populations that might not otherwise receive them, and to encourage third-party reimbursement for sealants. Today, sealant application is supported through several federally funded programs (e.g., Indian Health Service; Health Resources and Services Administration; Centers for Disease Control and Prevention) and is listed among covered services in all state Medicaid programs.[5] A 1994 workshop on Guidelines for Sealant Use produced recommendations for sealant use in both community-based and individual care programs.[96]

The findings of our systematic review are based on one study.[89] This study provided insufficient evidence to determine whether or not statewide or community-wide sealant promotion programs are effective in decreasing dental caries, because we could not determine from the data to what extent the programs contributed to a change in sealant use or a decrease in tooth decay.

Because we could not establish the effectiveness of these programs, we did not examine situations in which they would be applicable, barriers to implementation, or information about economic efficiency.

In conclusion, the Task Force found insufficient evidence to determine the effectiveness of statewide and community-wide sealant promotion programs in increasing sealant use or preventing tooth decay. Only one study qualified for the review, and the change in sealant use or reduction of related tooth decay could not be estimated from the data presented in that study.

Preventing or Controlling Oral and Pharyngeal Cancers

Each year, cancers of the oral cavity (mouth) or pharynx (throat) are diagnosed in about 30,000 Americans; about 8000 people die each year of these malignancies, which are mainly squamous cell carcinomas.[4,97,98] Tobacco use and excessive alcohol consumption together account for 90% of all oral cancers.[4,99] Oral and pharyngeal cancers are the 4th, 7th, and 14th most common cancers among African-American men, white men, and all women, respectively.[97] They are most often diagnosed at late stages and treated by methods (surgery, radiation therapy, and chemotherapy) that are often disfiguring and costly.[100] Overall relative five-year survival rates are about 50%, and mortality is nearly twice as high among some minorities (especially African-American men) as among whites.[98]

Since 1992, organized efforts to develop and implement a national strategic plan for preventing and controlling oral and pharyngeal cancers have been gaining momentum in the United States.[101] In 1996, a coalition of national, state, and local health agencies began promoting coordinated strategies in five areas: (1) advocacy, collaboration, and coalition building; (2) public health policy; (3) public education; (4) professional education and practice; and (5) data collection, evaluation, and research. Controversy, however, surrounds the conduct of interventions to prevent and control these cancers, including such issues as the roles of dental and medical practitioners in early detection, whether efforts to prevent tobacco use are more effective than early detection of cancers, and whether or not screening through oral examinations actually helps to prevent and control these cancers.

Population-Based Interventions for Early Detection of Pre-Cancers and Cancers: Insufficient Evidence to Determine Effectiveness

These programs educate the public about risk factors, symptoms, signs, and the value of early detection and train health workers to detect suspicious lesions. People at high risk of developing cancer, or those with cancer symptoms, are encouraged to examine themselves for suspicious lesions and to get a professional examination and follow-up. To help reach more people, such programs can also include examining people at the workplace, at home, at health fairs, in field clinics, or where people usually receive health care. Such examinations result in referrals of people with suspicious lesions for follow-up and treatment.

Effectiveness

- We found insufficient evidence to determine the effectiveness of population-based interventions for early detection of pre-cancers and cancers in reducing morbidity or mortality or improving the quality of life.
- Evidence was insufficient because no studies examined the effects of these programs on the stated outcomes.
- Insufficient evidence means that we were not able to determine whether or not the intervention works.

The findings of our systematic review are based on 19 studies (in 24 reports).[102-125] Although the studies looked at many aspects of the effects of population-based interventions for early detection of pre-cancers and cancers, none of them measured the three outcomes we had chosen to evaluate in this review: morbidity, mortality, and quality of life. The studies, therefore, provided insufficient evidence to determine whether or not these population-based interventions are effective in reducing cancer morbidity or mortality or in improving quality of life.

Because we could not establish the effectiveness of these programs, we did not examine situations in which the programs would be applicable, barriers to implementation, or information about economic efficiency.

In conclusion, the Task Force found insufficient evidence to determine the effectiveness of population-based interventions for early detection of pre-cancers and cancers in reducing cancer morbidity or mortality, or in improving the quality of life, because no studies in the review measured effectiveness in terms of those outcomes.

Preventing or Controlling Sports-Related Craniofacial Injuries

The consequences of sports-related injuries (e.g., bone fractures, tooth loss, concussions, brain damage) range from something as simple yet frustrating as a loss of game time to the much more serious events of paralysis and death. Helmets, facemasks, and mouthguards protect users from injuries to the head, face, and mouth. Protective equipment is mandatory in some professional sports. For example, baseball requires use of helmets, football requires helmets and facemasks, ice hockey requires helmets, and boxing requires mouthguards. In amateur sports, helmets, facemasks, and mouthguards are mandatory in boxing, football, ice hockey, and men's lacrosse and mouthguards are mandatory in women's field hockey. *Healthy People 2010*[4] established a developmental objective to increase the proportion of public and private schools that require the use of appropriate head, face, eye, and mouth protection for students participating in school-sponsored physical activities (Table 7–1).

Population-Based Interventions to Encourage Use of Helmets, Facemasks, and Mouthguards in Contact Sports: Insufficient Evidence to Determine Effectiveness

Population-based interventions to encourage the use of helmets, facemasks, and mouthguards when engaged in contact sports aim to prevent injuries to the head, face, and mouth. Rules of play concerning helmets, facemasks, goggles, and mouthguards vary by sport and position on the team. Intervention programs educate health professionals, parents, coaches, players, and officials of organized sports about the risk of injury and potential benefits of protective equipment, offer incentives for regular use of protective equipment at both practice and formal competition, and encourage the enforcement of rules of play involving safety equipment.

Effectiveness

- We found insufficient evidence to determine the effectiveness of population-based interventions in encouraging the use of helmets, facemasks, and mouthguards when engaging in contact sports.
- Evidence was insufficient because the reported effects of the intervention in increasing the use of protective equipment or decreasing related injuries were small and inconsistent.
- Insufficient evidence means that we were not able to determine whether or not the intervention works.

The findings of our systematic review are based on four studies.[126-129] An additional 13 studies were identified but did not meet our quality criteria and were excluded from the review.[130-142] To be able to recommend use of population-based interventions to encourage use of protective equipment in contact sports, the Task Force required that studies show increases in the use of such equipment or decreases in sports-related craniofacial injuries attributable to the intervention.

The four studies reported inconsistent and small effects of the intervention in increasing use of protective equipment or decreasing related injuries. The Task Force, therefore, found insufficient evidence to determine whether or not these interventions are effective in achieving the stated outcomes.

Because we could not establish the effectiveness of these interventions, we did not examine situations in which they would be applicable, barriers to implementation, or information about economic efficiency.

In conclusion, the Task Force found insufficient evidence to determine the effectiveness of population-based interventions to encourage use of helmets, facemasks, and mouthguards in contact sports, because available studies showed inconsistent and small effects.

IMPROVING ORAL HEALTH THROUGH USE OF THESE RECOMMENDATIONS

Public officials, community leaders, school systems, healthcare systems, and oral health practitioners can use the recommendations in this chapter to prevent and control dental caries. In this section, we provide information to help apply the recommended interventions to prevent dental caries in communities, along with the results of economic evaluations to estimate the resources needed to implement effective interventions where they are needed.

The Task Force found insufficient evidence to determine the effectiveness of interventions to prevent or control oral and pharyngeal cancers and sports-related craniofacial injuries, and therefore was not able to recommend for or against use of these interventions at this time. Users of the *Community Guide* who are developing or modifying organized efforts to prevent and control these conditions, however, can consider the findings presented in this chapter and the recommendations of other groups (described below), along with the need for additional research to fill gaps in our knowledge about the effectiveness of these promising interventions.

Preventing and Controlling Dental Caries

The Task Force has recommended community water fluoridation (CWF) and school-based or school-linked pit and fissure sealant delivery programs on the basis of strong evidence of effectiveness. To decide if CWF should be continued, expanded, or modified in their communities, public officials and water system operators should consider the recommendations and other evidence provided in this book along with such local information as the burden and cost of dental caries, resource availability, and the laws that regulate public water supplies.

Similarly, school systems, public officials, parents, and practitioners can use the recommendation for school-based sealant delivery programs as one factor in their decision to start, expand, or modify existing programs in their school districts. Other local factors include the overall burden and disparities in dental caries, especially in school districts with large proportions of vulnerable children who are less likely to receive dental sealants from private sources (e.g., children in low-income households). Some children of racial and ethnic minority groups have about three times more untreated decayed and missing teeth due to caries but are about one-third as likely to receive sealants.[8,11,143] In 2000, 29 states reported dental sealant programs serving 193,000 children, a number that represented only about 3% of poor children who could receive sealants.[144]

Community water fluoridation and school-based sealant programs should be considered in the context of other community-wide, provider-based, and individual strategies for preventing or controlling dental caries in communities.[5,12] Moreover, the results of the economic evaluations can also be used to help decision makers determine whether CWF and school-based sealant programs are affordable and wise expenditures that provide the worthwhile benefits of avoiding the often underestimated health consequences of dental caries.

Preventing and Controlling Oral and Pharyngeal Cancers

Users of the *Community Guide* who are developing or modifying organized efforts to reduce the burden of oral and pharyngeal cancers should consider the findings presented here together with recommendations of other groups.[101,145,146] For example, some experts have encouraged more widespread use of effective strategies to reduce tobacco use, an important cause of oral and pharyngeal cancers,[147–149] and other experts have encouraged clinicians to consider periodic oral examinations of people engaging in risk behaviors (tobacco use or excessive alcohol consumption) or manifesting suspicious symptoms.[145] We published a comparison of selected evidence reviews and recommendations on interventions to prevent oral and pharyngeal cancers in 2002,[6] and this article is also available at www.thecommunityguide.org/oral. Such comparisons can help readers of the *Community Guide* put the evidence and recommendations compiled by different authorities into a common framework that aids decision making.

In the absence of definitive recommendations on effective interventions to prevent and control oral and pharyngeal cancers in this report and other sources, users of this book may choose to advocate for new research studies on the effectiveness of various methods of oral examination (by dental care practitioners and other medical practitioners who must examine the mouth during the course of routine medical care) in detecting pre-cancers and in reducing sickness, disfigurement, and premature death from oral and pharyngeal cancers. Research questions identified through a systematic review of population-based interventions designed to prevent oral and pharyngeal cancers were published as part of the comprehensive evidence review conducted by the Task Force and previously published (see Truman et al., 2002[7] or www.thecommunityguide.org/oral/oral-rsch-quest.htm).

Preventing and Controlling Sports-Related Craniofacial Injuries

Users of the *Community Guide* who are developing or modifying organized efforts to prevent and control sports-related craniofacial injuries should consider the findings presented here together with findings and recommendations of other groups including the Office of the Surgeon General, American Dental Association, the American Academy of Pediatric Dentistry, the American Medical Association, and the American Academy of Pediatrics (see Table 5 in Gooch et al., 2002,[6] available at www.thecommunityguide.org/oral/oral-ajpm-c-compare-ev-rev.pdf). (Evidence of the efficacy of protective sports equipment in preventing injuries was not the focus of this review. Yet some investigators have observed that the frequency and severity of head, face, and oral injuries have decreased in some sports since the use of helmets, face-masks, and mouthguards became mandatory in selected organized contact sports [e.g., football and ice hockey].)[150,151] A comparison of selected evidence reviews and recommendations on interventions to prevent and control sports-related craniofacial injuries (see Table 6 in Gooch et al., 2002,[6] available at www.thecommunityguide.org/oral/oral-ajpm-c-compare-ev-rev.pdf) has revealed that the Surgeon General's report, policies and guidelines from selected medical and dental professional organizations, and mandatory rules of play from major governing bodies of organized sports all promote increased awareness and use of protective equipment in contact sports with risk of injury.

In the absence of definitive recommendations on effective use of protective head and face equipment to avoid injuries and death in contact sports, users of the *Community Guide* may choose to advocate for new research studies to fill the evidence gap. Research questions that were developed as previously described are available online at www.thecommunityguide.org/oral/oral-rsch-quest.htm.

CONCLUSION

This chapter summarizes Task Force conclusions and recommendations on interventions to prevent or control dental caries (tooth decay), oral (mouth) and pharyngeal (throat) cancers, and sports-related craniofacial injuries. The Task Force recommends both CWF and school-based or school-linked pit and fissure sealant delivery programs to help reduce dental caries. Evidence was insufficient to determine the effectiveness of population-based interventions for early detection of pre-cancers and cancers in reducing morbidity or mortality or improving the quality of life. Evidence was also insufficient to determine the effectiveness of population-based interventions to encourage the use of helmets, facemasks, and mouthguards in increasing the use of such equipment or decreasing sports-related craniofacial injuries. Details of these reviews have been published[6,7,152,153] and these articles, along with additional information about the reviews, are available at www.thecommunityguide .org/oral.

Acknowledgments

This chapter was written by the members of the systematic review development team: Benedict I. Truman, MD, MPH, Office of Minority Health, Office of the Director, Centers for Disease Control and Prevention (CDC), Atlanta, Georgia; Barbara F. Gooch, DMD, MPH, Division of Oral Health (DOH), National Center for Chronic Disease Prevention and Health Promotion (NCCDPHP), CDC, Atlanta; Iddrissu Sulemana, MPH, MA, Division of Epidemiology and Surveillance, National Immunization Program, CDC, Atlanta; Helen C. Gift, PhD, Division of Social Sciences, Brevard College, Brevard, North Carolina; Alice M. Horowitz, PhD, National Institute of Dental and Craniofacial Research (NIDCR), National Institutes of Health (NIH), Bethesda, Maryland; Caswell A. Evans, Jr., DDS, MPH, NIDCR/NIH, Bethesda; Susan O. Griffin, PhD, DOH/NCCDPHP/CDC, Atlanta; and Vilma G. Carande-Kulis, MS, PhD, Division of Prevention Research and Analytic Methods/Epidemiology Program Office (DPRAM/EPO)/CDC, Atlanta.

Consultants for the reviews were: Myron Allukian, Jr., DDS, MPH, Boston Public Health Commission, Boston, Massachusetts; Eugenio Beltran, DMD, DrPH, DOH/CDC, Atlanta; Aljernon Bolden, DMD, MPH, Boston University, Goldman School of Dental Medicine, Boston; Maria Teresa Canto, DDS, MPH, NIDCR/NIH, Bethesda; Timothy R. Collins, DDS, MPH, Los Angeles County Department of Health Services, Los Angeles, California; Stephen B. Corbin, DDS, MPH, Special Olympics, Inc., Washington, DC; Teresa A. Dolan, DDS, MPH, University of Florida College of Dentistry, Gainesville; Thomas F. Drury, PhD, NIDCR/NIH, Bethesda; Harold Goodman, DDS, MPH, Office of Oral Health, State of Maryland Department of Health and Mental Hygiene, Baltimore; Larry Hill, DDS, MPH, Cincinnati Health Department, Cincinnati, Ohio; Lori Hutwagner, MS, Division of Public Health Surveillance and Informatics, EPO/CDC, Atlanta; Amid I. Ismail, BDS, MPH, DrPH, University of Michigan School of Dentistry, Ann Arbor; Robert Isman, DDS, MPH, Office of Medi-Cal Dental Services, California Department of Health Services, Sacramento; William Kohn, DDS, MPH, DOH/NCCDPHP/CDC, Atlanta; Jayanth Kumar, DDS, MPH, New York State Health Department, Albany; Raymond A. Kuthy, DDS, MPH, University of Iowa College of Dentistry, Iowa City; Corinne E. Miller, DDS, PhD, Michigan Department of Community Health, Lansing; R. Gary Rozier, DDS, MPH, School of Public Health, University of North Carolina, Chapel Hill; Randy H. Schwartz, MSPH, American Cancer Society, Atlanta; Robert Selwitz, DDS, MPH, NIDCR/NIH, Bethesda; Mark Siegal, DDS, MPH, Bureau of Oral Health Services, Ohio State Health Department, Columbus; Janet Stansell, MLM, NCCDPHP/CDC, Atlanta; Scott L. Tomar, DMD, DrPH, University of Florida College of Dentistry, Gainesville; Steven Uranga McKane, DMD, MPH, SUM Consulting, West Hills, California; and B. Alex White, DDS, DrPH, Kaiser Permanente Center for Health Research, Portland, Oregon.

Articles included in the reviews were abstracted by: Dionne Johnson; Kim Johnson; and Virginia Noland.

References

1. Centers for Medicare and Medicaid Services. National health care expenditures projections: 2002–2012. Available at: www.cms.hhs.gov/statistics/nhe/projections-2002/proj2002.pdf. Accessed January 28, 2004.

2. Agency for Healthcare Research and Quality. Healthcare Cost and Utilization Project. Available at: http://www.ahrq.gov/data/hcup/hcupnet.htm. Accessed Nov. 1, 2001.

3. Burt CW, Overpeck MD. Emergency visits for sports-related injuries. Ann Emerg Med 2001;37(3):301–8.

4. U.S. Department of Health and Human Services. Healthy people 2010. 2nd ed. Washington, DC: U.S. Government Printing Office, 2000.

5. U.S. Department of Health and Human Services. Oral health in America: a report of the Surgeon General. Rockville, MD: Department of Health and Human Services, National Institute of Dental and Craniofacial Research, National Institutes of Health, 2000.

6. Gooch BF, Truman BI, Griffin SO, et al. A comparison of selected evidence reviews and recommendations on interventions to prevent dental caries, oral and pharyngeal cancers, and sport-related craniofacial injuries. Am J Prev Med 2002;23(1S):55–80.

7. Truman BI, Gooch BF, Sulemana I, et al. Reviews of evidence on interventions to prevent dental caries, oral and pharyngeal cancers, and sports-related craniofacial injuries. Am J Prev Med 2002;23(1S):21–54.

8. Kaste LM, Selwitz RH, Oldakowski RJ, et al. Coronal caries in the primary and permanent dentition of children and adolescents 1–17 years of age: United States, 1988–1991. J Dent Res 1996;75 spec no.:631–41.

9. Winn DM, Brunelle JA, Selwitz RH, et al. Coronal and root caries in the dentition of adults in the United States, 1988–1991. J Dent Res 1996;75 spec no.:642–51.

10. Brown LJ, Kaste LM, Selwitz RH, Furman LJ. Dental caries and sealant usage in U.S. children, 1988–1991: selected findings from the Third National Health and Nutrition Examination Survey. J Am Dent Assoc 1996;127(3):335–43.

11. Vargas CM, Crall JJ, Schneider DA. Sociodemographic distribution of pediatric dental caries: NHANES III, 1988–1994. J Am Dent Assoc 1998;129:1229–38.

12. Centers for Disease Control and Prevention. Recommendations for using fluoride to prevent and control dental caries in the United States. MMWR 2001;50(RR-14):1–42.

13. Centers for Disease Control and Prevention. Achievements in public health, 1900–1999: Fluoridation of drinking water to prevent dental caries. MMWR 1999; 48(41):933–40.

14. Centers for Disease Control and Prevention. Populations receiving optimally fluoridated public drinking water—United States, 2000. MMWR 2002;51(7):144–7.

15. Arnold FA Jr, Dean HT. Effect of fluoridated public water supply on dental caries prevalence. Public Health Rep 1956;71:652–8.

16. Attwood D, Blinkhorn AS. Trends in dental health of ten-year-old school children in south-west Scotland after cessation of water fluoridation. Lancet 1988;2(8605):266–7.

17. Backer-Dirks O. Some special features of the caries preventive effects of water fluoridation of drinking water in the Netherlands. Arch Oral Biol 1961;4(spec suppl): 187–92.

18. Beal JF, James PM. Dental caries prevalence in 5-year-old children following five and a half years of water fluoridation in Birmingham. Br Dent J 1971;130(7):284–8.

19. Beal JF, Clayton M. Fluoridation. A clinical survey in Corby and Scunthorpe. Public Health 1981;95(3):152–60.

20. Booth JM, Mitropoulos CM, Worthington HV. A comparison between the dental health of 3-year-old children living in fluoridated Huddersfield and non-fluoridated Dewsbury in 1989. Community Dent Health 1992;9(2):151–7.

21. Brown H, Poplove M. The Brantford-Sarnia-Stratford Fluoridation Caries Study: final survey, 1963. Can J Public Health 1965;56(8):319–24.

22. Ellwood RP, O'Mullane DM. The association between area deprivation and dental caries in groups with and without fluoride in their drinking water. Community Dent Health 1995;12(1):18–22.

23. Evans DJ, Rugg-Gunn AJ, Tabari ED. The effect of 25 years of water fluoridation in Newcastle assessed in four surveys of 5-year-old children over an 18-year period. Br Dent J 1995;178(2):60–4.

24. Fanning EA, Cellier KM, Somerville CM. South Australian kindergarten children: effects of fluoride tablets and fluoridated water on dental caries in primary teeth. Aust Dent J 1980;25(5):259–63.

25. Guo MK, Hsieh CC, Hong YC, Chen RS. Effect of water fluoridation on prevalence of dental caries in Chung-Hsing New Village, Taiwan, after 9 years. Taiwan I Hsueh Hui Tsa Chih—J Formosan Med Assoc 1984;83(10):1035–43.

26. Hardwick JL, Teasdale J, Bloodworth G. Caries increments over 4 years in children aged 12 at the start of water fluoridation. Br Dent J 1982;153(6):217–22.

27. Hawew RM, Ellwood RP, Hawley GM, Worthington HV, Blinkhorn AS. Dental caries in children from two Libyan cities with different levels of fluoride in their drinking water. Community Dent Health 1996;13(3):175–7.

28. Kalsbeek H, Kwant GW, Groeneveld A, Dirks OB, van Eck AA, Theuns HM. Caries experience of 15-year-old children in The Netherlands after discontinuation of water fluoridation. Caries Res 1993;27(3):201–5.

29. Kunzel W, Fischer T. Rise and fall of caries prevalence in German towns with different F concentrations in drinking water. Caries Res 1997;31(3):166–73.

30. Loh T. Thirty-eight years of water fluoridation—the Singapore scenario. Community Dent Health 1996;13(suppl 2):47–50.

31. Provart SJ, Carmichael CL. The relationship between caries, fluoridation and material deprivation in five-year-old children in County Durham. Community Dent Health 1995;12(4):200–3.

32. Rugg-Gunn A, Nicholas K. Caries experience of 5-year-old children living in four communities in North East England receiving differing water fluoride levels. Br Dent J 1981;150:9–12.

33. Seppa L, Karkkainen S, Hausen H. Caries frequency in permanent teeth before and after discontinuation of water fluoridation in Kuopio, Finland. Community Dent Oral Epidemiol 1998;26(4):256–62.

34. Slade GD, Spencer AJ, Davies MJ, Stewart JF. Influence of exposure to fluoridated water on socioeconomic inequalities in children's caries experience. Community Dent Oral Epidemiol 1996;24(2):89–100.

35. Tsutsui A, Yagi M, Horowitz AM. The prevalence of dental caries and fluorosis in Japanese communities with up to 1.4 ppm of naturally occuring fluoride. J Public Health Dent 2000;60(3):147–53.

36. Ast DB, Fitzgerald B. Effectiveness of water fluoridation. J Am Dent Assoc 1962; 65:581–8.

37. Blayney JR, Hill IN. Evanston Dental Caries Study. XXIV. Prenatal fluorides–value of waterborne fluorides during pregnancy. J Am Dent Assoc 1964;69:291–4.

38. Campagna L, Tsamtsouris A, Kavadia K. Fluoridated drinking water and maturation of permanent teeth at age 12. J Clin Pediatr Dent 1995;19(3):225–8.

39. Jones C, Taylor G, Woods K, Whittle G, Evans D, Young P. Jarman underprivileged area scores, tooth decay and the effect of water fluoridation. Community Dent Health 1997;14(3):156–60.

40. Kelman AM. Fluoridation—the Israel experience. Community Dent Health 1996; 13(suppl 2):42–6.

41. Margolis FJ, Reames HR, Freshman E, MaCauley CD, Mehaffey H. Fluoride. Ten-year prospective study of deciduous and permanent dentition. Am J Dis Child 1975; 129(7):794-800.

42. Rugg-Gunn A, Carmichael CL. Fluoridation in Newcastle and Northumberland: a clinical study of five year old children. Braz Dent J 1977;142:395-402.

43. Selwitz RH, Nowjack-Raymer RE, Kingman A, Driscoll WS. Prevalence of dental caries and dental fluorosis in areas with optimal and above-optimal water fluoride concentrations: a 10-year follow-up survey. J Public Health Dent 1995;55(2):85-93.

44. Weerheijm KL, Kidd EA, Groen HJ. The effect of fluoridation on the occurrence of hidden caries in clinically sound occlusal surfaces. Caries Res 1997;31(1):30-4.

45. McDonagh MS, Whiting PF, Wilson PM, et al. Systematic review of water fluoridation. BMJ 2000;321(7265):855-9.

46. Griffin SO, Gooch BF, Lockwood SA, Tomar SL. Quantifying the diffused benefit from water fluoridation in the United States. Community Dent Oral Epidemiol 2001; 29(2):120-9.

47. Birch S. The relative cost effectiveness of water fluoridation across communities: analysis of variations according to underlying caries levels. Community Dent Health 1990;7(1):3-10.

48. Doessel DP. Cost-benefit analysis of water fluoridation in Townsville, Australia. Community Dent Oral Epidemiol 1985;13(1):19-22.

49. Dowell TB. The economics of fluoridation. Br Dent J 1976;140(3):103-6.

50. Garcia AI. Caries incidence and costs of prevention programs. J Public Health Dent 1989;49(5 spec no.):259-71.

51. Kailis DG, Kailis SG, Stevenson TS, Wall C. Groote Eylandt studies. 2. Fluoridation of a small domestic water supply, C.M.S. Angurugu mission, Groote Eylandt, N.T., Australia. 1973-1974. Aust Dent J 1976;21(4):327-33.

52. Nelson W, Swint JM. Cost-benefit analysis of fluoridation in Houston, Texas. J Public Health Dent 1976;36(2):88-95.

53. Niessen LC, Douglass CW. Theoretical considerations in applying benefit-cost and cost-effectiveness analyses to preventive dental programs. J Public Health Dent 1984;44(4):156-68.

54. O'Keefe JP. A case study on the cost effectiveness of water fluoridation. Would fluoridation make economic sense in Montreal today? Ont Dent 1994;71(8):33-8.

55. Ringelberg ML, Allen SJ, Brown LJ. Cost of fluoridation: 44 Florida communities. J Public Health Dent 1992;52(2):75-80.

56. Bagramian RA. A 5-year school-based comprehensive preventive program in Michigan, U.S.A. Community Dent Oral Epidemiol 1982;10(5):234-7.

57. Bravo M, Baca P, Llodra JC, Osorio E. A 24-month study comparing sealant and fluoride varnish in caries reduction on different permanent first molar surfaces. J Public Health Dent 1997;57(3):184-6.

58. Burt BA, Berman DS, Silverstone LM. Sealant retention and effects on occlusal caries after 2 years in a public program. Community Dent Oral Epidemiol 1977;5(1):15-21.

59. Horowitz HS, Heifetz SB, Poulsen S. Retention and effectiveness of a single application of an adhesive sealant in preventing occlusal caries: final report after five years of a study in Kalispell, Montana. J Am Dent Assoc 1977;95(6):1133-9.

60. Klein SP, Bohannan HM, Bell RM, Disney JA, Foch CB, Graves RC. The cost and effectiveness of school-based preventive dental care. Am J Public Health 1985;75(4): 382-91.

61. McCune RJ, Bojanini J, Abodeely RA. Effectiveness of a pit and fissure sealant in the prevention of caries: three-year clinical results. J Am Dent Assoc 1979;99(4):619–23.

62. Messer LB, Calache H, Morgan MV. The retention of pit and fissure sealants placed in primary school children by Dental Health Services, Victoria. Aust Dent J 1997; 42(4):233–9.

63. Selwitz RH, Nowjack-Raymer R, Driscoll WS, Li SH. Evaluation after 4 years of the combined use of fluoride and dental sealants. Community Dent Oral Epidemiol 1995;23(1):30–5.

64. Songpaisan Y, Bratthall D, Phantumvanit P, Somridhivej Y. Effects of glass ionomer cement, resin-based pit and fissure sealant and HF applications on occlusal caries in a developing country field trial. Community Dent Oral Epidemiol 1995;23(1): 25–9.

65. Sterritt GR, Frew RA, Rozier RG. Evaluation of Guamanian dental caries preventive programs after 13 years. J Public Health Dent 1994;54(3):153–9.

66. Arrow P, Riordan PJ. Retention and caries preventive effects of a GIC and a resin-based fissure sealant. Community Dent Oral Epidemiol 1995;23(5):282–5.

67. Axelsson P, Paulander J, Svardstrom G, Tollskog G, Nordensten S. Integrated caries prevention: effect of a needs-related preventive program on dental caries in children. County of Varmland, Sweden: results after 12 years. Caries Res 1993;27(suppl 1):83–94.

68. Brown MA, Lawson RL, Malvitz DM, Calderone JJ, Mueller LA. Results from a school-based dental sealant program after ten years. 1999. Unpublished.

69. Carlsson A, Petersson M, Twetman S. Two-year clinical performance of a fluoride-containing fissure sealant in young schoolchildren at caries risk. Am J Dent 1997;10(3): 115–9.

70. Chestnutt IG, Schafer F, Jacobson AP, Stephen KW. The prevalence and effectiveness of fissure sealants in Scottish adolescents [letter]. Br Dent J 1994;177(4):125–9.

71. Clark DC, Berkowitz J. The relationship between the number of sound, decayed, and filled permanent tooth surfaces and the number of sealed surfaces in children and adolescents. J Public Health Dent 1997;57(3):171–5.

72. Fischman SL, English JA, Albino JE, et al. A comprehensive caries control program—design and evaluation of the clinical trial. J Dent Res 1977;56(spec no.): C99–C103.

73. Gray GB, Paterson RC. Management of fissure caries in the community dental services using sealant restorations: a field trial. Eur J Prosthodont Restor Dent 1998;6(1): 33–40.

74. Hardison JR. The use of pit-and-fissure sealants in community public health programs in Tennessee. J Public Health Dent 1983;43(3):233–9.

75. Heidmann J, Poulsen S, Mathiassen F. Evaluation of a fissure sealing programme in a Danish Public Child Dental Service. Community Dent Health 1990;7(4):379–88.

76. Heller KE, Reed SG, Bruner FW, Eklund SA, Burt BA. Longitudinal evaluation of sealing molars with and without incipient dental caries in a public health program. J Public Health Dent 1995;55(3):148–53.

77. Ismail AI, King W, Clark DC. An evaluation of the Saskatchewan pit and fissure sealant program: a longitudinal followup. J Public Health Dent 1989;49(4):206–11.

78. Ismail AI, Gagnon P. A longitudinal evaluation of fissure sealants applied in dental practices. J Dent Res 1995;74(9):1583–90.

79. Jones RB. The effects for recall patients of a comprehensive sealant program in a clinical dental public health setting. J Public Health Dent 1986;46(3):152–5.

80. Karlzen-Reuterving G, van Dijken JW. A three-year follow-up of glass ionomer cement and resin fissure sealants. ASDC J Dent Child 1995;62(2):108–10.

81. Klooz DN. A collaborative fissure sealant program in Niagara region. Ont Dent 1996;73(2):24–9.

82. Kumar JV, Davila ME, Green EL, Lininger LL. Evaluation of a school-based sealant program in New York State. J Public Health Manag Pract 1997;3(3):43–51.

83. Kuthy RA, Branch LG, Clive JM. First permanent molar restoration differences between those with or without dental sealants. J Dent Educ 1990;54(11):653–60.

84. Leal FR, Forgas-Brockmann L, Simecek J, Cohen ME, Meyer DM. A prospective study of sealant application in navy recruits. Mil Med 1998;163(2):107–9.

85. Lennon MA, O'Mullane DM, Taylor GO. A pragmatic clinical trial of fissure sealants in a community dental service programme for 6–10-year-old children. Community Dent Health 1984;1(2):101–9.

86. Mertz-Fairhurst EJ, Adair SM, Sams DR, et al. Cariostatic and ultraconservative sealed restorations: nine-year results among children and adults. ASDC J Dent Child 1995;62(2):97–107.

87. Morgan MV, Campain AC, Adams GG, Crowley SJ, Wright FA. The efficacy and effectiveness of a primary preventive dental programme in non-fluoridated areas of Victoria, Australia. Community Dent Health 1998;15(4):263–71.

88. Rock WP, Foulkes EE, Perry H, Smith AJ. A comparative study of fluoride-releasing composite resin and glass ionomer materials used as fissure sealants. J Dent 1996; 24(4):275–80.

89. Siegal MD, Garcia AI, Kandray DP, Giljahn LK. The use of dental sealants by Ohio dentists. J Public Health Dent 1996;56(1):12–21.

90. Simonsen RJ. Retention and effectiveness of dental sealant after 15 years. J Am Dent Assoc 1991;122(11):34–42.

91. Walker J, Floyd K, Jakobsen J. The effectiveness of sealants in pediatric patients. ASDC J Dent Child 1996;63(4):268–70.

92. Williams B, Laxton L, Holt RD, Winter GB. Fissure sealants: a 4-year clinical trial comparing an experimental glass polyalkenoate cement with a bis glycidyl methacrylate resin used as fissure sealants. Br Dent J 1996;180(3):104–8.

93. Calderone JJ, Mueller LA. The cost of sealant application in a state dental disease prevention program. J Public Health Dent 1983;43(3):249–54.

94. Leake JL, Martinello BP. A four-year evaluation of a a fissure sealant in a public health setting. J Can Dent Assoc 1976;42(8):409–15.

95. Morgan MV, Campain AC, Crowley SJ, Wright FA. An evaluation of a primary preventive dental programme in non-fluoridated areas of Victoria, Australia. Aust Dent J 1997;42(6):381–8.

96. Workshop on guidelines for sealant use: recommendations. The Association of State and Territorial Dental Directors, the New York State Health Department, the Ohio Department of Health and the School of Public Health, University of Albany, State University of New York. J Public Health Dent 1995;55(5 spec no):263–73.

97. American Cancer Society. Cancer facts and figures: estimated new cancer cases and deaths by sex for all sites, 2001. Available at: http://www3.cancer.org/cancerinfo. Accessed July 18, 2001.

98. Greenlee RT, Hill-Harmon B, Murray T, Thun M. Cancer statistics, 2001. CA: Cancer J Clin 2001;51(1):15–36.

99. American Cancer Society. Oral cancer. 4th ed. Silverman SJr, ed. Hamilton, Ontario, Canada: B.C. Decker, 1998.

100. Horowitz AM, Nourjah PA. Factors associated with having oral cancer examinations among U.S. adults 40 years or older. J Public Health Dent 1996;56(6):331–5.

101. Centers for Disease Control and Prevention. Preventing and controlling oral and pharyngeal cancer. Recommendations from a National Strategic Planning Conference. MMWR 1998;47(RR-14):1–12.

102. Banoczy J, Rigo O. Prevalence study of oral precancerous lesions within a complex screening system in Hungary. Community Dent Oral Epidemiol 1991;19(5):265–7.

103. Burzynski NJ, Firriolo FJ, Butters JM, Sorrell CL. Evaluation of oral cancer screening. J Cancer Educ 1997;12(2):95–9.

104. Clayman GL, Chamberlain RM, Lee JJ, Lippman SM, Hong WK. Screening at a health fair to identify subjects for an oral leukoplakia chemoprevention trial. J Cancer Educ 1995;10(2):88–90.

105. Downer MC, Evans AW, Hughes HC, Jullien JA, Speight PM, Zakrzewska JM. Evaluation of screening for oral cancer and precancer in a company headquarters. Community Dent Oral Epidemiol 1995;23(2):84–8.

106. Eversole LR, Silverman SJ, Tolley P, Polly M. The dental hygienist as a comprehensive head and neck cancer screener. Educ Dir Dent Aux 1980;5(4):25–32.

107. Fernandez GL, Sankaranarayanan R, Lence AJ, Rodriguez SA, Maxwell PD. An evaluation of the oral cancer control program in Cuba. Epidemiology 1995;6(4):428–31.

108. Ikeda N, Ishii T, Iida S, Kawai T. Epidemiological study of oral leukoplakia based on mass screening for oral mucosal diseases in a selected Japanese population. Community Dent Oral Epidemiol 1991;19(3):160–3.

109. Ikeda N, Downer MC, Ozowa Y, Inoue C, Mizuno T, Kawai T. Characteristics of participants and non-participants in annual mass screening for oral cancer in 60-year-old residents of Tokoname city, Japan. Community Dent Health 1995;12(2):83–8.

110. Jullien JA, Zakrzewska JM, Downer MC, Speight PM. Attendance and compliance at an oral cancer screening programme in a general medical practice. Eur J Cancer B Oral Oncol 1995;31B(3):202–6.

111. Jullien JA, Downer MC, Zakrzewska JM, Speight PM. Evaluation of a screening test for the early detection of oral cancer and precancer. Community Dent Health 1995;12(1):3–7.

112. Martin LM, Bouquot JE, Wingo PA, Heath CW Jr. Cancer prevention in the dental practice: oral cancer screening and tobacco cessation advice. J Public Health Dent 1996;56(6):336–40.

113. Mathew B, Sankaranarayanan R, Wesley R, Joseph A, Nair MK. Evaluation of utilisation of health workers for secondary prevention of oral cancer in Kerala, India. Eur J Cancer B Oral Oncol 1995;31B(3):193–6.

114. Mathew B, Sankaranarayanan R, Wesley R, Nair MK. Evaluation of mouth self-examination in the control of oral cancer. Iowa Dent J 1995;71(2):397–9.

115. Mathew B, Wesley R, Dutt SC, Amma S, Sreekumar C. Cancer screening by local volunteers. World Health Forum 1996;17(4):377–8.

116. Mathew B, Sankaranarayanan R, Sunilkumar KB, et al. Reproducibility and va-

lidity of oral visual inspection by trained health workers in the detection of oral precancer and cancer. Br J Cancer 1997;76(3):390–4.

117. Mehta FS, Gupta PC, Daftary DK, Pindborg JJ, Choksi SK. An epidemiologic study of oral cancer and precancerous conditions among 101,761 villagers in Maharashtra, India. Int J Cancer 1972;10(1):134–41.

118. Mehta FS, Gupta PC, Bhonsle RB, Murti PR, Daftary DK, Pindborg JJ. Detection of oral cancer using basic health workers in an area of high oral cancer incidence in India. Cancer Detect Prev 1986;9(3–4):219–25.

119. Prout MN, Morris SJ, Witzburg RA, Hurley C, Chatterjee S. A multidisciplinary educational program to promote head and neck cancer screening. J Cancer Educ 1992; 7(2):139–46.

120. Santana JC, Delgado L, Miranda J, Sanchez M. Oral Cancer Case Finding Program (OCCFP). Oral Oncol 1997;33(1):10–2.

121. Silverman S Jr, Bilimoria KF, Bhargava K, Mani NJ, Shah RA. Cytologic, histologic and clinical correlations of precancerous and cancerous oral lesions in 57,518 industrial workers of Gujarat, India. Acta Cytol 1977;21(2):196–8.

122. Suggs TF, Cable TA, Rothenberger LA. Results of a work-site educational and screening program for hypertension and cancer. J Occup Med 1990;32(3):220–5.

123. Warnakulasuriya KA, Nanayakkara BG. Reproducibility of an oral cancer and precancer detection program using a primary health care model in Sri Lanka. Cancer Detect Prev 1991;15(5):331–4.

124. Warnakulasuriya S, Ekanayake A, Stjernsward J, Pindborg JJ, Sivayoham S. Compliance following referral in the early detection of oral cancer and precancer in Sri Lanka. Community Dent Oral Epidemiol 1988;16(6):326–9.

125. Warnakulasuriya S, Pindborg JJ. Reliability of oral precancer screening by primary health care workers in Sri Lanka. Community Dent Health 1990;7(1):73–9.

126. Benson BWM, Meeuwisse WHM. Head and neck injuries among ice hockey players wearing full face shields vs half face shields. JAMA 1999;282(24):2328–32.

127. de Wet FA, Badenhorst M, Rossouw LM. Mouthguards for rugby players at primary school level. Iowa Dent J 1981;36(4):249–53.

128. Jolly KA, Messer LB, Manton D. Promotion of mouthguards among amateur football players in Victoria. Aust N Z J Public Health 1996;20(6):630–9.

129. Webster DA, Bayliss GV, Spadaro JA. Head and face injuries in scholastic women's lacrosse with and without eyewear. Med Sci Sports Exerc 1999;31(7):938–41.

130. Alexander D, Walker J, Floyd K, Jakobsen J. A survey on the use of mouthguards and associated oral injuries in athletics. Iowa Dent J 1995;81(2):41–4.

131. Brown KAE, Delrahim SB. Correlates of missed appointments in orofacial injury patients. Oral Surg Oral Med Oral Pathol Oral Radiol Endod 1999;87(4):405–10.

132. Castaldi CR. Sports-related oral and facial injuries in the young athlete: a new challenge for the pediatric dentist. Iowa Dent J 1986;8(4):311–6.

133. Chapman PJ. The prevalence of orofacial injuries and use of mouthguards in Rugby Union. Iowa Dent J 1985;30(5):364–7.

134. Chapman PJ. Orofacial injuries and the use of mouthguards by the 1984 Great Britain Rugby League touring team. Iowa Dent J 1985;19(1):34–6.

135. Cotton FR. Mouth protection: the healthy choice. Can Dent Hyg 1985;19(1):16–9.

136. Dennis CG, Parker DA. Mouthguards in Australian sport. Iowa Dent J 1972; 17(3):228–35.

137. Flanders RA. Project Mouthguard. Iowa Dent J 1995;64(2):67–9.

138. Garon MW, Merkle A, Wright JT. Mouth protectors and oral trauma: a study of adolescent football players. Iowa Dent J 1986;112(5):663–5.

139. Gassner R, Bosch R, Tuli T, Emshoff R. Prevalence of dental trauma in 6000 patients with facial injuries: implications for prevention. Oral Surg Oral Med Oral Pathol Oral Radiol Endod 1999;87(1):27–33.

140. McNutt T, Shannon SWJ, Wright JT, Feinstein RA. Oral trauma in adolescent athletes: a study of mouth protectors. Iowa Dent J 1989;11(3):209–13.

141. Seals RR Jr, Morrow RM, Kuebker WA, Farney WD. An evaluation of mouthguard programs in Texas high school football. Iowa Dent J 1985;110(6):904–9.

142. Yamada T, Sawaki Y, Tomida S, Tohnai I, Ueda M. Oral injury and mouthguard usage by athletes in Japan. Iowa Dent J 1998;14(2):84–7.

143. Burt BA. Trends in caries prevalence in North American children. Int Dent J 1994;44(4 suppl 1):403–13.

144. Association of State and Territorial Dental Directors. 2001 synopses of state and territorial dental public health programs. Available at: http://www.astdd.org/docs/state_synopsis_survey.pdf. Accessed December 9, 2003.

145. Hawkins RJ, Wang EE, Leake JL. Preventive health care, 1999 update: prevention of oral cancer mortality. The Canadian Task Force on Preventive Health Care. J Can Dent Assoc 1999;65(11):617–27.

146. Smith RA, Mettlin CJ, Davis KJ, Eyre H. American Cancer Society guidelines for the early detection of cancer. CA: Cancer J Clin 2000;50(1):34–49.

147. Fiore MC, Bailey WC, Cohen SJ, et al. Treating tobacco use and dependence. Clinical practice guideline. Rockville, MD: US Department of Health and Human Services, Public Health Service, 2000. Available at: http://www.surgeongeneral.gov/tobacco. Accessed July 13, 2000.

148. Hopkins DP, Briss PA, Ricard CJ, et al. Reviews of evidence regarding interventions to reduce tobacco use and exposure to environmental tobacco smoke. Am J Prev Med 2001;20(2S):16–66.

149. U.S. Preventive Services Task Force. Guide to clinical preventive services: report of the U.S. Preventive Services Task Force. 2nd ed. Baltimore: Williams & Wilkins, 1996.

150. Nowjack-Raymer RE, Gift HC. Use of mouthguards and headgear in organized sports by school-aged children. Public Health Rep 1996;3:82–6.

151. Ranalli DN. Prevention of sports-related traumatic dental injuries. Dent Clin North Am 2000;44(1):35–51.

152. Centers for Disease Control and Prevention. Promoting oral health: interventions for preventing dental caries, oral and pharyngeal cancers, and sports-related craniofacial injuries. MMWR 2001;50(RR-21):1–13.

153. Task Force on Community Preventive Services. Recommendations on selected interventions to prevent dental caries, oral and pharyngeal cancers, and sports-related craniofacial injuries. Am J Prev Med 2002;23(1S):16–20.

Chapter 8

Motor Vehicle Occupant Injury

*Insufficient evidence means that we were not able to determine whether or not the intervention works.

The Task Force approved the recommendations in this chapter in 1998 (child safety seats), 2000 (safety belts), and 2000–2002 (alcohol-impaired driving). The research on which the findings are based was conducted between 1966 and March 1998 (child safety seats); 1966–June 2000 (safety belts; alcohol-impaired driving; and 1966–December 2001 (mass media campaigns). This information has been previously published in the American Journal of Preventive Medicine [2001;21(4S):16–22, 23–30, 31–47, 48–65, 66–88; and 2004;27(1):57–65, 66] and the MMWR Recommendations and Reports series [2001; 50(no. RR-7):1–13]. No updates have been issued since journal publication.

Motor vehicle–related injuries are the leading cause of death among children and young adults in the United States[1,2] and the leading cause of death from unintentional injury for people of all ages.[2,3] More than 41,000 people in the United States die in motor vehicle crashes each year,[4] and another 3.5 million people sustain nonfatal injuries.[1] Crash injuries result in about 290,000 hospitalizations and 3.4 million emergency department visits annually.[2]

Viewed from a purely economic perspective, the societal burden of crash injuries and deaths is tremendous. Motor vehicle–related deaths and injuries cost the United States more than $230 billion annually, including $59 billion in property damage, $61 billion in lost productivity, and $33 billion in medical expenses.[5] Alcohol-related crashes contribute substantially to these costs, with a direct economic impact of about $51 billion in 2000 alone.[5]

Reduction of motor vehicle injuries remains a formidable public health challenge, despite sharp declines in motor vehicle–related death rates since 1925.[6] Three of the most important preventive measures to further reduce motor vehicle occupant injuries and deaths are use of child safety seats, use of safety belts, and deterrence of alcohol-impaired driving.[7,8]

This chapter provides recommendations on interventions to increase use of child safety seats, to increase use of safety belts, and to reduce alcohol-impaired driving. These areas were chosen because (1) use of child safety seats and safety belts are below national goals;[9] (2) 55% of traffic deaths are among motor vehicle occupants who were not properly restrained;[4] and (3) 41% of traffic deaths involve alcohol.[4] In addition, these three behaviors are modifiable risk factors that can be addressed using a variety of intervention strategies. Thus, reducing these three risk behaviors could dramatically reduce injuries to motor vehicle occupants.

OBJECTIVES AND RECOMMENDATIONS FROM OTHER ADVISORY GROUPS

The interventions recommended by the Task Force can be used to achieve objectives set out in *Healthy People 2010*[9] and by the National Highway Traffic Safety Administration (NHTSA; Table 8–1). In addition, the recommendations complement and add to information published by other groups. For example, the U.S. Preventive Services Task Force recommends counseling individual patients (including adults and parents of young children) to use occupant restraints (lap-shoulder safety belts and child safety seats), to wear helmets when riding motorcycles, and to refrain from driving while under the influence of alcohol or other drugs.[12] The American Academy of Pediatrics[13,14] (AAP; www.aap.org) suggests ways for pediatricians to implement office-based injury prevention counseling through The Injury Prevention Program (TIPP). The National Center for Injury Prevention and Control (Centers for Disease Control and Prevention; www.cdc.gov/ncipc/) makes recommenda-

Table 8-1. Selected *Healthy People 2010*[9] Objectives and NHTSA*
Goals Related to Motor Vehicle Occupant Injury

Healthy People 2010 Objective	*NHTSA Goal*
General	
Reduce deaths caused by motor vehicle crashes from 15.0 per 100,000 persons (1998 preliminary data, age adjusted to the year 2000 standard population) to 9.0 (Objective 15–15a)	Reduce the number of fatal and non-fatal injuries to no more than 1.0/100,000,000 vehicle miles traveled by 2008 (from 1.7 in 1996)[10]
Reduce deaths from 2 per 100 million vehicle miles traveled (in 1997) to 1 (15–15b)	
Reduce nonfatal injuries caused by motor vehicle crashes from 1270 per 100,000 persons (in 1997) to 1000 (21% improvement) (15–17)	
Child Safety Seat Use	
Increase use of child restraint devices for passengers up to 4 years of age from 92% (1998 preliminary data) to 100% (15–20)	Reduce child occupant fatalities (0–4 years) by 25% by 2005 (from 653 fatalities in 1996)[11]
Safety Belt Use	
Increase use of safety belts from 69% (in 1998) to 92% (33% improvement) (15–19)	Increase national seat belt use to 79% by 2004 (from 73% in 2001)[10]
Alcohol-Impaired Driving	
Reduce deaths caused by alcohol-related motor vehicle crashes from 6.1 per 100,000 persons (1997 baseline) to 4 per 100,000 (26–1a)	Reduce alcohol-related fatalities to no more than 0.53/100 million vehicle miles traveled by 2004 (from 0.63 in 2001)[10]
Reduce injuries caused by alcohol-related motor vehicle crashes from 122 per 100,000 persons (1997 baseline) to 65 per 100,000 (26–1b)	
Reduce the proportion of adolescents who report that they rode, during the previous 30 days, with a driver who had been drinking alcohol from 37% (in 1997) to 30% (26–6)	
Extend administrative license revocation laws, or programs of equal effectiveness, for persons who drive under the influence of intoxicants from 41 states (in 1998) to all states and the District of Columbia (26–24)	
Extend legal requirement for maximum blood alcohol concentration levels of 0.08% for motor vehicle drivers aged 21 years and older from 16 states (in 1998) to all states and the District of Columbia (26–25)	

*NHTSA: National Highway Traffic Safety Administration, U.S. Department of Transportation.

Reprinted from Am J Prev Med, Vol. 21, No. 4S, Task Force on Community Preventive Services, Recommendations to reduce injuries to motor vehicle occupants: increasing child safety seat use, increasing safety belt use, and reducing alcohol-impaired driving, p. 17, Copyright 2001, with permission from American Journal of Preventive Medicine.

tions through the MMWR (Morbidity and Mortality Weekly Report; www.cdc
.gov/mmwr/) on child safety seats, safety belts, and alcohol-impaired driving.
Recommendations are also available from NHTSA[15] (www.nhtsa.dot.gov),
the National Transportation Safety Board[16] (www.ntsb.gov), the American
Medical Association (www.ama-assn.org),[17] and the Department of Health
and Human Services (HHS; www.dhhs.gov).[9]

METHODS

Methods used for the reviews are summarized in Chapter 10. Specific methods used in the systematic reviews of motor vehicle occupant injury have been
described elsewhere[18] and are also available at www.thecommunityguide.org/
mvoi. Figure 8–1 depicts the conceptual framework used in these reviews.

ECONOMIC EFFICIENCY

A systematic review of economic evaluations was conducted for all recommended interventions, and a summary of each review is presented with the
related intervention. The methods used to conduct these economics reviews
are summarized in Chapter 11.

RECOMMENDATIONS AND FINDINGS

This section presents a summary of the findings of the systematic reviews conducted to determine the effectiveness of the selected interventions in this topic
area. Interventions are grouped into three categories: increasing child safety
seat use, increasing safety belt use, and reducing alcohol-impaired driving.

Increasing Child Safety Seat Use

For children up to four years of age, correctly installed child safety seats reduce injury-related hospitalization by 69%,[19] and they reduce the risk of death
by 70% for infants and by 47%-54% for toddlers (aged 1–4 years).[20] If all
children in this age group rode in safety seats, an additional 138 lives could
be saved each year and 20,000 injuries could be prevented.[4,21]

Nearly 30% of children under the age of four do not ride in a proper child
restraint, and are therefore at twice the risk of fatal and nonfatal injuries of
those riding restrained.[4,22,23] Of those children riding in safety seats, approximately 85% are improperly restrained.[24] Seating position imposes an additional risk factor: in passenger vehicles, children aged 12 years and younger
are 36% less likely to die in a crash if seated in the back seat.[25]

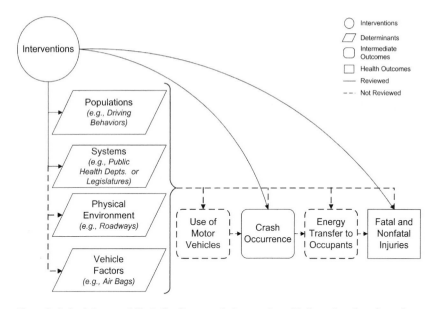

Figure 8–1. Logic framework illustrating the conceptual approach used in the systematic reviews of interventions to reduce injury to motor vehicle occupants. (Reprinted from Am J Prev Med, Vol. 21, No. 4S, Zaza S et al., Methods for conducting systematic reviews of the evidence of effectiveness and economic efficiency of interventions to reduce injuries to motor vehicle occupants, p. 25, Copyright 2001, with permission from American Journal of Preventive Medicine.)

Some groups of children are at greater risk than others. Child safety seat ownership and use are lower among rural populations and low-income families.[23,26-28] Although these families may not be able to afford safety seats, it may well be worthwhile to provide them for free or at a reduced cost, as 95% of low-income families who have safety seats use them.[21,29-31]

This chapter does not look at children who are too old or large to sit in child safety seats but who are too small to wear safety belts without the use of booster seats (generally children aged four to eight years).[32] Future updates of these reviews and recommendations should address this vulnerable population. Many of the studies reviewed were conducted when rates of child safety seat use were much lower than they are at present. Based on patterns observed with interventions to increase safety belt use, increased baseline usage rates could cause the effects of child safety seat interventions conducted in the future to be smaller than those reported in these reviews.[33]

Child Safety Seat Laws: Recommended (Strong Evidence of Effectiveness)

Child safety seat laws require children traveling in motor vehicles to be buckled into federally approved infant or child safety seats that are appropriate for the child's age and size. All states currently have child safety seat laws in place. The laws, which vary from state to state, specify the children they cover in terms of age, height, weight, or a combination of these factors.

Effectiveness

- Child safety seat laws are effective in reducing fatal injuries to children by approximately 35%.
- These laws are also effective in reducing all injuries to children by approximately 17%.
- These laws are also effective in increasing child safety seat use by approximately 13 percentage points.

Applicability

- These findings should be generally applicable in all U.S. communities.

The findings of our systematic review of child safety seat laws are based on nine studies evaluating the effectiveness of child safety seat laws that went into effect between 1978 and 1986 in the 50 states.[34-42] An additional 14 studies were identified but did not meet our quality criteria and were excluded from the review.[43-56] Two additional reports provided information on a study already included in our review.[57,58] All the laws allow for primary enforcement, which means that a driver can be stopped, cited, or fined simply for not restraining child passengers properly. The laws apply to children of various ages: some apply to children up to one year old and others apply to children up to five years old. Most laws do not specify a seating position, although one law applies only to children in the front seat. The various laws allow for penalties ranging from an oral warning to a $25 fine. No studies in this review examined other activities related to child safety seat laws, such as programs to lend seats to low-income families, levels of enforcement, or publicity about the law.

Child safety seat laws led to a 35% decrease in fatal injuries (range, 25.0% to 57.3%) and a 17.3% decrease in any type of injury (range, 10.5% to 35.9%). They also led to a 13 percentage point increase in child safety seat use (range, 5.0 to 35.0). The effect was the same for children of all ages covered by the law. Not enough information was available to determine how the other requirements of the laws (such as seating position or penalties) affect injury rates. These results show that child safety seat laws are effective in decreasing both fatal and nonfatal injuries and in increasing the use of the safety seats.

The results of these studies should be applicable to most child passengers in the United States. However, more specific information on applicability is not available because none of the studies looked at age, sex, race, socioeconomic status, or regional differences within states.

We did not find any other positive or negative effects of child safety seat laws, nor did we find any economic evaluations.

One barrier to strengthening or enhancing enforcement of these laws may be resistance to such changes by people who believe that the laws limit parental discretion.

In conclusion, the Task Force recommends maintaining or implementing child safety seat laws on the basis of strong evidence of their effectiveness in reducing injuries to children and increasing safety seat use. The findings of this review should be applicable in most communities in the United States.

Distribution and Education Programs: Recommended (Strong Evidence of Effectiveness)

Distribution and education programs provide free or low-cost child safety seats to parents, along with education about proper use of the seats. The idea behind such programs is that parents who cannot afford a safety seat or who have a poor understanding of the importance of the seat might be more likely to use it if they receive financial help in acquiring a safety seat and learn about the importance of using it.

Effectiveness

- Safety seat distribution and education programs are effective in reducing injuries by approximately 6%.
- These programs are also effective in increasing rates of correct child safety seat use by approximately 23 percentage points.
- The programs are also effective in increasing possession of child safety seats by approximately 51 percentage points.

Applicability

- These findings should be generally applicable across a range of settings and populations.

Other Effects

- A potential harm exists. The safety of seats that have been involved in crashes cannot be guaranteed, and such seats should be discarded. Programs must use new, not refurbished, seats and ensure that loaner seats that have been involved in crashes are discarded.

The findings of our systematic review of distribution and education programs are based on 10 studies that evaluated programs providing free loaner child safety seats, low-cost rentals, or direct giveaways to parents.[31,59–67] An additional seven studies were identified but did not meet our quality criteria and were excluded from the review.[29,68–73] The programs reviewed also gave parents information on how to use the seats correctly. This educational component varied considerably across programs in terms of content, length, intensity, and type of teaching method. Some programs simply provided lectures, brochures, or pamphlets on how to use the safety seat, whereas others used more active educational and behavioral techniques, such as discussions, problem solving, demonstrations, or rehearsal of correct use. These programs primarily focused on parents of infants rather than older children.

One program showed a relative decrease of 6.4% in fatal and nonfatal injuries of children up to age four. Measurements taken at the end of each of the 10 programs showed improvements in the correct use of child safety seats (median 22.6 percentage point increase; interquartile range, 4.0 to 62.3). Three programs also assessed safety seat use a second time, within a year of the first assessment, and found that the median increase had dropped to 6 percentage points (range, 2.1 decrease to 7.0 increase). In five studies, possession of child safety seats increased by 51 percentage points (range, 16.0 to 93.0). These results show that combining child safety seat distribution programs with education is effective in reducing injuries and in increasing both possession of safety seats and the proper use of those seats.

These results should be applicable to families of any socioeconomic status and ethnic background across the United States. The programs were effective in a variety of settings, including hospitals and clinics, as part of postnatal home visitation, and when provided by an automobile insurance company. However, only three reports described the effectiveness of such programs for children older than nine months.

These programs have a potential negative effect. By increasing the number of people with safety seats, the programs might also increase improper use of safety seats, particularly among new users. Intensive education and practice on proper use of safety seats, which were carried out in most of the studies included in this review, are important components of this intervention that guard against this potential misuse.

Warning: Programs that lend or give away safety seats must use new seats, not refurbished ones. The safety of seats that have been involved in crashes and then refurbished cannot be guaranteed, and such seats should be discarded.

We found economic evaluations of these programs, but none of them met our quality criteria. We did not, therefore, report results of these economic evaluations.

Potential barriers to implementation of child safety seat distribution and education programs include liability, the initial expense of purchasing seats, storage of seats, and training of personnel to provide education and distribute the seats. In addition, some child safety seats might be incompatible with certain vehicles.

In conclusion, the Task Force recommends programs that distribute child safety seats and educate recipients about proper use of the seats on the basis of strong evidence of effectiveness in (*1*) reducing injuries to infants and young children who are passengers in vehicles and (*2*) increasing both possession and correct use of safety seats. These findings should be applicable to most young child passengers (birth to age four) in the United States. Only new safety seats, not used or refurbished ones, should be distributed, because the safety of seats previously involved in crashes cannot be guaranteed.

Community-Wide Information and Enhanced Enforcement Campaigns: Recommended (Sufficient Evidence of Effectiveness)

Community-wide information and enhanced enforcement campaigns provide information about child safety seats and child automobile safety to an entire community (usually defined geographically). These campaigns use several approaches: mass media, publicity, safety seat displays in public places, and special law enforcement strategies, such as checkpoints, dedicated law enforcement officials, or alternative penalties (e.g., warnings instead of tickets).

Effectiveness

- These campaigns are effective in increasing child safety seat use by approximately 12 percentage points.

Applicability

- Our findings should be generally applicable in a variety of settings and populations, including populations of mixed socioeconomic status.

The findings of our systematic review are based on four studies that evaluated the effectiveness of community-wide information and enhanced enforcement campaigns.[74-77] An additional 10 studies were identified but did not meet our quality criteria and were excluded from the review.[78-87] We looked at campaigns that provided information on the importance and correct use of child safety seats through paid advertisements, public service announcements, commentaries by community leaders on local television and radio programs, newspaper articles and editorials, displays of safety seats in public locations, and direct mailings. In three studies conducted in states with existing child safety seat laws, the campaigns also incorporated special enforcement components, such as traffic checkpoints, assignment of law enforcement officers dedicated to enforcing the safety seat use law, and alternative penalties in place of citations (for example, informational warnings or vouchers to waive fines if a safety seat is purchased). The campaigns were conducted in cities, suburbs, and statewide. Numerous community organizations and government agencies—such as public safety and public health offices, schools, advocacy organizations, and parent groups—worked together to design and implement the campaigns.

In the four studies, a median 12.3 percentage point increase in safety seat use (range, 3.8 to 20.8) was measured from one to six months after the intervention began. Among campaigns that also included an enhanced law enforcement component, the two that used publicity to highlight the enhanced enforcement showed greater increases in safety seat use (20.8 and 13.1 percentage points) than the study that did not use publicity (4.4 percentage points). These results show that the combination of community-wide information campaigns and enhanced enforcement of safety seat laws is effective in increasing the use of child safety seats.

These results should be applicable to most communities in the United States, including those of mixed socioeconomic status. The studies were conducted in the United States, Canada, and Australia and involved populations at all socioeconomic levels. The campaigns were directed at parents of children from birth to 11 years of age. Two statewide campaigns most likely included urban, suburban, and rural populations, although this was not specified. None of the studies reported the racial or ethnic makeup of the study population.

Additional positive effects of enhanced enforcement may include increased detection and arrest for alcohol-impaired driving and other offenses and increased awareness of the importance of restraining child passengers. We did not find any negative effects.

We did not find any economic evaluations of the effects of these campaigns.

Although we hypothesized several barriers to implementing community-wide information and enhanced enforcement campaigns, we did not find any reported in the literature. Potential barriers could be the costs of developing and disseminating public information and educational material; airing television and radio announcements; enlisting the support and cooperation of the media, police departments, and other community leaders; and training enforcement personnel about the importance of enforcing child-restraint device laws. Another barrier might be the burden on court systems that need to handle additional offenders.

In conclusion, the Task Force recommends community-wide information combined with enhanced enforcement campaigns on the basis of sufficient evidence of effectiveness in increasing the use of child safety seats. The findings of this review should be applicable to most parents of children covered by child safety seat laws.

Incentive and Education Programs: Recommended (Sufficient Evidence of Effectiveness)

Incentive and education programs reward parents for obtaining and correctly using child safety seats or directly reward children for correctly using safety seats. These programs also include educational components of varying intensity.

Effectiveness

- These programs are effective in increasing child safety seat use in the short term (up to five months after the intervention) by approximately 10%.

Applicability

- Our findings should be generally applicable to a variety of populations and settings using a variety of rewards.

The findings of our systematic review are based on four studies.[88-91] One additional study was identified but did not meet our quality criteria and was excluded from the review.[92] In these studies, the rewards—ranging from inexpensive trinkets, stickers, or coupons for fast food meals or movies to relatively expensive prizes donated by community merchants—were distributed constantly over program periods ranging from one to five months. Parents had to show correct use of safety seats to receive rewards. In all programs, larger rewards were provided to randomly selected eligible participants. Some programs also gave smaller rewards to all eligible participants.

The programs all included educational components of varying intensity. Some programs simply provided information about the reward program itself, whereas others provided information about existing laws on safety seat use and the importance of using safety seats. The programs also varied in *how* they provided information: some used only brochures or other printed materials; others used more interactive educational and behavioral techniques, such as supervised practice of correct safety seat use, signed pledge cards, and educational videos.

Before they participated in these programs, parents and caregivers had low rates of safety seat use (median, 25.9%; range, 11.4% to 48.0%). The effectiveness of these programs in the short term was demonstrated by the increased use of safety seats (median 9.9 percentage points, range, 4.8 to 36.0) up to 4.5 months after the intervention. No studies in the review reported longer follow-up times.

These results should be applicable to a variety of populations and settings using a variety of rewards. Incentive and education programs were implemented in day care centers and as community-wide efforts in a variety of target populations (including parents of children of varying ages, all socio-economic groups, urban and rural populations, white and African-American populations), all showing similar increases in safety seat use.

A potential (but unmeasured) benefit might be that parents introduced to safety seats through these programs will continue to use them after the program has ended. We did not find any negative effects of these programs. None of the identified studies measured improper use of safety seats as a result of incentive and education programs.

We did not find any economic evaluations of these programs.

We did not identify any barriers to implementation of incentive and education programs. Potential barriers might include the costs of purchasing incentive rewards, training personnel to provide the education component, and garnering the support and participation of schools, day care centers, and other sites.

In conclusion, the Task Force recommends the combination of incentive and education programs on the basis of sufficient evidence that these programs increase use of child safety seats in the short term (up to five months). These findings should be applicable to most parents of young children in the United States.

Education Programs When Used Alone: Insufficient Evidence to Determine Effectiveness

Education programs provide information to parents, children, or professional groups about the importance of child safety seats and how to use them properly. A goal of providing information is to give people a cognitive foundation for behavior change and for instituting new policies.

This review excluded any child safety seat education programs delivered solely through one-on-one counseling of a patient by a primary care clinician. Those interventions have been reviewed and recommended in the *Guide to Clinical Preventive Services.*[12]

Effectiveness

- We found insufficient evidence to determine the effectiveness of education programs alone in increasing correct use of child safety seats.
- Evidence was insufficient because the educational interventions evaluated in these studies varied widely and the small number of available studies produced inconsistent results.

- Insufficient evidence means that we were not able to determine whether or not the intervention works.

The results of our systematic review are based on six studies that provided education to three different populations: parents, children, and professionals.[93-98] Ten additional studies were identified but did not meet our quality criteria and were excluded from the review.[47,99-107] Of the six studies reviewed, three that provided education to parents during the perinatal period found no evidence that perinatal programs increase correct use of safety seats. Parent education consisted of such activities and materials as a mock-up for practice with use of car safety seats, printed instructions or guidelines for new mothers, posters identifying safe versus unsafe seats, and a video from the Insurance Institute for Highway Safety about infants and children in crashes. One program providing education to children in a day care center increased knowledge about correct safety seat use but did not increase actual use. The education, a modified version of the "Riding with Bucklebear" program, used a real car seat and seat belts, a toy car with seat belts and a child safety seat, family figures represented by dolls, and pictures of desirable and undesirable behavior for riding in cars. Children learned songs about auto safety, watched a video, had brief lessons about safety, and played with Bucklebear. Training for police officers resulted in an increase in the number of citations issued for failure to use safety seats (from 0–10 to 10–20 per month) six months after the training period. Training for nursing or obstetrical directors in hospitals that offer newborn delivery services produced significant increases in the proportion of hospitals with written safety seat policies for newborns (62.3 percentage points higher than the baseline of 25.9%), hospitals with short-term loan programs for child safety seats (14.1 percentage point increase over a baseline of 58.8%), and hospitals with patient education programs (44.1 percentage point increase over a baseline of 51.2%). The variety of approaches used, the small number of studies of each approach, and the inconsistent improvement in correct use of child safety seats provided insufficient evidence to determine the effectiveness of this intervention.

Because we could not establish the effectiveness of these programs when used alone, we did not examine situations in which the programs would be applicable, information about economic efficiency, or possible barriers to implementation.

In conclusion, although education is a central component of many other interventions, the Task Force found insufficient evidence to determine the effectiveness of education programs alone in increasing proper use of child safety seats, because the small number of studies produced inconsistent results.

INCREASING SAFETY BELT USE

The use of safety belts is the single most effective means of reducing fatal and nonfatal injuries in motor vehicle crashes. Safety belt use is estimated to have saved 164,753 lives between 1975 and 2002.[108] In all types of crashes, manual lap-shoulder belts are approximately 45% effective in reducing fatalities in passenger cars and 60% effective in light trucks.[109,110] They are estimated to reduce the risk of serious injury to the head, chest, and extremities by 50% to 83%.[110] Lap belts alone are estimated to be 17% to 58% effective in preventing death in various seating positions compared with no restraints.[111-113]

Although safety belt use has risen dramatically in the United States over the past two decades, further increases in use remain a public health priority.[6,9,114] In 1983, only 14% of motor vehicle occupants wore safety belts.[115] That percentage rose to 51% by 1994, 69% by 1998, and 75% by 2002.[108] However, certain groups (e.g., teenagers, drinking drivers) consistently report lower than average usage rates.[116-119]

Airbags, although widely available, are considered only supplemental protection to safety belts. Airbags alone are 10% and 14% effective in reducing deaths and injuries, respectively, whereas airbags used with lap-shoulder belts reduce the risk of death by 50% and injury by 66% in front seats.[110]

Safety Belt Laws: Recommended (Strong Evidence of Effectiveness)

Safety belt laws—a critical component of efforts to increase safety belt use—require motor vehicle occupants to use safety belts. All current U.S. safety belt laws cover use by front seat occupants; other provisions, such as rear seat coverage, fines, affected age groups, type of enforcement, and exempted vehicles and drivers, vary by state. Every state except New Hampshire has some form of safety belt law.

Effectiveness

- Safety belt laws are effective in reducing fatal and nonfatal injuries by approximately 8%.
- These laws are also effective in increasing observed safety belt use by approximately 33 percentage points.
- These laws are also effective in increasing self-reported safety belt use by approximately 16 percentage points.

Applicability

- These findings should be generally applicable to adolescents and adults.

Other Effects

- Adults who use safety belts are also more likely to buckle up their child passengers.
- We found no evidence that drivers who use safety belts may be more likely to engage in risky driving behavior.

The findings of our systematic review of safety belt laws are based on 33 studies.[120-152] An additional 11 studies were identified but did not meet our quality criteria and were excluded from the review.[153-163] Two additional studies provided information on a study already included in our review.[164,165] The studies in the review showed that enactment of safety belt laws consistently increased safety belt use, whether use was self-reported (median 16 percentage point increase; range, 13 to 19) or observed (median 33 percentage point increase; interquartile range, 20 to 36). The research also showed that safety belt laws decrease fatal and nonfatal injuries by a median of 8% (interquartile range, 3% to 20%). After the systematic review had been completed, we found eight additional studies.[166-173] Although they were not included in the review, our preliminary analysis revealed that all eight studies also found that safety belt laws were effective.

These results should be applicable to adolescents and adults, as most of the studies looked at motor vehicle occupants who were at least 16 years old. Some studies looked at specific groups. Women consistently showed greater increases in safety belt use than men and usually began with higher usage rates. Older drivers also showed higher use rates. Adolescents had low use rates to begin with, but showed increases in safety belt use proportional to increases seen in other drivers after laws were enacted.

An additional benefit of safety belt laws is that adults who use safety belts are more likely to buckle up their child passengers. One study reported that a law mandating safety belt use in the front seat increased use by children aged 2–10 years in all seating positions within the vehicle.[142]

The decrease in fatal and nonfatal injuries associated with increased safety belt use is not as large as might be expected given the known effectiveness of safety belts in decreasing the risk of injury and death.[174,175] One explanation offered for this, and thus a potential negative effect of safety belt laws, is the concept of *risk compensation*,[176-178] which suggests that individuals compensate for reduced risk by acting more recklessly. According to this concept, when drivers wear safety belts they feel safer and will engage in more risky driving behaviors than they otherwise would. However, several studies[175,179,180] that looked at whether injury reductions associated with safety belt use are offset by injury increases associated with risky driving produced inconclusive results. In addition, no study has found a relationship between increased safety belt use and increased risky driving.[181-183] Thus, the concept that safety belt laws increase risky driving, thereby increasing crash or injury risks, is not supported by the available evidence.

We did not find any economic evaluations of the effects of these laws.

As with many legislative interventions, public opposition and the political climate are potential barriers to effective implementation. When states first began enacting safety belt laws, it was commonly argued that these laws interfered with personal freedom. However, NHTSA's 2000 Motor Vehicle Occupant Survey reported that 87% of individuals over the age of 16 support safety belt laws, with 67% supporting them "strongly" and 20% supporting them "somewhat."[118]

In conclusion, the Task Force recommends maintaining or implementing safety belt laws on the basis of strong evidence of their effectiveness in reducing fatal and nonfatal injuries and increasing both observed and self-reported safety belt use. These findings should be applicable to adolescents and adults in the United States.

Primary Enforcement Laws (vs. Secondary Enforcement Laws): Recommended (Strong Evidence of Effectiveness)

Primary enforcement laws allow police officers to stop a motorist solely for not wearing a safety belt. In contrast, secondary enforcement laws only allow a police officer to issue a safety belt citation after the motorist is stopped for another reason.

Although common in Europe, Great Britain, New Zealand, and Australia, primary enforcement laws are the exception, not the rule, in the United States. As of December 31, 2003, only 20 states, the District of Columbia, and Puerto Rico had enacted primary enforcement laws. Primary laws are thought to be more effective in getting drivers to buckle up. Police officers are more likely to write tickets if the law is primary. In addition to the greater freedom that officers have to enforce primary laws, they may also believe that such laws indicate that legislators, judges, and the general public view safety belt use as important. Therefore, primary laws are likely to generate stronger concerns among drivers that they will be caught and punished if they break the law.

Effectiveness (relative to secondary enforcement safety belt laws)

- Primary enforcement laws are effective in decreasing fatal injuries by approximately 8%.

- These laws are also effective in increasing observed safety belt use by approximately 14 percentage points.

Applicability

- These findings should be applicable to all U.S. drivers and passengers.

Other Effects

- We found no evidence that primary safety belt laws contribute to differential enforcement based on race, although this has been proposed as a potential harm.

For this systematic review, we included only studies that compared the effects of primary laws with those of secondary laws in the United States. The results of the review are based on 13 studies (in 12 reports), of which 9 compared states with primary laws to states with secondary laws and 4 evaluated the effect of changing from a primary law to a secondary law.[116,129,130,147,149,152,175,184–188] An additional two studies were identified but did not meet our quality criteria and were excluded from the review.[160,162] Five other studies provided information on studies already included in the review.[117,164,189–191] Primary laws were found to decrease fatal injuries (five studies: median 8% decrease; range, 3% to 14%); increase observed safety belt use (five studies: median increase of 14 percentage points; range, 12 to 23); and increase self-reported safety belt use (two studies: 1 and 22 percentage point increases).

These results should be applicable to all U.S. motorists. Studies were conducted in 49 states and the District of Columbia and looked at drivers and passengers of all ages.

According to one study,[187] when a primary enforcement law is passed, those who drive while intoxicated show a greater increase in safety belt use than other drivers. Two studies[116,147] also showed that passage of primary enforcement laws increased use among African-American and Hispanic populations more than it did among whites.

An additional benefit of safety belt laws is that adults who use safety belts are more likely to buckle up their child passengers (see Safety Belt Laws). One possible negative effect of primary safety belt laws is the potential for enforcement officers to stop drivers based purely on race or ethnicity. However, studies examining the issue have found no evidence that primary belt laws contribute to such differential enforcement or *racial profiling*.[116,188]

We did not find any economic evaluations of the effects of primary safety belt laws.

Perceived public opposition to primary safety belt laws presents a serious barrier to their implementation. Infringement on personal freedom and the potential for differential enforcement are the most frequently voiced concerns. To increase public acceptance, some states have included anti-harassment language in their primary safety belt laws.

Public support for primary safety belt laws appears to be strong. In 2000, 61% of the American public favored primary enforcement laws (in states with these laws, 70% supported them; in states with secondary laws, 53% supported primary laws).[118]

In conclusion, the Task Force recommends primary enforcement laws on the basis of strong evidence of their effectiveness in decreasing fatal injuries and increasing safety belt use. These findings should be applicable to all drivers in the United States.

Enhanced Enforcement: Recommended (Strong Evidence of Effectiveness)

Enhanced enforcement of safety belt laws can involve increasing the number of officers on patrol, increasing the number of citations issued for safety belt violations during regular patrols, conducting safety belt checkpoints, or a combination of these efforts. These programs are conducted in addition to normal enforcement practices and are usually publicized through media campaigns.

Enhanced enforcement programs are designed to increase public awareness of safety belt laws and the enforcement of these laws. Such heightened awareness is expected to increase the perceived risk of being detected and punished for failing to wear a safety belt, and thereby increase safety belt use and reduce injuries and deaths. Both the level of publicity and the visibility of enforcement may influence motorists' behavior and their perception of risks.

Enhanced enforcement programs are either intense efforts of short duration (called *waves* or *blitzes*) lasting for days or weeks, which may be repeated periodically, or maintenance of continuous enforcement levels over several weeks, months, or years. Enhanced enforcement programs are often referred to as *Selective Traffic Enforcement Programs* (STEPs) or *Special Traffic Enforcement Programs* (sTEPs).[192]

This review focused on enhanced enforcement programs that specifically targeted safety belt use and excluded studies of programs targeting multiple unsafe driving practices.

Effectiveness

- Enhanced enforcement is effective in decreasing both fatal and nonfatal injuries (by 7% and 15% in two studies).
- This activity is also effective in increasing observed safety belt use by approximately 16 percentage points.

Applicability

- These findings should be generally applicable to all U.S. motorists covered by safety belt laws.

Other Effects

- Enhanced enforcement may lead to increased arrests for other crimes, such as possession of weapons or drugs, impaired driving, or license violations.

The findings of our systematic review are based on 15 studies that looked at the effect of enhanced enforcement on fatal and nonfatal injuries and on safety belt use.[193-207] An additional two studies were identified but did not meet our quality criteria and were excluded from the review.[208,209] One additional study provided information on a study already included in our review.[210] Two studies that looked at fatal and nonfatal injuries combined found relative decreases of 7% and 15%, respectively, from enhanced enforcement programs. These programs also increased safety belt use by a median of 16 percentage points (interquartile range, 8 to 24). Increases in safety belt use were similar whether the program increased the number of officers on patrol or increased citations during regular patrols.

As for long-term effects, in the 11 programs that collected follow-up data, safety belt use decreased by a median of 6 percentage points (interquartile range, 0 to 8) in the months after enhanced enforcement programs ended, but still consistently remained higher than before the programs took place.

Overall, these findings show that enhanced enforcement is effective both in increasing the use of safety belts and in decreasing fatal and nonfatal injuries.

These results should be applicable to all U.S. motorists covered by safety belt laws. We reviewed a variety of enhanced enforcement programs in the United States and Canada, including city, county, state, provincial, and national programs. These programs varied in the amount of publicity they used, and were conducted both in states with primary safety belt laws and those with secondary laws. The programs may be less effective in urban areas. Studies in the United States that evaluated results by population density found greater increases in safety belt use in suburban and rural areas than in urban areas.

An additional positive effect of enhanced enforcement of safety belt laws is that it may lead to increased arrests for other crimes such as impaired driving, possession of weapons or drugs, or license violations. We did not identify any negative effects of enhanced enforcement programs.

We did not find any economic evaluations of enhanced enforcement programs.

One potential barrier to implementation of enhanced enforcement programs is the reluctance of state and community officials to implement such programs because of concerns about public opposition. However, two statewide telephone surveys conducted in California and North Carolina during such programs found that 70% and 87% of respondents, respectively, were in favor of enhanced enforcement programs to increase safety belt use. Another potential barrier is that police officers may be reluctant to participate in enhanced enforcement programs out of concern that they will be diverted from investigating more serious crimes. However, one study found that crime rates do not increase during enhanced enforcement campaigns. Additionally, interviews with both police and the public have revealed increasingly positive attitudes toward enhanced enforcement programs.[211]

In conclusion, the Task Force recommends enhanced enforcement of safety belt laws on the basis of strong evidence of their effectiveness in decreasing fatal and nonfatal injuries and in increasing observed safety belt use. These findings should be applicable to all motorists in the United States who are covered by safety belt laws.

REDUCING ALCOHOL-IMPAIRED DRIVING

The United States has made substantial progress in reducing alcohol-related traffic fatalities in recent decades. Since NHTSA began keeping records on alcohol involvement in fatal crashes in 1982, the proportion of alcohol-related traffic fatalities has declined from 57% to 41%.[4] Despite this progress, alcohol-related motor vehicle crashes continue to be a major public health problem, resulting in 17,448 deaths and 275,000 injuries in 2001.[4]

Since 1970, individual states and communities have used various approaches to reducing alcohol-impaired driving, most commonly laws to deter alcohol-impaired driving or to control the sale or public consumption of alcohol. By 1987, the minimum legal drinking age was 21 years in all states. As of July 12, 2004, 50 states, the District of Columbia, and Puerto Rico had lowered the illegal blood alcohol concentration (BAC) for drivers aged 21 years and older from 0.10 g/dL (grams per deciliter) to 0.08 g/dL (0.08%). Some states have also used sobriety checkpoints, enhanced enforcement of alcohol control policies, and training programs for servers of alcoholic beverages.

These systematic reviews looked at the effectiveness of laws and other community-based interventions in reducing alcohol-impaired driving and alcohol-related motor vehicle deaths. Of the 84 studies included in the reviews 59 were conducted in the United States and the remainder were conducted in Australia, Canada, New Zealand, France, and the Netherlands.

The review focused on interventions for which the primary goal is to reduce alcohol-impaired driving. Interventions intended to restrict access to alcohol (e.g., alcohol taxation, alcohol outlet zoning restrictions) or to address health outcomes of alcohol abuse or misuse other than alcohol-impaired driving were not reviewed. These topics may be included in a subsequent *Community Guide* review of interventions to prevent alcohol abuse and misuse.

The effectiveness of interventions to reduce alcohol-impaired driving may lie in their ability to increase drivers' perceived risk of detection and punishment, to reduce alcohol consumption in high-risk settings or among high-risk groups, and to foster a social norm in which drinking and driving is unacceptable.

0.08% Blood Alcohol Concentration Laws: Recommended (Strong Evidence of Effectiveness)

All U.S. states have long-standing laws prohibiting driving while impaired by alcohol. In 49 states, it is also illegal to operate a motor vehicle with a blood alcohol concentration (BAC) above a specified limit, regardless of whether the operator is visibly impaired. Originally, a BAC of 0.10% or 0.15% was considered illegal, but all states have since lowered the limit. At a BAC of 0.08%, all drivers are expected to experience impairment in driving-related skills.[212] In support of 0.08% BAC laws, the U.S. Congress included a provision in the Fiscal Year 2001 Department of Transportation and Related Agencies Appropriations Act[213] requiring states to implement 0.08% BAC laws by October 1, 2003, or risk losing federal highway construction funds. By that date, 45 states, the District of Columbia, and Puerto Rico had enacted laws lowering the illegal BAC to 0.08%. This review evaluates the effects of lowering the BAC limit from 0.10% to 0.08%.

The illegal BAC for drivers under the minimum legal drinking age of 21 is even lower. As of July 1998, all states had enacted laws for drivers up to 20 years old that establish BAC limits of 0.02% or less (see Lower Blood Alcohol Concentration Laws for Young or Inexperienced Drivers).

Effectiveness

- These laws are effective in reducing alcohol-related motor vehicle fatalities by approximately 7%.

Applicability

- Our findings should be applicable to all U.S. drivers.

The findings of our systematic review are based on nine studies that evaluated the effect of lowering the BAC to 0.08%.[214–222] All studies analyzed data from police reports of crashes. The studies showed a consistent reduction in alcohol-related motor vehicle fatalities (7% decrease; interquartile range, 4% to 15%) when measured 1 to 14 years after the law was passed (median 5 years). These results show that lowering the BAC limit to 0.08% is effective in reducing alcohol-related motor vehicle fatalities.

These results should be applicable to all drivers affected by 0.08% BAC laws. The studies used statewide fatal crash data, and the states studied are geographically diverse with varying population densities; we did not, however, find information on the effectiveness of these laws in various subgroups.

We did not find information on other positive or negative effects in this review, nor did we find any economic evaluations of the effects of 0.08% BAC laws.

One potential barrier to implementation of 0.08% BAC laws is the view held by some that the laws discourage *social drinkers* from driving after drinking small amounts of alcohol but do not deter *hard-core* drinkers from driving while incapacitated. However, our findings provide some evidence to counter this view: five studies[214,215,217,218,222] found that in most states, fatalities involving drivers with BACs of 0.10% or higher were reduced after 0.08% BAC laws were implemented.

In conclusion, the Task Force recommends the enactment and enforcement of 0.08% BAC laws on the basis of strong evidence of their effectiveness in reducing alcohol-related motor vehicle fatalities. These findings should be applicable to all U.S. drivers.

Minimum Legal Drinking Age Laws (Maintaining at 21 Years of Age): Recommended (Strong Evidence of Effectiveness)

Minimum legal drinking age (MLDA) laws specify an age below which it is illegal to purchase or publicly consume alcoholic beverages. This review assessed the effect of raising or lowering the MLDA on crashes and related fatal and nonfatal injuries.

In the United States, several states lowered their MLDA during the early 1970s. In response to an increase in motor vehicle deaths among young people, some of these same states later raised their MLDA. To address continuing concerns over youth drinking and driving, federal legislation was passed in 1984 that required states to adopt a minimum drinking age of 21 or lose highway funds. By 1987, all U.S. states had adopted laws establishing the MLDA of 21 years.

Effectiveness

- Raising the MLDA is effective in reducing fatal injury crashes by approximately 17% and fatal and nonfatal injury crashes combined by approximately 15%.

- Lowering the MLDA leads to approximately an 8% increase in fatal injury crashes and approximately a 5% increase in fatal and nonfatal injury crashes combined.

Applicability

- These findings should be applicable to all drivers 18–20 years of age.

Other Effects

- Raising the MLDA may lead to decreased alcohol consumption.
- Postulated increases in crash rates among newly eligible drinkers are not supported by the evidence.

The findings of our systematic review of MLDA laws are based on 33 studies (in multiple reports) that assessed the effects of raising or lowering the MLDA on motor vehicle crashes.[132,155,223–250] An additional 13 studies were identified but did not meet our quality criteria and were excluded from the review.[185,186,251–261] Three additional studies provided information on a study already included in our review.[262–264] The studies found that changes in the MLDA result in changes of 10% to 16% in alcohol-related crash outcomes for the targeted age groups: crashes decreased when the MLDA was raised (e.g., from 18 to 21 years) and increased when it was lowered (e.g., from 21 to 18 years).

These results should be applicable to drivers 18 to 20 years of age. They are based on studies from the United States, Australia, and Canada and may not apply to countries with different alcohol consumption or driving patterns.

An additional benefit of raising the MLDA is that it may decrease alcohol consumption. Raising the MLDA may also reduce the number of crashes involving adolescent drivers who are younger than the MLDA: some studies found that raising the MLDA led to an overall 6% relative decrease in crashes in this age group. However, the size of this effect was inconsistent across studies, with several showing no effect.

A possible negative effect of raising the MLDA is referred to as the *drinking experience* effect. Some researchers have proposed that when drivers who have not been legally allowed to drink reach the MLDA, their risk of alcohol-related crash involvement will dramatically increase because they are new to drinking and unfamiliar with its effects. However, it is difficult to estimate the drinking experience effect directly, and studies that attempted to do so have produced inconsistent results. One study examined the overall effect of raising the MLDA and found that, even with the drinking experience effect included, raising the MLDA substantially reduces fatal crashes.

We did not find any economic evaluations of the effects of these laws.

A potential barrier to strengthening or maintaining MLDA laws could be the belief held by some opponents of these laws that prohibition of drinking among young adults unjustly punishes them for the irresponsible behavior of the few who drink and drive.

In conclusion, the Task Force recommends maintaining or implementing the MLDA of 21 years on the basis of strong evidence of its effectiveness in reducing fatal and nonfatal injury crashes. These findings should be applicable to all 18–20-year-old drivers. An additional benefit of raising the MLDA may be a decrease in overall alcohol consumption in this age group.

Sobriety Checkpoints: Recommended (Strong Evidence of Effectiveness)

The primary goal of sobriety checkpoints is to reduce driving after drinking by increasing drinking drivers' perceived risk of being caught. Checkpoints therefore need to be highly visible and well publicized. The United States uses selective breath testing (SBT) checkpoints, at which law enforcement officials must have a reason to suspect that a driver who is stopped has been drinking before a breath test can be administered. Australia and some European countries use random breath testing (RBT) checkpoints, at which all drivers stopped are given breath tests. However, the potential for violating constitutional protections against unreasonable search and seizure prevents use of RBT checkpoints in the United States.

In the United States, law enforcement officers follow established procedures to properly conduct checkpoints.[265] These procedures include using objective criteria to determine checkpoint locations (e.g., the incidence of alcohol-related crashes in the area) and using a predetermined system for stopping cars (e.g., every third car that approaches the checkpoint).[266–268]

Effectiveness

- Selective breath testing checkpoints (used in the United States) are effective in reducing fatal and nonfatal injury crashes by approximately 20%.
- These checkpoints are also effective in reducing alcohol-impaired driving, alcohol-related crashes, and associated fatal and nonfatal injuries in a variety of settings and populations.

Applicability

- These findings should be applicable to all drivers in areas where sobriety checkpoints are permitted.

Other Effects

- Sobriety checkpoints also increase arrests of drivers for other offenses, such as driving with a suspended license or carrying weapons.

- Checkpoints have been criticized for potential inconvenience and intrusion on driver privacy, but their use was upheld by the U.S. Supreme Court.

The findings of our systematic review of sobriety checkpoints are based on 11 papers reporting on SBT checkpoints[266-276] and 12 studies (in 10 reports) on RBT checkpoints.[277-286] Nine papers included studies that did not meet our quality criteria and were excluded from the review.[282,287-294] Four additional papers provided information on studies already included in the review.[295-298] The use of both SBT and RBT checkpoints consistently resulted in fewer crashes. Selective breath testing checkpoints reduced fatal and nonfatal injury crashes by a median of 20% (range, 5% to 23%), and RBT checkpoints reduced these crashes by a median of 16% (interquartile range, 11% to 20%). These reductions were still evident over follow-up periods that ranged from 1 month to 10 years (median 14 months).

Checkpoints may also reduce drinking and driving in general. One study found that an RBT checkpoint program reduced the number of drivers with any detectable BAC level by 13% and the number of drivers with BACs above 0.08% by 24%.

Random breath testing checkpoints are more likely to detect drinking drivers than are SBT checkpoints, but passive alcohol sensors, which allow police to sample air in the car for alcohol vapors, can improve the detection rate at SBT checkpoints by approximately 50%.[299] If such technology becomes more widely used, the sensitivity in detecting drinking drivers at SBT checkpoints may approach that of RBT checkpoints.

These results should be applicable to all drivers in areas where sobriety checkpoints are permitted. The studies in our review generally assessed intensive enforcement and publicity campaigns, so the results may generalize best to these intensive interventions. Studies were conducted on interventions implemented at the city, county, state, and national levels, and were evaluated in rural areas, urban areas, and mixed rural and urban areas.

An additional benefit of sobriety checkpoints is that they can lead to increased arrests of drivers for other offenses, such as driving with a suspended license or carrying weapons. One negative effect of stopping drivers at checkpoints is the resulting inconvenience and intrusion on driver privacy. However, according to the U.S. Supreme Court, the brief intrusion of a properly conducted sobriety checkpoint is justified in the interest of reducing alcohol-impaired driving.[300] Some civil libertarian groups have also endorsed this position.

The findings of our systematic review of economic evaluations are based on four studies:[274,278,301,302] two[274,301] evaluated SBT checkpoints and two[278,302] evaluated RBT checkpoints. All studies conducted cost–benefit analyses. Of the four studies, three[278,301,302] reported annual net benefits and one[274] reported net benefits for the length of the intervention (nine months).

Selective Breath Testing Checkpoints. The first economic evaluation[301] modeled a one-year campaign conducted in a hypothetical community of 100,000 licensed drivers in the United States. The modeled campaign consisted of 156 checkpoints per year, each four hours in duration. The estimated annual total benefit from alcohol-related crashes averted was $9.2 million (in 1997 U.S. dollars). Estimated annual total costs of the intervention were $1.6 million. The estimated annual net benefit was $7.6 million (in 1997 U.S. dollars), resulting in a benefit-to-cost ratio of $6 per dollar invested.

The second study[274] evaluated a nine-month checkpoint campaign conducted in four California communities (a fifth community served as a comparison group and a sixth implemented roving driving while intoxicated [DWI] patrols). The program consisted of 18 checkpoints per community plus publicity campaigns and education programs. Total aggregated benefits of $3.86 million (in 1997 U.S. dollars) came from societal savings realized through avoided injuries and fatalities. Total costs of the intervention (aggregated for four communities) were $164,552. The aggregated net benefit was $3.7 million, resulting in a benefit-to-cost ratio of $23 per dollar invested.

In summary, from a societal viewpoint, the economic benefits of these interventions exceed the costs.

Random Breath Testing Checkpoints. The first study[278] was conducted three years after statewide RBT checkpoints were introduced in New South Wales, Australia. Annual total benefits were $228 million (in 1997 U.S. dollars). Annual total program costs were $4 million. The annual net benefit reported in the study was $224 million, resulting in a benefit-to-cost ratio of $57 per dollar invested.

The second study[302] modeled a proposed nationwide RBT checkpoint intervention in the Netherlands. The proposed intervention included a publicity component and incorporated a more efficient method of transporting offenders to police stations. Annual total benefits from cost savings in the reduction of alcohol-related injury and property damage were estimated at $31.4 million (in 1997 U.S. dollars). Annual total costs including materials and publicity were estimated at $15.6 million. The annual net benefit of the intervention was estimated to be $15.8 million, resulting in a benefit-to-cost ratio of $2 per dollar invested.

Although the U.S. Supreme Court allows SBT checkpoints,[300] their prohibition by some state courts presents a serious barrier to implementation. Where checkpoints are permitted, another important barrier is the concern police have over the low arrest rates.[291] Providing police officers with regular feedback on how checkpoints help reduce alcohol-related crashes may decrease their concerns.

In conclusion, the Task Force recommends the use of sobriety checkpoints on the basis of strong evidence of their effectiveness in reducing fatal and nonfatal crash injuries and in reducing alcohol-impaired driving and alcohol-related crashes. These findings should be applicable to all drivers in areas where sobriety checkpoints can be conducted.

Lower Blood Alcohol Concentration Laws for Young or Inexperienced Drivers: Recommended (Sufficient Evidence of Effectiveness)

Drinking and driving is especially dangerous for young people. A study of fatal crashes in the United States[303] estimated that 16–20-year-old male drivers with blood alcohol concentrations (BACs) between 0.08% and 0.10% were 24 times more likely to die in a motor vehicle crash than those who had not been drinking. Laws restricting the BAC of young drivers (under 21 years of age in the United States) to lower levels than those for adult drivers aim to prevent injury or death for these drivers, their passengers, and others using the road. As of July 1998, all 50 states had enacted lower BAC laws for young drivers. These laws are commonly referred to as *zero tolerance* laws.

Lower BAC laws may also be useful in populations other than young drivers. For example, the Centers for Disease Control and Prevention recommends that states consider enacting lower BAC laws for all drivers who transport children.[304]

Effectiveness

- Lower BAC laws are effective in reducing fatal crashes by approximately 17%.
- These laws are also effective in reducing fatal and nonfatal crashes (reported together) by approximately 10%.

Applicability

- Our findings should be applicable to all drivers affected by these laws (in the United States, those under 21 years of age).

Other Effects

- Lower BAC laws can result in underage drinking drivers with high BACs receiving only zero tolerance citations rather than being arrested for alcohol-impaired driving (as would drinking drivers over 20 years of age).

The findings of our systematic review of lower BAC laws for young or inexperienced drivers are based on six studies.[243,305–309] An additional three studies were identified but did not meet our quality criteria and were excluded from the review.[310-312] Two additional studies provided information on a study already included in our review.[313,314] The reviewed studies evaluated the number of motor vehicle crashes from 1 to 15 years after enactment of lower BAC laws (median 22 months) using the information in police reports. All six studies reported reductions in crashes. Three studies examined fatal crashes and reported declines of 24%, 17%, and 9%. Two studies examined fatal and nonfatal injury crashes and reported declines of 17% and 3.8%. One study examined crashes in which the investigating police officers believed that the driver had been drinking alcohol and reported a decline of 11%. These results show that lower BAC laws for young or inexperienced drivers are effective in reducing both fatal and nonfatal crashes.

These results should be applicable to all young and inexperienced drivers covered by lower BAC laws. This review did not address the effectiveness of lower BAC laws directed to other specific groups of drivers, such as commercial truck drivers and people convicted of driving while impaired. The states studied are geographically diverse, with both urban and rural populations represented.

A potential harm is that U.S. drivers under the age of 21 with high BACs could receive only zero tolerance citations for violating the lower BAC law, whereas adults with the same BAC would be arrested for the more serious offense of driving under the influence of alcohol (DUI). A study of California's 1994 lower BAC law[309] showed that about half of the potential DUI arrests among underage drivers were converted to less serious zero tolerance citations.

The findings of our systematic review of economic evaluations are based on one study.[315] The study, a cost–benefit analysis, applied previously published crash costs and used effectiveness data from other previously published studies to illustrate how these costs could be applied to lower BAC laws in the United States. The benefits from a reduction in alcohol-related crashes were estimated using the assumption that lower BAC laws reduce young drivers' alcohol-related crashes by 20%. The estimated benefit-to-cost ratio for lower BAC laws was $11 per dollar invested when violators received a six-month license suspension.

All U.S. states currently have lower BAC laws for drivers under 21 years of age, but several potential barriers to full enforcement of these laws exist.[309] Because young people are less likely than adults to drink in bars, police patrols that target bar neighborhoods are likely to miss underage drinking drivers. Also, officers may have difficulty identifying underage drinking drivers with low BACs because they may not show obvious signs of impairment. Finally, because of ambiguities, some state laws prohibit police officers from testing the BAC of an underage driver unless there is probable cause to believe that the driver's BAC is above the legal limit for adults.

In conclusion, the Task Force recommends maintaining or implementing lower BAC laws for young or inexperienced drivers on the basis of sufficient evidence of the effectiveness of the laws in reducing both fatal and nonfatal crashes. These findings should be applicable to all drivers affected by the laws (in the United States, all drivers under 21 years of age).

Intervention Training Programs for Servers of Alcoholic Beverages: Recommended Under Certain Conditions (Sufficient Evidence of Effectiveness)

People often drive after consuming alcohol in bars, clubs, and restaurants. Therefore, teaching bartenders and other servers of alcoholic beverages ways to prevent intoxication among their patrons may help to reduce alcohol-impaired driving.

Server intervention training programs can include teaching servers to offer patrons food with drinks, delay service to rapid drinkers, refuse service to intoxicated or underage patrons, and discourage intoxicated patrons from driving. These programs vary widely in terms of the content covered, instructional time, and the training method (e.g., face-to-face vs. videotaped). Some programs are offered in classroom settings by professional trainers, whereas others consist only of a video or written material that employees are encouraged to use on their own.[316] This training may be supplemented by role playing. Generally, the programs also involve education about alcohol beverage control (ABC) laws and identifying the signs of intoxication. Some programs also evaluate the alcohol serving policies of a drinking establishment and recommend changes to reduce intoxication, such as eliminating drink promotions, serving a variety of nonalcoholic beverages, or increasing the availability of food.[317]

As of January 1, 2000, 11 states had established mandatory server training programs for all licensed establishments and 10 states provided liability protection to establishments that voluntarily implemented server training.[318]

Factors other than server training can influence serving practices in licensed establishments. These factors include enforcement of existing ABC laws,[319] server liability (or dram shop) laws,[320] high-profile server liability cases,[320] and community coalitions to encourage responsible serving practices.[321] These factors can influence the degree of management support for server training and improvements in serving practices, which is thought to be essential for changing server behavior.[316,322–324]

Effectiveness

- This intervention is effective in reducing the level of intoxication in patrons when servers have received intensive, high-quality, face-to-face server training accompanied by strong and active management support.

Applicability

- The applicability of our findings is limited to the kinds of intensive, face-to-face, management-supported programs described here.
- Server training may not work when delivered by less intensive methods or in settings lacking strong management support.

Other Effects

- Decreased levels of intoxication may reduce other alcohol-related injuries, violence, and crime.

The findings of our systematic review of server intervention training programs are based on five studies.[323,325-328] Three additional studies were identified but did not meet our quality criteria and were excluded from the review.[329-331] Four additional reports provided information on studies already included in the review.[332-335]

The five studies in our review evaluated the effect of server training on server behaviors, patrons' BACs, and crash outcomes. Two studies looked at changes in server behaviors after relatively intensive (4½- to 6-hour) training programs and found significant improvements in appropriate serving practices. Three studies that evaluated patrons' BACs found that server training led to decreased intoxication. In one study, none of the pseudopatrons (research assistants posing as patrons) of trained servers reached BAC levels of 0.10%, but 45% of pseudopatrons of untrained servers did. A second study with less intensive server training (one to two hours) found decreases in the rate of intoxication of patrons leaving participating premises of 17% at a two-week follow-up and of 28% after three months; one establishment in this study had an unusually supportive manager, which may have accounted for much of this success. In a third study, conducted at a Navy enlisted club, an intensive 18-hour training course was supplemented by other policy changes, such as eliminating the sale of pitchers of drinks, resulting in a 33% decrease in the percentage of patrons with estimated BACs of 0.10% or greater. Although overall alcohol consumption did not substantially decrease, the rate of consumption did, suggesting that patrons drank more slowly but stayed in the establishment longer. A study that evaluated the effect of a statewide one-day mandatory server training program found that the training resulted in a decrease of 23% in single-vehicle nighttime injury crashes. Overall, these results show that intensive, high-quality, face-to-face training programs for servers of alcoholic beverages can be effective in reducing patron intoxication. It should not be assumed, however, that all kinds of training are effective.

Consistency of server training programs is essential to their effectiveness. Given the high employee turnover rate for servers, it is important to go beyond a *demonstration* training program. Training sessions should be offered on a continuing basis, and their quality should be consistent. Problems in staffing and scheduling training sessions can result in decreased quality of implementation.[327] Although less intensive server training programs (e.g., video-based) are easier and less expensive to implement, their effectiveness is not known.

The applicability of these results should be viewed with caution. Except for the study on mandatory server training,[326] all of the studies looked at drinking establishments whose managers volunteered to participate in the training programs. The managers who chose to participate may have been unusually supportive of the programs (and this may not be typical of managers). Three of the five programs evaluated were conducted in a small number of drinking establishments, were relatively time-intensive (longer than four hours), involved face-to-face training, and covered a broad curriculum including specific intervention practices. This contrasts with the types of training programs generally in use, which vary widely in intensity, mode of delivery, and content. Thus, the reviewed studies may reflect the best possible outcomes of server training. It is not clear that these findings are applicable to larger-scale community-wide programs, to programs with substantially different training methods or content, or to programs that do not recruit supportive managers. Additionally, follow-up periods were generally less than three months, so that long-term effects cannot be estimated.

The desirable effect of reduced alcohol-impaired driving can only be maintained if the affected patrons stop drinking or drink only in relatively safe environments after leaving the drinking establishment.[322] Ideally, servers at all drinking establishments within a community should receive training. In our review, only two studies evaluated community-wide server training programs. Thus, further research is needed on the fundamental question of whether server intervention training programs delivered community-wide are effective in decreasing intoxication and, ultimately, alcohol-impaired driving.

By reducing levels of intoxication, improved server practices may also provide the benefit of reducing the risk of other alcohol-related injuries, violence, and crime. Trained servers may also find that they get larger tips than before training. No negative effects of server training programs were noted.

We did not find any economic evaluations of server intervention training programs.

Resistance to server training by managers of drinking establishments is a potential barrier to effectively implementing this intervention. Although many managers of drinking establishments like the *concept* of server training,[331] they may also be concerned about a reduction in profits following training. This can erode crucial management support for improved server practices.[335] Although one study that examined gross receipts in bars found no noticeable reduction in profits following server training, this study was conducted at a Navy base enlisted club, and results may not be applicable to other types of drinking establishments. In addition to being concerned about profits, some managers also react negatively to the idea of "policing" their customers.[335]

Management support for server training programs could be increased by offering positive incentives (e.g., insurance discounts) to establishments that improve serving practices,[336] by strengthening or highlighting disincentives for irresponsible practices (e.g., stronger enforcement of ABC laws),[319] and by building broad community support for such programs.[331]

In conclusion, the Task Force recommends intensive, high-quality, face-to-face training for servers of alcoholic beverages when accompanied by strong and active management support, on the basis of sufficient evidence of the effectiveness of this kind of training in reducing the level of patron intoxication. These findings are limited to the intensive programs described here, and applicability to other situations should not be assumed.

Mass Media Campaigns: Recommended Under Certain Conditions (Strong Evidence of Effectiveness)

Mass media campaigns are typically carried out in conjunction with other programs and policies to prevent alcohol-impaired driving. Where adequate local resources can support a mass media campaign that is carefully planned, well executed, attains adequate audience exposure, and is supported by other prevention activities, this combination of activities can be effective in reducing alcohol-impaired driving.

Effectiveness

- Mass media campaigns can be effective in decreasing all crashes by approximately 13%.
- Campaigns can also be effective in decreasing injury crashes by approximately 10%.

Applicability

- These findings should be applicable to most people of driving age.

Mass media campaigns to deter alcohol-impaired driving are generally intended either to persuade people to avoid drinking and driving themselves or to motivate them to prevent others from drinking and driving. Key factors in the design of mass media campaigns are related to both the *content* and the *delivery* of the messages used. In terms of content, several themes are commonly used to motivate people, such as fear of arrest; fear of harming oneself, others, or property; a positive social norm in which drinking and driving don't mix; and portraying people who drink and drive as irresponsible and dangerous. Another aspect of content involves the actions suggested by the media campaign, including abstaining from or drinking in moderation when driving, using a designated driver, or taking the keys from someone who has had too much to drink. Content considerations also include how much anxiety the campaign should create: although arousing some anxiety is a good way to get people's attention, arousing too much anxiety or fear may cause people to stop listening to the message. The best combination may be arousing a degree of anxiety while providing solutions that people can use to protect themselves.

Optimal delivery of messages to the intended audience requires both control over when and where the ads appear and control over the quality of the ads themselves. To maximize exposure of target audiences to the message of the campaign, placement of ads is vital, and purchasing advertising space or time ensures control over placement; relying on free public service announcements leaves the scheduling of ads to media personnel who may not be concerned with the goals of the campaign. The messages to be delivered should be tested before the campaign is launched (*pretested*) to see which themes or concepts are most appropriate for target audiences. Conducting a campaign with untested messages can result in a diluted message, or the wrong message, being received.

The findings of our systematic review are based on eight studies (reported in six papers) that evaluated the effectiveness of mass media campaigns on fatal crashes, fatal and nonfatal injury crashes combined, crashes that damage property, and drivers' BACs.[337-342] Two additional studies were identified but did not meet our quality criteria and were excluded from the review.[343,344] Most of the reviewed campaigns pretested their messages, had high levels of audience exposure (achieved by using paid advertising), and conducted their mass media campaigns in conjunction with other local prevention efforts (e.g., enhanced law enforcement). The specific content of the messages varied.

We classified studies as focusing primarily on either the *legal consequences* or the *social and health consequences* of drinking and driving. Three of the evaluated campaigns focused on making the public aware of law enforcement activities and the legal consequences of drinking and driving. The remaining five studies focused on the social and health consequences of alcohol-impaired driving. Overall, the evaluated studies showed median decreases of 13% (interquartile range, 6% to 14%) in overall crashes and 10% (interquartile range, 6% to 15%) in injury crashes. We found no obvious difference in effect whether campaign messages focused on the legal consequences or the social and health consequences of drinking and driving, although it is conceivable that certain messages and modes of delivery may be more effective with one audience than another. Overall, these results show that mass media campaigns, under the conditions described here, can be effective in decreasing injury crashes.

These findings should be applicable to carefully planned and pretested mass media campaigns, with ads that reach the intended audience often enough, implemented in an environment with other ongoing prevention activities (e.g., grassroots activities, enhanced law enforcement efforts), and targeted to any audience of driving age.

Mass media campaigns may also raise awareness of the dangers that drinking and driving pose for a community, thereby helping to generate an interest in strengthening legislation. Some authors[345-347] believe that mass media campaigns may have greater impact when their goal is to change public policy rather than individual behavior.

The findings of our systematic review of economic evaluations of mass media campaigns are based on cost–benefit analyses conducted for two of the campaigns evaluated in this review.[341,348] The results have been adjusted to 1997 U.S. dollars. An analysis of the first 23 months of a campaign in Victoria, Australia, indicated that it cost US$403,174 per month for advertisement development, supporting media, media placement, and concept research.[349] Estimated savings from medical costs, productivity losses, pain and suffering, and property damage were US$8,324,532 per month, with US$3,214,096 of these savings accruing from averted medical costs.

A second analysis indicated that six-month campaigns in Wichita (using paid media) and Kansas City, Kansas (using public service announcements) had total costs of $454,060 and $322,660, respectively.[350] Costs for planning and evaluation research, message production, and media scheduling were included. Total savings from averted costs of insurance administration, premature funeral, legal and court, medical payments, property damage, rehabilitation, and employers' losses were estimated at $3,431,305 for the Wichita campaign and $3,676,399 in Kansas City.

In all three sites evaluated, the estimated societal benefits substantially exceeded the costs of developing and airing the campaign messages.

Those thinking about implementing a mass media campaign to reduce alcohol-related crashes are cautioned to do so only if the necessary resources and supports are in place. Campaigns implemented without adequate planning, pretesting of messages, ad placement, and support activities cannot be expected to reduce alcohol-related crashes.

In conclusion, on the basis of strong evidence of effectiveness in reducing alcohol-related crashes, injuries, and deaths, the Task Force recommends mass media campaigns that are carefully planned, well executed, attain adequate audience exposure, and are implemented in conjunction with other ongoing prevention activities. The findings of this review should be applicable to most people of driving age.

REDUCING INJURY TO MOTOR VEHICLE OCCUPANTS THROUGH USE OF THESE RECOMMENDATIONS

The recommendations in this chapter can be used in many ways to reduce injuries to motor vehicle occupants. States and communities can compare their current motor vehicle injury prevention activities with these recommendations, take steps to ensure that existing interventions are adequately implemented and funded, and consider implementing other recommended interventions.

These recommendations can be used to support or expand child safety seat distribution programs, bolster the use of incentives, and employ enhanced enforcement campaigns, all in conjunction with community-wide education efforts. For example, based on the recommendations, a community might concentrate on distribution of low-cost or no-cost child safety seats in low-income neighborhoods or seek local sponsorship to defray the costs of seats distributed to low-income families.

A comprehensive community program to reduce motor vehicle occupant injuries should include several interventions, such as legislation, enforcement, public education, training, and other community-oriented strategies. It is often useful to involve other partners in efforts to develop such a program. Potential partners include each state's Governor's Office of Highway Safety, directors of state injury control programs in health departments (www.stipda .org), local chapters of the National SAFE KIDS Campaign (www.safekids.org), the National Safety Council (www.nsc.org), and Mothers Against Drunk Driving (www.madd.org).

The Task Force recommended six state public health laws. Not all recommended laws are in effect in all states. Forty-nine states have laws requiring use of safety belts (New Hampshire has no such law), but only 20 states (plus

Washington, DC and Puerto Rico) had primary enforcement laws as of December 2003. As of December 2003, 45 states, plus Washington, DC and Puerto Rico, had enacted 0.08% BAC laws. Efforts such as those of the U.S. Congress, which included a provision in the 2001 Department of Transportation and Related Agencies Appropriations Act[213] requiring states to implement 0.08% BAC laws by October 2003 or risk losing federal highway construction funds, are major factors in getting such laws on the books. The Task Force recommendations can support efforts to adopt, maintain, or strengthen state or national laws or regulations. State injury control program directors can use the recommendations to develop testimony about the effectiveness of various traffic safety laws. State legislators can use the recommendations as they draft, debate, and vote on new or amended legislation. Advocacy and community groups, both local and national, can use the information to develop position statements for pending legislation. Health agencies can help educate the community about the importance and effectiveness of the laws and their enforcement. Health plans can publicize these findings among the populations they care for, and can apply them in their work with communities and in the work of their foundations.

CONCLUSION

This chapter summarizes Task Force conclusions and recommendations on interventions to reduce injuries to motor vehicle occupants. To increase proper use of child safety seats, the Task Force recommends child safety seat laws, distribution and education programs, incentive and education programs, and community-wide information and enhanced enforcement campaigns; insufficient evidence exists to determine the effectiveness of education programs when used alone in increasing the use of child safety seats. To increase the use of safety belts, the Task Force recommends safety belt laws, upgrading secondary to primary enforcement laws, and implementing enhanced enforcement efforts. To reduce alcohol-impaired driving, the Task Force recommends 0.08% blood alcohol concentration (BAC) laws, minimum legal drinking age laws (maintaining at 21 years of age), sobriety checkpoints, lower BAC for young or inexperienced drivers, intervention training programs for servers of alcoholic beverages under certain conditions, and mass media campaigns under certain conditions. Details of these reviews have been published[351–357] and these articles, along with additional information about the reviews, are available at www.thecommunityguide.org/mvoi.

Acknowledgments

This chapter was written by the members of the systematic review development team: Stephanie Zaza, MD, MPH, Division of Prevention Research and Analytic Methods, Epidemiology Program Office, Centers for Disease Control and Prevention (CDC), Atlanta, Georgia; David A. Sleet, PhD, MA, Division of Unintentional Injury Prevention (DUIP), National Center for Injury Prevention and Control (NCIPC), CDC, Atlanta; Ruth A. Shults, PhD, MPH, DUIP/NCIPC/CDC, Atlanta; Randy W. Elder, PhD, DUIP/NCIPC/CDC, Atlanta; Tho Bella Dinh-Zarr, PhD, MPH, DUIP/NCIPC/CDC, Atlanta; James L. Nichols, PhD, National Highway Traffic Safety Administration (NHTSA), Washington, DC; Richard Compton, PhD, NHTSA, Washington, DC; Robert S. Thompson, MD, Group Health Cooperative of Puget Sound, Seattle, Washington and the Task Force on Community Preventive Services.

Consultants for the reviews were: Julie C. Bolen, PhD, MPH, National Center for Chronic Disease Prevention and Health Promotion (NCCDPHP), CDC, Atlanta; Robert D. Brewer, MD, MSPH, NCCDPHP/CDC, Atlanta; Stephanie D. Bryn, MPH., Health Resources Services Administration, Rockville, Maryland; Forrest M. Council, PhD, University of North Carolina, Chapel Hill; Robert W. Denniston, MA, Substance Abuse and Mental Health Services Administration, Rockville, Maryland; Andrea C. Gielen, ScD, ScM, Johns Hopkins University, Baltimore, Maryland; Susan Gorcowski, MA, NHTSA, Washington, DC; Charles A. Hurley, BA, National Safety Council, Washington, DC; Bruce H. Jones, MD, MPH, NCIPC/CDC, Atlanta; Trudy A. Karlson, PhD, University of Wisconsin, Madison; Mark R. Kinde, MPH, Minnesota Department of Health, Minneapolis; David W. Lawrence, MPH, RN, San Diego State University, San Diego, California; Susan E. Martin, PhD, National Institute for Alcohol Abuse and Alcoholism, Rockville, Maryland; James A. McKnight, PhD, National Public Service Research Institute, Landover, Maryland; Angela D. Mickalide, PhD, CHES, National SAFE KIDS Campaign, Washington, DC; Lloyd F. Novick, MD, MPH, Onondaga County Department of Health, Syracuse, New York; Frederick P. Rivara, MD, MPH, University of Washington, Seattle; Carol W. Runyan, PhD, MPH, University of North Carolina, Chapel Hill; Richard J. Smith, MS, Health Resources and Services Administration, Rockville, Maryland; Patricia F. Waller, PhD, University of Michigan, Ann Arbor; Allan F. Williams, PhD, Insurance Institute for Highway Safety, Arlington, Virginia.

Articles included in the reviews were abstracted by: Jeanne Louisa Alongi; Patricia Bellas; Shannon Corbett-Perez; Ann Dellinger; Roberta A. Eidman; Irene Fischer; Jane Kattapong; David W. Lawrence; Shelley Levesque; John Oh; Dan Pallin; Matthew Patterson; Kyran Quinlan; Luann Rhodes; Eva Shipp; Ruth Shults; Daniel Sudakin; Stuart L. Usdan; L. J. David Wallace; Carol Ward; and Donna White.

References

1. National Center for Injury Prevention and Control. Working to prevent and control injury in the United States: fact book for the year 2000. Atlanta, GA: Centers for Disease Control and Prevention, 2000.

2. Centers for Disease Control and Prevention. Web-based Injury Statistics Query and Reporting System (WISQARS). Available at: http://www.cdc.gov/ncipc/wisqars. Accessed May 7, 2003.

3. Fingerhut LA, Warner M. Injury chartbook. Health, United States, 1996–97. Hyattsville, MD: National Center for Health Statistics, 1997.

4. National Highway Traffic Safety Administration. Traffic safety facts, 2002: a compilation of motor vehicle crash data from the Fatality Analysis Reporting System and the

General Estimates System. Washington, DC: U.S. Department of Transportation, National Highway Traffic Safety Administration, 2004. DOT HS 809 620.

5. Blincoe L, Seay A, Zaloshnja E, et al. The economic impact of motor vehicle crashes, 2000. Washington, DC: U.S. Department of Transportation, National Highway Traffic Safety Administration, 2002. DOT HS 809 446.

6. Centers for Disease Control and Prevention. Motor vehicle safety: a 20th century public health achievement. MMWR 1999;48(18):369–74.

7. Bolen JR, Sleet DA, Johnson VR, eds. Prevention of motor vehicle-related injuries: a compendium of articles from the Morbidity and Mortality Weekly Report 1985–1996. Atlanta, GA: National Center for Injury Prevention and Control, Centers for Disease Control and Prevention, 1997.

8. Sleet DA. Reducing motor vehicle trauma through health promotion programming. Health Educ Q 1984;11(2):113–25.

9. U.S. Department of Health and Human Services. Healthy people 2010. 2nd ed. Washington, DC: U.S. Government Printing Office, 2000.

10. U.S. Department of Transportation. DOT performance plan—FY 2004/ Highway safety. Available at: http://www.dot.gov/PerfPlan2004/safety_highway.html. Accessed July 9, 2003.

11. National Highway Traffic Safety Administration. Presidential initiative for increasing seat belt use nationwide: recommendations from the Secretary of Transportation. Washington, DC: U.S. Department of Transportation, National Highway Traffic Safety Administration, 1997. DOT HS 808 576.

12. U.S. Preventive Services Task Force. Guide to clinical preventive services: report of the U.S. Preventive Services Task Force. 2nd ed. Baltimore: Williams & Wilkins, 1996.

13. Committee on Injury and Poison Prevention, American Academy of Pediatrics. Selecting and using the most appropriate car safety seats for growing children: guidelines for counseling parents. Pediatrics 2002;109(3):550–3.

14. American Academy of Pediatrics Committee on Injury and Poison Prevention and Committee on Adolescence. The teenage driver. Pediatrics 1996;98(5):987–90.

15. National Highway Traffic Safety Administration. Integrated project teams reports (IPTs). Available at: http://www.nhtsa.dot.gov/IPTReports.html. Accessed January 14, 2004.

16. National Transportation Safety Board. We are all safer—NTSB-inspired improvements in transportation safety. 2nd ed. Available at: http://www.ntsb.gov/Publictn/1998/SR9801.pdf. Accessed April 1, 2003.

17. American Medical Association. Operating vehicles under the influence of alcohol or other drugs/underage drinking and driving. Available at: http://www.ama-assn.org/ama1/pub/upload/mm/388/underage_drnkndrive.pdf. Accessed March 5, 2004.

18. Zaza S, Carande-Kulis VG, Sleet DA, et al. Methods for conducting systematic reviews of the evidence of effectiveness and economic efficiency of interventions to reduce injuries to motor vehicle occupants. Am J Prev Med 2001;21(4S):23–30.

19. National Highway Traffic Safety Administration. Buckle Up America: The presidential initiative for increasing seat belt use nationwide. First report to Congress. Washington, DC: U.S. Department of Transportation, National Highway Traffic Safety Administration, 1998. DOT HS 808 667.

20. National Highway Traffic Safety Administration. Research note: revised estimates of child restraint effectiveness. Washington, DC: U.S. Department of Transportation, National Highway Traffic Safety Administration, 1996. Report No. 96.855.

21. Children's Safety Network. Childhood injury: cost and prevention facts. Child safety seats: how large are the benefits and who should pay? Landover, MD: Children's Safety Network: Economics and Insurance Resource Center, 1997.

22. Centers for Disease Control and Prevention. Air-bag associated fatal injuries to infants and children riding in front passenger seats—United States. MMWR 1995;44(45): 845–7.

23. Johnston C, Rivara FP, Soderberg R. Children in car crashes: analysis of data for injury and use of restraints. Pediatrics 1994;93(6):960–5.

24. Taft CH, Mickalide AD, Taft AR. Child passengers at risk in America: a national study of car seat misuse. Washington, DC: National SAFE KIDS Campaign, 1999.

25. Braver ER, Whitfield R, Ferguson SA. Seating positions and children's risk of dying in motor vehicle crashes. Inj Prev 1998;4(3):181–7.

26. Hazinski MF, Eddy VA, Morris JA. Children's traffic safety program: influence of early elementary school safety education on family seat belt use. J Trauma 1995;39(6): 1063–8.

27. National Highway Traffic Safety Administration. National Occupant Protection Use Survey (NOPUS) 2000: controlled intersection study. Washington, DC: U.S. Department of Transportation, National Highway Traffic Safety Administration, National Center for Statistics and Analysis, 2001. DOT HS 809 318.

28. National Highway Traffic Safety Administration. Rural and urban crashes: a comparative analysis. Washington, DC: U.S. Department of Transportation, National Highway Traffic Safety Administration, 1996. DOT HS 808 450.

29. Louis B, Lewis M. Increasing car seat use for toddlers from inner-city families. Am J Public Health 1997;87(6):1044–5.

30. National Highway Traffic Safety Administration. Strategies to increase the use of child safety seats by low-income families: a report to the Committees on Appropriations, U.S. House of Representatives, U.S. Senate. Washington, DC: U.S. Department of Transportation, National Highway Traffic Safety Administration, 1991.

31. Robitaille Y, Legault J, Abbey H, Pless IB. Evaluation of an infant car seat program in a low-income community. Am J Dis Child 1990;144(1):74–8.

32. Centers for Disease Control and Prevention. Motor-vehicle occupant fatalities and restraint use among children aged 4–8 years. United States, 1994–1998. MMWR 2000; 49(07):135–7.

33. Shults RA, Elder RW, Sleet DA, Thompson RS, Nichols JL. Primary enforcement seat belt laws are effective even in the face of rising belt use rates. Accid Anal Prev 2004; 36:491–3.

34. Evans WN, Graham JD. An estimate of the lifesaving benefit of child restraint use legislation. J Health Econ 1990;9:121–42.

35. Guerin D, MacKinnon DP. An assessment of the California child passenger restraint requirement. Am J Public Health 1985;75(2):142–4.

36. Rock SM. Impact of the Illinois child passenger protection act: a retrospective look. Accid Anal Prev 1996;28(4):487–92.

37. Wagenaar AC, Maybee RG, Sullivan KP. Michigan's compulsory restraint use policies: effects on injuries and deaths. Ann Arbor: University of Michigan Transportation Research Institute, 1987. UMTRI 87–10.

38. Margolis LH, Wagenaar AC, Liu W. The effects of a mandatory child restraint law on injuries requiring hospitalization. Am J Dis Child 1988;142:1099–103.

39. Seekins T, Fawcett SB, Cohen SH, et al. Experimental evaluation of public policy: the case of state legislation for child passenger safety. J Appl Behav Anal 1988;21(3): 233–43.

40. Sewell CM, Hull HF, Fenner J, Graff H, Pine J. Child restraint law effects on motor vehicle accident fatalities and injuries: the New Mexico experience. Pediatrics 1986; 78(6):1079–84.

41. Wagenaar AC, Webster DW, Maybee RG. Effects of child restraint laws on traffic fatalities in eleven states. J Trauma 1987;27(7):726–32.

42. Williams AF, Wells JK. Evaluation of the Rhode Island child restraint law. Am J Public Health 1981;71(7):742–3.

43. Agent KR. Usage rates and effectiveness of safety belts and child safety seats in Kentucky, 1988. Lexington: Kentucky Transportation Center, College of Engineering, University of Kentucky, 1988. KTC-88–6.

44. Agran PF, Dunkle DE, Winn DG. The effects of safety seat legislation on pediatric trauma. Washington, DC: U.S. Department of Transportation, Office of University Research, 1986. DOT/OST/P-34/86–044.

45. Agran PF, Dunkle DE, Winn DG. Effects of legislation on motor vehicle injuries to children. Am J Dis Child 1987;141:959–64.

46. Ain KB, Barrall DT, Perez RG, Ward HA. Patterns of automotive safety restraint use in Rhode Island: impact of the child passenger restraint law. R I Med J 1981;64:515–9.

47. Alvarez J, Jason LA. The effectiveness of legislation, education, and loaners for child safety in automobiles. J Community Psychol 1993;21:280–4.

48. Cunningham JL, Hughes EC, Philpot JW, Pentz CA. Parents' knowledge, attitudes and behavior about child passenger safety. Washington, DC: U.S. Department of Transportation, National Highway Traffic Safety Administration, 1981. DOT HS 805 947.

49. Hall WL. The North Carolina child passenger protection law: implementation and evaluation, July 1982–June 1985. Chapel Hill: University of North Carolina Highway Safety Research Center, 1985. 85–04-LE-304–01.

50. Montague RB. The introduction of child safety seat legislation in Virginia: types and levels of community response and effects on automobile accident statistics. Washington, DC: U.S. Department of Transportation, Office of University Research, 1984. DOT/OST/P-34/85/024.

51. Muller A. Is the Oklahoma child restraint law effective? [letter]. Am J Public Health 1986;76(10):1251–2.

52. O'Brien JF. Child safety restraint study: a study of the effects of child safety restraint legislation on the incidence and severity of motor vehicle accident injuries to children six years of age and younger (based on 1980–1982 and 1984–1985 accidents). Albany: New York State Department of Motor Vehicles, 1986. PB87–183554.

53. Partyka SC. Effect of child occupant protection laws on fatalities. Washington, DC: U.S. Department of Transportation, National Highway Traffic Safety Administration, 1989. DOT HS 807 453.

54. Rood DH, Kraichy PP. Evaluation of New York state's mandatory occupant restraint law. Volume 3: observational surveys of safety restraint use by children in New York State. Washington, DC: U.S. Department of Transportation, National Highway Traffic Safety Administration, 1986. DOT HS 806 972.

55. Williams AF. Evaluation of the Tennessee child restraint law. Am J Public Health 1979;69(5):455–8.

56. Williams AF, Wells JK. The Tennessee child restraint law in its third year. Am J Public Health 1980;71(2):163-5.

57. Wagenaar AC. Mandatory child restraint laws: impact on childhood injuries due to traffic crashes. J Safety Res 1985;16(1):9-21.

58. Wagenaar AC, Webster DW. Preventing injuries to children through compulsory automobile safety seat use. Pediatrics 1986;78(4):662-72.

59. Christophersen ER, Sullivan MA. Increasing the protection of newborn infants in cars. Pediatrics 1982;70(1):21-5.

60. Colletti RB. Longitudinal evaluation of a statewide network of hospital programs to improve child passenger safety. Pediatrics 1986;77(4):523-9.

61. Culler CJ, Cunningham JL. Compliance with the child passenger protection law: effects of a loaner program for low-income mothers. Washington, DC: U.S. Department of Transportation, National Highway Traffic Safety Administration, 1980. DOT HS 805 801.

62. Geddis DC, Appleton IC. Establishment and evaluation of a pilot child car seat rental scheme in New Zealand. Pediatrics 1986;77(2):167-72.

63. Hletko PJ, Robin SS, Hletko JD, Stone M. Infant safety seat use: reaching the hard to reach. Am J Dis Child 1987;141(12):1301-4.

64. Lindqvist KS. Does the use of child safety seats increase as the result of loan schemes? Accid Anal Prev 1993;25(4):421-9.

65. Reisinger KS, Williams AF. Evaluation of programs designed to increase the protection of infants in cars. Pediatrics 1978;62(3):280-7.

66. Saalberg JH, Morrison AJ. Restraint use and injury experience. In: Evaluation of the League General Insurance Company child safety seat distribution program; DOT HS 806 253. Washington, DC: U.S. Department of Transportation, National Highway Traffic Safety Administration, 1982:22-47.

67. Saalberg JH, Morrison AJ. Household survey. In: Evaluation of the League General Insurance Company child safety seat distribution program; DOT HS 806 253. Washington, DC: U.S. Department of Transportation, National Highway Traffic Safety Administration, 1982:63-120.

68. Berger LR, Saunders S, Armitage K, Schauer L. Promoting the use of car safety devices for infants: an intensive health education approach. Pediatrics 1984;74(1):16-9.

69. Hletko PJ, Hletko J, Shelness A, Nyberg J. The effect of an in-hospital maternity education program on observed correct crash restraint device use. 26th Annual Proceedings, American Association for Automotive Medicine, October 4-6, 1982:219-32.

70. Hletko PJ, Hletko J, Shelness A, Nyberg J. The effect of a toddler/child restraint device rental program on observed correct use. 27th Annual Conference Proceedings, American Association for Automotive Medicine, October 3-6, 1983:115-25.

71. Jarmark S, Ljungblom BA, Turbell T. Infant carriers—a trial in two counties. Linkoeping: National Swedish Road and Traffic Research Institute, 1988. 316A HS-040 518.VTI Rapport.

72. Moyes CD, Tustin RJ, McLean JF, Turner GR. Changing patterns in child restraint use [letter]. N Z Med J 1984;97(753):242.

73. Nichol KP, Cooney CE. The impact of a hospital-based educational loaner infant car seat program on infant car seat usage in a community. Travel Med Int 1984;2(3): 155-8.

74. Decina LE, Temple MG, Dorer HS. Increasing child safety-seat use and proper use among toddlers. Evaluation of an enforcement and education program. Accid Anal Prev 1994;26(5):667-73.

75. Heathington KW, Philpot JW, Perry RL. Impact of legislation and public information and education on child passenger safety. Transport Res Rec 1982;(844):62–70.

76. Lane JM, Milne PW, Wood HT. Evaluation of a successful rear seat belt publicity campaign. The 12th ARRB Conference, Hobart, Tasmania, August 27–31, 1984. Vermont South, Victoria, Australia: Australian Road Research Board, 1984:13–21.

77. Pless IB, Stulginskas J, Zvagulis I. Observed effects of media campaigns on restraint use. Can J Public Health 1986;77(1):28–32.

78. Boughton CJ, Johnston IR. The effects of radio and press publicity on the safe carriage of children in cars. Warrendale, PA: Society of Automotive Engineers, 1979. Report No. 790075.

79. Bowler MA, Torpey S. Community road safety program (Latrobe Valley). First 18 months of operation. Victoria, Australia: Road Traffic Authority, 1988. GR/88/3.

80. Cox RG, Fleming D. Selective enforcement campaign to increase the use of restraints by children in motor vehicles. Sydney, Australia: National Roads and Motorists' Association, 1981. UMTRI 47823.

81. Geddis DC. How children travel in cars in New Zealand. N Z Med J 1982;95:740–2.

82. Gielen AC, Radius S. Project KISS (Kids in Safety Seats): educational approaches and evaluation measures. Health Educ 1984;15(5):43–7.

83. Hall WL, Orr BT, Suttles DT, et al. Progress report on increasing child restraint usage through local education and distribution programs. Chapel Hill: University of North Carolina Highway Safety Research Center, 1983. UNC/HSRC-83-10-2.

84. Land G, Romeis JC, Gillespie KN, Denny S. Missouri's Take a Seat, Please! and program evaluation. J Public Health Manag Pract 1997;3:52–9.

85. McCooey EB, Feun L. TLC—tender loving care for tender living cargo: an innovative approach to child passenger safety in a local health department. Health Educ 1984;15(5):48–51.

86. National Highway Traffic Safety Administration. Evaluation of child safety seat enforcement strategies. Washington, DC: U.S. Department of Transportation, National Highway Traffic Safety Administration, 1989. DOT HS 807 479.

87. Wheeler YCH. Restraint use attitudes and knowledge prior to and following the 1993 rear seat child restraint use campaign in NSW amongst three non-English speaking background communities. New South Wales, Australia: Roads and Traffic Authority (NSW), Road Safety Bureau, 1994. Research Note RN 15/94.

88. Foss RD. Evaluation of a community-wide incentive program to promote safety restraint use. Am J Public Health 1989;79(3):304–6.

89. Roberts MC, Turner DS. Rewarding parents for their children's use of safety seats. J Pediatr Psychol 1986;11(1):25–36.

90. Roberts MC, Layfield DA. Promoting child passenger safety: a comparison of two positive methods. J Pediatr Psychol 1987;12(2):257–71.

91. Stuy M, Green M, Doll J. Child care centers: a community resource for injury prevention. J Dev Behav Pediatr 1993;14(4):224–9.

92. Liberato CP, Eriacho B, Schmiesing J, Krump M. SafeSmart safety seat intervention project: a successful program for the medically-indigent. Patient Educ Couns 1989; 13(2):161–70.

93. Arneson SW, Triplett JL. Riding with Bucklebear: an automobile safety program for preschoolers. J Pediatr Nurs 1990;5(2):115–22.

94. Christophersen ER, Sosland-Edelman D, LeClaire S. Evaluation of two comprehensive infant car seat loaner programs with 1-year follow-up. Pediatrics 1985;76(1):36–42.

95. Goebel JB, Copps TJ, Sulayman RF. Infant car seat usage. Effectiveness of a postpartum educational program. J Obstet Gynecol Nurs 1984;13(1):33–6.

96. Lavelle JM, Hovell MF, West MP, Wahlgren DR. Promoting law-enforcement for child protection: a community analysis. J Appl Behav Anal 1992;25(4):885–92.

97. Tietge NS, Bender SJ, Scutchfield FD. Influence of teaching techniques on infant car seat use. Patient Educ Couns 1987;9:167–75.

98. Wolf D, Tomek DJ, Stacy RD, Corbin DE, Greer DL. Promoting hospital discharge of infants in safety seats. J Community Health 1995;20(4):345–57.

99. Allen DB, Bergman AB. Social learning approaches to health education: utilization of infant auto restraint devices. Pediatrics 1976;58(3):323–8.

100. Bowman JA, Sanson-Fisher RW, Webb GR. Interventions in preschools to increase the use of safety restraints by preschool children. Pediatrics 1987;79(1):103–9.

101. Chang A, Dillman AS, Leonard E, English P. Teaching car passenger safety to preschool children. Pediatrics 1985;76(3):425–8.

102. Chang A, Hearey CD, Gallagher KD, English P, Chang PC. Promoting child passenger safety in children served by a health maintenance organization. Patient Educ Couns 1989;13:297–307.

103. Geddis DC, Pettengell R. Parent education: its effect on the way children are transported in cars. N Z Med J 1982;95:314–6.

104. Goodson JG, Buller C, Goodson WH III. Prenatal child safety education. Obstet Gynecol 1985;65(3):312–5.

105. Greenberg LW, Coleman AB. A prenatal and postpartum safety education program: influence on parental use of infant car restraints. J Dev Behav Pediatr 1982;3(1):32–4.

106. Miller JR, Pless IB. Child automobile restraints: evaluation of health education. Pediatrics 1977;59(6):907–11.

107. Williams AF, Wells JK, Ferguson SA. Development and evaluation of programs to increase proper child restraint use. J Safety Res 1997;28(2):69–73.

108. National Highway Traffic Safety Administration. Traffic safety facts 2002: occupant protection. Washington, DC: U.S. Department of Transportation, National Highway Traffic Safety Administration, 2002. DOT HS 809 610.

109. Evans L. The effectiveness of safety belts in preventing fatalities. Accid Anal Prev 1986;18:229–41.

110. National Highway Traffic Safety Administration. Fourth report to Congress: effectiveness of occupant protection systems and their use. Washington, DC: U.S. Department of Transportation, National Highway Traffic Safety Administration, 1999. DOT HS 808 919.

111. Kahane CJ. Fatality and injury reducing effectiveness of lap belts for back seat occupants. Warrendale, PA: Society of Automotive Engineers, 1987. Paper No. 870486.

112. Evans L. Traffic safety and the driver. New York: Van Nostrand Reinhold, 1991.

113. Padmanaban J, Ray R. Safety performance of rear seat occupant restraint systems. 36th STAPP Car Crash Conference Proceedings. Warrendale, PA: Society of Automotive Engineers, 1992. SAE pub. no. P-261.

114. Sleet DA, Lonero LP. Behavioral strategies for reducing traffic crashes. In: Bres-

low L, ed. Encyclopedia of public health. New York: Macmillan Reference USA/Gale Group Thomson Learning, 2002:184–7.

115. National Highway Traffic Safety Administration. Restraint system use in 19 U.S. cities. 1991 annual report. Washington, DC: U.S. Department of Transportation, National Highway Traffic Safety Administration, 1992. DOT HS 808 148.

116. Preusser DF, Preusser CW. Evaluation of Louisiana's safety belt law change to primary enforcement. Washington, DC: U.S. Department of Transportation, National Highway Traffic Safety Administration, 1997. DOT HS 808 620.

117. Ulmer RG, Preusser CW, Preusser DF. Evaluation of California's safety belt law change to primary enforcement. Washington, DC: U.S. Department of Transportation, National Highway Safety Traffic Administration, 1994. DOT HS 808 205.

118. Block A. 2000 Motor Vehicle Occupant Survey: Volume 2, seat belt report. Washington, DC: U.S. Department of Transportation, National Highway Traffic Safety Administration, 2001. DOT HS 809 389.

119. Grunbaum JA, Kann L, Kinchen SA, et al. Youth risk behavior surveillance—United States, 2001. MMWR 2002;51(SS-04):1–64.

120. Barancik JI, Kramer CF, Thode HC Jr, Harris D. Efficacy of the New York State seat belt law: preliminary assessment of occurrence and severity. Bull N Y Acad Med 1988;64:742–9.

121. Beaton SJ, Pearson GL, Arnegard RJ, Quinn KD. A field evaluation of the effectiveness of the Virginia safety belt law. Forensic Rep 1988;1:229–36.

122. Bernstein E, Pathak D, Rutledge L, Demarest G. New Mexico safety restraint law: changing patterns of motor vehicle injury, severity, and cost. Am J Emerg Med 1989; 7(3):271–7.

123. Brillhart BA, Jay HM. The impact of Texas state legislation on the use of safety belts. Rehabil Nurs 1988;13(3):146–9.

124. Campbell BJ, Stewart JR, Reinfurt DW. Change in injuries associated with safety belt laws. Accid Anal Prev 1991;23:87–93.

125. Chorba TL, Reinfurt D, Hulka BS. Efficacy of mandatory seat-belt use legislation. The North Carolina experience from 1983 through 1987. JAMA 1988;260(24):3593–7.

126. Cope JG, Johnson AW, Grossnickle WF. Behavior engineering proposals: 3. Effects on drivers and passengers of a mandatory use law for safety belts. Percept Mot Skills 1990;71:291–8.

127. Desai A, You MB. Policy implications from an evaluation of seat belt use regulation. Eval Rev 1992;16(3):247–65.

128. Dodson TB, Kaban LB. California mandatory seat belt law: the effect of recent legislation on motor vehicle accident related maxillofacial injuries. J Oral Maxillofac Surg 1988;46(10):875–80.

129. Escobedo LG, Chorba TL, Remington PL, Anda RF, Sanderson L, Zaidi AA. The influence of safety belt laws on self-reported safety belt use in the United States. Accid Anal Prev 1992;24:643–53.

130. Fielding JE, Knight KK, Goetzel RZ. The impact of legislation on self-reported safety belt use in a working population. J Occup Med 1992;34(7):715–7.

131. Kalfus GR, Ferrari JR, Arean P, et al. An examination of the New York mandatory seat belt law on a university campus. Law Hum Behav 1987;11(1):63–7.

132. Legge JS Jr. Reforming highway safety in New York State: an evaluation of alternative policy interventions. Soc Sci Q 1990;71(2):373–82.

133. Lestina DC, Williams AF, Lund AK, Zador P, Kuhlmann TP. Motor vehicle crash injury patterns and the Virginia seat belt law. JAMA 1991;265(11):1409–13.

134. Loeb PD. The effectiveness of seat belt legislation in reducing injury rates in Texas. Am Econ Rev 1995;85(2):81–4.

135. Loeb PD. Effectiveness of seat belt legislation in reducing various driver-involved injury rates in California. Accid Anal Prev 1993;25(2):189–97.

136. Lund AK, Pollner J, Williams AF. Preliminary estimates of the effects of mandatory seat belt use laws. Accid Anal Prev 1987;19(3):219–23.

137. Margolis LH, Bracken J, Stewart JR. Effects of North Carolina's mandatory safety belt law on children. Inj Prev 1996;2(1):32–5.

138. Pace BW, Thailer R, Kwiatkowski TG. New York State mandatory seatbelt use law: patterns of seatbelt use before and after legislation. J Trauma 1986;26(11):1031–3.

139. Preusser DF, Williams AF, Lund AK. The effect of New York's seat belt use law on teenage drivers. Accid Anal Prev 1987;19(2):73–80.

140. Preusser DF, Lund AK, Williams AF, Blomberg RD. Belt use by high-risk drivers before and after New York's seat belt use law. Accid Anal Prev 1988;20(4):245–50.

141. Reinfurt D. Evaluating the North Carolina safety belt wearing law. Accid Anal Prev 1990;22(3):197–210.

142. Russell J, Kresnow M, Brackbill R. Effect of adult belt laws and other factors on restraint use for children under age 11. Accid Anal Prev 1994;26:287–95.

143. States JD, Annechiarico RP, Good RG, et al. A time comparison study of the New York State safety belt use law utilizing hospital admission and police accident report information. Accid Anal Prev 1990;22(6):509–21.

144. Streff F, Wagenaar AC, Schultz RH. Reductions in police-reported injuries associated with Michigan's safety belt law. J Safety Res 1990;21:9–18.

145. Thyer BA, Robertson M. An initial evaluation of the Georgia safety belt use law: a nul MUL? Environ Behav 1993;25(4):506–13.

146. Tipton RM, Camp CC, Hsu K. Effects of mandatory seat belt legislation on self-reported seat belt use among male and female college students. Accid Anal Prev 1990; 22(6):543–8.

147. Ulmer RG, Preusser CW, Preusser DF, Cosgrove LA. Evaluation of California's safety belt law change from secondary to primary enforcement. J Safety Res 1995;26(4): 213–20.

148. Wagenaar AC, Wiviott MB. Effects of mandating seatbelt use: a series of surveys on compliance in Michigan. Public Health Rep 1986;101:505–13.

149. Wagenaar AC, Maybee RG, Sullivan KP. Mandatory seat belt laws in eight states: a time-series evaluation. J Safety Res 1988;19:51–70.

150. Wagenaar AC, Margolis LH. Effects of a mandatory safety belt law on hospital admissions. Accid Anal Prev 1990;22(3):253–61.

151. Williams AF, Wells JK, Lund AK. Shoulder belt use in four states with belt use laws. Accid Anal Prev 1987;19(4):251–60.

152. Winnicki J. Safety belt use laws: evaluation of primary enforcement and other provisions. Washington, DC: U.S. Department of Transportation, National Highway Traffic Safety Administration, 1995. DOT HS 808 324.

153. Adeyanju M. Public knowledge, attitudes, and behavior toward Kansas mandatory seatbelt use: implications for public health policy. J Health Soc Policy 1991;3(2):117–35.

154. Centers for Disease Control and Prevention. Safety-belt use and motor vehicle-related injuries—Navajo nation, 1988–1991. MMWR 1992;41(38):705–8.

155. Durant RF, Legge JS. Policy design, social regulation and theory building: lessons from the traffic safety policy arena. Polit Res Q 1993;46(3):641–56.

156. Geller ES. Intervening to increase children's use of safety belts. Alcohol Drugs Driving 1989;5:37–59.

157. Kuric J, Harrison C. Spinal cord injuries and a mandatory seat belt law. Sci Nurs 1989;6(2):29–31.

158. Latimer EA, Lave LB. Initial effects of the New York State auto safety belt law. Am J Public Health 1987;77(2):183–6.

159. Maguire B, Faulkner W. Safety belt laws and traffic fatalities. J Appl Sociol 1990; 7:49–61.

160. Maguire B, Faulkner WR, Mathers RA. Seat belt laws and traffic fatalities: a research update. Soc Sci J 1996;33(3):321–33.

161. Mortimer RG, Phillippo C. Before and after study reveals public attitude and ignorance toward mandatory seat belt use. Traffic Safety 1985;85:10–1, 25.

162. Nelson DE, Bolen J, Kresnow M. Trends in safety belt use by demographics and by type of state of safety belt law, 1987 through 1993. Am J Public Health 1998;88:245–9.

163. Petrucelli E. Seat belt laws: The New York experience—preliminary data and some observations. J Trauma 1987;27(7):706–10.

164. Escobedo LG, Chorba TL, Remington PL, Anda RF, Sanderson L, Zaidi AA. State laws and the use of car safety seat belts. N Engl J Med 1991;325(22):1586–7.

165. Reinfurt DW, Stewart JR, Weaver NL, Green AM. Occupant restraint monitoring program. Chapel Hill: University of North Carolina Highway Safety Research Center, 1991. No. HSRC-PR183.

166. Asch P, Levy D. An evaluation of the New Jersey safety belt use law. Newark, NJ: Rutgers University, Bureau of Economic Research, 1989.

167. Carter E, Schonfeld P. Safety belt use and highway safety in Maryland. Washington, DC: Transportation Research Board, 1991. Transportation Research Record, No. 1325.

168. Curtis C, Lovrich NP. Report to the Washington State Legislature: The impact of the 1986 mandatory safety belt use law. Pullman: Division of Governmental Studies and Services, Washington State University, 1988.

169. Datta TK, Guzek P. Restraint system use in 19 U.S. cities—1989 annual report. Washington, DC: U.S. Department of Transportation, National Highway Traffic Safety Administration, 1990. DOT HS 807 595.

170. Hall WL, Tolbert WG, Cox CL, Lowrance JC. Comprehensive program for increasing use of safety seats and seat belts for children and young adults: final report 1992. Chapel Hill: University of North Carolina Highway Safety Research Center, 1993. UNC/HSRC-93/3/1.

171. Highway Loss Data Institute. Insurance Special Report: insurance injury loss experience in eight states with seat belt laws, 1983–1986 models. Washington, DC: Highway Loss Data Institute, 1988. HLDI A-28, HS-040 523.

172. Rock SM. Impact of the Illinois seat belt use law on accidents, deaths, and injuries. Eval Rev 1992;16:491–507.

173. Stoke CB. An observational survey of safety belt and child safety seat use in Virginia: the 1990 update. Charlottesville: Virginia Transportation Research Council, 1992. VTRC 92 R22.

174. Graham JD. Injuries from traffic crashes: meeting the challenge. Annu Rev Public Health 1993;14:515–43.

175. Evans WN, Graham JD. Risk reduction or risk compensation? The case of mandatory safety-belt use laws. J Risk Uncertain 1991;4:61–73.

176. Richens J, Imrie J, Copas A. Condoms and seatbelts: the parallels and the lessons. Lancet 2000;355(9201):400–3.

177. Wilde GJ. Risk homeostasis theory: an overview. Inj Prev 1998;4:89–91.

178. Hedlund J. Risky business: safety regulations, risk compensation, and individual behavior. Inj Prev 2000;6(2):82–9.

179. Asch P, Levy D, Shea D, Bodenhorn H. Risk compensation and the effectiveness of safety belt use laws: a case study of New Jersey. Policy Sci 1991;24:181–97.

180. Garbacz C. More evidence on the effectiveness of seat belt laws. Appl Econ 1992; 24:313–5.

181. Lund AK, Zador P. Mandatory belt use and driver risk taking. Risk Anal 1984; 4(1):41–53.

182. O'Neill B, Lund AK, Zador P, Ashton S. Mandatory belt use and driver risk taking: an empirical evaluation of the risk-compensation hypothesis. In: Evans L, Schwing RC, eds. Human behavior and traffic safety (GM symposium series). New York: Plenum Press, 1985:93–118.

183. Evans L, Wasielewski P, Von Buseck CR. Compulsory seat belt usage and driver risk-taking behavior. Hum Factors 1982;24(1):41–8.

184. Campbell BJ. The association between enforcement and seat belt use. J Safety Res 1988;19:150–63.

185. Houston DJ, Richardson LE, Neeley GW. Legislating traffic safety: a pooled time series analysis. Soc Sci Q 1995;76:328–45.

186. Houston DJ, Richardson LE, Neeley GW. Mandatory seat belt laws in the states: a study of fatal and severe occupant injuries. Eval Rev 1996;20(2):146–59.

187. Lange JE, Voas RB. Nighttime observations of safety belt use: an evaluation of California's primary law. Am J Public Health 1998;88(11):1718–20.

188. Solomon MG, Nissen WJ. Evaluation of Maryland, Oklahoma, and the District of Columbia's seat belt law change to primary enforcement. Washington, DC: U.S. Department of Transportation, National Highway Traffic Safety Administration, 2000. DOT HS 809 213.

189. Campbell BJ. The relationship of seat belt law enforcement to level of belt use. Chapel Hill: University of North Carolina Highway Safety Research Center, 1987. No. HSRC-TR72.

190. Hoxie P, Skinner D. Effects of mandatory seat belt use laws on highway fatalities in 1985. Washington, DC: U.S. Department of Transportation, National Highway Traffic Safety Administration, 1987. DOT HS 807 083.

191. Wagenaar AC, Maybee RG, Sullivan KP. Effects of mandatory seat belt laws on traffic fatalities in the first eight states enacting seat belt laws. Ann Arbor: University of Michigan Transportation Research Institute, 1987. UMTRI-87-18.

192. National Highway Traffic Safety Administration. Steps for conducting sTEPs. Washington, DC: U.S. Department of Transportation, National Highway Traffic Safety Administration, 1995. DOT HS 808 458.

193. Dussault C. Effectiveness of a Selective Traffic Enforcement Program combined with incentives for seat belt use in Quebec. Health Educ Res 1990;5(2):217–23.

194. Hagenzieker MP. Enforcement or incentives? Promoting safety belt use among military personnel in the Netherlands. J Appl Behav Anal 1991;24:23–30.

195. Jonah BA, Dawson NE, Smith GA. Effects of a selective traffic enforcement program on seat belt usage. J Appl Psychol 1982;67:89–96.

196. Jonah BA, Grant BA. Long-term effectiveness of selective traffic enforcement programs for increasing seat belt use. J Appl Psychol 1985;70(2):257–63.

197. Lund AK, Stuster J, Fleming A. Special publicity and enforcement of California's belt use law: making a "secondary" law work. J Criminal Justice 1989;17:329–41.

198. Malenfant JE, Van Houten R. The effects of nighttime seat belt enforcement on seat belt use by tavern patrons: a preliminary analysis. J Appl Behav Anal 1988;21(3): 271–6.

199. Mortimer RG, Goldsteen K, Armstrong RW, Macrina D. Effects of incentives and enforcement on the use of seat belts by drivers. J Safety Res 1990;21:25–37.

200. Roberts DS, Geller ES. A statewide intervention to increase safety belt use: adding to the impact of a belt use law. Am J Health Promot 1994;8(3):172–4.

201. Rood DH. Selective Traffic Enforcement Program for occupant restraints: final report. Albany: Institute for Traffic Safety Management and Research, State University of New York at Albany, 1987.

202. Solomon MG, Nissen WJ, Preusser DF. Occupant protection Special Traffic Enforcement Program evaluation. Washington, DC: U.S. Department of Transportation, National Highway Traffic Safety Administration, 1999. DOT HS 808 884.

203. Streff FM, Molnar LJ, Christoff C. Increasing safety belt use in a secondary enforcement state: evaluation of a three-county special enforcement program. Accid Anal Prev 1992;24(4):369–83.

204. Watson REL. The effectiveness of increased police enforcement as a general deterrent. Law Soc Rev 1986;20(2):293–9.

205. Williams AF, Reinfurt D, Wells JK. Increasing seat belt use in North Carolina. J Safety Res 1996;27(1):33–41.

206. Williams AF, Lund AK, Preusser DF, Blomberg RD. Results of a seat belt use law enforcement and publicity campaign in Elmira, New York. Accid Anal Prev 1987;19(4): 243–9.

207. Williams AF, Hall WL, Tolbert WG, Wells JK. Development and evaluation of pilot programs to increase seat belt use in North Carolina. J Safety Res 1994;25(3):167–75.

208. Jones R, Joksch H, Lacey J, Wiliszowski C, Marchetti L. Site report: Knoxville, Tennessee field test of combined speed, alcohol and safety belt enforcement strategies. Washington, DC: U.S. Department of Transportation, National Highway Traffic Safety Administration, 1995. DOT HS 808 243.

209. Mounce NH, Brackett RQ, Womack KN. Evaluation on six occupant protection selective traffic enforcement programs in Texas. Washington, DC: U.S. Department of Transportation, National Highway Traffic Safety Administration, 1990. Contract No. DTNH22–89-C-05192.

210. Williams AF, Preusser DF, Blomberg RD, Lund AK. Seat belt use law enforcement and publicity in Elmira, New York: A reminder campaign. Am J Public Health 1987; 77(11):1450–1.

211. National Highway Traffic Safety Administration. 1998 Motor Vehicle Occupant Safety Survey. Volume 2: seatbelt report. Washington, DC: U.S. Department of Transportation, National Highway Traffic Safety Administration, 2000. DOT HS 809 051.

212. Moskowitz H, Fiorentino D. A review of the literature on the effects of low doses of alcohol on driving-related skills. Washington, DC: U.S. Department of Transportation, National Highway Traffic Safety Administration, 2000. DOT HS 809 028.

213. Department of Transportation and Related Agencies Appropriations Act, 2001, Pub. L. No. 106–346, 2000.

214. Apsler R, Char AR, Harding WM, Klein TM. The effects of .08 BAC laws. Washington, DC: U.S. Department of Transportation, National Highway Traffic Safety Administration, National Center for Statistics and Analysis, 1999. DOT HS 808 892.

215. Foss RD, Stewart JR, Reinfurt DW. Evaluation of the effects of North Carolina's 0.08% BAC law. Chapel Hill: University of North Carolina Highway Safety Research Center, 1998. DOT HS 808 893.

216. Hingson R, Heeren T, Winter M. Lowering state legal blood alcohol limits to 0.08%: the effect on fatal motor vehicle crashes. Am J Public Health 1996;86(9):1297–9.

217. Hingson R, Heeren T, Winter M. Effects of recent 0.08% legal blood alcohol limits on fatal crash involvement. Inj Prev 2000;6(2):109–14.

218. Johnson D, Fell J. The impact of lowering the illegal BAC limit to .08 in five states. 39th Annual Proceedings, Association for the Advancement of Automotive Medicine, October 16–18, 1995, Chicago, 1995:45–64.

219. Research and Evaluation Associates. The effects following the implementation of an 0.08 BAC limit and administrative per se law in California. Washington, DC: U.S. Department of Transportation, National Highway Traffic Safety Administration, National Center for Statistics and Analysis, 1991. DOT HS 807 777.

220. Rogers PN. The general deterrent impact of California's 0.08% blood alcohol concentration limit and administrative per se license suspension laws, vol. 1. Sacramento: California Department of Motor Vehicles, Research and Development Section, 1995. No. CAL-DMV-RSS-95-158.

221. Scopatz RA. Methodological study of between-states comparisons, with particular application to .08% BAC law evaluation. Paper presented at the Transportation Research Board 77th annual meeting. Washington, DC, January 11–15, 1998.

222. Voas RB, Tippets AS, Fell J. The relationship of alcohol safety laws to drinking drivers in fatal crashes. Accid Anal Prev 2000;32:483–92.

223. Brown DB, Maghsoodloo SA. A study of alcohol involvement in young driver accidents with the lowering of the legal age of drinking in Alabama. Accid Anal Prev 1981; 13(4):319–22.

224. Chaloupka FJ, Saffer H, Grossman M. Alcohol control policies and motor vehicle fatalities. J Legal Stud 1993;22:161–86.

225. Cook PJ, Tauchen G. The effect of minimum drinking age legislation on youthful auto fatalities. J Legal Stud 1984;13:169–90.

226. Decker MD, Graitcer PL, Schaffner W. Reduction in motor vehicle fatalities associated with an increase in the minimum drinking age. JAMA 1988;260(24):3604–10.

227. Dee TS. State alcohol policies, teen drinking and traffic fatalities. J Public Econ 1999;72(2):289–315.

228. DuMouchel W, Williams AF, Zador P. Raising the alcohol purchase age: its effects on fatal motor vehicle crashes in twenty-six states. J Legal Stud 1987;16(1):249–66.

229. Ferreira J, Sickerman A. The impact of Massachusetts reduced drinking age on auto accidents. Accid Anal Prev 1976;8:229–39.

230. Figlio DN. Effect of drinking age laws and alcohol-related crashes: time-series evidence from Wisconsin. J Policy Anal Manage 1995;14(4):555–66.

231. Hingson R, Scotch N, Mangione T, et al. Impact of legislation raising the legal drinking age in Massachusetts from 18 to 20. Am J Public Health 1983;73:163–9.

232. Hoskin AF, Yalung Mathews D, Carraro BA. Effect of raising the legal minimum drinking age on fatal crashes in 10 states. J Safety Res 1986;17(3):117–21.

233. Lillis R, Williams T, Williford W. The impact of the 19-year-old drinking age in New York. Advances in Substance Abuse 1987;suppl 1, Control Issues in Alcohol Abuse Prevention: Strategies for States and Communities:133–46.

234. Males M. Minimum purchase age for alcohol and young-driver fatal crashes: a long-term view. J Legal Stud 1986;15(1):181–211.

235. Naor EM, Nashold RD. Teenage driver fatalities following reduction in the legal drinking age. J Safety Res 1975;7:74–9.

236. O'Malley PM, Wagenaar AC. Effects of minimum drinking age laws on alcohol use, related behaviors and traffic crash involvement among American youth: 1976–1987. J Stud Alcohol 1991;52(5):478–91.

237. Ruhm CJ. Alcohol policies and highway vehicle fatalities. J Health Econ 1996; 15(4):435–54.

238. Saffer H, Grossman M. Drinking age laws and highway mortality rates: cause and effect. Econ Inq 1987;25:403–17.

239. Saffer H, Grossman M. Beer taxes, the legal drinking age, and youth motor vehicle fatalities. J Legal Stud 1987;16:351–74.

240. Saffer H, Chaloupka F. Breath testing and highway fatality rates. Appl Econ 1989;21(7):901–12.

241. Smith DI, Burvill PW. Effect on traffic safety of lowering the drinking age in three Australian states. J Drug Issues 1986;16:183–98.

242. Smith RA, Hingson RW, Morelock S, et al. Legislation raising the legal drinking age in Massachusetts from 18 to 20: effect on 16 and 17 year olds. J Stud Alcohol 1984; 45:534–9.

243. Voas RB, Tippetts AS, Fell J. The United States limits drinking by youth under age 21: does this reduce fatal crash involvements? 43rd Annual Proceedings, Association for the Advancement of Automotive Medicine, September 20–21, 1999. Barcelona (Sitges), Spain, 1999:265–78.

244. Wagenaar AC. Raising the legal drinking age in Maine: impact on traffic accidents among young drivers. Int J Addict 1983;18:365–77.

245. Wagenaar AC, Maybee R. Legal minimum drinking age in Texas: effects of an increase from 18 to 19. J Safety Res 1986;17(4):165–78.

246. Wagenaar AC. Preventing highway crashes by raising the legal minimum age for drinking: the Michigan experience 6 years later. J Safety Res 1986;17(3):101–9.

247. Whitehead PC, Craig J, Langford N, MacArthur C, Stanton B, Ferrence RG. Collision behavior of young drivers: impact of the change in the age of majority. J Stud Alcohol 1975;36:1208–23.

248. Williams AF, Rich RF, Zador PL. The legal minimum drinking age and fatal motor vehicle crashes. J Legal Stud 1975;4:219–39.

249. Williams AF, Zador PL, Harris SS, Karpf RS. The effect of raising the legal minimum drinking age on involvement in fatal crashes. J Legal Stud 1983;12:169–79.

250. Womble K. Impact of minimum drinking age laws on fatal crash involvements: an update of the National Highway Traffic Safety Administration analysis. J Traffic Safety Educ 1989;37(1):4–5.

251. Asch P, Levy DT. Does the minimum drinking age affect traffic fatalities? J Policy Anal Manage 1987;6(2):180–92.

252. Asch P, Levy DT. Young driver fatalities: the roles of drinking age and drinking experience. South Econ J 1990;57:512–20.

253. Bako G, Mackenzie WC, Smith ESO. The effect of legislated lowering of the drinking age on total highway accidents among young drivers in Alberta, 1970–1972. Can J Public Health 1976;67:161–3.

254. Colon I, Cutter HSG. The relationship of beer consumption and state alcohol and motor vehicle policies to fatal accidents. J Safety Res 1983;14:84–9.

255. Colon I. The alcohol beverage purchase age and single-vehicle highway fatalities. J Safety Res 1984;15:159–62.

256. Legge JS Jr, Park J. Policies to reduce alcohol-impaired driving: evaluating elements of deterrence. Soc Sci Q 1994;75(3):594–606.

257. MacKinnon DP, Woodward JA. The impact of raising the minimum drinking age on driver fatalities. Int J Addict 1986;21(12):1331–8.

258. Robertson LS. Blood alcohol in fatally injured drivers and the minimum legal drinking age. J Health Polit Policy Law 1989;14(4):817–25.

259. Vingilis E, Smart RG. Effects of raising the legal drinking age in Ontario. Br J Addict 1981;76:415–25.

260. Wilkinson JT. Reducing drunken driving: which policies are most effective? South Econ J 1987;54:322–34.

261. Zylman R. Fatal crashes among Michigan youth following reduction of legal drinking age. Q J Stud Alcohol 1974;35:283–6.

262. Arnold R. Effect of raising the legal drinking age on driver involvement in fatal crashes: the experience of thirteen states. Washington, DC: U.S. Department of Transportation, National Highway Traffic Safety Administration, 1985. DOT HS 806 902.

263. Wagenaar AC. Effects of an increase in the legal minimum drinking age. Public Health Policy 1981;2:206–24.

264. Wagenaar AC. Effects of the raised legal drinking age on motor vehicle accidents in Michigan. HSRI Res Rev 1981;11(4):1–8.

265. National Highway Traffic Safety Administration. The use of sobriety checkpoints for impaired driving enforcement. Washington, DC: U.S. Department of Transportation, National Highway Traffic Safety Administration, 1990. DOT HS 807 656.

266. Voas RB, Rhodenzer E, Lynn C. Evaluation of Charlottesville checkpoint operation: final report, December 30, 1983 to December 31, 1984. Washington, DC: U.S. Department of Transportation, National Highway Traffic Safety Administration, 1985. US DOT Contract no. DTNH 22–83-C-05088.

267. Lacey JH, Jones RK, Smith RG. Evaluation of checkpoint Tennessee: Tennessee's statewide sobriety checkpoint program. Washington, DC: U.S. Department of Transportation, National Highway Traffic Safety Administration, 1999. DOT HS 808 841.

268. Mercer GW, Cooper PJ, Kristiansen LA. A cost/benefit analysis of a 5-month intensive alcohol-impaired driving road check campaign. 40th Annual Proceedings of the Association for the Advancement of Automotive Medicine, Vancouver, British Columbia, October 7–9, 1996:283–92.

269. Castle SP, Thompson JD, Spataro JA, et al. Early evaluation of a statewide sobriety checkpoint program. 39th Annual Proceedings, Association for the Advancement of Automotive Medicine, October 16–18, 1995, Chicago, 1995:65–78.

270. Jones R, Joksch H, Lacey J, Wiliszowski C, Marchetti L. Site report: Wichita, Kansas field test of combined speed, alcohol, and safety belt enforcement strategies.

Washington, DC: U.S. Department of Transportation, National Highway Traffic Safety Administration, 1995. DOT HS 808 244.

271. Lacey JH, Stewart JR, Marchetti LM, Popkin CK, Murphy PV. Enforcement and public information strategies for DWI (driving-while-intoxicated) general deterrence: ARREST DRUNK DRIVING—the Clearwater and Largo, Florida experience. Chapel Hill: University of North Carolina Highway Safety Research Center, 1986.

272. Levy DT, Asch P, Shea D. An assessment of county programs to reduce driving while intoxicated. Health Educ Res 1990;5(2):247–56.

273. Mercer GW. The relationships among driving while impaired charges, police drinking-driving roadcheck activity, media coverage and alcohol-related casualty traffic accidents. Accid Anal Prev 1985;17(6):467–74.

274. Stuster JW, Blowers PA. Experimental evaluation of sobriety checkpoint programs. Washington, DC: U.S. Department of Transportation, National Highway Safety Traffic Administration, 1995. DOT HS 808 287.

275. Voas RB, Holder HD, Gruenewald PJ. The effect of drinking and driving interventions on alcohol-involved traffic crashes within a comprehensive community trial. Addiction 1997;92(suppl. 2):S221-S236.

276. Wells JK, Preusser DF, Williams AF. Enforcing alcohol-impaired driving and seat belt use laws, Binghamton, NY. J Safety Res 1992;23(2):63–71.

277. Armour M, Monk K, South D, Chomiak G. Evaluation of the 1983 Melbourne random breath testing campaign: interim report, casualty accident analysis. Melbourne, Australia: Victoria Road Traffic Authority, 1985. N8–85.

278. Arthurson RM. Evaluation of random breath testing. Sydney: Traffic Authority of New South Wales, 1985. Research Note RN 10/85.

279. Cameron M, Diamantopolou K, Mullan N, Dyte D, Gantzer S. Evaluation of the country random breath testing and publicity program in Victoria, 1993–1994. Melbourne, Australia: Monash University Accident Research Center, 1997. Report 126.

280. Cameron MH, Cavallo A, Sullivan G. Evaluation of the random breath testing initiative in Victoria, 1989–1991: multivariate time series approach. Melbourne, Australia: Monash University Accident Research Centre, 1992. Report 38.

281. Hardes G, Gibberd RW, Lam P, Callcott R, Dobson AJ, Leeder SR. Effects of random breath testing on hospital admissions of traffic-accident casualties in the Hunter Health Region. Med J Aust 1985;142(12):625–6.

282. Henstridge J, Homel R, Mackay P. The long-term effects of random breath testing in four Australian states: a time series analysis. Canberra, Australia: Federal Office of Road Safety, 1997. No. CR 162.

283. Homel R, Carseldine D, Kearns I. Drink-driving countermeasures in Australia. Alcohol Drugs Driving 1988;4(2):113–44.

284. McCaul KA, McLean AJ. Publicity, police resources and the effectiveness of random breath testing. Med J Aust 1990;152(6):284–6.

285. McLean AJ, Clark MS, Dorsch MM, Holubowycz OT, McCaul KA. Random breath testing in South Australia: effects on drink-driving. Adelaide, South Australia: NHMRC Road Accident Research Unit, University of Adelaide, 1984. HS 038 357.

286. Ross HL, McCleary R, Epperlein T. Deterrence of drinking and driving in France: an evaluation of the law of July 12, 1978. Law Soc Rev 1981;16:345–74.

287. Armstrong BK, Howell CM. Trends in injury and death in motor vehicle acci-

dents in Australia in relation to the introduction of random breath testing. Aust Drug Alcohol Rev 1988;7(3):251–9.

288. Dunbar JA, Penttila A, Pikkarainen J. Drinking and driving: success of random breath testing in Finland. BMJ 1987;295(6590):101–3.

289. Hendrie D, Cooper L, Ryan G, Kirov C. Review of the random breath testing program in Western Australia in 1996/1997. Nedlands, Western Australia: Road Accident Prevention Research Unit, Department of Public Health, the University of Western Australia, 1998. Research Report RR67.

290. Lacey JH, Marchetti LM, Stewart JR, et al. Enforcement and public information strategies for DWI general deterrence: the Indianapolis, Indiana experience. Washington, DC: U.S. Department of Transportation, National Highway Traffic Safety Administration, 1988. DOT HS 807 434.

291. Lacey JH, Jones RK. Assessment of changes in DWI enforcement/level: final report. Washington, DC: U.S. Department of Transportation, National Highway Traffic Safety Administration, 1991. DOT HS 807 690.

292. Levy D, Shea D, Asch P. Traffic safety effects of sobriety checkpoints and other local DWI programs in New Jersey. Am J Public Health 1989;79(3):291–3.

293. Paciullo G. Random breath testing in New South Wales. Med J Aust 1983;1:620–1.

294. Vingilis E, Salutin L. A prevention programme for drinking and driving. Accid Anal Prev 1980;12:267–74.

295. Homel R. The impact of random breath testing in New South Wales, December 1982 to February 1983. Med J Aust 1983;(i):616–9.

296. Homel R. Drink-driving law enforcement and the legal blood alcohol limit in New South Wales. Accid Anal Prev 1994;26(2):147–55.

297. Levy D. Methodologies for the evaluation of local traffic safety programs: with an application to New Jersey DWI programs. Eval Program Plann 1988;11(3):255–66.

298. Vingilis E, Salutin L, Chan G. R.I.D.E. (Reduce Impaired Driving in Etobicoke): a driving-while-impaired countermeasure programme, one-year evaluation. Toronto: Addiction Research Foundation, 1979.

299. Lund AK, Jones IS. Detection of impaired drivers with a passive alcohol sensor. In: Noordzij PC, Roszbach R, eds. Alcohol, drugs, and traffic safety. Proceedings of the 10th International Conference on Alcohol, Drugs, and Traffic Safety, Amsterdam, September 9–12, 1986. Amsterdam: Elsevier, 1987:379–82.

300. *Michigan Department of State Police v. Sitz.* No. 88-1897, Supreme Court of the United States. 1990.

301. Miller TR, Galbraith MS, Lawrence BA. Costs and benefits of a community sobriety checkpoint program. J Stud Alcohol 1998;59:462–8.

302. Wesemann P. Costs and benefits of police enforcement in the Netherlands. In: Perrine MW, ed. Alcohol, drugs, and traffic safety. Proceedings of the 11th International Conference on Alcohol, Drugs and Traffic Safety, Chicago, October 24–27, 1989. Chicago: National Safety Council, 1990:142–50.

303. Zador PL, Krawchuk SA, Voas RB. Alcohol-related relative risk of driver fatalities and driver involvement in fatal crashes in relation to driver age and gender: an update using 1996 data. J Stud Alcohol 2000;61:387–95.

304. Quinlan KP, Brewer RD, Sleet DA, Dellinger AM. Child passenger deaths and injuries involving drinking drivers. JAMA 2000;(283)17:2249–52.

305. Blomberg RD. Lower BAC limits for youth: evaluation of the Maryland .02 law. Washington, DC: U.S. Department of Transportation, National Highway Traffic Safety Administration, 1992. DOT HS 807 860.

306. Haque MO, Cameron M. Effect of the Victorian Zero BAC legislation on serious casualty accidents: July 1984–December 1985. J Safety Res 1989;20(3):129–37.

307. Hingson R, Heeren T, Winter M. Lower legal blood alcohol limits for young drivers. Public Health Rep 1994;109(6):738–44.

308. Maisey GE. The effect of lowering the statutory alcohol limit for first year drivers from 0.08 to 0.02 gm/100 ml (monograph). Perth: Western Australia Police Department, Research and Statistic Section, 1984. Research Report 84/2.

309. Voas RB, Lange JE, Tippetts AS. Enforcement of the zero tolerance law in California: a missed opportunity? 42nd Annual Proceedings, Association for the Advancement of Automotive Medicine, October 5–7, 1998. Charlottesville, VA. 1998:369–83.

310. Lacey JH, Jones RK, Wiliszowski CH. Zero tolerance laws for youth: four states' experience. Washington, DC: U.S. Department of Transportation, National Highway Traffic Safety Administration, 2000. DOT HS 809 053.

311. Smith DI. Effect of low proscribed blood alcohol levels (BALs) on traffic accidents among newly-licensed drivers. Med Sci Law 1986;26(2):144–8.

312. Streff FM, Hopp ML. Evaluation of Michigan's under age 21 zero-tolerance alcohol-impaired driving law. Ann Arbor: University of Michigan Transportation Research Institute, 1997. UMTRI 97–50.

313. Hingson R, Heeren T, Morelock S. Effects of Maine's 1982 .02 law to reduce teenage driving after drinking. Alcohol Drugs Driving 1989;5(1):25–36.

314. Hingson R, Heeren T, Howland J, Winter M. Reduced BAC limits for young people (impact on night fatal crashes). Alcohol Drugs Driving 1991;7(2):117–27.

315. Miller TR, Lestina DC, Spicer RS. Highway crash costs in the United States by driver age, blood alcohol level, victim age, and restraint use. Accid Anal Prev 1998;30(2):137–50.

316. Toomey TL, Kilian GR, Gehan JP, Perry CL, Jones-Webb R, Wagenaar AC. Qualitative assessment of training programs for alcohol servers and establishment managers. Public Health Rep 1998;113(2):162–9.

317. Geller ES, Elder JP, Hovell MF, Sleet DA. Behavior change approaches to deterring alcohol-impaired driving. In: Ward W, Lewis FM, eds. Advances in health education and promotion, Vol. 3. London: Jessica Kingsley, 1991:45–68.

318. Alcohol Epidemiology Program. Alcohol policies in the United States: highlights from the 50 states. Minneapolis: University of Minnesota Press, 2000.

319. McKnight AJ, Streff FM. The effect of enforcement upon service of alcohol to intoxicated patrons of bars and restaurants. Accid Anal Prev 1994;26(1):79–88.

320. Holder H, Wagenaar A, Saltz RF, Mosher J, Janes K. Alcoholic beverage server liability and the reduction of alcohol-related problems: evaluation of dram shop laws (final report). Washington, DC: U.S. Department of Transportation, National Highway Traffic Safety Administration, 1990. DOT HS 807 628.

321. Hauritz M, Homel R, McIlwain G, Burrows T, Townsley M. Reducing violence in licensed venues through community safety action projects: the Queensland experience. Contemp Drug Probl 1998;25:511–51.

322. Single E. Server intervention: a new approach to the prevention of impaired driving. Health Educ Res 1990;5(2):237–45.

323. Saltz RF. The role of bars and restaurants in preventing alcohol-impaired driving: an evaluation of server intervention. Eval Health Prof 1987;10(1):5–27.

324. Saltz RF. Research needs and opportunities in server intervention programs. Health Educ Q 1989;16(3):429–38.

325. Gliksman L, McKensie D, Single E, Douglas R, Brunet S, Moffatt K. The role of alcohol providers in prevention: an evaluation of a server intervention programme. Addiction 1993;88(9):1195–203.

326. Holder HD, Wagenaar AC. Mandated server training and reduced alcohol-involved traffic crashes: a time series analysis of the Oregon experience. Accid Anal Prev 1994;26(1):89–97.

327. Lang E, Stockwell T, Rydon P, Beel A. Can training bar staff in responsible serving practices reduce alcohol-related harm? Drug Alcohol Rev 1998;17(1):39–50.

328. Russ NW, Geller ES. Training bar personnel to prevent drunken driving: a field evaluation. Am J Public Health 1987;77(8):952–4.

329. Howard-Pitney B, Johnson MD, Altman DG, Hopkins R, Hammond N. Responsible alcohol service: a study of server, manager, and environmental impact. Am J Public Health 1991;81(2):197–9.

330. McKnight AJ. Factors influencing the effectiveness of server-intervention education. J Stud Alcohol 1991;52(5):389–97.

331. Saltz RF, Stanghetta P. A community-wide responsible beverage service program in three communities: early findings. Addiction 1997;92(suppl 2):s237-s249.

332. Geller ES, Russ NW, Delphos WA. Does server intervention training make a difference? Alcohol Health Res World 1987;11(4):64–9.

333. McKnight AJ. Development and field test of a responsible alcohol service program. Volume III: final results. Washington, DC: U.S. Department of Transportation, National Highway Traffic Safety Administration, 1989. DOT HS 807 449.

334. Saltz RF. Server intervention: will it work? Alcohol Health Res World 1986; 10(4):12–9.

335. Stockwell TR, Rydon P, Lang E, Beel AC. An evaluation of the "Freo Respects You" responsible alcohol service project. Perth, Western Australia: National Centre for Research into the Prevention of Drug Abuse, Division of Health Sciences, Curtin University of Technology, 1993. NDRI Technical Report No. T40.

336. Peters J. Beyond server training: An examination of future issues. Alcohol Health Res World 1986;10(4):24–7.

337. Cameron M, Vulcan P. Evaluation review of the supplementary road safety package and its outcomes during the first two years. Auckland, New Zealand: Land Transport Safety Authority, 1998.

338. Epperlein T. Initial deterrent effects of the crackdown on drinking drivers in the state of Arizona. Accid Anal Prev 1987;19(4):285–303.

339. Lastovicka JL. Highway safety mass media youth project. Washington, DC: U.S. Department of Transportation, National Highway Traffic Safety Administration, 1987. Contract DTNH22–85-C-15404.

340. McLean AJ, Kloeden CN, McCaul KA. Drink-driving in the general night-time driving population, Adelaide 1989. Aust J Public Health 1991;15(3):190–3.

341. Newstead S, Cameron M, Gantzer S, Vulcan A. Modelling of some major factors influencing road trauma trends in Victoria 1989–1993. Victoria, Australia: Monash University Accident Research Centre, Victoria, 1995:74.

342. Worden JK, Waller JA, Riley TJ. The Vermont public education campaign in alcohol and highway safety: A final review and evaluation. Waterbury: Vermont Department of Mental Health, 1975. CRASH Report No. I-5.

343. Macpherson T, Lewis T. New Zealand drink-driving statistics: the effectiveness of road safety television advertising. Marketing Bull 1998;9:40–51.

344. Tay R. Effectiveness of the anti-drink driving advertising campaign in New Zealand. Road Transport Res 1999;8(4):3–15.

345. DeJong W. A review of national television PSA campaigns for preventing alcohol-impaired driving, 1987–1992. J Public Health Policy 1995;16(1):59–80.

346. Wallack L. Drinking and driving: toward a broader understanding of the role of the mass media. J Public Health Policy 1984;5:471–96.

347. Yanovitzky I, Bennett C. Media attention, institutional response, and health behavior change: the case of drunk driving, 1978–1996. Communic Res 1999;26:429–53.

348. Murry JP, Stam A, Lastovicka JL. Evaluating an anti-drinking and driving advertising campaign with a sample survey and time series intervention analysis. J Am Stat Assoc 1993;88(421):50–6.

349. Cameron MH, Haworth N, Oxley J, Newstead SV, Le T. Evaluation of Transport Accident Commission road safety advertising. Melbourne, Australia: Monash University Accident Research Centre, 1993. Report No. RN52.

350. Murry JP Jr, Stam A, Lastovicka JL. Paid- versus donated-media strategies for public service announcement campaigns. Public Opin Q 1996;60:1–29.

351. Centers for Disease Control and Prevention. Motor-vehicle occupant injury: strategies for increasing use of child safety seats, increasing use of safety belts, and reducing alcohol-impaired driving. A report on recommendations of the Task Force on Community Preventive Services. MMWR 2001;50(RR-7):1–13.

352. Task Force on Community Preventive Services. Recommendations to reduce injuries to motor vehicle occupants: increasing child safety seat use, increasing safety belt use, and reducing alcohol-impaired driving. Am J Prev Med 2001;21(4S):16–22.

353. Zaza S, Carande-Kulis VG, Sleet DA, et al. Methods for conducting systematic reviews of the evidence of effectiveness and economic efficiency of interventions to reduce injuries to motor vehicle occupants. Am J Prev Med 2001;21(4S):23–30.

354. Zaza S, Sleet DA, Thompson RS, Sosin DM, Bolen JC, Task Force on Community Preventive Services. Reviews of evidence regarding interventions to increase use of child safety seats. Am J Prev Med 2001;21(4S):31–47.

355. Dinh-Zarr TB, Sleet DA, Shults RA, et al. Reviews of evidence regarding interventions to increase use of safety belts. Am J Prev Med 2001;21(4S):48–65.

356. Shults RA, Elder RW, Sleet DA, et al. Reviews of evidence regarding interventions to reduce alcohol-impaired driving. Am J Prev Med 2001;21(4S):66–88.

357. Elder RW, Shults RA, Sleet DA, et al. Effectiveness of mass media campaigns for reducing drinking and driving and alcohol-involved crashes: a systematic review. Am J Prev Med 2004;27(1):57–65.

Chapter 9

Violence

*Insufficient evidence means that we were not able to determine whether or not the intervention works.

The Task Force approved the recommendations in this chapter in 2001–2002. The research on which the findings are based was conducted prior to December 2001. Findings on home visitation and firearms laws have been published in the MMWR Recommendations and Reports series [2003:52(RR-14):1–20] and findings on therapeutic foster care have also been published [2004:53(RR- 10):1–8]. Expanded reports on the findings summarized in this chapter are being submitted to the American Journal of Preventive Medicine for publication in a special supplement.

Reducing violence-related injury and death is a major goal of public health. Violence-related injuries and deaths can result from both interpersonal violence and suicidal behavior. The consequences of violence also make it an important public health concern. Among people of all ages, 20,308 deaths from homicide and 30,622 deaths from suicide were reported in 2001.[1] Although interpersonal violence has declined substantially since the mid-1990s, in 2002 there were 2.3 incidents of violent crime (assault, robbery, and rape, but not murder[2]) for every 100 people in the United States 12 years of age and older.

Violent crimes by and against juveniles (people under 18 years of age) are a major focus of our systematic reviews of violence prevention. Over the past 25 years, juveniles have been involved as offenders in at least 25% of serious violent victimizations.[3] Rates of arrest for violent crimes peak in the late teen years.[3] In a survey, victims estimated that more than one-third of the perpetrators of violent crime were 20 years of age or younger.[2] In 1994, 33% of juvenile homicide victims were killed by a juvenile offender.[3]

In 2000, 16- to 19-year-olds in the United States were also more likely to be victims of violent crime than any other age group.[2] Since at least 1976, people between the ages of 18 and 24 years have experienced the highest rates of homicide.[3] Youth under the age of 15 years in the United States are five times as likely to be murdered as are their counterparts in 25 other industrialized nations combined.[4] In 1999, 4.2% of juveniles were reported to be victims of maltreatment (abuse or neglect).[5] Violent victimization of women, including threats of rape and sexual assault, is highest among women 16–19 years of age.[2]

Rates of suicide also rise substantially during adolescence, reaching a plateau among people aged 35 to 44 years and rising substantially again only after age 74.[6] The rate of suicide among children under the age of 15 in the United States is twice that of the combination of 25 industrialized nations noted above.[4]

OBJECTIVES AND RECOMMENDATIONS FROM OTHER ADVISORY GROUPS

Home Visitation

In 1991, the U.S. Advisory Board on Child Abuse and Neglect recommended universal home visitation,[7] but its recommendation was not accepted by the Department of Health and Human Services or implemented by Congress. In contrast to the findings of the Task Force review reported here, some government reviews have found home visitation effective for preventing youth violence. The recent report on *Youth Violence* by the Surgeon General[8] concludes that nurse home visitation "has shown significant long-term effects on violence, delinquency, and related risk factors in a number of studies." The Office of Justice Programs' review, *Preventing Crime. What Works, What Doesn't, What's Promising,*[9] also gives a high rating to early home visitation by nurses, other professionals, and trained paraprofessionals for preventing crime and its risk factors. The Centers for Disease Control and Prevention (CDC) cites the home visitation approach among the best practices for preventing youth violence.[10] Violence-specific objectives in *Healthy People 2010*[11] that might be related to home visitation are included in Table 9-1. (It should be noted that home visitation may also affect health-related outcomes other than violence. As noted, these outcomes are not systematically reviewed here, and corresponding goals and objectives are not included in Table 9-1.)

Other governments have also reviewed home visitation programs. The Canadian Task Force on Preventive Health Care recommends early childhood home visitation programs for preventing child maltreatment in disadvantaged families.[12] It notes that the strongest evidence exists for the nurse-delivered programs (as used in the program by Olds et al.[13]), which start prenatally and continue for two years after the child is born.

Finally, nonprofit organizations have assessed the benefits of home visitation. The Center for the Study and Prevention of Violence recommends nurse home visitation for preventing child abuse and neglect and child violence, among other benefits. It cites the program designed by Olds et al.[13] as a model "Blueprint" program that meets its highest standards of evidence in terms of experimental design, substantial effect, replication, and sustainability. Similarly, Developmental Research and Programs, Inc., cites several early home visitation programs[14] (including the nurse home visitation program by Olds et al.[15] and the Syracuse Family Development Research Program[16]) among its recommended preventive strategies.

Therapeutic Foster Care

The Surgeon General's 2001 report on *Youth Violence*[8] recommended therapeutic foster care as a model program for preventing further violence among violent or seriously delinquent adolescents. In contrast to the findings of the Task Force review reported here, the Surgeon General's 1999 report on *Mental Health*[17] endorsed therapeutic foster care for children with emotional problems without clearly specifying age limits; this report also noted the standards of the Foster Family-Based Treatment Association (www.ffta.org/products.html).

Similarly, the Center for the Study and Prevention of Violence recommends therapeutic foster care as a cost-effective alternative to group or residential treatment, incarceration, or hospitalization for adolescents who have prob-

Table 9–1. Selected *Healthy People 2010*[11] Objectives Related to Violence Prevention

Objective	Population	Baseline	2010 Objective
Injury Prevention			
Reduce hospitalization for nonfatal head injuries per 100,000 population (Objective 15–1)	All	60.6 (1998[a])	45.0
Reduce hospitalization for nonfatal spinal cord injuries per 100,000 population (15–2)	All	4.5 (1998[a])	2.4
Reduce firearm-related deaths per 100,000 population (15–3)	All	11.3 (1998[a])	4.1
Reduce the proportion of persons living in homes with firearms that are loaded and unlocked (15–4)	All	19% (1998[a])	16%
Reduce nonfatal firearm-related injuries per 100,000 population (15–5)	All	24.0 (1997[a])	8.6
Reduce nonfatal poisonings per 100,000 population (15–7)	All	348.4 (1997[a])	292
Reduce deaths caused by poisoning per 100,000 population (15–8)	All	6.8 (1998[a])	1.5
Reduce deaths caused by suffocation per 100,000 population (15–9)	All	4.1 (1998[a])	3.0
Reduce hospital emergency department visits per 1,000 population (15–12)	All	131 (1997[a])	126
Unintentional Injury Prevention			
Reduce deaths caused by unintentional injuries per 100,000 population (15–13)	All	35.0 (1998[a])	17.5
Reduce nonfatal unintentional injuries (15–14)	All	Developmental	
Violence and Abuse Prevention			
Reduce homicides per 100,000 population (15–32)	All	6.5 (1998[a])	3.0
Reduce maltreatment of children per 1000 children aged <18 years (15–33a)	Children	12.9[b] (1998)	10.3
Reduce child maltreatment fatalities per 100,000 children aged <18 years (15–33b)	Children	1.6[b] (1998)	1.4
Reduce the rate of physical assault by current or former intimate partners per 1000 persons aged ≥12 years (15–34)	Adolescents/ adults	4.4 (1998)	3.3
Reduce the annual rate of rape or attempted rape per 1000 persons aged ≥12 years (15–35)	Adolescents/ adults	0.8 (1998)	0.7
Reduce sexual assault other than rape per 1000 persons aged ≥12 years (15–36)	Adolescents/ adults	0.6 (1998)	0.4

Table 9–1. *Continued*

Objective	Population	Baseline	2010 Objective
Reduce physical assaults per 1000 persons aged ≥12 years (15–37)	Adolescents/ adults	31.1 (1998)	13.6
Reduce physical fighting among adolescents (students in grades 9 through 12) fighting during the previous 12 months) (15–38)	Adolescents	36% (1999)	32%
Reduce weapon carrying by adolescents on school property (students in grades 9 through 12 carrying during the past 30 days) (15–39)	Adolescents	6.9% (1999)	4.9%
Mental Health and Mental Disorders			
Reduce the suicide rate per 100,000 population (18–1)	All	11.3 (1998[a])	5.0
Reduce the rate of suicide attempts by adolescents (12-month average) among adolescents in grades 9 though 12 (18–2)	Adolescents	2.6% (1999)	1.0%

[a]Age adjusted to year 2000 standard population.

[b]Note that objective 15–33a is per 1000 children under 18 years of age, whereas objective 15–33b is per 100,000 children under 18 years of age. Comparable objectives would be reduction of child maltreatment to 1290 per 100,000 children under 18 years of age and reduction of child maltreatment fatalities to 1.6 per 100,000.

lems with chronic antisocial behavior, emotional disturbance, and delinquency.[18] The Center also cites evidence of the effectiveness of therapeutic foster care for younger children. The Center recommends the program designed by Chamberlain[19] as a model "Blueprint" program that meets its highest standards of evaluation evidence.

Violence-specific objectives in *Healthy People 2010*[11] that might be related to therapeutic foster care are included in Table 9–1.

Firearms Laws

Firearms-specific objectives in *Healthy People 2010*[11] are included in Table 9–1.

METHODS

Methods used for the reviews are summarized in Chapter 10. Specific methods used in the systematic reviews of violence prevention have been described elsewhere[20-22] and are available at www.thecommunityguide.org/violence.

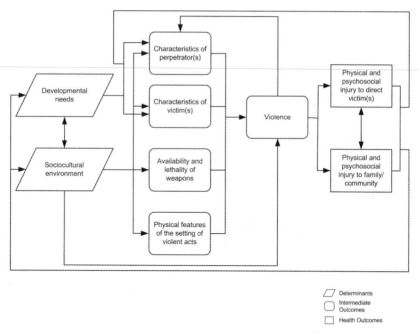

Figure 9–1. Logic framework illustrating the conceptual approach used in systematic reviews of violence prevention.

The logic framework depicting the conceptual approach used in these reviews is presented in Figure 9–1.

ECONOMIC EFFICIENCY

A systematic review of available economic evaluations was conducted for the recommended interventions, and a summary of each review is presented with the related intervention. The methods used to conduct these economics reviews are summarized in Chapter 11.

RECOMMENDATIONS AND FINDINGS

The three sections that follow present a summary of the findings of the systematic reviews conducted to determine the effectiveness of the selected interventions in preventing violence.

Early Childhood Home Visitation

In early childhood home visitation programs, parents and children are visited at home during the child's first two years of life by trained personnel who provide some combination of information, support, or training about child health, development, and care. Home visitation has been used to meet a wide range of objectives, including improvement of the home environment, family development, and the prevention of child behavior problems. Early childhood home visitation has been used to address a variety of public health goals for both visited children and their parents, including violence reduction, other health outcomes (e.g., rates of vaccination) and health-related outcomes such as educational achievement, problem-solving skills, and greater access to resources (e.g., social services, education, and employment opportunities).[23,24]

Our systematic review of the effectiveness of early childhood home visitation for preventing violence focused on violence by and against juveniles. We defined home visitation as a program that includes visitation of parent(s) and child(ren) in their home by trained personnel who convey information about child health, development, and care; offer support; provide training; or deliver any combination of these services. Visitors can be nurses, social workers, other professionals, or paraprofessionals (people with no formal training, who are trained specifically by and for the home visitation program; they may be community peers). For purposes of this review, visits had to occur during at least part of the child's first two years of life, but could begin during pregnancy and continue after the child's second birthday. Although we were prepared to review programs in which participation in home visitation programs was either voluntary or mandated (e.g., by a court), we found no program in which participation was mandated.

In the United States, home visitation programs have generally been offered to specific groups, such as low-income; minority; young; less educated; first-time mothers; substance abusers; children at risk of abuse or neglect; and low-birthweight, premature, disabled, or developmentally compromised infants. (Home visitation programs are common in Europe and are most often universal [i.e., made available to all childbearing families, regardless of the estimated risk of child-related health or social problems].[25]) Visitation programs are often *two-generational*,[26] addressing problems and introducing interventions of mutual benefit to parents and children. Programs may include (but are not limited to) one or more of the following components: training of parent(s) on prenatal and infant care; training on parenting to prevent child abuse and neglect; developmental interaction with infants and toddlers; family planning assistance; development of problem-solving and life skills; educational and work opportunities; and linkage with community services. Home visitation programs may be complemented by the provision of day care; parent group meetings for support, instruction, or both; advocacy; transportation; or other services. When such services are provided in addition to home visitation, we refer to the program as *multicomponent*.

We reviewed studies of home visitation that assessed any of four violent outcomes, whether or not violence was the primary target or outcome of the visitation.

1. Violence against the child, specifically maltreatment (which includes all forms of child abuse and neglect).
2. Intimate partner violence.
3. Violence by the visited parent, other than child maltreatment or intimate partner violence.
4. Violence by the visited child, against self or others, including violence in school, delinquency, crime, or other observed or reported violent behavior.

Early Childhood Home Visitation to Prevent Violence Against the Child (Maltreatment [Abuse or Neglect]): Recommended (Strong Evidence of Effectiveness)

In 1999, 4.2% of children under the age of 18 in the United States were reported to be victims of maltreatment. One-third of those reports were investigated by child protective services and were not confirmed. Further complicating this picture, national survey data indicate that cases of maltreatment are substantially underreported.[27-29] Child maltreatment can include physical, sexual, or emotional abuse; physical, emotional, or educational neglect; or any combination. Not only is child maltreatment a form of violence in and of itself, but it is associated with adverse consequences among maltreated children, such as early pregnancy, drug abuse, school failure, mental illness, suicidal behavior, and chronic diseases.[30-32] Although the relationship is not well understood, children who have been physically abused are more likely to perpetrate aggressive behavior and violence later in their lives, even when other risk factors for violent behavior have been ruled out.[33] Abuse and neglect are both associated with poverty and single-parent households; for reasons such as this, many home visitation programs in the United States are directed to poorer, minority, and single-parent families.

Effectiveness

- Early childhood home visitation is effective in reducing child maltreatment by approximately 39%.
- Programs using nurses or mental health workers were more effective than those using paraprofessionals.
- Beneficial effects were found principally in programs lasting two years or longer.

- These programs should be applicable to most families at risk, as defined above.

We reviewed evidence about the effects of home visitation on the subsequent maltreatment (abuse or neglect) of visited children. We included studies in the review only if they reported at least one of these outcome measures: reports from child protective services; abuse or neglect reported or observed by parents or others; emergency room visits or hospitalizations for injury or ingestion; reported injury; or out-of-home placement. We looked for but did not find any qualifying studies about other forms of child victimization, such as bullying.

The results of our systematic review are based on 21 studies (with 26 intervention arms, in 20 reports).[34-53] One additional study (representing one intervention arm) had limitations in the quality of execution and was excluded from the review.[54]

Intervention arms assessed the effects of home visitation on abuse or neglect (reported by child protective services or by home visitors); on rates of injury, trauma, or the ingestion of poison (from records of emergency room visits, other medical or hospital records, or mothers' reports); and on out-of-home placement. Most studies assessed maltreatment, injury, or trauma at the end of the intervention (follow-ups, 10 months to 3 years). One study[50] assessed abuse and neglect 15 years after the intervention began (i.e., when the children were 15 years of age). Overall, the intervention group had a lower rate of abuse or neglect, injury or trauma, or out-of-home placement than the comparison group (median change −38.9%; interquartile range, −74.1% to +24.0%), indicating that these programs are effective in reducing child maltreatment.

In investigating the hypothesis that home visitation can reduce or prevent maltreatment, a bias may be encountered. The presence of a home visitor who might observe maltreatment and is legally required to report it may actually increase the reported observations of maltreatment among home-visited children. Adjusting for the presence of this reporting bias tends to strengthen results showing that home visiting decreases child maltreatment.

We found that professional visitors (i.e., nurses and mental health workers) produced more beneficial results than paraprofessionals. We also found that programs that lasted two years or longer tended to show more beneficial results than shorter programs, regardless of the professional status of the visitor.

We looked for, but did not find, any substantial or consistent differences in effect based on randomized versus nonrandomized assignment to treatment group; whether programs were initiated prenatally or postnatally; or whether program components were home visitation only or home visitation plus additional services such as child care, pediatric care, free transportation, or parent support groups.

These results should be applicable to at-risk families in a variety of settings. All studies were conducted in the United States, except for one in Canada. Most programs targeted people believed to benefit most from such program components as support in parenting and life skills, prenatal care, and case management. Home visitation programs were conducted with teenage parents; single mothers; families of low socioeconomic status (SES); families with very-low-birthweight infants; parents previously investigated for child maltreatment; and parents with alcohol, drug, or mental health problems. No reviewed study assessed the effectiveness of home visitation in preventing violence in the general population.

An analysis of the effects of one program on intimate partner violence[55] suggests that parental partner violence may hinder the beneficial effects of home visitation on child abuse; therefore, partner violence may need to be addressed before home visitation programs can be effective in reducing child maltreatment in the home.

Other potential benefits were identified in one study.[50] That study reported consistently beneficial, but statistically nonsignificant, effects for visited mothers, including decreases in the number of subsequent pregnancies (a risk factor for child abuse), in months receiving Aid to Families with Dependent Children (AFDC), in months receiving food stamps, and in problems related to illicit substance use. The study also found a small increase in time employed. Statistically significant results for these outcomes were, however, found only in a subsample (40% of the total sample) that included only single mothers of low SES.

Consequences for the visited children other than violent behavior or victimization were less clear at 15-year follow- up.[15] For example, this study found decreases in the incidence of drug use, in the number of sexual partners, and in the number of long-term school suspensions, but also reported increases in the incidence of alcohol use and in the number of visited children who ever had sex. Among the children of low SES single mothers, home visitation was generally associated with desired results, including a significant reduction in the number of sex partners; nonsignificant reductions in the use of drugs, alcohol, and cigarettes; an increase in the number of short-term suspensions; and a (desirable) decrease in the number of long- term school suspensions.

Other possible beneficial effects of the home visitation programs mentioned in the literature include improved social, emotional, and physical development of visited children; higher rates of vaccination; better access to, and use of, medical care; improved family planning; improved home environment; and a higher level of education and professional achievement attained by the parents.[23,24]

We identified one economic evaluation of a home visitation intervention to reduce child abuse and neglect.[56] This study, carried out in a semi-rural county in upstate New York, evaluated the net benefits of a nurse home visitation program provided to first-time mothers. Of the mothers in the study, 61% were of low SES and 24% were either unmarried or under 19 years of age. Home visits by a registered nurse began before the child was born and lasted until the child reached two years of age. The visits began on a weekly basis; by 20 months after delivery, visits were made every six weeks. Program content included parent education, the strengthening of family support (by encouraging other family members and friends to become involved in the home visit and in child care), and the linking of families with other health and human services. Goals included improvement of the child's health, reduction of child abuse, and improvement of the mother's own life course.

The costs and benefits analyzed for this intervention were limited to government costs and benefits, not those of program participants, the healthcare system, or society at large. Program costs considered were through the child's second birthday and included nurse salaries and fringe benefits; nurse training; part-time secretary; part-time supervisor; taxicab; linked services such as the Women, Infants, and Children (WIC) nutritional supplementation program; supplies; and overhead. The benefits considered were through the child's fourth birthday and included reduced use of government services (i.e., AFDC, Child Protective Services, Food Stamps, and Medicaid) and newly generated tax revenues from mothers returning to work.

Authors reported results for a subsample of low-income mothers as well as for the whole sample. For the low-income subsample, governmental benefits more than offset program costs, for a net benefit to government of $350.61 per low-income family (adjusted to 1997 dollars). Including benefits attributable only to reduced need for child maltreatment services (3% of total benefits) was not enough to offset program costs in the low-income subsample (i.e., costs exceeded benefits). For the whole sample, governmental costs exceeded benefits, which resulted in a net benefit of -$3,081 per family (adjusted to 1997 dollars). Benefits attributable to reduced child maltreatment were not specified for the whole sample. Including benefits beyond those of the government, such as averted healthcare costs, productivity losses, and other possible benefits associated with reduced child maltreatment would likely result in greater net benefits.

For the above program, adjusted nurse visitation direct costs—including salaries, fringe benefits, part-time supervisor and secretary, overhead, travel, and supplies—were estimated to be $6286 per family in 1997 dollars over the two-year intervention period. In a 1998 follow-up investigation,[13] program costs were reestimated to be $7000 per family (in 1997 dollars). This estimate was based on the original study design but was calculated to serve 100 families with four full-time nurse specialists, each taking on no more than 25 cases. In addition to the full-time nurses, the new estimate includes a part-time secretary and nurse supervisor; comprehensive office and program materials, including cell phones; liability insurance; medical supplies; general staff development; and mileage. In most cases, training and technical assistance, including a computer and network fees, were also necessary at program outset (but were not included in the base case analysis). Such start-up costs were estimated to increase program costs to $8000 per family during the first three years of the program.

Another study with a less intensive intervention (i.e., five visits over 18 months) was conducted at the Hospital of the University of Pennsylvania in Philadelphia.[36] Early discharge and home visitation were carried out only if the infant's physical condition and environment met specified criteria (e.g., clinically well, stable maintenance of body temperature, and adequate home care facilities) and if parental consent was given. Program costs of nurse home visitation for very-low-birthweight infants who had been discharged early were estimated and included pre- and post-discharge nurse time, telephone, and travel expenses. Average program costs (adjusted to 1997 dollars) were estimated to be $958 per family. Infants included in the study were born between October 1982 and December 1984 and received post-discharge follow-up care by either a full- time or part-time specialist with a master's degree in nursing. Pre-discharge visits established a relationship between the nurse and parents to facilitate training and information exchange to prevent abuse and neglect. Post-discharge visits provided further instruction and assessment of both infant and parent well-being. Nurses also contacted the parents by telephone during the first eight weeks after discharge and were on call to address immediate concerns. The large difference between this program cost estimate and that provided by Olds et al.[13] is most likely due to program duration and frequency of visits as well as additional program costs included in the estimate.

Barriers to implementing home visitation interventions include difficulties in the retention of study participants and program staff.[23] Because home interventions have generally been targeted to families of low SES, in challenging life circumstances with few resources, it is understandable that such families might be overwhelmed with other problems and might lack sustained interest in or ability to commit to regular home visitation; they might also be hard to reach and retain in the program because of frequent life transitions.[57]

Home visiting personnel (especially when paraprofessional lay visitors are used) may be hard to recruit, train, and retain due to low pay and difficult work conditions. It has also been noted that paraprofessional visitors may require more training and supervision than professionals (e.g., nurses).

In conclusion, the Task Force found strong evidence that early childhood home visitation programs are effective in preventing child maltreatment, reducing reported maltreatment by approximately 39%. In addition, programs delivered by professional visitors (nurses or mental health workers) seemed to produce greater effects than those delivered by paraprofessionals. Beneficial results were seen in programs lasting two years or longer, whether delivered by paraprofessionals or by professionals.

Early Childhood Home Visitation to Prevent Intimate Partner Violence: Insufficient Evidence to Determine Effectiveness

Although intimate partner violence victimizes men as well as women in the United States, women are three times more likely than men to be victims.[58] One out of four women in the United States will be the victim of partner violence: 7.7% will be victims of rape and 22.1% will be victims of other physical assaults.[58] Home visitation programs have the potential to reduce violence between visited parents by improving parental life skills, strengthening family social support, and facilitating links to community services.

Effectiveness

- We found insufficient evidence to determine the effectiveness of home visitation in reducing intimate partner violence.
- Evidence was insufficient because the only study included in the review did not report a statistically significant effect of the intervention on intimate partner violence.
- Insufficient evidence means that we were not able to determine whether or not the intervention works.

In our systematic review of the evidence of the effect of home visitation on violence between the parents of visited children, we included only studies that measured reported and observed partner victimization or arrests and convictions for partner assault. The results of our review are based on one study,[59] a 15-year follow-up to the study by Olds et al.[13] Among the wide range of outcomes examined was the incidence of domestic violence in the families of visited children over the 15-year follow-up period. No significant difference in the incidence of domestic violence between the intervention and control groups was found. This single study provided insufficient evidence to determine whether or not home visitation programs are effective in reducing violence between the parents of visited children.

Because we could not establish the effectiveness of this intervention on partner violence, we did not examine situations where it would be applicable, information about economic efficiency, or possible barriers to implementation.

In conclusion, we found insufficient evidence to determine the effectiveness of home visitation in reducing violence between the parents of visited children, because only a single study qualified for the review and this study failed to find any significant changes.

Early Childhood Home Visitation to Prevent Violence by Visited Parents (Other Than Child Maltreatment or Intimate Partner Violence): Insufficient Evidence to Determine Effectiveness

Some home visitation programs try to reduce violence by visited parents by facilitating the development of parental life skills, strengthening family social support, and facilitating links to community services. We looked at what effects the visits had on the violent behavior of parents of visited children.

Effectiveness

- We found insufficient evidence to determine the effectiveness of home visitation in reducing violence by visited parents.
- Evidence was insufficient because, in the single qualifying study, statistically significant changes were found only in a subsample of the studied population.
- Insufficient evidence means that we were not able to determine whether or not the intervention works.

In our systematic review of the effect of home visitation on parental violence in the visited home (other than child maltreatment and intimate partner violence, addressed separately in this chapter), we included only studies that measured reported and observed violence, arrests or convictions for violent crime (from self-reports or official reports), or general arrests and convictions.

The results of our review are based on one study,[50] a 15-year follow-up to the Elmira study by Olds et al.[60] Nearly half of the mothers in the study had been teenagers when home visitation began. The study reported statistically nonsignificant reductions in arrests and convictions for mothers in the intervention group compared with mothers in the control group. However, in a subsample of mothers who were single and of low SES at the time of visitation, the study reported statistically significant reductions in maternal arrests and convictions. Although the findings from this subsample are encouraging, the single study provides insufficient evidence to determine whether or not home visitation programs are effective in reducing violence by visited parents.

Because we could not establish the effectiveness of this intervention, we did not examine situations where it would be applicable, information about economic efficiency, or possible barriers to implementation.

In conclusion, the Task Force found insufficient evidence to determine the effectiveness of home visitation interventions in preventing parental violence. Although statistically significant changes were found in a subsample of the population in the only study in the review, the findings for the total sample were not statistically significant.

Early Childhood Home Visitation to Prevent Violence by Visited Children: Insufficient Evidence to Determine Effectiveness

Juveniles commit violence at a higher rate than any other age group in the United States.[3] Risk factors for chronic violence include low socioeconomic status (SES), abusive parents, and poor parent–child relations, including harsh, lax, or inconsistent discipline. Early childhood home visitation might lead to the reduction of later violence by the visited child by addressing several of these risk factors, including parenting skills and opportunities for parents to improve the conditions of their families.

Effectiveness

- We found insufficient evidence to determine the effectiveness of home visitation in reducing violence by visited children.
- Evidence was insufficient because findings from the small number of available studies were inconsistent.
- Insufficient evidence means that we were not able to determine whether or not the intervention works.

In our systematic review of the effect of home visitation on the later violent behavior of children who were home-visited early in their lives, we included only studies that measured reported and observed violence or violent crime; official records of arrests, convictions, or delinquency; externalizing behavior (in which psychological problems are acted out); and conduct disorder (in which young people violate the basic rights of others or societal norms). Prevention of youth suicide was not included because we found no studies that assessed this outcome.

The findings of our systematic review are based on four studies that reported the effects of home visitation programs on violence by the visited children.[15,16,61,62] One study[15] examined criminal and delinquency outcomes in 15-year-olds whose nurse home visitation began prenatally and continued through the first two years of their lives. Self-reported delinquency (i.e., committing acts that are explicitly violent or have violent connotations [threat of violence or the violation of property and its owners]) was the principal outcome in this study because it referred to self-reported behavior, unaffected by the social processes of arrest or conviction. In the total sample, statistically nonsignificant changes were found in self-reported major delinquent acts and in arrests of subjects as reported by subjects' mothers; a statistically significant decrease was found in self-reported arrests and convictions. Among the children of single mothers of low SES, home visitation was associated with a nonsignificant decrease in major delinquent acts and with significant decreases in self-reported arrests and convictions, as well as arrests reported by the child's mother.

Another study[16] of a multicomponent home visitation program assessed delinquent and violent outcomes when visited children had reached 13–16 years of age. Using probation processing as an indicator of serious crime, the study found a significant reduction in this measure among the intervention group. Further, it appears that the offenses committed by comparison subjects were more serious than those committed by home-visited subjects and that 2 (out of 54) subjects in the comparison group committed violent crimes, whereas none of 65 subjects in the intervention group committed such crimes.

The other two studies reported only externalizing behavior (from the Externalizing subscale of the Child Behavior Checklist[63]) when the children were five years old[62] and nine years old.[61] Both studies reported no significant differences between intervention and comparison groups.

Although the number of studies is sufficient to draw a conclusion about the effectiveness of home visitation in preventing later violence by visited children, the inconsistent findings provide insufficient evidence on which to base a recommendation.

Because we could not establish the effectiveness of this intervention, we did not examine situations where it would be applicable, information about economic efficiency, or possible barriers to implementation.

In conclusion, although the number of studies in the review would be sufficient to determine the effectiveness of home visitation in preventing later violence by visited children, the study findings are inconsistent. Two studies found no significant differences in outcomes between intervention and control populations, one study found a beneficial effect, and one had mixed results. Because of these mixed findings, the evidence is insufficient to determine the effectiveness of home visitation interventions in preventing child violence.

Therapeutic Foster Care

In therapeutic foster care programs, children and adolescents who cannot live at home are placed in homes with foster parents trained to provide a structured environment that teaches social and emotional skills. Program personnel work closely with foster parents and may also collaborate with teachers, probation officers, employers, and others in the youth's environment to ensure pro-social learning and behavior. Program youth are monitored at home, in school, and during leisure activities. Although *therapeutic foster care* is known by many names, 10 common components are:[64]

1. Treating only one or two children in homes of carefully selected substitute (*foster*) families;
2. Low caseloads for each program staff member: responsible for only 5–15 youth and their foster families;
3. Close, treatment-oriented supervision of the foster parents to promote a therapeutic relationship with each child;
4. Providing thorough documentation of treatment services for each child;
5. Recognizing the professional nature of the work of treatment parents through intensive training before and during the child's stay, good pay, and regular performance evaluations;
6. Providing strong support services for treatment parents;
7. Making crisis intervention services readily available;
8. Providing a liaison to the child's school, teachers, and counselors;
9. Providing medical services, including health screening for the foster child; and
10. Coordinating the various aspects of care for each child.

We reviewed studies of the effects of therapeutic foster care on the violent behavior of (1) adolescents with chronic delinquency and (2) children with severe emotional disturbance.

Therapeutic Foster Care for the Reduction of Violence by Chronically Delinquent Adolescents: Recommended (Sufficient Evidence of Effectiveness)

In the programs in our review, older juveniles (12–18 years of age) with a history of chronic delinquency, who had been mandated to out-of-home care but were sufficiently safe to be treated in the community, were placed in therapeutic foster care. Program personnel collaborated closely and daily with foster families throughout the program (average length, six to seven months).

Effectiveness

- Programs that involve special training of foster parents, monitoring of the young people under their care, and close involvement of case workers were effective in reducing the violent behavior of these adolescents.

Applicability

- Applicability of these programs to settings and groups other than those studied cannot be assumed.

The findings of our systematic review are based on three studies by the same team of researchers, which assessed the effects of therapeutic foster care on incarcerations one year after the intervention, arrests for violent crimes one and two years after the intervention, and self-reported felony assaults one year after the intervention, respectively.[65–67] Two other studies by the same team did not evaluate violent outcomes and were therefore excluded from the review.[68,69]

In the first study, measuring rates of incarceration for all crimes of male and female adolescents (12–18 years old), those in therapeutic foster care showed significantly greater reductions than did matched controls in the two years following treatment. Additionally, more than twice the proportion of young people in therapeutic foster care completed the program than did controls. The second study compared the number of arrests for violent crimes one year before and one year after treatment among boys and girls 12–18 years old. Although the aggressive behavior of the girls increased significantly during the program and that of the boys diminished, one year after the program both girls and boys showed large and significant reductions in arrests for violent crimes. The third study, of boys 12–17 years old, showed that, although both the boys in therapeutic foster care and those in regular group homes had high rates of referral to court for delinquency after the intervention, after controlling for demographics and criminal backgrounds those in the treatment group had significantly fewer felony assaults than did the controls. Researchers also demonstrated that the family management practices of therapeutic foster care (including discipline, supervision, and positive relationships between adults and children), as well as the separation of juveniles from their delinquent peers, had a clear effect on the subsequent reduction in the boys' violent behavior.

The applicability of these findings to other settings should be viewed with caution. All three studies were conducted by the same research team in the same geographic area. The programs were intensive, including training for the foster parents, weekly parent group meetings, case workers on call at all times, and monitoring of juveniles' school, work, and leisure activities. Additionally, the young people in these programs were predominantly white; no study has evaluated the effects, if any, of differences in ethnic or racial backgrounds. In the studies reviewed, two characteristics of the young people's backgrounds did appear to limit the effectiveness of therapeutic foster care: being victims of sexual abuse and coming from homes where parents had a history of crime or chronic drug abuse.

Potential benefits, beyond the measured reductions in criminal behavior, may result from therapeutic foster care. Young people who went through these programs were taught responsible family behavior and improved their school attendance and homework performance, as well as their relations with teachers and peers. Additionally, program participants, after returning home, lived there nearly twice as long as controls.

A potential harm should be noted in the fact that the problem behaviors of girls in one study increased during the first six months of therapeutic foster care.

The findings of our systematic review of economic evaluations of therapeutic foster care programs for chronically delinquent juveniles are based on two studies.[18,70] One study[18] assessed program costs for therapeutic foster care, analyzing only those program costs incurred by the government (state and local), and included the costs of personnel (i.e., case manager, program director, therapists, recruiter, and foster parent trainer) and foster parent stipends, as well as additional health services (e.g., mental health care). Average program costs were $18,837 per youth (in 1997 dollars). This study, however, lacked sufficient detail on program costs and sensitivity analyses of important study parameters.

The second study was an incremental cost–benefit analysis[70] of a therapeutic foster care program compared with standard group care. Incremental program costs were $1912 (in 1997 dollars) per youth. Total net benefits (benefits minus costs) ranged from $20,351 to $81,664 per youth. This estimated range does not include benefits to program youth, such as increased earnings and improved life course outcomes. Although the study included many details on program benefits, insufficient details on program costs were provided.

For foster parents, the rigors of therapeutic foster care, in contrast to regular group home care, can present barriers to the implementation of these programs. Recruiting, training, and retaining foster families willing to work with the demands of the program present the major obstacles. Young people must be monitored at all times, and parents are expected to adhere closely to the relatively strict program guidelines. Providing training and support to the parents, along with an increased monthly stipend, did increase retention rates of families in the programs.[71]

In conclusion, the Task Force found sufficient evidence to recommend therapeutic foster care for adolescents (12–18 years of age) with chronic delinquency as a means of reducing violent behavior. These results, based on carefully structured programs conducted by the same research team, in the same geographic area, may not be applicable to other groups or settings if programs fail to maintain the key elements of the reviewed programs.

Therapeutic Foster Care for the Reduction of Violence by Children with Severe Emotional Disturbance: Insufficient Evidence to Determine Effectiveness

In these programs, clusters of five foster parent families cooperated in the care of five children (5–13 years old) with severe emotional disturbance (SED). Programs were conducted for an average length of 18 months.

Effectiveness

- We found insufficient evidence to determine the effectiveness of therapeutic foster care in reducing the violent behavior of children with SED.
- Evidence was insufficient because too few studies were available and those studies showed inconsistent, largely undesirable, findings.
- Insufficient evidence means that we were not able to determine whether or not the intervention works.

The findings of our systematic review are based on two studies of children with SED.[72,73] One study,[72] of boys and girls 6–12 years old, assessed the effects of cluster therapeutic foster care on *conduct disorder* (a measure of defiant behavior and physical aggression, not equivalent to the psychiatric diagnosis of conduct disorder). The other study,[73] of boys and girls 6–13 years old, focused on *externalizing behavior* as assessed in the Externalizing subscale of the Child Behavior Checklist.[63] The first study reported an increase in conduct disorders associated with cluster therapeutic foster care compared with the control program for girls and a negligible effect for boys; neither effect was statistically significant. The second study reported a small, statistically nonsignificant increase in externalizing behavior among children following the intervention. These results, therefore, provide insufficient evidence to determine whether or not therapeutic foster care is effective in reducing the violent behavior of children with SED.

Because we could not establish the effectiveness of this intervention, we did not examine situations where it would be applicable, information about economic efficiency, or possible barriers to implementation.

In conclusion, the Task Force found insufficient evidence to determine the effectiveness of therapeutic foster care in reducing the violent behavior of children with SED. Too few studies were available, and study findings were inconsistent and mostly in the undesirable direction.

Firearms Laws

Although rates of firearm-related injuries in the United States have declined since 1993, they remained the second leading cause of injury mortality in 2001.[1] In that year, an average of 81 firearm-related deaths occurred each day, including those resulting from suicide, homicide, legal intervention, and unintentional injury. From 1993 to 2000, fatal assaultive violence was highest among people 20–24 years of age; for all age groups, rates among males were approximately five times rates among females.[74] It is estimated that one-fourth of violent crimes—murder, aggravated assault, rape, and robbery—committed in 1999 (a total of 1,430,693) were committed with a firearm.[2] In 1998, for each firearm-related death, two nonfatal firearm-related injuries were treated in hospital emergency departments.[74] Rates of firearm-related homicide, suicide, and unintentional death in the United States exceed those of 25 other high-income nations (i.e., 1996 GNP≥$US9636 per capita) for which data are available.[75] In 1994, the cost of firearm-related violence in the United States was estimated to be approximately $100 billion annually, of which at least $15 billion was attributable to violence against youth.[76]

Approximately 4.5 million new firearms are sold each year in the United States, including 2 million handguns. In addition, estimates of annual secondhand firearms transactions range from 2 to 4.5 million.[77,78] Further, it is estimated that approximately a half million firearms are stolen annually.[78] Thus, the total number of firearms transactions approaches 9.5 million per year.

Our systematic review examined firearms laws as one of many approaches to the reduction of firearm-related violence.[79,80] The manufacture, distribution, sale, acquisition, storage, transportation, carrying, and use of firearms in the United States are regulated by a complex array of federal, state, and local laws and regulations. We focused on assessing the effects of selected federal and state laws on violence-related public health outcomes, including violent crimes, suicide, and unintentional injuries; we also noted related effects on other outcomes, such as property crime, the apprehension of criminals, and school expulsion. We were unable to find sufficient evidence to determine the effectiveness of any of the eight firearms laws or aspects of firearms laws reviewed: bans on specified firearms or ammunition; acquisition restrictions; waiting periods for firearm acquisition; firearm registration and licensing of firearm owners; *shall issue* concealed weapons carry laws;

child access prevention (CAP) laws; zero gun tolerance in school laws; and combinations of firearms laws.

Bans on Specified Firearms or Ammunition: Insufficient Evidence to Determine Effectiveness

Bans on firearms and ammunition prohibit the acquisition and possession of certain categories of firearms (e.g., machine guns or assault weapons) or ammunition. They can also include prohibitions on the importation or manufacture of specified firearms. Bans may be federal, state, or local and can be combined with additional firearm regulations, such as requirements for safe storage, age restrictions on acquisition, or restrictive licensing requirements for firearms dealers. Bans are intended to decrease the availability of certain types of firearms to potential offenders and thus reduce the capacity of such offenders to perpetrate crime.[81]

Bans are usually imposed on the types of firearms or ammunition thought either to be particularly dangerous and not well suited for hunting or self-defense (e.g., semi-automatic and fully automatic assault weapons) or disproportionately involved in crime (such as cheap, low-quality, small-caliber handguns often referred to as *Saturday night specials*). Sometimes, especially in high-crime urban settings, bans may include a broad spectrum of firearms (e.g., the ban enacted in Washington, DC, in 1976 on the purchase, sale, transfer, and possession of handguns by civilians unless the handguns were previously owned and registered[82]).

Bans commonly exempt firearms owned prior to implementation of the ban (i.e., the weapons are *grandfathered*), although such bans may require the registration of grandfathered firearms. Grandfathering is a critical element in bans insofar as it can allow stocks of the banned items to remain available after the ban goes into effect.

Effectiveness

- We found insufficient evidence to determine the effectiveness of bans on specified firearms and ammunition in preventing violence.
- Evidence was insufficient because of the small number of studies, limitations in study design and execution, and inconsistent results.
- Insufficient evidence means that we were not able to determine whether or not the intervention works.

The findings of our systematic review are based on nine reports.[81-89] Five studies that evaluated the 1976 Washington, DC, ban on handguns reached inconsistent conclusions about the effect of the law in reducing homicide. One study found a decrease in suicide, but this finding was inconsistent with that of another study in the review. Findings of a study of the effect on homicide of the 1994 Federal Violent Crime Control Act (banning large assault weapons and large-capacity ammunition magazines) suggested that the ban had a beneficial effect. Other studies (including two that looked at Saturday night specials) found inconsistent effects or did not measure a health-related outcome. This small number of studies, with limitations in the quality of study design and execution as well as inconsistent results, provided insufficient evidence to determine whether or not these laws are effective in reducing violence.

Because we could not establish the effectiveness of the laws reviewed, we did not examine circumstances in which they would be applicable, information about economic efficiency, or possible barriers to implementation.

In conclusion, the Task Force found insufficient evidence to determine the effectiveness of bans on specified firearms and ammunition in preventing violence. The number of available studies was small, some studies had limitations in their design or execution, and results across studies were inconsistent.

Acquisition Restrictions: Insufficient Evidence to Determine Effectiveness

Acquisition restrictions attempt to deny the purchase of firearms by people with certain characteristics that indicate high risk for illegal or other harmful use of firearms. These characteristics may relate to criminal backgrounds, such as a felony conviction or indictment, a domestic violence restraining order, being a fugitive from justice, or having been convicted on drug charges; personal situations, such as being judged to be "mentally defective," being an illegal immigrant, or having a dishonorable military discharge; and other factors, including being a minor.

Although restrictions on such factors as age are easy to confirm, conducting a background check is not always a successful process. Records are not always available, and laws limit the time allowed to research records that do exist.

Effectiveness

- We found insufficient evidence to determine the effectiveness of acquisition restrictions in preventing violence.
- Evidence was insufficient because of the small number of studies, limitations in study design and execution, and inconsistent results.
- Insufficient evidence means that we were not able to determine whether or not the intervention works.

The findings of our systematic review are based on four studies that assessed the effects of acquisition restrictions on violence.[85,90-92] Studies examined the effects of restrictions based on felony convictions (on violent crime overall and on homicide and suicide); restrictions based on misdemeanor convictions on overall violent crime; and the effect of restrictions on people who were minors, were "mentally defective," or abused drugs or alcohol on specific violent crimes, suicide, and unintentional injury. Overall, results showed inconsistent effects or were not statistically significant, thereby providing insufficient evidence to determine whether or not acquisition restrictions are effective in preventing violence.

Because we could not establish the effectiveness of the laws reviewed, we did not examine circumstances in which they would be applicable, information about economic efficiency, or possible barriers to implementation.

One potential benefit of acquisition restrictions can be the capture of people for whom warrants are outstanding. One potential harm can be denying purchase to an eligible applicant because of incorrect initial information about relevant restrictions.

In conclusion, the Task Force found insufficient evidence to determine the effectiveness of acquisition restrictions in preventing violence. The number of available studies was small, some studies had limitations in their design or execution, and results across studies were inconsistent.

Waiting Periods for Firearm Acquisition: Insufficient Evidence to Determine Effectiveness

Waiting periods for firearm acquisition require a specified delay between application for and acquisition of a firearm. This requirement is usually imposed to allow time to check the applicant's background or to provide a *cooling-off* period for people at risk of committing an impulsive crime or suicide. Waiting periods can be combined with requirements in addition to background checks, such as a requirement for safety training.

The interim Brady Handgun Violence Prevention Act,[93] a federal law that went into effect in 1994, mandated a background check and a five-day waiting period for handgun purchasers. In 1998, this waiting period expired and was replaced by a mandatory computerized National Instant Criminal Background Check System (www.fbi.gov/hq/cjisd/nics/index.htm) required not only for handguns, but also for all firearm purchases, and allowing dealers to sell a firearm if the Federal Bureau of Investigation (FBI) reports no adverse evidence to the dealer within three days of application. However, some states have longer waiting periods for handgun or long firearm purchases.

Effectiveness

- We found insufficient evidence to determine the effectiveness of waiting periods for firearm acquisition in reducing suicide, homicide, aggravated assault, robbery, rape, or unintentional firearm-related injury death.
- Evidence was insufficient because of the small number of available studies, limitations in study design and execution, and inconsistent effects.
- Insufficient evidence means that we were not able to determine whether or not the intervention works.

The findings of our review are based on seven studies on the effects of waiting periods on violent outcomes.[85,90,94–98] One study was conducted in Queensland, Australia; the rest of the studies were conducted in the United States.

Studies evaluating the effects of waiting periods on homicide had mixed results, some showing a reduction in homicide and others an increase; none of the results were statistically significant. Studies evaluating the effects of waiting periods on suicide (measuring long firearm purchase, handgun purchase [and the Brady Law five-day waiting period], and both long firearm and handgun purchases) also showed mixed results. Evidence of the law's effects on aggravated assault, robbery, rape, and unintentional firearm-related injury death were also inconsistent in direction, and none were statistically significant.

Several studies suggested the presence of a partial *substitution effect* for suicide, in which decreases in firearm-related suicide are accompanied by smaller increases in non-gun suicide. No such substitution effects were found for homicide, aggravated assault, or robbery.

Overall, these results provided insufficient evidence to determine whether or not waiting periods are effective in reducing suicide, homicide, aggravated assault, robbery, rape, or unintentional firearm-related injury deaths.

Because we could not establish the effectiveness of the laws reviewed, we did not examine circumstances in which they would be applicable, information about economic efficiency, or possible barriers to implementation.

Although concerns are sometimes voiced about the possibility that waiting periods may give criminals (who acquire firearms by illegal means and avoid the waiting period) an advantage over law-abiding citizens (who may lack means of self-defense during the waiting period), we found no evidence to support or dispute this.

In conclusion, the Task Force found insufficient evidence to determine the effectiveness of waiting periods in preventing suicide, homicide, aggravated assault, robbery, rape, or unintentional firearm-related injury death because of the small number of available studies, limitations in study design and execution, and effects that were inconsistent in direction and lacked statistical significance.

Firearm Registration and Licensing of Firearm Owners:
Insufficient Evidence to Determine Effectiveness

Registration requires that a record of the owners of specified firearms be created and retained.[99] Licensing requires an individual to obtain a license or other form of authorization or certification that allows the purchase or possession of a firearm.[99] Licensing and registration requirements are often combined with other firearms regulations, such as safety training or safe storage requirements.

Effectiveness

- We found insufficient evidence to determine the effectiveness of firearm registration and licensing of firearm owners in preventing violence.
- Evidence was insufficient because the small number of available studies had limitations in design and execution as well as inconsistent results.
- Insufficient evidence means that we were not able to determine whether or not the intervention works.

The registration practices of states and the federal government vary widely.[100] The Firearm Owners Protection Act of 1986[101] specifically precludes the federal government from establishing and maintaining a national registry of firearms and their owners. Likewise, no federal firearm licensing requirements or provisions for individual purchasers exist. However, several states have laws that require the licensing of firearm owners or registration of firearms, and recorded information is kept in centralized registries. Some states have laws requiring registration of handguns. Licensing and registration may serve as instruments for the control of illegal firearms ownership, transfer, and use[102,103] and may also deter illegal acquisition and use.

The findings of our systematic review are based on five studies on the effects of licensing on violent outcomes,[85,96–98,103] two[85,103] of which also reported on the effects of registration. One study collected data in 1980 (and one year before and after), one in 1978, one in 1969–1970, and one in 1960 and 1970; one assessed firearms retrieved from crimes during a one-year period (1997–1998). Evidence of the effects of licensing and registration on diverse outcomes was inconsistent, with half of the studies showing decreases in violence and half showing increases. These findings provided insufficient evidence to determine whether or not firearm registration or licensing of firearm owners is effective in preventing violence.

Because we could not establish the effectiveness of the laws reviewed, we did not examine circumstances in which they would be applicable, information about economic efficiency, or possible barriers to implementation.

Several benefits have been associated with the licensing of firearms owners and the registration of firearms, including enhanced law enforcement and the tracing of illegal firearms to their source.[102,104] A harm associated with licensing and registration is the threat to the privacy and perceived rights of owners.[105]

In conclusion, the Task Force found insufficient evidence to determine the effectiveness of firearm registration and licensing of owners in preventing violence. Only a small number of studies was available, with limitations in their design and execution and inconsistent results.

Shall Issue Concealed Weapons Carry Laws: Insufficient Evidence to Determine Effectiveness

Shall issue concealed weapons carry laws (shall issue laws) require authorities to issue permits to carry concealed weapons to any qualified applicant. Prior to 1977, only 8 states had shall issue laws; as of 2000, 31 states had them.[106] In contrast, some states have *may issue* laws—in which the issuing authority has the discretion to issue or deny a firearms permit based on such criteria as the perceived need or moral character of the applicant—and some states completely prohibit the carrying of concealed weapons. State laws vary as to who can receive a carry permit, but generally disqualify someone who has had a prior felony conviction or a conviction on a drug charge in the past three years, who has been committed to a mental hospital in the past five years, who is a fugitive from justice, or who is too young. State laws also differ substantially in terms of firearms safety training, permit fees, and places where firearms may not be carried.[107]

Effectiveness

- We found insufficient evidence to determine the effectiveness of shall issue laws in preventing homicide, aggravated assault, robbery, rape, or homicide of police.
- Evidence was insufficient because too few qualifying studies were available for each outcome of interest.
- Insufficient evidence means that we were not able to determine whether or not the intervention works.

Two principal hypotheses, not mutually exclusive, have been proposed to predict the effects of shall issue laws. Because the laws allow for self-defense, some believe that potential criminals may be deterred by fear of an armed victim.[108] If so, publicity about the law and the fact that individuals could be carrying concealed firearms is likely to be more important in reducing violence than the actual number of firearms carried. Others have reasoned that the presence of more firearms can both increase rates of unintended and intended injury in spontaneous confrontations and lead potential criminals to carry and use more lethal firearms more often.[109] If this is correct, the actual number of additional firearms carried is important. In a survey on the attitudes of imprisoned felons,[110,111] felons claim to be deterred from committing a crime if they think victims might be armed, but they also carry firearms to deter violence by victims. Therefore, shall issue laws may have contrary effects on firearms behavior—both deterring and escalating firearms carrying among perpetrators.

The findings of our systematic review are based on four studies of the effects of shall issue laws on violent outcomes.[85,112–114] An additional eight studies were identified but did not meet our quality criteria and were excluded from the review.[108,115–121]

Analysis of available data was hampered by the methods used to collect data (at the county, state, and federal levels), the types of data (e.g., versus arrests), and the sources of data reporting. Because of concerns about the reliability of county-level crime data for research purposes,[122] we did not consider any of the county-level studies in our assessment of the effects of shall issue laws on violence.

The four qualifying studies of shall issue laws included one study that examined national effects on homicide using Vital Statistics reports (from the National Center for Health Statistics [NCHS] of the CDC); one study that used both Vital Statistics and FBI Uniform Crime Report (UCR) data to examine the effects of shall issue and other firearms laws on multiple violent outcomes; one study that used Vital Statistics to assess the effects of shall issue laws in five selected counties; and one study that used state-level UCR data to assess the effects of shall issue laws on homicides in which police are the victims. Thus, three qualifying studies assessed homicide as an outcome, one assessed police as homicide victims, and one assessed multiple other violent outcomes.

The limited amount of available evidence showed no consistent trends and provided insufficient evidence to determine whether or not shall issue laws are effective in preventing violence. Two studies suggested a reduction in homicide associated with shall issue laws at the national level and a third suggested mixed effects, with an overall increase in homicide associated with the laws. The study of police as homicide victims showed a small, statistically nonsignificant decline in the homicide of police associated with shall issue laws. (Over the past three decades, a mean of 83 police have been the victims of homicide per year—0.6% of all U.S. homicides. We consider this separate from homicide in the general population.)

Because we could not establish the effectiveness of the laws reviewed, we did not examine circumstances in which they would be applicable, information about economic efficiency, or possible barriers to implementation.

In conclusion, the Task Force found insufficient evidence to determine the effects of shall issue laws on homicide, aggravated assault, robbery, rape, and homicide of police because too few qualifying studies were available for each outcome of interest.

Child Access Prevention Laws: Insufficient Evidence to Determine Effectiveness

Child access prevention (CAP) laws are designed to limit children's access to and use of firearms. The laws require firearm owners to store their firearms locked, unloaded, or both. In some states, firearm owners are liable not simply when firearms are improperly stored, but also when a child uses the owner's improperly stored firearm to threaten or harm him- or herself or another person.

Child access prevention laws are relatively recent: Florida passed the first in 1989, and after the shootings at Columbine High School in April 1999, two more states adopted CAP laws and they were under consideration in six more states.[123] By 2000, 16 states had adopted CAP laws.[106] In three CAP law states (Florida, Connecticut, and California) violation of CAP laws is a felony; in the rest of CAP law states it is a misdemeanor.

Effectiveness

- We found insufficient evidence to determine the effectiveness of CAP laws in preventing violence.
- Evidence was insufficient because only a small number of studies, with limitations in the quality of execution, was available.
- Insufficient evidence means that we were not able to determine whether or not the intervention works.

The findings of our systematic review are based on three studies of the effect of CAP laws;[95,124,125] all examined the outcome of unintentional firearm-related injury deaths, and one examined firearm-related and non-firearm-related suicides and homicides. On the untested assumption that locked and unloaded firearms may hinder rapid access to firearms for self-defense, one study examined multiple outcomes, including violent crimes (i.e., homicide, aggravated assault, robbery, and rape) committed with and without firearms, as well as firearm-related suicides. All studies assessed outcomes among juveniles; one study also examined effects on older age groups.

All the studies presented a common challenge for our analysis: the law is intended to reduce injuries *caused* by juveniles, but the studies all assess juvenile *victims*. As a result, the assessment of the effects of CAP laws on outcomes other than suicide may be biased. None of the studies assessed levels of publicity, awareness, or enforcement of CAP laws.

One study indicated that the reduction in unintentional firearm-related injury death among juveniles less than 15 years of age was statistically significant in states that prosecute CAP law violations as a felony, and was not significant in states in which the crime is a misdemeanor. However, another study, including data from three additional states that had passed CAP laws and three more years of follow-up, confirmed the earlier finding on states with misdemeanor prosecution but showed that the effect of the law on unintentional firearm-related injury death among juveniles less than 15 years of age is statistically significant in Florida (a state with a felony sanction) but not in the other two felony states.

One study indicated a reduction in firearm-related suicide among juveniles less than 15 years of age associated with CAP laws. Studies of homicide, assault, robbery, and rape indicate mixed results, with two showing reductions in firearm-related homicide among juveniles less than 15 years of age and in assault at all ages and three showing increases in total homicide, robbery, and rape at all ages. (Only the findings on robbery and rape are statistically significant.) Overall, too few studies examined each outcome to determine the effectiveness of CAP laws in preventing violence.

Because we could not establish the effectiveness of the laws reviewed, we did not examine circumstances in which they would be applicable, information about economic efficiency, or possible barriers to implementation.

In conclusion, the Task Force found insufficient evidence to determine the effectiveness of CAP laws in preventing violence or unintentional firearm-related injury and other violent outcomes because of the small number of available studies, all with limitations in the quality of execution.

Zero Tolerance of Firearms in Schools: Insufficient Evidence to Determine Effectiveness

The Gun-Free Schools Act, passed in 1994,[126] stipulates that each state receiving federal funds under the Act must have a law requiring local education agencies to expel a student from school for at least one year if the student is found in possession of a firearm at school. (This expulsion requirement can be modified on a case-by-case basis.) Expulsion may lead to alternative school placement or to *street* placement (full expulsion, with no formal education, for a specified length of time), after which students are generally allowed to return to their regular schools.

Effectiveness

- We found insufficient evidence to determine the effectiveness of zero tolerance of firearms in schools in preventing violence.
- Evidence was insufficient because we found no studies of these laws.
- Insufficient evidence means that we were not able to determine whether or not the intervention works.

The carrying of weapons in schools appears to have declined steadily during the 1990s, as did involvement in physical fights on school property.[127,128] However, the proportion of high school students who reported being threatened or injured with a weapon on school property in the past year remained steady over this period, at 7% to 9%. The rate of serious violent crimes at or on the way to school peaked in 1994 and declined from then until at least 2000.[128] And, whether or not metal detectors are a viable approach to reducing the presence of guns in schools, few schools use them: in 1996–1997, 4% of public schools reported random, hand-held metal detector checks on students, and in 1% of schools students were required to pass through metal detectors every day.[129] By our estimate, it appears that less than 4.4% of firearms carried in schools were detected in association with the Gun-Free Schools Act.[20]

In our systematic review, we found no study that attempted to evaluate the effects of zero tolerance of firearms in schools on violence, nor did we find a study measuring the specific effect of the Gun-Free Schools Act on firearm carrying in schools. Therefore, the evidence was insufficient to determine whether or not zero tolerance is effective in preventing violence or in reducing the carrying of firearms in schools. We did, however, find one study[130] of the effectiveness of metal detector programs in reducing the carrying of firearms in schools. (Although firearms detection is not explicitly required in the Gun-Free Schools Act, the effectiveness of the law may depend on the ability to detect firearms.) The rate of carrying firearms to, from, or in school was half as great in schools with metal detector programs as in schools without the programs, although the rate of weapon carrying elsewhere was the same.

Because we could not establish the effectiveness of the laws reviewed, we did not examine circumstances in which they would be applicable, information about economic efficiency, or possible barriers to implementation.

A major potential, albeit unintended, harm of the Gun-Free Schools Act of 1994, particularly if firearm detection becomes more effective, is the street expulsion of thousands of students with low school achievement and high risk of violence. Even though the specific effect of firearm-related expulsion is not known, expulsion can result in a life course with fewer opportunities for (legal) employment, fewer resources, and a greater likelihood of criminal behavior and imprisonment.[131,132] The resulting lower productivity and increased criminal activity may well have high societal costs.[131] One review for the U.S. Department of Education[133] indicates that alternative schools for violent students may be effective and cost effective in reducing violent behavior and enhancing emotional development for youth suspended or expelled from school; however, the review also notes that alternative schools may stigmatize their students and increase discrimination against them.

In conclusion, the Task Force found insufficient evidence to determine the effectiveness of zero tolerance of firearms in schools in preventing violence because no studies of zero tolerance were identified. A single study measured the effect of a school metal detector program on firearm-carrying behavior but not specifically on violence.

Combinations of Firearms Laws: Insufficient Evidence to Determine Effectiveness

The process that makes firearms available includes manufacture or import, distribution, acquisition, storage, and carrying. Because of the complexity and diversity of the manufacture, distribution, and use of firearms in the United States, laws that attempt to reduce violence by targeting single aspects of the firearms process may be ineffective. We examined whether combinations of laws are more effective in reducing violence than individual laws.

Effectiveness

- We found insufficient evidence to determine the effectiveness of combinations of firearms laws in preventing violence.
- Evidence was insufficient because the available studies showed inconsistent findings.
- Insufficient evidence means that we were not able to determine whether or not the intervention works.

The findings of our systematic review are based on three kinds of evidence: studies of the effects of comprehensive national laws, cross-national studies of firearms laws, and *index studies* (in which law types within jurisdictions are categorized and counted, and the counts compared with rates of specific forms of violence within the same jurisdictions).

Our review of comprehensive national laws focused on two such laws: the Gun Control Act of 1968 (Public Law 90–618) in the United States (two studies[96,134]) and the Criminal Law Amendment Act of 1977 in Canada (10 studies[135–144]). A study of the Gun Control Act of 1968 showed results in opposite directions (an increase in homicide, adjusted for new firearms, and a decrease in homicide, adjusted for the total firearm stock). The best study of the comprehensive Canadian firearms law indicated decreased rates of homicide but increased rates of firearm-related suicide.

In the cross-national studies of comprehensive laws, the effects of more and less comprehensive firearms regulations on violence were assessed by comparing regions within the United States and Canada (three studies[145-147]). One study found an association between the degree of firearms regulation and firearm-related aggravated assault and homicide, but not of other forms of interpersonal violence. The second study found that the degree of regulation was associated with lower rates of firearm-related suicide and higher rates of other forms of suicide. The third study indicated no association between national levels of firearms regulation and rates of homicide.

The index studies compared degrees of firearms regulation and violent outcomes among U.S. states and cities. Our findings are based on six index studies.[85,96,97,148-150] Two additional studies were identified but did not meet our quality criteria and were excluded from the review.[98,151] Index studies yielded heterogeneous results about homicide, rape, aggravated assault, robbery, and unintentional firearm-related injury death. Only for suicide did all index studies show a reduction associated with a greater amount of regulation: two of five results were statistically significant.

Overall, these results provided insufficient evidence to determine whether these combinations of laws are effective in preventing violence.

Because we could not establish the effectiveness of the combinations of laws reviewed, we did not examine circumstances in which they would be applicable, information about economic efficiency, or possible barriers to implementation.

In conclusion, based on national law assessments, international comparisons, and index studies, the Task Force found insufficient evidence to determine whether the degree or intensity of firearms regulation is associated with decreased (or increased) violence. Current evidence is inconsistent and, in general, methodologically inadequate to draw conclusions about causal effects.

REDUCING VIOLENCE THROUGH USE OF THESE RECOMMENDATIONS

Many environmental, community, family, and personal risk factors for the development of violent behaviors are recognized.[152,153] The two interventions recommended by the Task Force in this review—early childhood home visitation for the prevention of child maltreatment and therapeutic foster care for the reduction of violence by chronically delinquent adolescents—offer opportunities to reduce the development of serious violent behavior by carrying out family-level interventions at two critical developmental phases. Home visitation programs of two or more years' duration may prevent the initiation of a form of violence that is detrimental for all immediately involved and, in addition, has severe long-term personal and societal consequences and costs for direct victims and others. In turn, therapeutic foster care may serve to end or slow the development of chronically violent behaviors that have already been initiated and that have long-term consequences for adolescent perpe- trators, for their families and communities, and for society more broadly.

The median effect of home visitation programs—a 39% reduction in rates of child maltreatment in comparison to programs with minimal services, but not including home visits—indicates the enormous potential of these pro- grams. The population that might benefit is a large one. In 1999, 33% of the 3.6 million births in the United States were to single mothers, 12% were to teen mothers, and 22% were to mothers with less than a high school educa- tion;[154] 43% of births—approximately 1.7 million—were to mothers with at least one of these characteristics (B. Hamilton, National Center for Health Statistics, personal communication, Sept. 9, 2002). In addition, some home visitation programs are designed to address other populations at risk, such as poor single mothers.

The median effect of therapeutic foster care—on the order of a 70% re- duction in rates of violence among chronically delinquent adolescent partici- pants, compared with the usual care in group homes—also indicates the great potential of such programs. The population that might be served by these programs is also large, though difficult to estimate; it is likely to be on the order of tens or hundreds of thousands of adolescents. Countering the development of chronically violent behaviors by means of therapeutic foster care would clearly require both extensive societal commitment to support such programs and the commitment of individual families and communities to undertake the daily work of therapeutic foster care, which is undoubtedly both challenging and rewarding. Here again, the benefits are likely to sub- stantially reward the societal investment.

Decisions about choosing programs to address the problem of violence clearly depend on the magnitude of the problem in the decision makers' com- munities, other problems they face and their priorities, and the resources they have or may call upon. For both programs recommended here, in addi- tion to financial resources, personnel to implement the program and adapt it to local needs and personnel to deliver the program (i.e., trained home visi- tors and trained therapeutic foster care families) will be needed. In Europe, home visitation programs are common, well established, and financed by na- tional and local governments; integrated with other health and social service programs; and most often universal (i.e., made available to all childbearing families, regardless of the estimated risk of child-related health or social problems).[25] Researchers have suggested that, in the United States, programs such as Medicaid might serve as a foundation for a national program of early childhood home visitors directed at needy populations.[25]

CONCLUSION

This chapter summarizes Task Force conclusions and recommendations on interventions to reduce violent behavior, primarily among juveniles. To prevent violence directed at children (maltreatment [abuse or neglect]), the Task Force recommends home visitation during early childhood. Insufficient evidence exists at this time to determine the effectiveness of early childhood home visitation to prevent intimate partner violence, violence by visited parents (other than child maltreatment or intimate partner violence), or violence by visited children. The Task Force recommends therapeutic foster care for the reduction of violence by chronically delinquent adolescents, but evidence was insufficient to determine the effectiveness of therapeutic foster care for the reduction of violence by children with severe emotional disturbance.

The Task Force also reviewed possible ways to reduce the injury and premature death associated with improper use of firearms, but found insufficient evidence to determine the effectiveness of any of eight approaches: bans on specified firearms or ammunition; acquisition restrictions; waiting periods for firearm acquisition; firearm registration and licensing of firearm owners; shall issue concealed weapon carry laws; child access prevention laws; zero tolerance of firearms in schools; and combinations of firearms laws.

Insufficient evidence should not be interpreted as evidence of ineffectiveness, but rather as lack of current knowledge about whether an intervention is effective or not. Details of these reviews have been published[20-22,155-157] and these articles, along with additional information about the reviews, are available at www.thecommunityguide.org/violence.

Acknowledgments

This chapter was written by members of the systematic review development team: Robert A. Hahn, PhD, MPH, Division of Prevention Research and Analytic Methods (DPRAM), Epidemiology Program Office (EPO), Centers for Disease Control and Prevention (CDC), Atlanta; Oleg O. Bilukha, MD, PhD, DPRAM/EPO/CDC, Atlanta; Jessica S. Lowy, MPH (therapeutic foster care only), DPRAM/EPO/CDC, Atlanta; Susan Snyder, PhD, DPRAM/EPO/CDC, Atlanta; Alex Crosby, MD, MPH, Division of Violence Prevention, National Center for Injury Prevention and Control (NCIPC), CDC, Atlanta; Mindy T. Fullilove, MD, New York State Psychiatric Institute, Columbia University, New York, New York and the Task Force on Community Preventive Services; Farris Tuma, ScD; and Eve K. Moscicki, ScD, MPH, National Institute of Mental Health, Bethesda, Maryland; Akiva Liberman, PhD, National Institute of Justice, Department of Justice, Washington, DC.

Consultants for all reviews were: Laurie M. Anderson, PhD, DPRAM/EPO/CDC, Olympia, Washington; Carl Bell, MD, Community Mental Health Council, Chicago, Illinois; Red Crowley, Men Stopping Violence, Atlanta, Georgia; Sujata Desai, PhD, NCIPC/CDC, Atlanta; Deborah French, Colorado Department of Public Health and Environment, Denver; Darnell F. Hawkins, PhD, JD, University of Illinois at Chicago; Danielle LaRaque, MD, Harlem Hospital Center, New York, New York; Barbara Maciak, PhD, MPH, EPO/CDC, Detroit, Michigan; James Mercy, PhD, NCIPC/CDC, Atlanta; Suzanne Salzinger, PhD, New York State Psychiatric Institute, New York, New York; Patricia Smith, Michigan Department of Community Health, Lansing.

Articles included in the reviews were abstracted by: Oleg O. Bilukha; Robert A. Hahn; and Melissa Stigler.

References

1. Arias E, Anderson RN, Hsiang-Ching K, Murphy SL, Kochanek KD, Division of Vital Statistics. Deaths: final data for 2001. Natl Vital Stat Rep 2003;52(3):1–115.

2. Maguire K, Pastore AL, eds. Sourcebook of criminal justice statistics 2002. U.S. Department of Justice, Bureau of Justice Statistics. Washington, DC: U.S. Government Printing Office, 2003.

3. Snyder HN, Sickmund M. Juvenile offenders and victims: 1999 national report. Washington, DC: U.S. Department of Justice, Office of Juvenile Justice and Delinquency Prevention, 1999.

4. Rates of homicide, suicide, and firearm-related death among children—26 industrialized countries. MMWR 1997;46(5):101–5.

5. U.S. Department of Health and Human Services, Administration on Children, Youth and Families. Child maltreatment 1999. Washington, DC: U.S. Government Printing Office, 2001.

6. Minino AM, Arias E, Kochanek KD, Murphy SL, Smith BL. Deaths: final data for 2000. Natl Vital Stat Rep 2002;50(15):1–120.

7. Krugman RD. Universal home visiting: a recommendation from the U.S. Advisory Board on Child Abuse and Neglect. Future Child 1993;3(3):184–200.

8. Youth violence: a report of the Surgeon General. Washington, DC: Department of Health and Human Services, 2001.

9. Sherman LW, Gottfredson DC, MacKenzie DL, Eck J, Reuter P, Bushway SD. Preventing crime: what works, what doesn't, what's promising. A report to the United States Congress (NCJ 171676). Washington, D.C.: U.S. Department of Justice, Office of Justice Programs, 1997.

10. Thornton TN, Craft CA, Dahlberg LL, Lynch BS, Baer K. Best practices of youth violence prevention: a sourcebook for community action. Atlanta, GA: Centers for Disease Control and Prevention, 2000.

11. U.S. Department of Health and Human Services. Healthy people 2010. 2nd ed. Washington, DC: U.S. Government Printing Office, 2000.

12. MacMillan HL, Feightner JW, Goldbloom R, et al. Preventive health care, 2000 update: Prevention of child maltreatment. Can Med Assoc J 2000;163(11):1451–8.

13. Olds DL, Hill P, Mihalic SF, O'Brien R. Prenatal and infancy home visitation by nurses. In: Elliott DS, ed. Blueprints for violence prevention. Boulder: Center for the

Study and Prevention of Violence, Institute of Behavioral Science, University of Colorado at Boulder, 1998.

14. Communities That Care prevention strategies: a research guide to what works. Seattle: Developmental Research and Programs, 2000.

15. Olds DL, Henderson CR Jr, Cole R, et al. Long-term effects of nurse home visitation on children's criminal and antisocial behavior: 15-year follow-up of a randomized controlled trial. JAMA 1998;280(14):1238–44.

16. Lally JR, Mangione PL, Honig AS. The Syracuse University Family Development Research Program: long-range impact of an early intervention with low-income children and their families. In: Powell DR, ed. Parent education as early childhood intervention: emerging directions in theory, research and practice. Norwood, NJ: Ablex, 1988:79–104.

17. Mental health: a report of the Surgeon General. Washington, DC: Department of Health and Human Services, 1999.

18. Chamberlain P, Mihalic SF. Blueprints for violence prevention. Book eight: multidimensional treatment foster care. Boulder: Center for the Study and Prevention of Violence, Institute of Behavioral Science, University of Colorado at Boulder, 1998.

19. Chamberlain P. Family connections: treatment foster care for adolescents with delinquency. Eugene, OR: Castalia, 1994.

20. Hahn RA, Bilukha O, Crosby A, et al. Firearms laws and the reduction of violence: a systematic review. Am J Prev Med 2005; in press.

21. Bilukha O, Hahn RA, Crosby A, et al. The effectiveness of early childhood home visitation in preventing violence: a systematic review. Am J Prev Med 2005; in press.

22. Hahn RA, Lowy J, Bilukha O, et al. The effectiveness of therapeutic foster care for the prevention of violence: a systematic review. Am J Prev Med 2005; in press.

23. Barnett WS. Long-term effects of early childhood programs on cognitive and school outcomes. Future Child 1995;5(3):25–50.

24. Yoshikawa H. Long-term effects of early childhood programs on social outcomes and delinquency. Future Child 1995;5(3):51–75.

25. Kamerman SB, Kahn A. Home health visiting in Europe. Future Child 1993;3(3):39–52.

26. St. Pierre RG, Layzer JI, Barnes HV. Two-generation programs: design, cost, and short-term effectiveness. Educ Child Dev 1995;5(3):76–93.

27. National Research Council. Understanding child abuse and neglect. Washington, DC: National Academy Press, 1993.

28. Office of Juvenile Justice and Delinquency Prevention. Juvenile offenders and victims: 1999 national report. Washington, DC: U.S. Department of Justice, 1999.

29. Sedlak AJ, Broadhurst DD. Third national incidence study of child abuse and neglect. Washington, DC: U.S. Department of Health and Human Services, Administration for Children and Families, National Center on Child Abuse and Neglect, 1996.

30. Dube SR, Anda RF, Felitti VJ, Chapman DP, Williamson DF, Giles WH. Childhood abuse, household dysfunction, and the risk of attempted suicide throughout the life span: findings from the Adverse Childhood Experiences study. JAMA 2001;286(24):3089–96.

31. Kelley BT, Thornberry TP, Smith CA. In the wake of child maltreatment. Washington, DC: Office of Juvenile Justice and Delinquency Prevention, U.S. Department of Justice, 1997.

32. Felitti VJ, Anda RF, Nordenberg D, et al. Relationship of childhood abuse and

household dysfunction to many of the leading causes of death in adults. The Adverse Childhood Experiences (ACE) Study. Am J Prev Med 1998;14(4):245–58.

33. Dodge KA, Bates JE, Pettit GS. Mechanisms in the cycle of violence. Science 1990;250(4988):1678–83.

34. Barth RP. An experimental evaluation of in-home child abuse prevention services. Child Abuse Negl 1991;15:363–75.

35. Brayden R, Altemeier W, Dietrich M, et al. A prospective study of secondary prevention of child maltreatment. J Pediatr 1993;122:511–6.

36. Brooten D, Kumar S, Brown LP, et al. A randomized clinical trial of early hospital discharge and home follow-up of very-low-birth-weight infants. N Engl J Med 1986; 315(15):934–9.

37. Caruso Whitney GA. Early intervention for high-risk families: reflecting on a 20-year-old model. In: Albee GW, Gullotta TP, eds. Primary prevention works. Thousand Oaks, CA: Sage, 1997:68–86.

38. Dawson P, Van Doornick WJ, Robinson JL. Effects of home- based, informal social support on child health. J Dev Behav Pediatr 1989;10(2):63–7.

39. Duggan A, Windham A, McFarlane E, et al. Hawaii's healthy start program of home visiting for at-risk families: evaluation of family identification, family engagement, and service delivery. Pediatrics 2000;105(1 pt 3):250–9.

40. Flynn L. The adolescent parenting program: improving outcomes through mentorship. Public Health Nurs 1999;16(3):182– 9.

41. Gray JD, Cutler CA, Dean JG, Kempe CH. Prediction and prevention of child abuse and neglect. J Soc Issues 1979;35:127– 39.

42. Hardy JB, Street R. Family support and parenting education in the home: an effective extension of clinic-based preventive health care services for poor children. J Pediatr 1989;115(6):927–31.

43. Honig AS, Morin C. When should programs for teen parents and babies begin? Longitudinal evaluation of a teen parents and babies program. J Prim Prev 2001;21(4):447–54.

44. Huxley P, Warner R. Primary prevention of parenting dysfunction in high risk cases. Am J Orthopsychiatry 1993;63(4):582–8.

45. Katzev A, Pratt C, Henderson T, McGuigan W. Oregon's Healthy Start effort: 1997–98 status report. Corvallis: Oregon State University Family Policy Program, 1999.

46. Kitzman H, Olds DL, Henderson CR Jr, et al. Effect of prenatal and infancy home visitation by nurses on pregnancy outcomes, childhood injuries, and repeated childbearing: a randomized controlled trial. JAMA 1997;278(8):644–52.

47. Larson CP. Efficacy of prenatal and postnatal home visits on child health and development. Pediatrics 1980;66:191– 7.

48. Marcenko MO, Spence M, Samost L. Outcomes of a home visitation trial for pregnant and postpartum women at-risk for child placement. Child Youth Serv Rev 1996;18: 243–59.

49. Mulsow MH, Murry VM. Parenting on edge: economically stressed, single, African American adolescent mothers. J Fam Issues 1996;17(5):704–21.

50. Olds DL, Eckenrode J, Henderson CR Jr, et al. Long-term effects of home visitation on maternal life course and child abuse and neglect: fifteen-year follow-up of a randomized trial. JAMA 1997;278(8):637–43.

51. Siegel E, Bauman KE, Schaefer ES, Saunders MM, Ingram DD. Hospital and home

support during infancy: impact on maternal attachment, child abuse and neglect, and health care utilization. Pediatrics 1980;66(2):183–90.

52. Velasquez J, Christensen M, Schommer B. Intensive services help prevent child abuse. MCN Am J Matern Child Nurs 1984;9:113–7.

53. Wagner MM, Clayton SL. The Parents as Teachers program: results from two demonstrations. Future Child 1999;9(1):91–115.

54. Armstrong KA. A treatment and education program for parents and children who are at-risk of abuse and neglect. Child Abuse Negl 1981;5:167–75.

55. Eckenrode J, Ganzel B, Henderson CR Jr, et al. Preventing child abuse and neglect with a program of nurse home visitation: the limiting effects of domestic violence. JAMA 2000;284(11):1385–91.

56. Olds DL, Henderson CR Jr, Phelps C, Kitzman H, Hanks C. Effect of prenatal and infancy nurse home visitation on government spending. Med Care 1993;31(2):155–74.

57. Spoth R, Redmond C, Hockaday C, Shin CY. Family programs: barriers to participation in family skills preventive interventions and their evaluation. A replication and extension. Fam Relat 1996;43:247–54.

58. Maguire K, Pastore AL. Sourcebook of criminal justice statistics—1999. Maguire K, Pastore AL, eds. Washington, DC: U.S. Department of Justice, Bureau of Justice Statistics, 2000.

59. Eckenrode J. What works in nurse home visiting programs. In: Alexander G, Curtis PA, Kluger MP, eds. What works in child welfare. Washington, DC: Child Welfare League of America, 2000:35–43.

60. Olds DL, Henderson CR Jr, Tatelbaum R, Chamberlin R. Improving the life-course development of socially disadvantaged mothers: a randomized trial of nurse home visitation. Am J Public Health 1988;78(11):1436–45.

61. Achenbach TM, Howell CT, Aoki MF, Rauh VA. Nine-year outcome of the Vermont intervention program for low birth weight infants. Pediatrics 1993;91:45–55.

62. St. Pierre RG, Layzer JI. Using home visits for multiple purposes: the Comprehensive Child Development Program. Future Child 1999;9(1):134–51.

63. Achenbach TM, Edelbrock C. Manual for the Child Behavior Checklist and Revised Child Behavior Profile. Burlington: University of Vermont, Department of Psychiatry, 1983.

64. Meadowcroft P. Treating emotionally disturbed children and adolescents in foster homes. Child Youth Serv 1989;12(1–2):23–43.

65. Chamberlain P. Comparative evaluation of specialized foster care for seriously delinquent youth. Community Altern Int J Fam Care 1990;2(2):21–36.

66. Chamberlain P, Reid JB. Differences in risk factors and adjustment for male and female delinquents in treatment foster care. J Child Fam Stud 1994;3(1):23–39.

67. Chamberlain P, Reid JB. Comparison of two community alternatives to incarceration for chronic juvenile offenders. J Consult Clin Psychol 1998;66(4):624–33.

68. Chamberlain P, Reid JB. Using a specialized foster care community treatment model for children and adolescents leaving the state mental hospital. J Community Psychol 1991;19(3):266–76.

69. Chamberlain P, Friman PC. Residential programs for antisocial children and adolescents. In: Stoff DM, Breiling J, Maser JD, eds. Handbook of antisocial behavior. New York: Wiley, 1997:416–24.

70. Aos S, Phipps P, Barnoski R, Lieb R. The comparative costs and benefits of programs to reduce crime. Olympia: Washington State Institute for Public Policy, 2001.

71. Chamberlain P, Moreland S, Reid K. Enhanced services and stipends for foster parents: effects on retention rates and outcomes for children. Child Welfare1992;71(5): 387–401.

72. Rubinstein JS, Armentrout JA, Levin S, Herald D. The Parent-Therapist Program: alternate care for emotionally disturbed children. Am J Orthopsychiatry 1978;48(4): 654–62.

73. Evans ME, Armstrong MI, Kuppinger AD, Huz S, McNulty TL. Preliminary outcomes of an experimental study comparing treatment foster care and family-centered intensive case management. In: Epstein MH, Kutash K, Duchnowski A, eds. Outcomes for children and youth with emotional and behavioral disorders and their families: programs and evaluation best practices. Austin, TX: Pro-Ed, 1998:543–80.

74. Gotsch KE, Annest JL, Mercy JA, Ryan GW. Surveillance for fatal and nonfatal firearm-related injuries—United States, 1993–1998. In: CDC Surveillance Summaries, April 13, 2001. MMWR 2001;50(no. SS-2):1–34.

75. Krug EG, Dahlberg LL, Mercy JA, Zwi AB, Lozano R. World report on violence and health. Geneva: World Health Organization, 2002.

76. Cook PJ, Ludwig J. The costs of gun violence against children. Future Child 2002; 12(2):87–99.

77. Bureau of Alcohol Tobacco and Firearms. Commerce in firearms in the United States. Washington, DC: U.S. Department of the Treasury, Bureau of Alcohol, Tobacco and Firearms, 2000.

78. Cook PJ, Molliconi S, Cole TB. Regulating gun markets. J Criminal Law Criminol 1995;86(1):59–92.

79. Kellermann AL, Lee RK, Mercy JA, Banton JG. The epidemiologic basis for the prevention of firearm injuries. Annu Rev Public Health 1991;12:17–40.

80. Powell EC, Sheehan KM, Christoffel KK. Firearm violence among youth: public health strategies for prevention. Ann Emerg Med 1996;28(2):204–12.

81. Vernick JS, Webster DW, Hepburn LM. Effects of Maryland's law banning Saturday night special handguns on crime guns. Inj Prev 1999;5(4):259–63.

82. Loftin C, McDowall D, Wiersema B, Cottey TJ. Effects of restrictive licensing of handguns on homicide and suicide in the District of Columbia. N Engl J Med 1991; 325(23):1615–20.

83. Britt CL, Bordua DJ, Kleck G. A reassessment of the D.C. gun law: some cautionary notes on the use of interrupted time series designs for policy impact assessment. Law Soc Rev 1996;30(2):361–80.

84. Jones ED. The District of Columbia's "Firearms Control Regulation Act of 1975": the toughest handgun control law in the United States—or is it? Ann Am Acad Polit Soc Sci 1981;455:138–49.

85. Kleck G, Patterson EB. The impact of gun control and gun ownership levels on violence rates. J Quant Criminol 1993;9:249–87.

86. McDowall D, Loftin C, Wiersema B. Using quasi- experiments to evaluate firearm laws: comment on Britt et al.'s reassessment of the D.C. gun law. Law Soc Rev 1996; 30(2): 381–91.

87. Nicholson R, Garner A. The analysis of the Firearms Control Act of 1975: handgun control in the District of Columbia. Washington, DC: United States Conference of Mayors, 1980.

88. Roth JA, Koper CS. Impacts of the 1994 assault weapons ban: 1994–1996. Washington, DC: U.S. Department of Justice, 1999.

89. Weil DS, Knox RC. The Maryland ban on the sale of assault pistols and high-capacity magazines: estimating the impact in Baltimore. Am J Public Health 1997;87(2): 297–8.

90. Ludwig J, Cook PJ. Homicide and suicide rates associated with implementation of the Brady Handgun Violence Prevention Act. JAMA 2000;284(5):585–91.

91. Wintemute GJ, Wright MA, Drake C, Beaumont JJ. Subsequent criminal activity among violent misdemeanants who seek to purchase handguns. JAMA 2001;285(8): 1019–26.

92. Wright MA, Wintemute GJ, Rivara FP. Effectiveness of denial of handgun purchase to persons believed to be at high risk for firearm violence. Am J Public Health 1999;89(1):88–90.

93. Brady Handgun Violence Prevention Act, Pub. L. 103–159, 18 U.S.C. §922, 1993.

94. Cantor CH, Slater PJ. The impact of firearm control legislation on suicide in Queensland: preliminary findings. Med J Aust 1995;162(11):583–5.

95. Lott JR, Whitley JE. Safe-storage gun laws: accidental deaths, suicides, and crime. J Law Econ 2001;44(2):659–90.

96. Magaddino JP, Medoff MH. An empirical analysis of federal and state firearm control laws. In: Kates DB, ed. Firearms and violence. Cambridge, MA: Ballinger, 1984: 225–58.

97. DeZee MR. Gun control legislation: impact and ideology. Law Policy Q 1983;5: 367–79.

98. Murray D. Handguns, gun control laws and firearm violence. Soc Probl 1975;23: 81–92.

99. DeFrancesco S, Vernick JS, Weitzel MM, LeBrun EE. Gun policy glossary: policy, legal and health terms. Baltimore: The Johns Hopkins Center for Gun Policy and Research, 2000.

100. U.S. Department of Justice. Survey of state procedures related to firearm sales, midyear 2000. Washington, DC: Bureau of Justice Statistics, U.S. Department of Justice, 2000.

101. Firearm Owners Protection Act, Pub. L. 99–308, 18 U.S.C. §926, 1986.

102. Bureau of Alcohol Tobacco and Firearms. Following the gun: enforcing federal laws against firearms traffickers. Washington, DC: U.S. Department of the Treasury, Bureau of Alcohol, Tobacco and Firearms, 2000.

103. Webster DW, Vernick JS, Hepburn LM. Relationship between licensing, registration, and other gun sales laws and the source state of crime guns. Inj Prev 2001;7:184–9.

104. Teret SP. The firearm injury reporting system revisited. JAMA 1996;275(1):70.

105. National Rifle Association of America Institute for Legislative Action. Fact sheet: licensing and registration. Available at: http://www.nraila.org/FactSheets.asp?FormMode=Detail&ID=28. Accessed on February 13, 2003.

106. Vernick JS, Hepburn LM. State and federal gun laws: trends for 1970–1999. In: Cook PJ, Ludwig J, eds. Evaluating gun policy. Washington, DC: Brookings Institution Press, 2003:345– 402.

107. Bureau of Alcohol Tobacco and Firearms. State laws and published ordinances—firearms. Washington, DC: U.S. Department of the Treasury, Bureau of Alcohol, Tobacco and Firearms, 2000.

108. Lott JR. More guns, less crime: understanding crime and gun-control laws. 2nd edition. Chicago: University of Chicago Press, 2000.

109. Webster DW, Vernick JS, Ludwig J, Lester KJ. Flawed gun policy research could endanger public safety. Am J Public Health 1997;87(6):918–21.

110. Wright JD, Rossi PH. The armed criminal in America: a survey of incarcerated felons. Washington, DC: National Institute of Justice, 1985.

111. Wright JD, Rossi PH. Armed and considered dangerous: a survey of felons and their firearms. Hawthorne, NY: Aldine de Gruyter, 1986.

112. Ludwig J. Concealed-gun-carrying laws and violent crime: evidence from state panel data. Int Rev Law Econ 1998;18:239–54.

113. McDowall D, Loftin C, Wiersema B. Easing concealed firearms laws: effects on homicide in three states. J Criminal Law Criminol 1995;86(1):193–206.

114. Mustard DB. The impact of gun laws on police deaths. J Law Econ 2001;44(2): 635–58.

115. Ayres I, Donohue JJ III. Nondiscretionary concealed weapons laws; a case study of statistics, standards of proof, and public policy. Am Law Econ Rev 1999;6(1/2): 436–70.

116. Black DA, Nagin D. Do right-to-carry laws deter violent crime? J Leg Stud 1998; 27:209–19.

117. Dezhbakhsh H, Rubin PH. Lives saved or lives lost? The effects of concealed-handgun laws on crime. AEA Papers Proc 1998;88(2):468–74.

118. Duggan M. More guns, more crime. J Polit Econ 2001;109(5):1086–114.

119. Moody CE. Testing for the effects of concealed weapons laws: specification errors and robustness. J Law Econ 2001;44(2):799–813.

120. Olson DE, Maltz MD. Right-to-carry concealed weapon laws and homicide in large U.S. counties: the effect on weapon types, victim characteristics, and victim-offender relationship. J Law Econ 2001;44(2):747–70.

121. Plassmann F, Tideman TN. Does the right to carry concealed handguns deter countable crimes? Only a count analysis can say. J Law Econ 2001;44(2):771–98.

122. Maltz MD, Targonski J. A note on the use of county- level UCR data. J Quant Criminol 2002;18(3):297–318.

123. Gun violence prevention update. New York: Funder's Collaborative for Gun Violence Prevention, 2001.

124. Webster DW, Starnes M. Reexamining the association between child access prevention gun laws and unintentional shooting deaths of children. Pediatrics 2000;106(6): 1466–9.

125. Cummings P, Grossman DC, Rivara FP, Koepsell TD. State gun safe storage laws and child mortality due to firearms. JAMA 1997;278(13):1084–6.

126. Pub. L. No. 103–382—October 20, 1994, Gun-Free Schools Act, 20 USC 8921, Section 14601, 1994.

127. Brener ND, Simon TR, Krug EG, Lowry R. Recent trends in violence-related behaviors among high school students in the United States. JAMA 1999;282(5):440–6.

128. U.S. Departments of Education and Justice. Indicators of school crime and safety, 2001. Washington, DC: National Center for Education Statistics, Bureau of Justice Statistics, 2001. NCJ 190075.

129. U.S. Departments of Education and Justice. Indicators of school crime and

safety, 1998. Washington, DC: National Center for Education Statistics, Bureau of Justice Statistics, 1998. NCJ 172215.

130. Violence-related attitudes and behaviors of high school students—New York City. MMWR 1993;42(40):773-7.

131. Bagley C, Pritchard C. The billion dollar cost of troubled youth: prospects for cost-effective prevention and treatment. Int J Adolesc Youth 1998;7(3):211-25.

132. Peng SS. High school dropouts: a national concern. Washington, DC: National Center for Education Statistics, 1985.

133. Alternative education programs for violent and chronically disruptive students: best practices. Washington, DC: Safe and Drug-Free Schools Program, U.S. Department of Education, 1996.

134. Zimring FE. Firearms and federal law: The Gun Control Act of 1968. J Leg Stud 1975;4:133-98.

135. Carrington PJ, Moyer S. Gun availability and suicide in Canada: testing the displacement hypothesis. Stud Crime Crime Prev 1994;3:168-78.

136. Carrington PJ, Moyer S. Gun control and suicide in Ontario. Am J Psychiatry 1994;151(4):606-8.

137. Leenaars AA, Lester D. Effects of gun control on homicide in Canada. Psychol Rep 1994;75(1 pt 1):81-2.

138. Lester D, Leenaars AA. Suicide rates in Canada before and after tightening firearm control laws. Psychol Rep 1993;72:787-90.

139. Mauser G, Holmes RA. An evaluation of the 1977 Canadian firearms legislation. Eval Rev 1992;16(6):603-17.

140. Mundt RJ. Gun control and rates of firearms violence in Canada and United States. Can J Criminol 1990;32:137-54.

141. Programme Evaluation Section. A statistical analysis of the impacts of the 1977 firearms control legislation. Ottawa, Canada: Department of Justice, 1996.

142. Rich CL, Young JG, Fowler RC, Wagner J, Black NA. Guns and suicide: possible effects of some specific legislation. Am J Psychiatry 1990;147(3):342-6.

143. Scarff E. Evaluation of the Canadian gun control legislation. Ottawa, Canada: Minister of Supply and Services, 1983.

144. Sproule CF, Kennett D. The use of firearms in Canadian homicides 1972-1982: the need for gun control. Can J Criminol 1988;30:31-7.

145. Centerwall BS. Homicide and the prevalence of handguns: Canada and the United States, 1976 to 1980. Am J Epidemiol 1991;134(11):1245-60.

146. Sloan JH, Rivara FP, Reay DT, Ferris JAJ, Path MRC, Kellermann AL. Firearm regulations and rates of suicide: a comparison of two metropolitan areas. N Engl J Med 1990;322(6):369-73.

147. Sloan JH, Kellermann AL, Reay DT, et al. Handgun regulations, crime, assaults, and homicide: a tale of two cities. N Engl J Med 1988;319(19):1256-62.

148. Boor M, Blair JH. Suicide rates, handgun control laws, and sociodemographic variables. Psychol Rep 1990;66:923-30.

149. Geisel M, Roll R, Wettick R. The effectiveness of state and local regulation of handguns. Duke Law J 1969;43 :647-73.

150. Medoff MH, Magaddino JP. Suicides and firearm control laws. Eval Rev 1983; 7(3):357-72.

151. Lester D, Murrell ME. The preventive effect of strict gun control laws on suicide and homicide. Suicide Life Threat Behav 1982;12(3):131–40.

152. Hawkins JD, Herrenkohl TI, Farrington DP, et al. Predictors of youth violence. Washington, DC: Office of Juvenile Justice and Delinquency Prevention, U.S. Department of Justice, 2000. Juvenile Justice Bulletin, NCJ 179065.

153. Lipsey MW, Wilson DB. Effective intervention for serious juvenile offenders: a synthesis of research. In: Loeber R, Farrington DP, eds. Serious and violent juvenile offenders: risk factors and successful interventions. Thousand Oaks, CA: Sage, 1998: 313–45.

154. Eberhardt MS, Ingram DD, Makuc DM, et al. Health, United States, 2001, with urban and rural chartbook. Hyattsville, MD: National Center for Health Statistics, 2001.

155. Hahn RA, Bilukha OO, Crosby A, et al. First reports evaluating the effectiveness of strategies for preventing violence: early childhood home visitation. MMWR 2003; 52(RR- 14):1–9.

156. Task Force on Community Preventive Services. Recommendations to reduce violence through early childhood home visitation, therapeutic foster care, and firearms laws. Am J Prev Med 2005; in press.

157. Centers for Disease Control and Prevention. Therapeutic foster care for the prevention of violence. A report on recommendations of the Task Force on Community Preventive Services. MMWR 2004;53(RR-10):1–8.

Part III

Methodological
Background

Chapter 10

Methods Used for Reviewing Evidence and Linking Evidence to Recommendations

Establishing an explicit process for reviewing evidence and linking evidence to recommendations serves to enhance the credibility of those recommendations. This chapter discusses the established methods and process by which evidence is identified, assessed, summarized, and linked to recommendations in the *Community Guide.* Here, we outline the steps in our process, discuss a few updates and lessons learned, and briefly discuss the rationale for our approach.

This chapter is not a manual for conducting systematic reviews, although detailed information on *Community Guide* methods can be found elsewhere.[1,2] The aim of this chapter is to help users to better understand our methods of developing reviews and recommendations and, therefore, to enhance the credibility of *Community Guide* recommendations. These methods are not the only possible approach, nor are they presented as the best conceivable approach. They reflect various real-life constraints on time, personnel, and other resources that affect the conduct of systematic reviews. Nonetheless, with them, we have generated a large number of credible and transparent findings and recommendations across diverse areas of public health. These *Community Guide* methods have evolved over time and will continue to adapt to enhancements in systematic review methodology, in translating evidence into recommendations, and in meeting user needs.

The methods and process of *Community Guide* reviews are overseen and directed by the independent, nonfederal Task Force on Community Preventive Services, which also makes the evidence-based recommendations. The Task Force's independence helps to insulate the scientific process from real or perceived political pressure. The diversity of expertise on the Task Force well qualifies its members to make the inevitable judgment calls in conducting a review (e.g., Which outcomes should be considered to represent success? How much diversity can be tolerated in a group of related but not identical interventions? What constitutes *consistency* of results?). Task Force members are also well suited to making the inevitable trade-offs in making recommendations (e.g., How much benefit is required to outweigh occasional harms?).

Once a general topic has been selected by the Task Force, the first steps in conducting a review are:

- Set priorities for topics to review
- Convene a systematic review development team

After selecting topics, the systematic review development team:

- Develops a conceptual model for each topic and intervention and specifies the outcomes that will be used to determine if the interventions are effective (that is, the extent to which they actually achieve important goals in promoting health or reducing disease, injury, and impairment).
- Identifies and defines priority interventions.
    - We have defined an *intervention* to be any activity (or group of related activities) intended to prevent disease or promote health in a group of people.
- Systematically searches for and retrieves scientific literature that may provide evidence of the effectiveness of the selected interventions.
- Rates the quality of the studies (both in terms of study design and execution).
- Summarizes the size of any observed effects and the strength of the body of evidence for each intervention across the studies according to the number of studies, their quality, and the size and consistency of effect among the studies. In this step we also consider whether, among all of the available studies, any common threats to validity exist that might reduce confidence in the results.
- Translates the strength of evidence into a recommendation.

The steps are described in more detail in this chapter.

METHODS AND PROCESS FOR DEVELOPING *COMMUNITY GUIDE* REVIEWS AND RECOMMENDATIONS

Select Topics

The Task Force chooses broad topics for review on the basis of the public health burden of the problem; how preventable it is; how it relates to other public health initiatives; and the current level of research and practice activity in public health, clinical, and other settings.[3] The agenda-setting process incorporates input from interested others. For example, the first round of priority setting by the Task Force benefited from information provided by subject matter experts from the Centers for Disease Control and Prevention (CDC) and elsewhere in the Department of Health and Human Services.[3]

Convene a Team

The systematic review development team (the team) of 6–12 people meets frequently to direct the review, and 10–30 additional consultants provide opinions and expertise as needed. Generalists on the team (including staff, Task Force members, and methodologists) ensure that diverse viewpoints are reflected, that reviews are conducted and communicated in a consistent manner, that rigorous review methods are applied, and that the results can be understood by generalist audiences. Subject matter experts (e.g., experts in the substantive scientific area, experts in the practical implementation of programs and policies, or experts in the particular populations or settings involved) ensure that the questions are relevant to practice, that the information is complete and accurate, and that the reviews and recommendations are conceptually sound. The independence of the Task Force is complemented by the involvement of staff of federal, state, and local agencies, which may have opportunities to act on the results. All of the various collaborators provide valuable and complementary contributions that help to enhance the quality of the reviews and the credibility of the findings, as well as helping to assure that results are useful and used.

Develop a Conceptual Model

We organize our reviews using conceptual models—easy-to-understand diagrams that describe relationships between causes of public health problems (determinants), interventions, intermediate outcomes (such as changes in behavior), and health outcomes. Rather than strictly adhering to one theory, we have used various theories and other conceptual background to inform the development of our conceptual models and to reflect thinking that is relevant to a broad spectrum of public health topics, interventions, and approaches.

We use two types of conceptual models at different stages of the review process. We develop a *logic framework* (Figure 10–1 is one example of a logic framework) early in the systematic review process to illustrate the broad public health context in which a set of interventions might act. Logic frameworks show the "big-picture" relationships among social, environmental, and biological determinants, outcomes, strategic points for action, and interventions. By providing an easy-to-understand visual representation of the overall topic area, logic frameworks help us to consider interventions that might be used to address important public health issues, set priorities among the interventions, and help us determine which outcomes need to be considered, including important benefits and harms.

The next step is to develop an *analytic framework* (Figure 10–2 is one example of an analytic framework, related to the logic framework in Figure 10–1) for each intervention to be reviewed, which expands on a portion of the logic framework. Analytic frameworks depict in more detail the complex relationships between preventive interventions and outcomes. They are used to map the plan for evaluating interventions, and they guide the search for

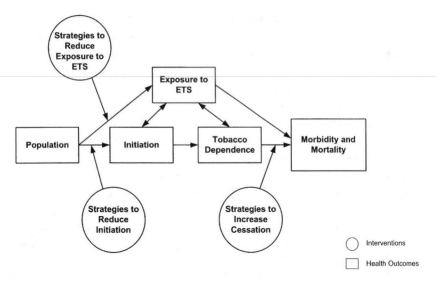

Figure 10–1. Example of a logic framework illustrating the conceptual approach used in the tobacco reviews. (ETS = environmental tobacco smoke.) (Reprinted from Am J Prev Med, Vol. 20, No. 2S, Hopkins DP et al., Reviews of evidence regarding interventions to reduce tobacco use and exposure to environmental tobacco smoke, p. 18, Copyright 2001, with permission from American Journal of Preventive Medicine.)

evidence. Analytic frameworks are also useful for identifying exactly which interventions will be assessed in the systematic review and which outcomes will be used to assess the success (or effectiveness) of an intervention. Generally, to consider an intervention effective, we require that it either shows improvements in health or leads to changes in behaviors or other factors that have been shown to result in better health. For example, we determined that tobacco use cessation and improved vaccine coverage are clearly related to better health and used them as acceptable markers for success in our reviews. In contrast, knowledge and attitudes are usually considered to be important but are not considered, independently, to translate into improvements in population health. Analytic frameworks are also useful to make certain that we do not overlook important outcomes and that we have targeted the appropriate types of evidence for search and retrieval.

We continue to use the analytic frameworks after a review is completed to communicate our findings. For example, we can use the frameworks to illustrate the numbers of studies and strength of evidence linking interventions to particular outcomes, to highlight gaps in knowledge where further research is needed, and to help users choose interventions that are good matches for particular local problems.

In general, we develop logic and analytic frameworks and intervention categories early in the review process and use them to guide the reviews. However, this process allows for adding important questions as they arise.

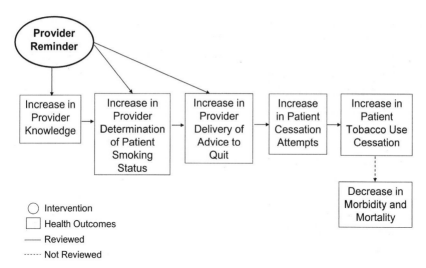

Figure 10–2. Example of an analytic framework illustrating the relationships between the intervention and outcomes. Provider reminders are one of the interventions in the larger category of strategies to increase tobacco use cessation.

Define and Group Interventions

We usually consider four aspects of each intervention:[2]

1. The type of intervention (including content, activities, and breadth of focus);
2. How the intervention is delivered (e.g., who delivers it; time period, frequency, and duration);
3. Who is targeted (e.g., general population, high-risk group, professional group); and
4. Where the intervention is delivered (e.g., setting).

We also most typically look at the effectiveness of interventions in achieving particular outcomes (e.g., home visiting interventions to promote vaccination probably have different effects from home visiting interventions to prevent violence). The title used for a particular type of intervention usually highlights one or more of these dimensions (e.g., the name "School-Based Education to Reduce Tobacco Use" is based on the setting [schools] and the outcome [tobacco use], although the other dimensions also apply).

To perform *Community Guide* reviews and make recommendations, we define a set of *like* interventions on which to focus a particular review. We determine whether related interventions can be grouped together on the basis of their similarity (in terms of the four dimensions described above and the outcomes addressed) and on whether a single conclusion can be drawn about how the intervention affects one or more outcomes of interest. We sometimes consider other factors as well, such as depth of available literature or the theoretical basis for making the case that the interventions are substantially similar. The process of grouping interventions can be a challenge because no two community interventions are exactly alike and because nomenclature used in available studies can vary widely.

The strategy for grouping interventions should allow fair, understandable, and valid evaluations of various kinds of interventions. It is important to avoid combining too broadly—that is, comparing results from interventions that differ in important ways in terms of their conceptual basis or the evidence they provide. At the same time, it is important to avoid groupings that are too narrow, which can inhibit our ability to draw conclusions and compare and contrast results. We find that some prudent combination of information about similar but not identical interventions is needed to be able to draw useful conclusions.

Select Interventions to Evaluate

Topics addressed in *Community Guide* systematic reviews are very broad, and the intervention reviews are time-consuming and resource intensive. For these reasons, it is necessary to set priorities for which interventions to review.

The process of selecting interventions for review involves developing the logic framework, deciding whether any areas of the logic framework will be excluded from further consideration (e.g., because an area was already covered in another review), developing a candidate list of interventions, and setting priorities using some type of voting procedure among the team and the consultants. The Task Force approves or modifies the resulting priorities.

Priority-setting criteria are next adapted for a particular review. Teams consider the following issues: potential to reduce the burden of disease and injury; potential to increase healthy behaviors and reduce unhealthy behaviors; potential to increase the implementation of effective but not widely used interventions; potential to phase out widely used, less effective interventions in favor of more effective or more cost-effective options; and current level of interest among providers and decision makers. Other priority-setting criteria may be added as relevant and appropriate.

Occasionally, review teams may engage in formal scoring and weighting of the criteria. One or more rounds of this process results in a prioritized list of interventions. Although this process for selecting interventions is systematic, it is dependent on judgment. A different group of participants might choose a different set of interventions. Nonetheless, selecting topics and interventions using a process that is as broad, open, and transparent as possible should maximize the likelihood that the reviews and the resulting recommendations will be useful to a broad audience.

Systematically Search for and Retrieve Evidence

Once intervention priorities have been set, we engage in a thorough search for relevant information in the scientific literature. Performing this search systematically increases the validity and generalizability of results. Searches are designed to be as comprehensive as possible to reduce the likelihood that the review will evaluate a biased selection of studies.

To search for evidence, we:

- Determine which types of documents are relevant to the study question
- Identify relevant systematic or narrative reviews, and then identify additional studies from the reference sections of these reviews
- Determine which databases are most likely to yield the appropriate document types
- Determine the search parameters and inclusion criteria
- Conduct the search
- Read titles and abstracts of the resulting document list to determine potential relevance
- Obtain potentially relevant documents
- Review documents to confirm that they meet inclusion criteria
- Review documents for additional references

At a minimum, *Community Guide* reviews include recent intervention studies published in journals. Government and other technical reports can also be included. If, after the first attempts at a search, the evidence found for a particular intervention is sparse or nonexistent, other document types, such as dissertations, books, or abstracts, may be considered. This process systematically identifies readily available evidence. It is not possible for any review to include all evidence that might be retrieved if unlimited resources were available.

We are charged with producing public health recommendations applicable in the United States. Including studies from more countries can increase the amount of available literature and may also increase the number of approaches that have been evaluated, but can potentially reduce applicability to the United States. To date, all of our reviews have included U.S. studies, most have included studies from other developed countries, and a few have included studies from developing countries. For most reviews, we have been willing to assume that public health interventions in developed countries might translate to the United States if adapted appropriately. When we have limited ourselves to U.S. studies, we have generally done so because the local social context is believed to have important effects on intervention effectiveness. For example, for some of our reviews of interventions related to violence prevention, the social context was thought to differ substantially between the United States and other developed countries, so we reviewed only

U.S. studies. On the other hand, for most interventions we have argued that the developing world context has been sufficiently different from that of the United States to preclude inclusion of studies from the developing world in our reviews.

Given resource constraints, to date we have limited our reviews to studies published in English. If, in the future, our subject matter experts suggest that additional key references are published in a different language, we will seek to have the relevant studies translated.

Assess Individual Studies

To ensure consistency, reduce bias, and improve validity and reliability in *Community Guide* systematic reviews, a standardized abstraction form and procedure has been developed[2] and is available at www.thecommunityguide .org/methods/abstractionform.pdf. The form guides reviewers through the process of summarizing studies. It captures important descriptive information about each intervention; identifies qualitative and quantitative results; assesses suitability of study design; and documents important threats to validity.[2] Each included study is read and summarized by at least two reviewers. When reviewers have differences in opinion, team members reconcile those differences. The abstraction form balances flexibility for the evaluation of papers reflecting different study designs and intervention types with the necessity of a common, systematic approach to the reviews to maximize validity and reliability.

Assess and Summarize Bodies of Evidence

Summarizing Evidence of Effectiveness

We characterize study designs in terms of suitability and quality of execution. Three possible categories describe suitability: greatest, moderate, or least suitable design. These categories are based on the presence or absence of study design characteristics that affect our confidence that the intervention being evaluated really caused the effects or outcomes being measured (internal validity).[1]

Quality of study execution is assessed on the basis of six characteristics (descriptions of the study population and the intervention, sampling of the study population, measurement of exposures and outcomes, data analysis, interpretation of results, and other threats that have not already been addressed in the other categories) and limitations in any of these characteristics, as defined by the *Community Guide*,[2] are noted. (Details of scoring quality limita-

tions are available at www.thecommunityguide.org/methods/scoring-rules
.htm.) Each study is categorized as having good, fair, or limited quality of execution based on the number of limitations. Performance in the quality do-
mains can either affect our confidence that the intervention being evaluated
really caused the effects or outcomes being measured (internal validity) or
our confidence that the study results can be generalized to populations and
contexts beyond the particular ones included in the studies themselves (external validity).

To give decision makers information about what to expect, we summarize
the information across studies in a variety of ways. Results across a group of
related studies are always discussed qualitatively (that is, using tables and
text). Sometimes, we perform no other summary. Results are also summarized using graphs and quantitative methods when possible and when such
an analysis is useful. In addition, we strive to make a statement about the
typical size of the effect and how much that effect has varied across studies.
We usually calculate an average effect using an easily understandable effect
measure (either the mean or the median) as our best estimate of changes that
will occur if the intervention is used.

Determining whether studies can be combined is a judgment that depends
on several characteristics of the body of evidence. Sometimes we conclude
that *no combination* across studies is feasible or desirable. We would reach
this conclusion in cases where there are too few studies; the interventions or
components of the interventions are too varied to allow meaningful over-
arching conclusions; measured outcomes within the body of evidence are too
diverse to allow assessment of the overall effectiveness of selected interventions; or the quality of individual studies is too poor or the problems with the
body of evidence overall are too severe to allow confidence in any measured
effect. It is hoped that this conclusion and its rationale will lead to improvements in future research.

Sometimes, *qualitative combination* is feasible and useful but quantitative
summary is not. In this case we cannot produce a mean or median effect size.
Such a conclusion might read, for example, "All of the qualifying studies
showed improvements in the health outcomes evaluated; however, the diversity of health outcomes studied precluded the calculation of a 'typical' effect." At other times, quantitative summaries are not thought to provide substantial added value for decision making. For example, "All qualifying studies
showed increased measures of knowledge" is frequently as useful as "Knowledge measures generally increased by an average of 1 standard deviation with
a 95% confidence interval of .6 to 1.6."

We often use *"simple" quantitative combination*. Where quantitative results are available from studies with reasonable quality and conceptual similarity, we find it useful to transform study results to a common scale (e.g.,

percentage point changes). This allows us to describe the size of the changes associated with the interventions and also to describe the distribution of results using plots and simple descriptive statistics (e.g., median and range). This has the added benefit of providing additional empirical data on the similarity or difference in results across studies, thus providing additional data to inform decisions on whether the interventions and the results are sufficiently similar to combine and, if so, to present a *typical* effect size. If the results are not sufficiently similar, we attempt to explain the variations using stratified analyses. For example, studies could be stratified by characteristics of the study (e.g., the length of follow-up), characteristics of the intervention (e.g., duration), characteristics of the population (e.g., sex of the study population), or characteristics of the context (e.g., type of setting in which the intervention occurred).

We sometimes combine study results using the formal statistical procedures of *meta-analysis,* which involves converting study results to a common metric, calculating a confidence interval for each result, and calculating a summary estimate of effect across the group of studies that is weighted by the precision of each study. For example, a study with a narrow confidence interval (higher precision) would typically carry greater weight in the overall average. Additional variables that may affect the study results can be controlled through procedures called *meta-regression,* in which intervention and other study characteristics are used in a statistical model to explain variability in outcomes. The statistical details of these techniques are beyond the scope of this chapter but are available in other sources.[4]

The choice between *simple* quantitative combination and formal statistical procedures involves a range of pros and cons. Simple quantitative combination has the potential advantages of being easier to implement and understand, and of allowing more studies to be included (because we need not exclude studies, for example, that do not report information on the variability of results). Formal statistical procedures also have potential advantages: they may give greater weight to more precise results, and they use formal rules for deciding when an effect is significantly different from no effect. For ease of interpretation and simplicity of calculation, we have tended to err toward use of the simplest analytic strategy that will adequately represent the available data.

Finally, the body of evidence of the effectiveness of an intervention is characterized as strong, sufficient, or insufficient on the basis of the number of available studies, the strength of their design and execution, and the size and consistency of reported effects (Table 10–1).

One can achieve sufficient or strong evidence in a variety of ways. For example, sufficient or strong evidence can be achieved through one or two very well designed and executed studies with few threats to validity. Alternatively,

Table 10–1. Assessing the Strength of a Body of Evidence on Effectiveness of Population-Based Interventions in the *Guide to Community Preventive Services*

Evidence of Effectiveness[a]	Execution (Good or Fair[b])	Design Suitability (Greatest, Moderate, or Least)	Number of Studies	Consistent[c]	Effect Size[d]	Expert Opinion[e]
Strong	Good	Greatest	At least 2	Yes	Sufficient	Not used
	Good	Greatest or moderate	At least 5	Yes	Sufficient	Not used
	Good or fair	Greatest	At least 5	Yes	Sufficient	Not used
	(Meets design, execution, number, and consistency criteria for sufficient but not strong evidence)				Large	Not used
Sufficient	Good	Greatest	1	Not applicable	Sufficient	Not used
	Good or fair	Greatest or moderate	At least 3	Yes	Sufficient	Not used
	Good or fair	Greatest, moderate, or least	At least 5	Yes	Sufficient	Not used
Expert Opinion	Varies	Varies	Varies	Varies	Sufficient	Supports a recommendation
Insufficient[f]	A. Insufficient designs or execution	Insufficient designs or execution	B. Too few studies	C. Inconsistent	D. Small	E. Not used

[a]The categories are not mutually exclusive; a body of evidence meeting criteria for more than one of these should be placed in the highest possible category.

[b]Studies with limited execution are not used to assess effectiveness.

[c]Generally consistent in direction and size of effect

[d]Sufficient and large effect sizes are defined on a case-by-case basis and are based on Task Force opinion.

[e]Expert opinion will not be routinely used in the *Community Guide* but can affect the classification of a body of evidence as shown.

[f]Reasons for a determination that evidence is insufficient will be described as follows: A. Insufficient designs or executions, B. Too few studies, C. Inconsistent, D. Effect size too small, E. Expert opinion not used. These categories are not mutually exclusive, and one or more of them will occur when a body of evidence fails to meet the criteria for strong or sufficient evidence.

Reprinted from Am J Prev Med, Vol. 18, No. 1S, Briss PA et al., Developing an evidence-based *Guide to Community Preventive Services*—methods, p. 40, Copyright 2000, with permission from American Journal of Preventive Medicine.

and more commonly, a group of individually less persuasive studies can provide sufficient or strong evidence taken together, especially if their flaws are not overlapping.

Summarizing Other Effects

Interventions designed to lead to health outcomes sometimes result in what we refer to as *other effects,* that is, important outcomes of the intervention that are side effects rather than the primary effects used to assess effectiveness. Other effects may be intentional or incidental and can relate to either health or non-health outcomes. They can include *harms* (for example, sobriety checkpoints may compromise motorist privacy) or *benefits* (for example, workplace smoking bans may reduce the risk of fire and workplace cleaning costs).

Community Guide reviewers identify potentially important other effects and systematically search for and evaluate the strength of evidence supporting these, following the same process used for assessing effectiveness. Identifying important other effects may affect the Task Force recommendations. For example, credible evidence that harms outweigh benefits will lead to recommendations that interventions not be used.

In reviews to date, available data on either the harms or side benefits of community interventions has been sparse. Our efforts to summarize other effects have thus been used mainly in developing directions for future research rather than recommendations.

Assessing the Applicability of Available Effectiveness Data

To help users determine the likelihood that reviewed interventions will apply to their local populations and settings, *Community Guide* reviews provide information on the applicability of bodies of evidence and resulting recommendations. By studying the conceptual basis of the intervention and the variability or robustness of empirical findings across different contexts, we find that we can generally describe applicability using one of these four conclusions.

- Review findings are likely to be applicable across a broad range of settings, populations, or intervention characteristics.
- Review findings are likely to be applicable across a broad range of settings, populations, or intervention characteristics, assuming that the intervention is appropriately adapted to the population of interest.
- Review findings are applicable only to populations or settings that have been included in the studies, and broader applicability is uncertain.

- Review findings are applicable only to the populations or settings included in the studies.

These categories have been developed to provide a structure for decisions and to link the decisions to supporting conceptual and empirical information. They should not be thought of as a hierarchical grading scheme—that is, the first category is not "better" than the last. Rather, they are intended to help users assess the extent to which the findings may apply to their local situations.

Economic Evaluations

Interventions to improve health are typically constrained by scarce or limited resources. Decision makers seek useful information about the resources required for various interventions, and the return that can be expected relative to the cost of an intervention, to help them allocate resources to produce maximum improvements in health. Whenever economic data on recommended interventions are available, the review team collects, abstracts, adjusts, and summarizes results from economic studies to support decision making. We do this to make economic information more available and comparable across studies. (The rationale, utility, procedures, and instruments for summarizing economic information are discussed further in Chapter 11.) However, economic information on public health interventions reviewed to date has been sparse.

Summarizing Barriers to Implementation of Interventions

Community Guide reviews provide information on barriers that might impede implementation of interventions. Examples of such barriers include political opposition to smoking restrictions by smokers and the tobacco industry, difficulty passing legislation on vaccination requirements, or state constitutional prohibitions against sobriety checkpoints to reduce alcohol-impaired driving.

Each recommended intervention evaluated in a *Community Guide* review includes a description of barriers to implementation that have been encountered or that the systematic review development team thinks likely to be encountered when implementing particular interventions. This information can come from reviewed studies, additional evidence searches specific to barriers (although research descriptions of barriers have been sparse), or the opinion of review team members who are subject matter experts. Knowledge of barriers can help decision makers select interventions or help practitioners anticipate potential problems so that they can find ways to work around barriers early in the implementation process.

Translating Evidence into Recommendations

The *Community Guide* provides systematic, evidence-based recommendations to diverse public health audiences. The recommendations highlight which interventions are most appropriate and effective for promoting health and preventing disease and injury in communities based on the aggregated evidence of public health research.

After reviewing the findings from a systematic review, the Task Force either recommends use of the intervention or finds that evidence is insufficient to determine whether or not the intervention is effective. The Task Force's recommendations primarily address evidence of the effectiveness of interventions, but other factors, such as applicability, barriers, and economic evidence, are sometimes incorporated.

Using Effectiveness Data to Formulate Recommendations

Recommendations are primarily driven by effectiveness data, which the *Community Guide* systematically summarizes using the guidelines shown in Table 10–1. Evidence for the effectiveness of interventions is determined to be strong, sufficient, or insufficient to determine effectiveness based on the number of available studies, the suitability of their designs and quality of execution, and the consistency and size of reported effects.

In general, a direct relationship exists between strength of evidence and strength of recommendation, as shown in Table 10–2. Although the recommendation language described here has evolved slightly from previous versions,[1] neither the process of developing recommendations nor the intent of the recommendations has changed.

Table 10–2. Relationship Between Strength of Evidence of Effectiveness and Recommendations

Strength of Evidence of Effectiveness	*Recommendation*
Strong	The intervention is recommended on the basis of strong evidence of effectiveness
Sufficient	The intervention is recommended on the basis of sufficient evidence of effectiveness
Insufficient information	Available studies do not provide sufficient evidence to determine the effectiveness of the intervention
Sufficient or strong evidence of ineffectiveness or harm	Use of the intervention is discouraged based on sufficient or strong evidence
Insufficient empirical information, supplemented by expert opinion	The intervention is recommended on the basis of expert opinion

The consistency of results also affects recommendations. When evidence of effectiveness is inconsistent and the inconsistency can be attributed to certain characteristics of the population, setting, or intervention, recommendations can be targeted to a specific context. For example, some interventions may be appropriate for urban populations but not for rural populations, or for use in health department clinics but not in managed care organizations.

All else being equal (e.g., strength of evidence and consistency of findings), a large effect size can strengthen a body of evidence. Conversely, a small effect size can weaken a body of evidence. The Task Force also has the option of making a recommendation based solely on expert opinion, but has not done so to date.

Other Factors

As described above, *Community Guide* reviews also collect and evaluate information on the applicability of findings to various populations and settings and on the intervention's other effects (that is, side effects). These factors can affect the recommendations. In contrast, economic impact and barriers that have been observed when implementing interventions, although included in systematic reviews for the consideration of users, do not generally influence Task Force recommendations.

Applicability

The Task Force makes judgments about the contexts in which the recommendations apply. These judgments are based on (1) a conceptual understanding of the intervention in question, (2) what the research evidence says about the consistency or variability of results of the intervention across different intervention characteristics, and (3) the characteristics of the settings and populations. In most cases, *Community Guide* recommendations have been thought to apply to a wide range of populations and settings, but, at times, recommendations are targeted to a specific context. For example, some diabetes interventions have been recommended for people with type 1 but not type 2 diabetes, or vice versa, and standing orders to promote vaccinations have been recommended for adults but not for children.

Other Effects

Documented harms to health that outweigh benefits will lead to recommendations against use of interventions. However, because harms are frequently understudied relative to benefits, postulated serious harms that have not yet been adequately studied may lead to recommendations for further research rather than to practice recommendations (even if the intervention has been found to be effective in changing some outcomes). There may also be cases in which an intervention is effective in some populations but harmful to one or more other populations. In such cases, the Task Force may make a more narrowly targeted recommendation than would otherwise be made or may recommend against use of the intervention.

Economic Analyses

Economic information does not routinely influence *Community Guide* recommendations, because the availability and quality of data are often limited. Additionally, different users will bring different values to bear in terms of how and whether economic information should be incorporated into decision making.

Barriers to Intervention Implementation

Each intervention evaluated in a *Community Guide* systematic review includes information on barriers that have been encountered when implementing interventions. This information is primarily provided for decision makers to consider when selecting interventions and does not typically influence recommendations.

The Role of Task Force Opinion and Judgment

Although *Community Guide* reviews are explicit and systematic, an element of judgment is always involved. The same is true for the development of recommendations. Many Task Force decisions (including, for example, intervention definitions and outcomes used to define success) influence the resulting recommendations. A different group of decision makers could reach different conclusions.

Another area in which Task Force judgment may be influential is where evidence is insufficient to determine the effectiveness of an intervention. In such cases, the Task Force has reserved the option of making recommendations based solely on expert opinion. However, after more than 170 reviews, the Task Force has not yet elected to exercise this option.

Summarizing Evidence Gaps

Community Guide systematic reviews identify and assess existing evidence to provide a basis for public health decisions. An important additional benefit of these reviews is identification of areas where this evidence is lacking or is of poor quality. Identifying these evidence gaps or research needs— questions that remain to be answered about a given topic area— can help researchers and funding agencies focus their efforts on areas most in need of further study (i.e., research agendas). For each intervention evaluated, whether or not evidence was already sufficient for a recommendation, we identify remaining evidence gaps. Where evidence of effectiveness of an intervention is sufficient or strong, remaining questions about effectiveness, applicability, other effects, economic consequences, and barriers are summarized. Where evidence of effectiveness of an intervention is insufficient, remaining questions about only effectiveness and other effects are summarized. Applicability issues are summarized only if they affect the assessment of effectiveness. The team decides if it is premature to identify research gaps in economic evaluations or barriers before effectiveness is demonstrated.

For each category of evidence, issues that emerge from the review are identified, based on the informed judgment of the team. Several factors influence that judgment. When a conclusion is drawn about evidence, the team decides if additional issues remain. Specifically:

- If effectiveness was demonstrated by using some but not all outcomes, all other possible outcomes are not necessarily listed as research gaps.
- If the available evidence was thought to be generalizable, we do not necessarily identify all subpopulations or settings where studies had not been done.
- Within each body of evidence, the team considers whether there are general methods issues that would improve future studies in that area.

(See Chapter 12 for a more complete discussion of research needs.)

CONCLUSION

The rigorous systematic reviews and Task Force recommendations in the *Community Guide* are designed to make a vast range of current scientific evidence accessible and useful to decision makers who are responsible for selecting appropriate health interventions for their communities. Information in these reviews and recommendations includes systematically derived and communicated information on:

- High-priority health topics
- Conceptual models that identify important public health outcomes, high-priority interventions to achieve them, and the proposed ways in which the interventions should work
- The empirical studies that have measured the success of these programs, including
  - The quality of those studies, individually and collectively
  - The size and variability of reported effects, including changes in intermediate and health outcomes and costs
  - Likely applicability of the findings across different intervention characteristics and community contexts

- Barriers to implementation, and
- Task Force recommendations about using or not using an intervention.

In this way, the *Community Guide* contributes to the scientific basis for effective public health practice that should be used in conjunction with information about local needs, resources, priorities, and barriers. *Community Guide* recommendations and reviews also help researchers and those who support research to identify gaps and redundancies in what we know and to develop an appropriate public health research agenda.

Acknowledgments

This chapter was written by Peter A. Briss, MD, MPH, Community Guide Branch, Division of Prevention Research and Analytic Methods (DPRAM), Epidemiology Program Office (EPO), Centers for Disease Control and Prevention (CDC), Atlanta, Georgia; Patricia Dolan Mullen, DrPH, Center for Health Promotion and Prevention Research, University of Texas–Houston, School of Public Health; and David P. Hopkins, MD, MPH, Community Guide Branch, DPRAM/EPO/CDC, Atlanta.

References

1. Briss PA, Zaza S, Pappaioanou M, et al. Developing an evidence-based Guide to Community Preventive Services— methods. Am J Prev Med 2000;18(1S):35–43.
2. Zaza S, Wright-de Aguero L, Briss PA, et al. Data collection instrument and procedure for systematic reviews in the Guide to Community Preventive Services. Am J Prev Med 2000;18(1S):44–74.
3. Zaza S, Lawrence RS, Mahan CS, et al. Scope and organization of the Guide to Community Preventive Services. Am J Prev Med 2000;18(1S):27–34.
4. Cooper H, Hedges LV, eds. The handbook of research synthesis. New York: Russell Sage Foundation, 1994.

Chapter 11

Understanding and Using
the Economic Evidence

THE IMPORTANCE OF ECONOMICS TO HEALTH POLICY DECISION MAKING

Obtaining evidence on the effectiveness of public health interventions is a critical first step in selecting those interventions most likely to improve population health or prevent disease. However, in addition to knowing "What works and what is the size of the impact?" policymakers need other information to answer the question "What is the best choice of interventions for our program?" Public health decision makers, faced with limited resources, must routinely make decisions about how to prioritize public health problems and related interventions and choose among several alternatives. In making such choices, decision makers can benefit by knowing the financial resources required to implement each effective intervention and how dollars invested compare to outcomes achieved. Economic evaluations provide this information by comparing the costs and consequences of public health interventions (policies, programs, and other activities) (see Table 11–1). This chapter addresses the rationale and value of systematic reviews of economic evaluations, describes the methods used by the *Community Guide* to conduct such reviews, and provides information to help decision makers interpret review findings.

OVERVIEW OF ECONOMIC EVALUATION METHODS

Four main methods are used in economic evaluations: cost analysis (CA), cost–effectiveness analysis (CEA), cost–utility analysis (CUA), and cost–benefit analysis (CBA). Table 11–2 includes a brief description of these methods, what they compare, and the economic summary measures they produce.

Cost Analysis

Cost analysis involves the systematic collection and assessment of costs associated with an intervention. These costs are typically expressed as dollars or dollars per person served by the program. For example, a multicomponent intervention program to promote child vaccinations might cost $23 per child[1] in the area served. Cost analyses can be conducted alone, but they are often

Table 11–1. Successful Use of Economic Data in Public Health: Three Examples from the Centers for Disease Control and Prevention

RTI International, in collaboration with economists from the National Center for Chronic Disease Prevention and Health Promotion (NCCDPHP, CDC), developed a life-time economic model to assess the cost-effectiveness of screening for undiagnosed diabetes. This work resulted in the adoption of a diabetes screening policy by the state Diabetes Control Programs and a major change in the screening policy of the American Diabetes Association (ADA).

Economists from the National Center for Infectious Diseases (NCID, CDC) published the first economic estimates of the potential impact of the next influenza pandemic. The estimates of impact have been incorporated into the U.S. national influenza pandemic response plan.

NCCDPHP economists developed SAMMEC (Smoking-Attributable Mortality, Morbidity, and Economic Costs), a Web-based computational program available at www.cdc.gov /tobacco/sammec. SAMMEC allows the user to estimate the health and health-related economic consequences of smoking to adults and infants in terms of the number of annual deaths, years of potential life lost, medical expenditures, and productivity losses among adults due to smoking, as well as smoking-attributable infant deaths and excess neonatal healthcare costs. This tool is widely used by both public health departments and policymakers.

combined with measures of intervention effectiveness in a CEA or CBA. Cost analysis takes into account the costs incurred to develop and implement an intervention, including direct costs, indirect costs, and intangible costs. Direct costs represent the value of resources used specifically for the intervention. These costs may be characterized as medical or non-medical. Direct medical costs can include costs such as clinical services, diagnostic tests, and medications. Direct non-medical costs can be costs such as those associated with a mass media campaign, including media development, training, materials, and the cost of advertising. Indirect costs include the resources that are forgone to participate in an intervention, typically measured as lost wages or lost leisure time. Economic value can be assigned to each unit of time lost from normal activities. Intangible costs, such as the pain, grief, or suffering associated with an intervention, can also be considered, but they are difficult to quantify and are seldom included in an economic evaluation.

Financial costs should be distinguished from the broader concept of economic costs. Financial costs are the actual dollar costs expended for services, typically the actual costs of care, but in a public health context these also include program costs. Examples of financial costs include staff salaries, rent, and supplies. In addition to financial cost expenditures, economic costs include the opportunity costs or value of a resource for which there is no direct monetary expenditure (the value of the benefit that could be derived from the next best use of that resource) and the value of intangibles. Examples of opportu-

Table 11–2. Overview of Economic Evaluation Methods

Economic Evaluation Method	Comparison	Measurement of Health Effects	Economic Summary Measure
Cost analysis	Used to compare net costs of different programs for planning and assessment	Dollars	Net cost Cost of illness
Cost–effectiveness analysis	Used to compare interventions that produce a common health effect	Health effects, measured in natural units	Cost-effectiveness ratio Cost per case averted Cost per life-year saved
Cost–utility analysis	Used to compare interventions that have morbidity and mortality outcomes	Health effects, measured as years of life, adjusted for quality of life	Cost per quality-adjusted life year (QALY)
Cost–benefit analysis	Used to compare different programs with different units of outcomes (health and nonhealth)	Dollars	Net benefit or cost Benefit-to-cost ratio

nity costs include the value of volunteer time, space in the local public health department, and donated materials and supplies. Economic costs or financial costs can be used to compare alternative interventions, though economic and financial costs cannot be directly compared.

Cost analysis can include cost-of-illness (COI) estimates, which take into account the direct costs (medical and non-medical) and indirect costs associated with a health condition. Cost-of-illness analyses are a type of burden-of-disease measure. Cost-of-illness estimates can be incidence-based (reflecting total lifetime costs of a disease or illness) or prevalence-based (reflecting total costs of a disease in a specific time frame—for example, one year, divided by the number of cases). Cost analyses that include COI are presented as net costs, which are calculated by subtracting the cost of the illness (or injury) averted from total program costs. For example, the COI of an intervention for women with established diabetes that provides preconception care in addition to prenatal care[2] would include the total program costs less the cost of the illness averted (congenital anomalies). The result is often expressed in terms of dollars per person covered by the intervention—in this case, net cost per program enrollee. Results are sometimes also expressed as net costs per population (such as the population of a state or of the United States).

Cost–Effectiveness Analysis

Cost–effectiveness analysis (CEA) compares the costs of an intervention or policy with the measures of health improvement that are gained. These might be expressed as dollars per additional life-year saved. For example, an intensive mass media program to promote smoking cessation might cost $138 per life year saved.[3] With CEA, health improvements are measured in natural units (e.g., cases of disease prevented or number of lives saved). The summary measure for CEA is the cost-effectiveness (CE) ratio, which measures the net cost of the intervention or program relative to its health effects. In other words, it is the cost per unit of health effect (e.g., cost per year of life saved). Often, two CE ratios are reported: the incremental CE ratio, which compares a given intervention to another effective intervention, and the average CE ratio, which uses a *no-program* comparison.[4] For example, if in an effort to improve oral health within a community a public health practitioner compared a community water fluoridation program to a school-based fissure sealant delivery program, this would require an incremental CE ratio. If the community water fluoridation program was the only intervention under consideration, then this would indicate a no-program comparison, necessitating an average CE ratio.

Cost–effectiveness analysis is most useful for comparing interventions that address the same health problem. The effectiveness of an intervention can be measured using intermediate outcomes (e.g., number of people who stop smoking) or final outcomes (e.g., cases of disease prevented or years of life saved). Intermediate measures are usually of value only where they are clearly linked to final outcomes. For example, percentage reduction in tobacco smoking is considered an acceptable intermediate measure of effectiveness because it has been clearly linked to decreases in lung cancer and improvements in life expectancy. Use of final outcomes is generally preferable, since it permits a more complete assessment of the economic value of the intervention. However, for many issues, final outcomes can be difficult to quantify and expensive to assess (e.g., if they are rare or occur far in the future).

Cost–Utility Analysis

Cost–utility analysis (CUA) is a special type of CEA that compares costs of an intervention or policy with one particular measure of health improvement, the quality-adjusted life year (QALY). The QALY is an effort to take into account measures of both mortality and morbidity. For example, a year lived in perfect health may count as 1 QALY, whereas a year spent living with a serious illness might count as only 0.6 QALY. The advantage of these measures is that they allow direct comparison on the same scale of different types of health effects. Results of CUAs are typically expressed as cost/QALY saved. For example, a mass media program to promote smoking cessation might cost $151 per QALY saved,[5] where some of the improvement is attributable to reduced mortality and the remainder is attributable to a better quality of life. Two other measures of health improvement often associated with CUA are the disability-adjusted life year (DALY) and the healthy life year (HeaLY). However, neither of these alternatives is widely used in practice. (For more information about QALYs and related measures, see[4,6,7].)

Cost–Benefit Analysis

Cost–benefit analysis (CBA) takes into account all costs and consequences (which can include both benefits and harms) associated with an intervention and expresses them in dollar terms. These dollar terms are adjusted to their current or present value through a mechanism known as *discounting*. Discounting is a method used to make the value of costs and benefits comparable regardless of when they occur. Typically, costs in prevention effectiveness studies are incurred at or near the beginning of the intervention, whereas the benefits are spread out over several years. The two most commonly used summary measures for CBA are net benefits (present value of benefits less harms, minus cost of prevention) and benefit–cost ratio (present value of benefits divided by present value of costs). For example, if the present value of the benefits of an exercise program is $1100 per participant and the present value of associated costs is $450 per participant, then the net benefits are $650 per participant. The benefit–cost ratio of this intervention would be $1100 / $450 or 2.44.[8] Benefits of public health interventions, found in CBAs, CEAs, and CUAs, are often expressed in terms of increased life expectancy, decreased morbidity, averted medical costs, and increased worker productivity. In addition, CBA can capture important non-health effects (such as the increased value of housing with good sanitation systems), and the costs of harms related to an intervention can be factored into the analysis as well. For example, a potential harm could be loss in productivity incurred by a business associated with an on-site occupational health clinic. As a general rule, if the benefits exceed the cost (that is, if the benefit–cost ratio is greater than 1 or the net benefit is greater than 0), the program is considered to provide good economic value.

WHAT TYPES OF ECONOMIC EVALUATIONS CAN BE USED FOR WHAT PURPOSES?

The context in which a decision is made determines what type of economic evaluation is most useful and appropriate. If lawmakers need to allocate resources to interventions in two different sectors of the economy, such as education and health, the outcomes of interest must be converted to a common unit (such as dollars) to make the interventions comparable. A cost–benefit analysis is appropriate here. Public health policymakers often must decide how to allocate limited funds to address diverse public health issues that have different outcomes with respect to survival and quality of life (e.g., alcohol-impaired driving, HIV, and diabetes). Cost–utility analysis is an appropriate technique to use when making such decisions because it allows diverse health outcomes to be converted to a common unit, QALYs (see Cost–Utility Analysis above). Public health practitioners must often decide between two interventions that affect the same outcome, such as reducing initiation of tobacco use. In this circumstance, they can use cost-effectiveness analysis to compare the cost and outcomes of two or more interventions designed to reduce tobacco use.

COMMUNITY GUIDE METHODS FOR SYSTEMATIC REVIEW OF ECONOMIC EVALUATIONS

For each intervention recommended by the Task Force on Community Preventive Services (the Task Force), a systematic review is conducted to assess the quality of existing relevant economic evaluations and to summarize the findings. The lack of standardized methods and reporting of economic data hampers the use of data on costs and financial benefits in evidence-based reviews of effectiveness. To improve the comparability and usefulness of the very limited body of economic evidence, the economic data presented by the Task Force are abstracted and adjusted using the standardized economic abstraction form developed as part of the *Community Guide* initiative. The objective is to make economic research more accessible to decision makers and other stakeholders in order to help them use resources in the most efficient way to achieve a given health improvement at the lowest cost.

In this section we briefly describe *Community Guide* methods for systematic reviews of economic evaluations. These methods follow the same basic steps as the reviews of evidence of effectiveness and include a systematic search for economic evidence, assessment of individual studies (data abstraction and quality assessment), and a summary of the body of evidence.

The first step is to conduct a systematic search of the literature to find studies on intervention effectiveness that include economic evaluations (such as CA, CBA, CEA, or CUA). A study must meet certain criteria, determined by the Task Force, to be included in the review. It must be a primary study (not a review), published in English, and conducted in an established market economy (a developed country, as defined by the World Bank). The study must also include sufficient detail to abstract and adjust economic results.

Finally, the study must have been published within a relevant time frame such that the costs and the intervention effectiveness are thought to be reasonably applicable to the current U.S. context.

Studies that meet the inclusion criteria are subjected to data abstraction, cost adjustment, and quality assessment by two independent reviewers. Disagreements are resolved between the two reviewers. To abstract the data, reviewers use a standardized form (available at www.thecommunityguide.org/methods/econ-abs-form.pdf) to guide them through the process of summarizing studies. The abstraction form captures important information about each study, including study characteristics, intervention description, type of economic evaluation, costs and benefits, and data sources. Abstracted economic data are converted to a common currency (U.S. dollars). Costs are then adjusted for inflation with reference to a base year. Studies are also adjusted, when possible, to reflect a discount rate of 3% over the relevant time horizon.

After the data are abstracted, the quality of the study is assessed across five categories: study design, measurement of costs, measurement of outcomes, evidence of effectiveness, and analysis. Based on this assessment, study quality is characterized as very good, good, satisfactory, or unsatisfactory. Results of unsatisfactory studies are excluded from further review. Studies that contain fatal flaws, as determined by the reviewers, are also considered unsatisfactory and are excluded from the review. For example, if a CEA of a smoking cessation program evaluated the outcome of quitting smoking for only one week following the intervention, the study would be considered to have a fatal flaw, because this is an insufficient time period to assess the cost-effectiveness of the intervention. For more details on the methods used in our systematic reviews, see Carande-Kulis et al.[9] The economic data abstraction form and quality assessment scale can be found on the *Community Guide* website at www.thecommunityguide.org/methods/econ-abs-form.pdf.

HOW TO INTERPRET AND USE ECONOMIC RESULTS

Although systematic reviews of economic evaluations can provide useful summaries of published information on costs and benefits of interventions, decision makers should interpret any summary economic measures with caution. In this section, we provide information on how to use and interpret economic evaluations in the *Community Guide*. The design of the economic study—study parameters, including study perspective, methods, and time frame—is important and should be taken into account when interpreting results (see details below). The parameters can be used to identify costs after the program has been completed or they can be used when the program is in effect to *frame* (define the context of) the study. Other important considerations in

interpreting and using the results of economic analysis are the baseline prevalence of disease risk factors, the nature and scale of the intervention, the target population, and the setting in which the intervention was delivered.

Study Parameters

The parameters of an economic evaluation, including study perspective, analytic methods, relevant time frame, audience for the evaluation, and other
key issues, determine what types of data are included and analyzed in the
study. Study parameters affect the applicability of study results to different
situations and populations, and should be taken into consideration when interpreting and using study results. One important parameter is the perspective (the viewpoint from which the analysis is conducted), which determines
the costs and health outcomes included in the analysis. For example, a study
conducted from a government perspective includes only those costs and benefits experienced by the government and may not account for costs or benefits relevant to a health insurance purchaser.

Table 11–3 illustrates the types of costs included in a typical CEA from four
perspectives: society as a whole, the insurer or other payer, the employer, and
the client. Direct medical costs that are not covered by an insurer or an employer, such as deductibles and co-payments, are incurred by the client.
These non-covered payments would be included in the client perspective.
However, the societal perspective would include all direct medical costs, both

Table 11–3. Examples of Costs Included in a Typical Cost–Effectiveness Analysis,
Based on the Perspective of the Analysis

	Perspective			
Cost	Societal	Insurer/ Payer	Employer	Client
Direct medical	Yes	Yes[a]	Yes[a]	Yes[b]
Direct non-medical (e.g., trans-portation, day care)	Yes	No	No	Yes
Indirect (e.g., time lost from work)	Yes[c]	No	Yes[c]	Yes[c]
Intangible (e.g., pain and suffering)	Yes[c]	No	No	Yes[c]

[a]Covered payments.

[b]Out-of-pocket payments.

[c]If not incorporated in the effect measure.

Adapted from Farnham PG, Haddix AC. Study design. In: Haddix AC, Teutsch SM, Corso PS, eds. Prevention effectiveness: a guide to decision analysis and economic evaluation. 2nd ed. New York: Oxford University Press, 2003:11–27.

covered and non-covered. Although decision makers need to consider the relevance of the perspective to their own situations, they also need to appreciate the societal perspective so that they can assess the full consequences of decisions. For example, if an employer wants to determine whether to provide reimbursement for vaccination as an employee benefit and a program to encourage employees to be vaccinated, the employer's perspective would obviously be a significant consideration, since the organization's net profit might be affected. Costs would include healthcare system and provider charges reimbursed by the employer as well as productivity losses due to employees' absence from work. However, as a corporate citizen, the employer may also be interested in the societal perspective: does this program provide good value from the perspective of the general population by enhancing the health and attractiveness of the local community? From the societal perspective, all costs and benefits would be taken into account, regardless of who pays or who receives them. By considering multiple perspectives, the employer has a better understanding of a program's overall financial impact.

The time frame of an economic study is also important in interpreting economic findings. The *time frame* is the period during which the intervention or treatment is delivered along with any necessary follow-up. In contrast, the *analytic horizon* (or *time horizon*) refers to the entire period during which the costs and benefits are measured. If all the important results of an intervention can be measured in the short term, then the analytic horizon will be short. For most prevention programs, the analytic horizon should be sufficient to assess all of the benefits of the program. However, it is important to note that health effects may be realized long after the intervention has concluded and may span a person's lifetime. For example, consider a tobacco cessation program. With such a program, the time frame during which the intervention is delivered may be relatively short, possibly one year or less. However, the analytic horizon would include the lifetime of the (former) smoker to account for the period over which the benefits of reducing tobacco-related illnesses (e.g., cancer or heart disease) are realized. The value of the benefits that accrue during the analytic horizon must be included in the economic analysis.

Additional Considerations

Decision makers should also consider the current prevalence of risk factors, the nature and scale of the intervention at start-up versus maintenance phase, the target population, and the setting in which the intervention was delivered. The prevalence of risk factors has economic implications. For example, a mass media smoking cessation intervention aimed at a large population will have both higher costs and greater potential benefits in settings with high smoking prevalence than a telephone smoking cessation counseling intervention. A program may have high intervention costs, but through economies of scale, the cost per person of the program might be less than if it were aimed at a smaller population. In addition, costs may vary by geographic region, which could also affect the applicability of an economic evaluation. Decision makers should consider all of these factors, which affect the costs of interventions and the potential returns on investments. Other factors to consider include the feasibility of implementing an intervention, the acceptability of the intervention to a population, ethical and political concerns, and regulatory and legal issues.[3]

Limitations of Economic Evaluations

The usefulness of economic findings may be limited by aspects of the methods of economic evaluation. One issue is the various methods for measuring costs and benefits. The lack of one standardized method of measurement may limit the comparability of studies. Significant progress in this area has recently been made with the publication of several books that provide guidelines for conducting economic evaluations of health care,[6,7,10] public health programs,[4] and HIV prevention.[11]

Another issue is the highly variable quality of published economic evaluations. Such variation in quality was apparent in assessing economic evidence associated with most interventions. For example, when we reviewed economic evaluations of vaccine programs in schools, one evaluation, which received a "very good" quality score, reported quantities and costs of resources attributable to personnel, communications, transportation, advertising, overhead, follow-up, supplies, medication, diagnostic procedures, outpatient services, and disease complications, all from a societal perspective. This study also calculated income lost due to illness and death. The summary measures were reported as cost per life-year saved and cost per child vaccinated. In comparison, a second study failed to specify the study perspective, did not report quantities of resources separately from resource prices, omitted volunteer time, and neglected to discount future costs and outcomes. The resulting "unsatisfactory" quality score led to its exclusion from the overall review of the intervention. To improve quality, checklists have been developed to assess adherence of an economic evaluation to specific quality standards.[12] *The Community Guide* uses a quality assessment scale (on p. 31 at www.the communityguide.org/methods/econ-abs-form.pdf) to determine if studies meet minimum quality requirements for inclusion in a review. This scale also identifies areas of deficiencies in study quality.

Specific economic measures also raise concerns about appropriate interpretations. For example, important limitations of CE ratios have been described.[4] These ratios sometimes indicate that an intervention is both more costly and more effective than comparable interventions. For example, the most cost-effective approach to hepatitis B vaccination (in terms of cost per case prevented) might be vaccination of selected healthcare workers. However, that would have only a minor impact on the overall burden of hepatitis B. Universal newborn vaccination may have a higher cost per case prevented, but it prevents many more cases. In such cases, decisions have to be made about the reallocation of resources away from another program. However, CE ratios do not provide information on the opportunity costs of such decisions.[13] Many researchers also question the appropriateness of different types of health-related quality-of-life measures that are used in CUA. Some measures are based on general improvements in health, and others are based on disease-specific health improvements.[14-17] Such differences can make it impractical to compare one QALY with another. Therefore, prior to making comparisons between prevention strategies targeting different diseases or health problems, the decision maker should be aware of the methodology used to derive the QALYs.

A challenge in the greater use of economic evaluation to support decisions is the continued debate about what represents *good economic value.*[18-20] Differences in study perspective and methodology can greatly affect study results. Therefore, a judgment about the relative economic value of an intervention requires the economic evaluation of other interventions by similar methods, but such evaluations are not usually available. Finally, economic evaluations can present challenging ethical issues, such as equity concerns: Who "wins" and who "loses" in an economic evaluation? Does a particular economic evaluation favor the concerns of the younger members of a population at the expense of the elderly?[21] Another area of concern is that health values (preferences) are generally elicited from a small segment of a population and may not be representative of the population as a whole.[22] Attempts are made to address these challenges and concerns through the derivation and use of QALYs. However, the success of these attempts may be considered subjective.

GAPS IN THE ECONOMIC DATA ABOUT PREVENTIVE SERVICES

We conduct systematic reviews of economic data in the hope of providing useful summaries for decision makers. However, we frequently find that no economic evaluations are available for interventions recommended by the Task Force (economic evidence was available for only about half of the interventions recommended by the Task Force as of February 2004, and the available evidence was frequently just a single study).[23] These gaps in our knowledge are created because so few studies exist, and available studies often do not fit the intervention recommended by the Task Force or do not meet the quality requirements for inclusion in the review.

Evidence gaps can also be seen in a positive light. Because interventions chosen for Task Force review address important health issues, evidence gaps guide the research agenda for future economic evaluations of public health prevention programs.

SUMMARY OF ECONOMIC EVALUATION IN PUBLIC HEALTH DECISION MAKING

There is a great deal of interest in determining the economic impact of health promotion and disease prevention.[24] Despite the inconsistencies in the methods employed in many published, peer-reviewed economic evaluation studies to date, researchers have applied methods of economic evaluation to virtually all areas of public health.[25,26] As the number of economic studies has increased over time, the opportunity to summarize and compare economic information to inform public health decision making has increased as well. One of the goals of the *Community Guide* is to help decision makers and other stakeholders to use resources wisely through careful assessment of the value of public health prevention interventions. Economic evaluations provide explicit descriptions of the costs and consequences of different courses of action in public health. They also provide a framework for thinking about costs, benefits, and the *structure* of a decision. Although these evaluations have limitations that need to be assessed carefully, they are nonetheless a useful tool for public health decision making. Systematic reviews of economic evaluations contribute to that goal by summarizing a body of economic evidence, adjusting economic data to facilitate study comparisons, raising awareness of the limitations and applicability of the existing evidence, and guiding a research agenda for future economic evaluations of public health prevention programs. By summarizing and interpreting economic studies, systematic reviews make economic information available in a more useful and accessible form. The real value of economic information is that it can improve the efficiency of public health programs, furthering the public health mission by making the greatest possible improvement in the health of a population using available resources.

Glossary

Analytic horizon The period of time after an intervention ends, during which costs and outcomes accrue and are measured.

Cost analysis (CA) An economic evaluation technique that involves the systematic collection, categorization, and analysis of program costs.

Cost–benefit analysis (CBA) An analysis that compares both costs and benefits in dollar terms.

Cost–effectiveness analysis (CEA) An analysis used to compare the cost of alternative interventions that produce a common health effect.

Cost–utility analysis (CUA) A type of cost– effectiveness analysis that uses years of life saved combined with quality of life during those years as a health outcome measure.

Costs The value of resources (people, buildings, equipment, and supplies) used to produce a good or service.

Economic costs The value of resources, including opportunity costs, often used to compare alternative interventions.

Final outcomes The ultimate outcome of interest, such as diseases averted or years of life saved.

Financial costs The actual dollar costs for services, typically the actual costs of care.

Intermediate outcomes The near-term effects of a policy, program, or intervention, such as persons screened or cases prevented.

Opportunity costs The value of the alternatives given up in order to use the resource as the program so chooses.

Perspective The viewpoint of the bearers of the costs and benefits of an intervention (e.g., society, government, healthcare providers, business, or clients).

Productivity loss Costs associated with the decrease in production and income attributable to a disease, disability, or death.

Time frame The period during which the intervention or treatment is delivered, including any follow-up.

Acknowledgments

This chapter was written by Glenda A. Stone, PhD, Division of Hereditary Blood Disorders, National Center on Birth Defects and Developmental Disabilities, Centers for Disease Control and Prevention (CDC), Atlanta, Georgia; Angela B. Hutchinson, PhD, MPH, Prevention Research Branch, Division of HIV/AIDS Prevention, CDC, Atlanta; Phaedra S. Corso, PhD, Prevention Development and Evaluation Branch, Division of Violence Prevention, National Center for Injury Prevention and Control, CDC, Atlanta; Steven M. Teutsch, MD, MPH, Outcomes Research and Management, Merck & Co., Inc., West Point, Pennsylvania; Jonathan E. Fielding, MD, MPH, MBA, Los Angeles Department of Health Services, University of California School of Public Health, Los Angeles, and the Task Force on Community Preventive Services; Vilma G. Carande-Kulis, PhD, MS, Division of Prevention Research and Analytic Methods (DPRAM), Epidemiology Program Office (EPO), CDC, Atlanta; and Peter A. Briss, MD, MPH; Community Guide Branch, DPRAM/EPO/CDC, Atlanta.

References

1. Briss PA, Rodewald LE, Hinman AR, et al. Reviews of evidence regarding interventions to improve vaccination coverage in children, adolescents, and adults. Am J Prev Med 2000;18(1S):97–140.

2. Elixhauser A, Weschler JM, Kitzmiller JL, et al. Cost- benefit analysis of precon-

ception care for women with established diabetes mellitus. Diabetes Care 1993;16(8): 1146-57.

3. Secker-Walker RH, Worden JK, Holland RR, Flynn BS, Detsky AS. A mass media programme to prevent smoking among adolescents: costs and cost effectiveness. Tob Control 1997;6:207-12.

4. Haddix AC, Teutsch SM, Corso PS, eds. Prevention effectiveness: a guide to decision analysis and economic evaluation. 2nd ed. New York: Oxford University Press, 2003.

5. Hopkins DP, Briss PA, Ricard CJ, et al. Reviews of evidence regarding interventions to reduce tobacco use and exposure to environmental tobacco smoke. Am J Prev Med 2001;20(2S):16-66.

6. Drummond MF, O'Brien BJ, Stoddart GL, Torrance GW. Methods for the economic evaluation of health care programmes. 2nd ed. New York: Oxford University Press, 1997.

7. Gold MR, Siegel JE, Russell LB, Weinstein MC. Cost- effectiveness in health and medicine. New York: Oxford University Press, 1996.

8. Kahn EB, Ramsey LT, Brownson R, et al. The effectiveness of interventions to increase physical activity: a systematic review. Am J Prev Med 2002;22(4S):73-107.

9. Carande-Kulis VG, Maciosek MV, Briss PA, et al. Methods for systematic reviews of economic evaluations for the Guide to Community Preventive Services. Am J Prev Med 2000;18(1S):75-91.

10. Petitti DB. Meta-analysis, decision analysis, and cost- effectiveness analysis: methods for quantitative synthesis in medicine. 2nd ed. New York: Oxford University Press, 2000.

11. Holtgrave DR, ed. Handbook of economic evaluation of HIV prevention programs. New York: Plenum, 1998.

12. Chiou CF, Hay JW, Wallace JF, et al. Development and validation of a grading system for the quality of cost- effectiveness studies. Med Care 2003;41(1):32-44.

13. Donaldson C, Currie G, Mitton C. Cost effectiveness analysis in health care: contraindications. BMJ 2002;325(7369):891-4.

14. Dowie J. Decision validity should determine whether a generic or condition-specific HRQOL measure is used in health care decisions. Health Econ 2002;11(1):1-8.

15. Feeny D. Commentary on Jack Dowie, "Decision validity should determine whether a generic or condition-specific HRQOL measure is used in health care decisions." Health Econ 2002;11(1):13-6.

16. Gold MR, Franks P, McCoy KI, Fryback DG. Toward consistency in cost-utility analyses: using national measures to create condition-specific values. Med Care 1998; 36(6):778-92.

17. Guyatt G. Commentary on Jack Dowie, "Decision validity should determine whether a generic or condition-specific HRQOL measure is used in health care decisions." Health Econ 2002;11(1):9-12.

18. Laupacis A, Feeny D, Detsky AS, Tugwell PX. How attractive does a new technology have to be to warrant adoption and utilization? Tentative guidelines for using clinical and economic evaluations. Can Med Assoc J 1992;146(4):473-81.

19. Stone PW, Teutsch S, Chapman RH, Chaim B, Goldie SJ, Neumann PJ. Cost-utility analyses of clinical preventive services: published ratios, 1976-1997. Am J Prev Med 2000;19(1):15-23.

20. Tengs TO, Adams ME, Pliskin JS, et al. Five-hundred life-saving interventions and their cost-effectiveness. Risk Anal 1995;15(3):369-90.

21. Williams A. Intergenerational equity: an exploration of the "fair innings" argument. Health Econ 1997;6(2):117–32.

22. Sampietro-Colom L, Phillips VL, Hutchinson AB. Eliciting women's preferences in health care: a review of the literature. Int J Technol Assess Health Care 2004;20(2): 145–155.

23. Corso PS, Schofield A, Briss PA, Carande-Kulis VG. Economic efficiency of population-based interventions: exposing the gaps. Unpublished.

24. Corso PS, Thacker SB, Koplan JP. The value of prevention: experiences of a public health agency. Med Decis Making 2002;22(5 suppl):S11–S16.

25. Owens DK. Analytic tools for public health decision making. Med Decis Making 2002;22(5 suppl):S3–S10.

26. Sencer DJ, Axnick NW. Utilization of cost/benefit analysis in planning prevention programs. Acta Med Scand 1975(Suppl 576):123–9.

Chapter 12

Continuing Research Needs

In the introduction to this book, three possible results of a *Community Guide* systematic review were described: an intervention is found to be effective, it is found to be ineffective or harmful, or insufficient evidence is available to determine its effectiveness. This chapter addresses the ways in which the *Community Guide* might inform public health intervention research by identifying the areas where insufficient evidence is found or where there is conflicting evidence. We also discuss specific measures to improve the quality of intervention research. This chapter is intended to serve as a guide for organizations that fund public health intervention research and for researchers themselves. Because the information in this chapter is based entirely on our review process, it is not a comprehensive summary of the entire field of intervention research. We hope, however, that it will help a range of organizations set research agendas and contribute to improving research quality.

IMPROVING THE QUALITY OF PUBLIC HEALTH INTERVENTION RESEARCH

In the course of developing the *Community Guide,* we learned a great deal about the quality of public health intervention research and how it could be improved. This section describes lessons learned that might contribute to the overall public health intervention research agenda. The numerous partners involved in the *Community Guide* provided a wide range of insights, ideas, and examples about how their organizations use the *Community Guide.* These examples serve as the basis for this section.

Evaluate High-Priority Interventions in High-Priority Topics

The topics chosen and reported in this book and at www.thecommunityguide .org are high-priority public health issues. The process of identifying them emphasized a preventable public health burden. The list of review topics was finalized by the Task Force on Community Preventive Services only after a process that included extensive input from broad multidisciplinary teams drawn from the Centers for Disease Control and Prevention (CDC), the National Institutes of Health (NIH), the U.S. Department of Health and Human

Services (HHS), state and local public health departments, the healthcare delivery sector, purchasers of health care, and others. Once topics were selected, we also used a process of broad stakeholder input to determine which interventions to review within those topics.

Thus, the *Community Guide* provides information on interventions that address problems widely held to be among the most important ones that public health must address. When the science base for these interventions is sparse or of low quality, the reviews can provide systematically collected and evaluated information on promising but understudied topics with important public health implications. For example, some topics have an extensive evidence base (e.g., reducing tobacco use), while other critical public health areas (e.g., the sociocultural environment, obesity prevention) are relatively understudied. The reviews can also reduce repetition of research beyond that needed for appropriate replication, making it easier to allocate limited research resources to the issues where additional information might make a greater difference. Researchers and research funding organizations can use the *Community Guide* to inform their priority setting among research questions.

Develop or Adapt a Conceptual Model for the Intervention

Each intervention to be implemented and tested should have a conceptual or theoretical model like those illustrated in this book. Such models can improve the quality of research by making the conceptual or theoretical basis of the intervention explicit, by specifying hypotheses to be tested, and by documenting outcomes to be measured. For these reasons, research funding organizations should require applicants to specify a conceptual model. The *Community Guide* methods (summarized in Chapter 10) and the individual chapters provide examples of such a conceptual modeling process.

Measure Outcomes That Credibly Reflect Intervention Effectiveness

Each of our reviews defines which outcomes are thought to represent the *success* of the intervention. For these reviews, intervention effectiveness is usually assessed according to health outcomes (e.g., injury rates), established proxies for health outcomes (e.g., vaccine coverage rates), or health behaviors with established links to health outcomes (e.g., seat belt use or tobacco use). Intermediate outcomes (e.g., knowledge, attitudes, process measures, or environmental characteristics) are important mediators, but they do not always correlate well with the ultimate goal of improving health behaviors and health outcomes. The individual chapters of this book can provide researchers and research funding organizations with key health, proxy, or behavioral outcome measures for individual interventions identified by large multidisciplinary teams of experts on the methodology and subject matter.

Conduct Research on Understudied Interventions

We have found great variability in the number of evaluations performed on each intervention, from no evaluations to as many as several dozen. The smaller the number of high-quality evaluations of interventions, the greater the need for additional studies, unless the findings are remarkably persuasive. Therefore, by identifying understudied areas, the *Community Guide* can help to increase the impact of limited research resources.

For every intervention reviewed, a list of the major remaining research needs was developed by the review team. Topic-specific lists have been published as part of the scientific review articles[1-12] and are not repeated in this book, although we identify cross-cutting research needs later in this chapter. The process for summarizing research gaps has been described elsewhere[13] and is summarized in Chapter 10.

Consider Harms as Well as Benefits

When making recommendations, the Task Force attempts to balance the benefits of public health interventions with potential harms. Some interventions may not pose a credible risk of harms. Even when harms are possible, however, potential negative effects are studied much less frequently than potential benefits. Where harms are a concern and have not been studied, they should be studied to better assess the net benefit of the intervention.

Perform Evaluations Appropriate to the Stage of Progress of the Field

Different types of intervention studies are more or less appropriate, depending on the stage of development of a particular field, such as cancer prevention and control. As a field matures, the research focus may shift over time. In the early stages of public health research in a given area, researchers define the problem epidemiologically and identify risk factors that are possible targets for intervention. Later, they develop theory-based interventions and a taxonomy of those that are promising. This stage is followed by evaluating the effectiveness of the interventions and assessing the applicability, efficiency, and barriers to implementing effective interventions.

Each of our reviews presents background information and conceptual models that help to show the stage of progress of a given field. In addition, each review of an individual intervention provides information about what is already known and what remains to be studied about the intervention's effectiveness, applicability, efficiency, and barriers to implementation.

Assess Intervention Effectiveness Using the Most Suitable Study Design Possible

Suitability is the appropriateness of the study design for measuring effectiveness. Designs that best limit biases and confounding are considered to be of greater suitability and generally result in greater confidence in the findings. However, such designs (including randomized controlled trials) are often not feasible or ethical in evaluating population-based interventions such as those reviewed here. In addition, designs of greater suitability can limit the external validity of a study (our confidence that the study results can be generalized to populations and contexts beyond the particular ones included in the studies themselves). For example, a study in which specially selected volunteers are assigned to an intervention under conditions in which they are closely monitored by study staff may not translate well to routine practice. It is often therefore reasonable to use a design of lesser suitability if it has advantages with respect to external validity that compensate for any disadvantages with respect to internal validity (our confidence that the intervention being evaluated really caused the effects or outcomes being measured). In addition, if designs with greater suitability are not feasible or appropriate, the use of the best possible design should not impede one's ability to draw conclusions. Non-comparative study designs (i.e., studies without a concurrent or other comparison group), although useful for some questions, are not appropriate for evaluating intervention effectiveness. The reviews in this volume include studies with a range of suitable study designs to ensure a comprehensive assessment of the effectiveness of population-based interventions.[14]

Conduct and Describe Effectiveness Studies in Ways That Minimize Potential Threats to Internal Validity

The Task Force and its methods work group[14] developed a standard taxonomy of important quality indicators that are applicable to diverse study designs and intended to help minimize threats to internal and external validity.[15] This taxonomy forms the basis for the following recommendations on study design, execution, and dissemination of intervention evaluation studies:

1. Describe the study population in terms of person, place, time, and other relevant characteristics.
2. Describe the intervention in enough detail so that it can be replicated. If journal space is a limiting factor, consider supplementary reports or supporting Internet publications.

3. Describe the selection of the study population. Choose this population in ways that minimize selection bias or threats to external validity (e.g., minimize unnecessary exclusions).
4. Measure exposure to the intervention and its relevant outcomes in reliable and valid ways. Document reliability and validity of both exposure and outcome measures.
5. Conduct statistical tests where appropriate. Choose appropriate statistical tests and perform them correctly.
6. Ensure high follow-up rates.
7. Minimize confounding through study design and analytic techniques.
8. Minimize and explain other potential biases.

Additional advice about assessing quality[16,17] and improving reporting for randomized[18] and non-randomized studies[19] is available elsewhere.

Maximize the External Validity of Effectiveness Studies

The advice above primarily addresses the internal validity of studies that evaluate intervention effectiveness. External validity is also important, especially for population-based research. In addition to steps 1 and 3 above, external validity may be enhanced by performing additional research in new populations or contexts, thus complementing rather than duplicating existing research.

Maximize Credibility and Comparability of Economic Studies

Our reviews involve a concerted effort to systematically include and review all information about the economic impact of each recommended intervention (see Chapter 11). Unfortunately, economic evaluations of population-based interventions are rare, and there is considerable variation in the quality and comparability of those that have been published. Enormous gaps in this research area provide ample opportunity for researchers and research funding organizations to explore new areas of public health intervention research. The *Community Guide* process includes innovative methods for systematic reviews and adjustments of economic research, building on the work of the Panel for Cost Effectiveness in Medicine.[20] In addition, our method of conducting economic reviews is unique in its use of quality-scoring criteria for assessing the appropriateness of methods, the validity of results, and the completeness of reporting.[21,22]

Describe Implementation Processes for Effective Interventions

In developing and communicating findings, we are often asked to provide information about how to implement interventions. Although this is beyond the current scope of the *Community Guide* and information on this topic is available elsewhere,[23] this is nonetheless a critical aspect of public health that has been surprisingly underemphasized. Research on the steps needed to implement interventions, and on the identification of and methods for overcoming barriers to intervention implementation, is needed to provide public health programs with adequate information for implementing effective interventions. In addition, researchers, funders, government agencies, voluntary organizations, and others should work together to make their intervention materials and processes widely available (e.g., on the Internet). This would go á long way toward reducing the need to "reinvent the wheel" each time an intervention is implemented.

CROSS-CUTTING RESEARCH NEEDS IDENTIFIED
THROUGH THE *COMMUNITY GUIDE* REVIEW PROCESS

Each *Community Guide* review leads to the identification of specific questions related to intervention research, which we publish in the scientific review articles.[1-12] In this chapter we identify a number of cross-cutting research needs that have emerged in two or more reviews. These questions will not apply to all interventions, but are issues that come up frequently and are generally worth considering systematically. Intervention studies designed and reported with these questions in mind should provide useful answers. In each section, a specific representative question from a review is presented as an example.

Questions Pertaining to Methods

As the reviews were carried out, we uncovered a number of questions about the process of synthesizing intervention research consistently. In this section, we identify general questions that can be answered using rigorous scientific techniques. We do not include questions that resulted from poor execution or reporting of intervention evaluations.

Several issues related to study outcomes emerged during these reviews. In some cases, further research is necessary to determine "What is the public health importance of the outcomes under study?" Questions about the process by which interventions are presumed to affect final outcomes also frequently arose, such as:

- What theoretical or conceptual basis links the outcome measures with the intervention under study?
- To what extent are proximal outcomes predictive of or related to health outcomes? For example, in some interventions provided for children, desired outcomes are far in the future.

Other methodological challenges are related to the improvement of measurement in evaluation research:

- When interventions are implemented, to what extent is the target population exposed?
- How do we improve the measurement (reliability, validity, sensitivity, specificity) of outcome and exposure measures?

Finally, several questions were raised about potential ways of improving future research syntheses:

- How much can a specific intervention vary (e.g., content, materials, setting) and still be assumed to belong to the same class of interventions? For example:

    Even though disease and case management [for diabetes] were found effective in the managed care setting for improving glycemic control and provider monitoring of certain important outcomes, several important research gaps were identified in this review. One of the most pressing needs is to better define effective interventions. Disease management has multiple component interventions. To make optimal use of resources, however, only the interventions that contribute most to positive outcomes should be implemented, and these interventions need to be defined.[8]

- How can meta-analytic and information synthesis techniques be improved for summarizing studies, explaining variability across studies, or both?
- How can reporting of studies be improved to facilitate the inclusion of studies involving research synthesis and meta-analysis?

Questions Pertaining to the Interventions

Effectiveness

Several key questions about an intervention's effectiveness could be better answered if researchers considered them in the design and reporting of intervention studies.

- How do various intervention characteristics (e.g., content, specificity, method of delivery, frequency of delivery) contribute to effectiveness? For example:

    Which neighborhood features (e.g., sidewalks, parks, traffic flow, proximity to shopping) are the most crucial in influencing [physical] activity patterns?[7]

- Do multiple prevention messages act synergistically or do they contradict one another?
- What is the relationship between the level of program intensity and the level of program effectiveness?
- What are the minimum requirements for duration and intensity of interventions to achieve effectiveness?
- What are the optimal requirements for duration and intensity of interventions to achieve maximum effectiveness?
- Are interventions with a strong theoretical basis more likely to be effective than others?
- How is effectiveness of the intervention affected by the baseline rate of the risk factor or disease under study?
- What are the most and least effective combinations of services in multi-component interventions?
- What is the minimal combination of core components required for intervention effectiveness?
- Can components of multicomponent interventions that don't contribute to overall intervention effectiveness be identified and eliminated to maintain effectiveness and increase efficiency?

Applicability

Several issues in data collection and reporting might strengthen conclusions about applicability. For example:

- Do the effects of these interventions vary by key social or demographic variables (e.g., gender, age, race, ethnicity, or socioeconomic status)?
- What is the effectiveness of the intervention in reducing racial and ethnic disparities?
- How do cultural characteristics of the target population contribute to increased or decreased effectiveness?
- Do the effects of these interventions vary by different implementation settings? For example:

  How do different practice settings (e.g., independent private practice settings versus [health] management organization settings) contribute to increased or lessened effectiveness of various interventions?[4]

- Does intervention effectiveness vary by urban or rural setting?
- Does intervention effectiveness vary depending on who delivers the intervention (e.g., physicians vs. others; lay health workers vs. others; people of particular demographics or backgrounds vs. others)?
- What theoretical or conceptual basis suggests that effectiveness might vary by different population or setting characteristics?

Other Benefits or Harms

Potential harms of interventions are frequently not studied or not reported. The same applies to unanticipated beneficial effects. Without better information about the full range of intervention consequences, it is difficult to assess the net benefit of the intervention. It may be helpful to ask questions like:

- Does the intervention result in unintended harms? For example:

   If mixed-income housing developments are effective in beginning a process of revitalization that attracts higher-income households to a neighborhood, to what extent does this revitalization and the related increases in housing costs ultimately push poor families out of the area?[2]

- Does the intervention result in unanticipated positive (beneficial) side effects?

Questions Pertaining to Diffusion, Dissemination, Implementation, and Sustainability of Interventions

To promote and implement effective interventions that can ensure a sustained positive impact on communities, research questions such as the following should be addressed:

- What are the most effective ways of disseminating research findings?
- What are the most effective ways of communicating findings so that they will be useful and used?
- How can we help communities with priority setting and planning?
- How can a more strategic approach be applied to the selection of interventions so that they are more likely to reach important goals?
- What information and actions are most important in gaining community or political support for interventions?
- How do community coalitions affect or influence the delivery and effectiveness of interventions?
- To ease implementation of interventions, what strategies are effective in reducing barriers?
- What is the nature and role of *opinion leaders* or *champions* in implementing and sustaining an intervention?
- What kinds of community involvement in intervention design contribute to sustainability of community-based interventions?
- What is the pattern of effectiveness of the intervention over time (e.g., continuing improvement, deterioration)? For example:

   What effects do these interventions [to reduce alcohol-impaired driving] have on long-term changes in social norms about drinking and driving?[10]

- How long does the effect of the intervention endure after the intervention itself is completed?
- What are the most effective ways to maintain the effects of the intervention?
- What effects do these interventions have on long-term changes in social norms?
- How can community-wide efforts become embedded in the regular activities of local organizations, government, and institutions?

Questions Pertaining to Economic Methods, Measurement, and Studies

Our systematic reviews of the economic literature on population-based interventions identified a consistent lack of information across all of the topics reviewed. Thus, the research questions in this section are basic economic efficiency questions that need to be answered for nearly all population-based interventions. For a set of examples of economic research questions, see Table 12–1.

- What are the costs (e.g., economic, productivity, or opportunity costs) of these interventions?
- What is the cost benefit, cost utility, or cost effectiveness of these interventions?
- Which specific characteristics of these interventions contribute to economic efficiency?
- How do the opportunity costs of multicomponent interventions compare with those of single-component interventions?
- What combinations of components in multicomponent interventions are most cost-effective?
- How does cost or cost effectiveness vary by context?
- What are the most cost-effective combinations of intervention components?

Table 12–1. Example of Economic Research Questions

Available economic information was limited to a single study of mass media campaigns (to prevent youth tobacco use initiation). Therefore, considerable research is warranted regarding the following questions:

- Are the costs and cost-effectiveness, net cost, or net benefit of mass media campaigns similar to or substantially different from those that have been previously reported?
- How do the costs per tobacco user averted by this intervention compare with other tobacco prevention interventions?
- How do specific characteristics of mass media campaigns contribute to economic efficiency?
- What combinations of components in multicomponent interventions are most cost-effective?

CONCLUSION

The basic premise of the *Community Guide* is that decisions about intervention selection should be informed, at least in part, by existing scientific understanding of the effectiveness and applicability of those interventions. Our process of conducting systematic reviews also identifies gaps in the evaluation of high-priority interventions and policies, either lack of available research or ways in which the available research can be improved. The fact that these gaps exist is not an indictment of public health research: scientific research is always built piece by piece, and new opportunities will always exist to build on the work that has already been done. Recognition of these gaps confirms that a data-based decision-making process can be applied to how our research resources—most importantly time and funding—are spent to fill those gaps and improve quality efficiently. Researchers, research organizations, and funders of public health intervention research who need to take a strategic approach to answering those needs should find this chapter helpful.

Acknowledgments

This chapter was written by Peter A. Briss, MD, MPH, Community Guide Branch, Division of Prevention Research and Analytic Methods, Epidemiology Program Office, Centers for Disease Control and Prevention (CDC), Atlanta, Georgia; Barry Portnoy, PhD, Office of Disease Prevention, Office of the Director, National Institutes of Health (NIH), Rockville, Maryland; Martina Vogel-Taylor, MT, Office of Disease Prevention, Office of the Director, NIH, Rockville; and Stephanie Zaza, MD, MPH, Steps Program Office, National Center for Chronic Disease Prevention and Health Promotion, CDC, Atlanta.

References

1. Anderson LM, Shinn CM, Fullilove MT, et al. The effectiveness of early childhood development programs: a systematic review. Am J Prev Med 2003;24(3S):32–46.
2. Anderson LM, St Charles J, Fullilove MT, et al. Providing affordable family housing and reducing residential segregation by income: a systematic review. Am J Prev Med 2003;24(3S):47–67.
3. Anderson LM, Scrimshaw SC, Fullilove MT, Fielding JE, Normand J, Task Force on Community Preventive Services. Culturally competent healthcare systems: a systematic review. Am J Prev Med 2003;24(3S):68–79.
4. Briss PA, Rodewald LE, Hinman AR, et al. Reviews of evidence regarding interventions to improve vaccination coverage in children, adolescents, and adults. Am J Prev Med 2000;18(1S):97–140.
5. Dinh-Zarr TB, Sleet DA, Shults RA, et al. Reviews of evidence regarding interventions to increase use of safety belts. Am J Prev Med 2001;21(4S):48–65.
6. Hopkins DP, Briss PA, Ricard CJ, et al. Reviews of evidence regarding interventions

to reduce tobacco use and exposure to environmental tobacco smoke. Am J Prev Med 2001;20(2S):16–66.

7. Kahn EB, Ramsey LT, Brownson R, et al. The effectiveness of interventions to increase physical activity: a systematic review. Am J Prev Med 2002;22(4S):73–107.

8. Norris SL, Nichols PJ, Caspersen CJ, et al. The effectiveness of disease and case management for people with diabetes: a systematic review. Am J Prev Med 2002;22(4S): 15–38.

9. Norris SL, Nichols PJ, Caspersen CJ, et al. Increasing diabetes self-management education in community settings: a systematic review. Am J Prev Med 2002;22(4S): 39–66.

10. Shults RA, Elder RW, Sleet DA, et al. Reviews of evidence regarding interventions to reduce alcohol-impaired driving. Am J Prev Med 2001;21(4S):66–88.

11. Truman BI, Gooch BF, Sulemana I, et al. Reviews of evidence on interventions to prevent dental caries, oral and pharyngeal cancers, and sports-related craniofacial injuries. Am J Prev Med 2002;23(1S):21–54.

12. Zaza S, Sleet DA, Thompson RS, Sosin DM, Bolen JC, Task Force on Community Preventive Services. Reviews of evidence regarding interventions to increase use of child safety seats. Am J Prev Med 2001;21(4S):31–47.

13. Zaza S, Carande-Kulis VG, Sleet DA, et al. Methods for conducting systematic reviews of the evidence of effectiveness and economic efficiency of interventions to reduce injuries to motor vehicle occupants. Am J Prev Med 2001;21(4S):23–30.

14. Briss PA, Zaza S, Pappaioanou M, et al. Developing an evidence-based Guide to Community Preventive Services— methods. Am J Prev Med 2000;18(1S):35–43.

15. Zaza S, Wright-de Aguero L, Briss PA, et al. Data collection instrument and procedure for systematic reviews in the Guide to Community Preventive Services. Am J Prev Med 2000;18(1S):44–74.

16. Agency for Healthcare Research and Quality. Systems to rate the strength of scientific evidence. Available at: www.ahcpr.gov/clinic/epcsums/strengthsum.pdf. Accessed May 12, 2003.

17. Deeks JJ, Dinnes J, D'Amico R, et al. Evaluating non- randomised intervention studies. Health Technol Assess 2003;7(27):1–186.

18. Moher D, Schulz KF, Altman D, CONSORT Group. The CONSORT statement: revised recommendations for improving the quality of reports of parallel-group randomized trials. JAMA 2001;285(15):1987–91.

19. Des Jarlais DC, Lyles C, Crepaz N, the TREND Group. Improving the reporting quality of nonrandomized evaluations of behavioral and public health interventions: the TREND statement. Am J Public Health 2004;94(3):361–6.

20. Gold MR, Siegel JE, Russell LB, Weinstein MC. Cost- effectiveness in health and medicine. New York: Oxford University Press, 1996.

21. Carande-Kulis VG, Maciosek MV, Briss PA, et al. Methods for systematic reviews of economic evaluations for the Guide to Community Preventive Services. Am J Prev Med 2000;18(1S):75–91.

22. Economic evaluation abstraction form, version 3.0. Available at: http://www.the communityguide.org/methods/econ-abs-form.pdf. Accessed September 9, 2003.

23. Work Group on Health Promotion and Community Development at the University of Kansas in Lawrence. Community Tool Box. Available at: http://ctb.ku.edu. Accessed April 7, 2004.

Glossary

The definitions in this glossary apply to words and phrases as used in the *Guide to Community Preventive Services.* A separate definition is provided for words that appear in italics in a given definition. For example, the definition of **Body of evidence** contains the two terms *qualifying studies* and *Community Guide,* both of which can also be found in this Glossary.

In addition to the economic terms listed in this Glossary, Chapter 11 contains its own glossary of economics terms used in that chapter.

Adapted/Adapting See *Tailoring* and *Targeting*

Aggregate/aggregated studies An approach to evaluating studies that consolidates a number of studies on the basis of similarities such as location, study population, the period of study, and data analyzed. Each aggregate study, although composed of two or more studies, is analyzed as if it were a single study.

Analytic framework (See also *Logic framework*) A diagram that shows hypothesized links between an intervention and related *intermediate outcomes, health outcomes,* and other *effects.* An analytic framework expands on a specific portion of a *logic framework,* and is used to plan evaluations of *interventions* and to guide the search for evidence.

Applicability A judgment about the populations and/or settings in which a recommended activity could be implemented successfully, based on the populations and settings represented in the studies reviewed and conceptual information about the intervention. The *Community Guide* provides information on applicability for all recommended activities. (See also *External validity.*)

Arm See *Intervention arm.*

Before-and-after studies In contrast to studies with an *intervention group* and a *comparison group,* before-and-after studies are conducted within a single group. Outcomes are measured before and after the intervention.

Benefit-to-cost ratio A measure, from a cost–benefit analysis, of the total benefits of an intervention divided by the total costs.

Body of evidence The complete set of *qualifying studies* in a *Community Guide* systematic review.

Clinical setting Setting in which the primary purpose is the delivery of medical care in a one-on-one provider-patient relationship. Can include private office practices, managed care facilities (e.g., HMOs, PPOs, community health centers), clinics, or hospitals. (See also *Community setting.*)

Community A group of individuals sharing one or more characteristics such as geographic location (e.g., a neighborhood), culture, age, or a particular risk factor. In the *Guide to Community Preventive Services,* for the purposes of evaluating whether interventions make communities healthier, we have chosen to apply the broadest possible use of *community.*

Community-based intervention An *intervention* conducted within and by members of a particular community (e.g., grassroots efforts, efforts by a local civic group). Can be done in conjunction with an outside group (e.g., nonprofit organization, research group).

Community Guide The *Guide to Community Preventive Services.*

Community Guide *reference case* A standard set of methodological practices for performing cost–effectiveness analyses , as recommended by the Panel on Cost-effectiveness in Health and Medicine (Gold MR, Siegel JE, Russel LB, Weinstein MC. Cost-effectiveness in health and medicine: report of the Panel on Cost-effectiveness in Health and Medicine. New York: Oxford University Press, 1996).

Community-oriented intervention An *intervention* meant to improve the *health* or reduce injury or impairment of people in a *community.* Community-oriented interventions include but are not limited to *community-based interventions.*

Community setting Setting for which the primary purpose is *not* medical care, for example, geographic communities, schools, churches, homeless shelters, worksites, libraries. (See also *Clinical setting.*)

Comparison group A group that is not exposed to a particular *intervention;* the control group, used to determine what would have happened if the intervention had not been carried out. The *intervention group* is exposed to the intervention.

Consultants, consultation team A group of 10–30 people, with special knowledge in the field under review, who work in consultation with the *systematic review development team,* providing opinion and expertise in support of a *systematic review.*

Coordination team See *Systematic review development team.*

Cost analysis The most basic type of *economic evaluation.* It is the systematic collection, categorization, and analysis of all of the costs associated with an intervention.

Cost–benefit analysis A type of *economic evaluation* that measures both costs and benefits (i.e., positive and negative consequences) associated with an *intervention* in dollar terms.

Cost–effectiveness analysis An analysis used to compare the cost of alternative *interventions* that produce a common *health effect* (e.g., cost per injury averted or *life-years saved*).

Cost-saving An *intervention, program,* or *policy* is said to be cost-saving if the costs averted by the intervention exceed the costs of the program.

Cost–utility analysis A type of *cost–effectiveness analysis* that uses *life-years saved* adjusted for quality of life during those years as a *health outcome* measure. These measures are called *quality-adjusted life-years (QALYs).*

Determinants Factors hypothesized to affect *outcomes,* such as demographic and population factors; environmental factors; or aspects of a particular social, economic, educational, healthcare, or cultural system.

Development team See *Systematic review development team.*

Econometric methods Applying statistical methods to the study of economic data.

Economic efficiency Achieving the greatest improvement in *health* using the available resources.

Economic evaluation An assessment of the economic impact of an *intervention, program,* or *policy.*

Effect The change in an *outcome* that results from an *intervention.*

Effect measure The measurement used to describe the *effect* and the *effect size*.

Effect size The magnitude of the *effect*.

Effectiveness The degree to which an *intervention* achieves a desired *outcome* in practice.

External validity The ability to generalize study results to populations and contexts beyond the particular ones included in the studies themselves. (See also *Applicability.*)

Guide to Clinical Preventive Services (*Clinical Guide*) The clinical counterpart to the *Guide to Community Preventive Services*, prepared and published by the *U.S. Preventive Services Task Force (USPSTF)*. The *Clinical Guide*, widely used by primary care providers, health policy makers, and others, provides current and scientifically defensible information from published clinical research on the *effectiveness* of different preventive services and the quality of evidence upon which conclusions are based.

Guide to Community Preventive Services (*Community Guide*) The body of evidence and recommendations approved by the Task Force on Community Preventive Services, including this book; the website, www.thecommunityguide.org; and articles published in scientific journals. See the Introduction for a full explanation of the scope of the *Community Guide.*

Health Positive physical, mental, psychological, and social function and the absence of disease, injury, or impairment.

Health indicator A measure of the *health* of people in a *community*, such as infant mortality rates, rates of obesity, or incidence of diabetes.

Health outcome The change in *health* that is hypothesized to result from the intervention (e.g., reduced morbidity or mortality or increased physical, mental, or psychological function). In *Community Guide systematic reviews*, health outcomes to be measured are defined in the planning stages of the review.

Healthcare providers Individuals from any of several professional groups (e.g., physicians, nurses, and others) who provide direct healthcare services to individual clients or patients.

Healthcare systems Systems for delivering healthcare that may include, for example, hospitals, clinics, health maintenance organizations (HMOs), and community health centers.

Inclusion criteria Characteristics of a study that make it appropriate for inclusion in a particular *Community Guide systematic review*. A study that is included must also meet the *quality criteria* before it can become part of the *body of evidence*.

Insufficient evidence to determine effectiveness A *body of evidence* that does not provide enough information for the Task Force to determine whether or not an *intervention* is *effective*. A finding of "insufficient evidence" indicates the need for additional research into the effectiveness of the intervention; it does not mean that the intervention doesn't work, but rather that we can't tell yet if it works.

Intermediate outcome One in a series of *effects* that results from an *intervention* and may lead to a *health outcome*. For example, in an educational intervention designed to reduce skin cancer incidence, intermediate outcomes could be covering-up behavior or seeking shade. In a *Community Guide systematic review*, an intermediate outcome considered to have a strong and established link to a *health outcome* may serve as a *recommendation outcome.*

Internal validity Whether the intervention being evaluated really caused the effects or outcomes being measured.

Intervention In the *Community Guide,* an intervention is any kind of planned activity or group of activities (including programs, policies, and laws) designed to prevent disease or injury or promote *health* in a group of people.

Intervention arm In a study in which two or more groups are compared, each group that receives an *intervention* is an arm.

Intervention group A group of people exposed to an intervention. (See also *Comparison group.*)

Intervention, multicomponent An *intervention* that includes more than one activity. For example, mass media campaigns to motivate young people to remain tobacco-free can be combined or coordinated with additional intervention activities, such as increases in tobacco product excise taxes, school-based education, and other community-wide educational activities.

Life-years saved A measure of the improvement in *health* that results from an *intervention.*

Logic framework (See also *Analytic framework*) A diagram that illustrates the public health context in which a specific disease prevention or health promotion activity takes place. Logic frameworks show relationships between social, environmental, and biological *determinants* and *outcomes,* and strategic points at which action can be taken to change the *outcome.*

Multicomponent intervention (See *Intervention, multicomponent*)

Net benefit A measure from a *cost–benefit analysis,* calculated as the value of the benefits gained minus the costs (including, for example, *program* costs and harms).

Net cost The total *program* costs minus the cost of averted disease and the cost of averted productivity losses.

Other effects Outcomes or effects other than those anticipated as a possible result of the *intervention.* These can be positive (beneficial) effects (e.g., smoking bans and restrictions might reduce cleaning costs or fire risks as well as improving health) or negative (harmful) effects (e.g., programs to reduce the costs of vaccines have been hypothesized to reduce the impetus to develop new vaccines).

Outcome (See also *Health outcome, Intermediate outcome,* and *Recommendation outcome*) The desired result of implementing an *intervention.*

% A change expressed with the percent (%) symbol represents a relative difference. For example, if 50% of participants had already quit smoking at the beginning of the study, a 10% improvement over this baseline would result in a total of 55% who had quit (the 50% baseline plus 10% of that baseline, which is 5%).

Percentage point A percentage point change represents an absolute difference. For example, if 50% of participants had already quit smoking at the beginning of the study, an increase of 10 percentage points would mean that a total of 60% had quit at the end of the study (because 50% + 10 percentage points = 60%).

Policy A set of organizational rules (including but not limited to laws) intended to promote health or prevent disease.

Program An institutionalized system of *intervention* activities.

QALY or quality-adjusted life year An effort to take into account measures of both illness and (premature) death. For example, a year lived in perfect health may count as 1 QALY, whereas a year spent living with a serious illness might count as only 0.6 QALY.

Qualifying studies In a *Community Guide systematic review,* all studies that meet the *in-*

clusion criteria are then rated on the quality of the study design and execution. Studies that meet these *quality criteria* become the qualifying studies for that review.

Quality criteria Characteristics used by a *systematic review development team* to establish the likely validity of the results by assessing how well a study was performed.

Recommendation outcome An *outcome* on which the *Task Force* will base a recommendation, usually either a *health outcome* or a well-established proxy for a health outcome. Decisions about which outcomes will be recommendation outcomes are made at the beginning of a review by members of the *systematic review development team* and the *Task Force on Community Preventive Services*.

Strategy A larger category under which a group of related interventions is organized. For example, the strategy of increasing child safety seat use includes child safety seat laws, community-wide information and enhanced enforcement campaigns, distribution and education programs, incentive and education programs, and education programs when used alone.

Strong evidence of effectiveness A body of evidence that meets the requirements for strong evidence set forth in Table 10–1 of Chapter 10, Methods Used for Reviewing Evidence and Linking Evidence to Recommendations.

Sufficient evidence of effectiveness A body of evidence that meets the requirements for sufficient but not strong evidence set forth in Table 10–1 of Chapter 10, Methods Used for Reviewing Evidence and Linking Evidence to Recommendations.

Systematic review A process by which a body of literature is reviewed and assessed using systematic methods that are intended to reduce bias in the review process and improve understandability.

Systematic review development team The group of 6–10 people that directs the *Community Guide systematic review*. Also referred to as the coordination team, review team, or development team. These teams typically include subject matter experts, a Task Force member, an economist, a research assistant, and others with special knowledge of the subject.

Tailoring (see also *Targeting*) An intervention or program is tailored when it is adapted to address characteristics of individuals. For example, tailoring a health behavior change program means adapting that program to address the individual needs of each participant.

Target population The population or community to which a given intervention is directed.

Targeting (see also *Tailoring*) An intervention or program is targeted when it is adapted to address characteristics of groups. For example, point-of-decision prompts (signs placed near elevators that encourage people to take the stairs to increase their physical activity or to lose weight) can be more effective when they address the needs of the people likely to see them.

Task Force on Community Preventive Services, the Task Force (See also *U.S. Preventive Services Task Force*) A 15-member non-federal panel initiated in 1996 by the Director, Centers for Disease Control and Prevention (CDC), under the auspices of the U.S. Public Health Service. The mission of this task force is to carry out systematic reviews of prevention interventions that can be carried out in *communities* and to develop recommendations based on the findings of these reviews. The Task Force findings are presented in the *Guide to Community Preventive Services* (the *Community Guide*).

Team See *Systematic review development team*.

U.S. Preventive Services Task Force (USPSTF) (See also *Task Force on Community Preventive Services*) A non-federal panel, commissioned by the U.S. Public Health Service in 1984 and 1990, charged with developing recommendations for clinicians on the appropriate use of preventive interventions, based on systematic reviews of evidence of clinical effectiveness. The USPSTF findings are presented in the *Guide to Clinical Preventive Services* (the *Clinical Guide*).

Appendix

The Guide to Community Preventive Services (*Community Guide*) encompasses population-based interventions across a range of topics using a variety of strategies—from laws to policies to education to changes in the systems that deliver health care—that can be applied in a wide variety of settings. This Appendix provides a comprehensive listing of all findings included in this book, presented in alphabetical order by topic.

It is important to note that "insufficient evidence to determine effectiveness" means that we were not able to determine whether or not the intervention works.

Cancer (Chapter 4)

Area of Focus	*Intervention*	*Finding*
Preventing skin cancer by reducing exposure to ultraviolet radiation and increasing sun-protective behaviors	**In Specific Settings**	
	Educational and policy interventions in primary schools	Recommended for improving children's sun-protective covering-up behavior
	Educational and policy interventions in recreational and tourism settings	Recommended for improving adult sun-protective covering-up behavior
		Insufficient evidence to determine effectiveness in improving children's sun-protective behaviors
	Educational and policy interventions in child care centers	Insufficient evidence to determine effectiveness
	Educational and policy interventions in secondary schools and colleges	Insufficient evidence to determine effectiveness
	Programs in outdoor occupational settings	Insufficient evidence to determine effectiveness
	Programs in healthcare system and provider settings	Insufficient evidence to determine effectiveness
	In Diverse Settings	
	Interventions oriented to children's parents and caregivers	Insufficient evidence to determine effectiveness
	Mass media campaigns alone	Insufficient evidence to determine effectiveness
	Community-wide multicomponent programs, including comprehensive community-wide interventions	Insufficient evidence to determine effectiveness
Promoting informed decision making for cancer screening	Informed decision making interventions to promote cancer screening	Insufficient evidence to determine effectiveness

Diabetes (Chapter 5)

Area of Focus	Intervention	Finding
In the health-care system	Disease management	Recommended
	Case management	Recommended
Diabetes self-management education (DSME)	DSME in community gathering places	Recommended for adults with type 2 diabetes
	DSME in the home	Recommended for adolescents with type 1 diabetes
		Insufficient evidence to determine effectiveness for people of all ages with type 2 diabetes
	DSME in summer camps	Insufficient evidence to determine effectiveness
	DSME at the worksite	Insufficient evidence to determine effectiveness
	Educating school personnel about diabetes	Insufficient evidence to determine effectiveness

Motor Vehicle Occupant Injury (Chapter 8)

Area of Focus	Intervention	Finding
Increasing child safety seat use	Child safety seat laws	Recommended
	Distribution and education programs	Recommended
	Community-wide information and enhanced enforcement campaigns	Recommended
	Incentive and education programs	Recommended
	Education programs when used alone alone	Insufficient evidence to determine effectiveness
Increasing safety belt use	Safety belt laws	Recommended
	Primary enforcement laws (vs. secondary enforcement laws)	Recommended
	Enhanced enforcement	Recommended
Reducing alcohol-impaired driving	0.08% blood alcohol concentration (BAC) laws	Recommended
	Minimum legal drinking age laws	Recommended (maintaining at 21 years of age)
	Sobriety checkpoints	Recommended
	Lower BAC for young or inexperienced drivers	Recommended
	Intervention training for servers of alcoholic beverages	Recommended (under certain conditions)
	Mass media campaigns	Recommended (under certain conditions)

Oral Health (Chapter 7)

Area of Focus	Intervention	Finding
Preventing or controlling dental caries	Community water fluoridation	Recommended
	School-based or school-linked pit and fissure sealant delivery programs	Recommended
	Statewide or community-wide sealant promotion programs	Insufficient evidence to determine effectiveness
Preventing or controlling oral and pharyngeal cancers	Population-based interventions for early detection of pre-cancers and cancers	Insufficient evidence to determine effectiveness
Preventing or controlling sports-related craniofacial injuries	Population-based interventions to encourage use of helmets, facemasks, and mouthguards in contact sports	Insufficient evidence to determine effectiveness

Physical Activity (Chapter 2)

Area of Focus	Intervention	Finding
Informational approaches to increasing physical activity	Community-wide campaigns	Recommended
	Point-of-decision prompts	Recommended
	Mass media campaigns	Insufficient evidence to determine effectiveness
	Classroom-based health education focused on providing information	Insufficient evidence to determine effectiveness
Behavioral and social approaches to increasing physical activity	School-based physical education	Recommended
	Individually-adapted health behavior change programs	Recommended
	Social support interventions in community settings	Recommended
	College-based health education and physical education	Insufficient evidence to determine effectiveness
	Classroom-based health education focused on reducing television viewing and video game playing	Insufficient evidence to determine effectiveness
	Family-based social support	Insufficient evidence to determine effectiveness
Environmental and policy approaches to increasing physical activity	Creation of or enhanced access to places for physical activity combined with informational outreach activities	Recommended
	Point-of-decision prompts	Recommended

Area of Focus	*Intervention*	*Finding*
Early childhood development	Comprehensive, center-based, early childhood development programs for low-income children	Recommended to improve children's readiness for school and to reduce retention in grade and placement in special education
		Insufficient evidence to determine effectiveness for these outcomes:
		• Behavioral assessments of child's social interaction and social risks (e.g., teen pregnancy, teen fatherhood, high school drop out, unemployment, use of social services)
		• Use of child health screening, preventive services, dental care
		• Parental educational attainment, parental employment, access to health services
Housing	Tenant-based rental assistance programs	Recommended to improve family safety
		Insufficient evidence to determine effectiveness for these outcomes:
		• Substandard housing conditions that pose health and safety risks
		• Behavioral problems in school and at home, delinquent acts, arrests for violent crime, arrests for property crime
		• Self-reported symptoms of depression and anxiety by household head
		• Self-rated health status as good or excellent compared to fair or poor
		• Child needing medical attention for accidents or asthma, child use of preventive services
	Mixed income housing developments	Insufficient evidence to determine effectiveness
Culturally competent health care	Programs to recruit and retain staff who reflect the cultural diversity of the community served	Insufficient evidence to determine effectiveness
	Use of interpreter services or bilingual providers for clients with limited English proficiency	Insufficient evidence to determine effectiveness
	Cultural competency training for healthcare providers	Insufficient evidence to determine effectiveness
	Use of linguistically and culturally appropriate health education materials	Insufficient evidence to determine effectiveness
	Culturally specific healthcare settings	Insufficient evidence to determine effectiveness

Tobacco (Chapter 1)

Area of Focus	Intervention	Finding
Reducing tobacco use initiation	Increasing the unit price for tobacco products	Recommended
	Mass media education campaigns, when combined with other interventions	Recommended
	Restricting Minors' Access to Tobacco Products	
	Community mobilization, when combined with additional interventions (stronger local laws directed at retailers, active enforcement of retailer sales laws, retailer education with reinforcement) to restrict minors' access to tobacco products	Recommended
	Sales laws directed at tobacco retailers to reduce illegal sales to minors when implemented alone	Insufficient evidence to determine effectiveness
	Laws directed at minors' purchase, possession, or use of tobacco products when implemented alone	Insufficient evidence to determine effectiveness
	Active enforcement of sales laws directed at retailers when implemented alone	Insufficient evidence to determine effectiveness
	Retailer education with reinforcement and information on health consequences when implemented alone	Insufficient evidence to determine effectiveness
	Retailer education without reinforcement when implemented alone	Insufficient evidence to determine effectiveness
	Community education about minors' access to tobacco products when implemented alone	Insufficient evidence to determine effectiveness
Increasing tobacco use cessation— interventions appropriate for communities	Increasing the unit price for tobacco products	Recommended
	Mass media education campaigns combined with other interventions	Recommended
	Mass media education—cessation series	Insufficient evidence to determine effectiveness
	Mass media education—cessation contests	Insufficient evidence to determine effectiveness
Increasing tobacco use cessation— interventions appropriate for healthcare systems	Healthcare provider reminder systems	Recommended
	Healthcare provider reminder systems with provider education, with or without client education	Recommended
	Reducing client out-of-pocket costs for effective cessation therapies	Recommended

Tobacco (Chapter 1) *(continued)*

Area of Focus	*Intervention*	*Finding*
	Multicomponent interventions that include client telephone support	Recommended
	Healthcare provider education alone	Insufficient evidence to determine effectiveness
	Healthcare provider feedback and assessment	Insufficient evidence to determine effectiveness
Reducing exposure to environmental tobacco smoke (ETS)	Smoking bans and restrictions	Recommended
	Community education to reduce exposure to ETS in the home	Insufficient evidence to determine effectiveness

Vaccine-Preventable Diseases: Universally Recommended Vaccines (Chapter 6, Section I)

Area of Focus	Intervention	Finding
Increasing community demand for vaccines	Client reminder and recall systems	Recommended
	Multicomponent interventions that include education	Recommended
	Vaccination requirements for child care, school, and college attendance	Recommended
	Community-wide education when used alone	Insufficient evidence to determine effectiveness
	Clinic-based education when used alone	Insufficient evidence to determine effectiveness
	Client or family incentives	Insufficient evidence to determine effectiveness
	Client-held medical records	Insufficient evidence to determine effectiveness
Enhancing access to vaccination services	Reducing out-of-pocket costs	Recommended
	Expanding access in healthcare settings	Recommended as part of a multicomponent intervention
		Insufficient evidence to determine effectiveness when used alone
	Vaccination programs in women, infants, and children (WIC) settings	Recommended
	Vaccination programs in schools	Recommended
	Home visits	Recommended
	Vaccination programs in child care centers	Insufficient evidence to determine effectiveness
Provider- or system-based interventions	Provider reminder and recall systems	Recommended
	Assessment plus feedback for vaccination providers	Recommended
	Standing orders	Recommended for adults
		Insufficient evidence to determine effectiveness for children
	Provider education only	Insufficient evidence to determine effectiveness

Vaccine-Preventable Diseases: Targeted Vaccines (Chapter 6, Section II)

Area of Focus	*Intervention*	*Finding*
Increasing community demand for targeted vaccinations	Clinic-based client education when used alone	Insufficient evidence to determine effectiveness
	Client reminder systems when used alone	Insufficient evidence to determine effectiveness
	Community-wide education when used alone	Insufficient evidence to determine effectiveness
	Client or family incentives when used alone	Insufficient evidence to determine effectiveness
	Vaccination requirements when used alone	Insufficient evidence to determine effectiveness
Enhancing access to targeted vaccination services	Reducing client out-of-pocket costs when used alone	Insufficient evidence to determine effectiveness
	Expanding access in healthcare settings when used alone	Insufficient evidence to determine effectiveness
Provider- or system-based interventions	Provider reminder systems when used alone	Recommended
	Provider education when used alone	Insufficient evidence to determine effectiveness
	Standing orders when used alone	Insufficient evidence to determine effectiveness
	Assessment plus feedback for vaccination providers when used alone	Insufficient evidence to determine effectiveness
Multiple interventions implemented in combination	One or more interventions to enhance access to vaccination services *plus* At least one provider- or system-based intervention *and/or* At least one intervention to increase community demand for vaccination services	Recommended

Violence (Chapter 9)

Area of Focus	Intervention	Finding
Early childhood home visitation	Early childhood home visitation	Recommended for prevention of violence against the child (maltreatment [abuse or neglect])
		Insufficient evidence to determine effectiveness in preventing:
		• Intimate partner violence
		• Violence by visited parents (other than child maltreatment or intimate partner violence)
		• Violence by visited children
Therapeutic foster care	Therapeutic foster care	Recommended for the reduction of violence by chronically delinquent adolescents
		Insufficient evidence to determine effectiveness in reducing violence by children with severe emotional disturbance
Firearms laws	Bans on specific firearms or ammunition	Insufficient evidence to determine effectiveness
	Acquisition restrictions	Insufficient evidence to determine effectiveness
	Waiting periods for firearm acquisition	Insufficient evidence to determine effectiveness
	Firearm registration and licensing of firearm owners	Insufficient evidence to determine effectiveness
	"Shall issue" concealed weapon carry laws	Insufficient evidence to determine effectiveness
	Child access prevention (CAP) laws	Insufficient evidence to determine effectiveness
	Zero tolerance of firearms in schools	Insufficient evidence to determine effectiveness
	Combinations of firearms laws	Insufficient evidence to determine effectiveness

Index

Note: Page numbers followed by f and t refer to figures and tables, respectively.